Effective Management

in Nursing

Second Edition

EFFECTIVE MANAGEMENT IN NURSING

SECOND EDITION

Eleanor J. Sullivan, PhD, RN
School of Nursing
University of Minnesota
Minneapolis, Minnesota

Phillip J. Decker, PhD
College of Business Administration
Western Kentucky University
Bowling Green, Kentucky

ADDISON-WESLEY PUBLISHING COMPANY
Health Sciences Division, Menlo Park, California
Reading, Massachusetts · Menlo Park, California · New York
Don Mills, Ontario · Wokingham, England · Amsterdam · Bonn
Sydney · Singapore · Tokyo · Madrid · Bogota · Santiago · San Juan

Sponsoring Editor: Nancy Evans
Production Supervisor: Wendy Earl
Production Coordinator: Richard Mason, Bookman Productions
Copy Editor: Carol Dondrea
Cover Design: Michael Rogondino
Interior Design: Wendy Calmenson
Composition: G & S Typesetters, Inc.

Library of Congress Cataloging in Publication Data

Sullivan, Eleanor J., 1938–
  Effective management in nursing.

  Includes bibliographies and index.
  1. Nursing services—Administration.   2. Nursing services—
Canada—Administration.   I. Decker, Phillip J.   II. Title.   [DNLM:
1. Administrative Personnel—nurses' instruction.   2. Nursing.
3. Nursing Care—organization & administration.   WY 105 S949e]
RT89.S85   1987   362.1'73'068   87-19559
ISBN 0-201-12781-4

  BCDEFGHIJ-BA-891098

Addison-Wesley Publishing Company
Health Sciences Division
2727 Sand Hill Road
Menlo Park, California 94025

This book is dedicated to:

Eleanor's grandmother, Alice Reed Clore, Nursing Class of 1914, who inspired Eleanor to enter the nursing profession; Rusti Moore, who introduced Phil to Nursing; Wendy, Colleen, Sean, Brad, and Pat, Eleanor's children; Martha Goodrich, Phil's mother; and Shirley Martin, who continues to inspire.

Foreword

Never before in the history of health care has there been so much change as exists in this field today. Moreover, the dramatic changes of the past few years are likely to continue in the foreseeable future. At the same time the nursing profession has its own cycles of change and commotion. We continue to debate many important issues regarding nursing practice, the educational preparation for practice, the organization of our profession, the scientific basis of nursing and health care, and the management of nursing and health care services.

The position of nurses and nursing within the health care system is important, in large part because the vast majority of direct patient care is provided by nurses. Beyond the provision of direct patient care, however, nurses in institutions hold a position of crucial importance: they are the interface between patient care and institutional operations. While nurses are the around-the-clock providers of patient care in institutions, they also interact on a continual and usually reciprocal basis with operational, support, and administrative components of those organizations.

Simply stating the importance of the nursing manager would be nothing new. The role of the nursing manager as norm-setter, value-transmitter, and director of both routine and non-routine services and operations has been described in nursing and organization literature. As nursing practice has evolved, so has the role of the nursing manager. However, even more different than the *content* of that role is the current *context* of nursing practice and nursing management. The effectiveness of the nursing manager is based first and foremost on a thorough understanding and appreciation of nursing practice and the scientific base for that practice. In addition, an effective nursing manager requires extensive knowledge and skill in understanding and manipulating the environments in which nurses practice.

Due to the integration of the *content* and *context* of nursing practice, the role of the nursing manager presents an interesting composite of demands. The nursing manager is responsible for the work of a group of clinical practitioners in the context of a largely bureaucratic environment; the potential sources of conflict may be compared to those of scientists in industry. Health care institutions still reflect a predominantly bureaucratic orientation, though in recent years there has been some movement toward open-system designs, with greater attention paid to the blend of technology, structure, and environment. However, the emphasis of professional nursing on client or patient-centered care implies flexibility in routines and the exercise of discretionary judgment. The greater the demand for flexibility and judgment by the nurse, the greater the potential conflict between that nurse and the rules and procedures of a bureaucratic institution.

A decade ago the health care environment was already highly complex and demanding for both practitioners and managers. However, the introduction of the prospective payment system in this decade has added many new variables and challenges. This new system has shaken the foundations of a heavily regulated health care environment. Although this environment is not yet deregulated, the phenomenon of a "marketplace" is certainly more evident now than it was a few years ago. As a result, more attention has been paid to costs of services and quality of care.

In the increasingly competitive health care environment, every manager is required to pay attention to the perceived "value" of services provided, that is, access to care, and the quality and costs of those services. The nursing manager also faces increasing pressure to improve the professional level of nursing practice, so as to ensure that practice is based on scientific knowledge directed toward designated goals and objectives, and to ensure at all times that the operations of an institution are compatible with strategic directions and decisions.

Eleanor Sullivan and Phillip Decker have produced a very timely and excellent work focusing on these concepts and the effective performance of the nurse manager in this environment. This welcome addition to the nursing management literature details the wide range of knowledge and skills essential for effectiveness in nursing management in today's changing environment. Application of these concepts by every nursing manager will help to promote the provision of adequate nursing care for the people we serve.

Sue T. Hegyvary, Ph.D., F.A.A.N.
Professor and Dean
School of Nursing
University of Washington

Contents

Part Four Human Resource Management Skills

Part Five   Basic Survival Skills

Preface

The nursing profession's first priority is competent and safe patient care. This philosophy gives direction to nurses' activities and provides a basis for intellectual, practical, and ethical decision making. By adroitly managing resources and by providing leadership to staff, the nurse manager assures the best possible environment for providing high-quality patient care.

Effective Management in Nursing is based on the above philosophical commitment. It is designed for use in a first course in nursing management, taught either in the undergraduate or graduate curriculum or in the nursing service setting. Additionally, any new nurse manager will find this book a practical guide to essential management concepts and skills.

While revised and updated throughout, this second edition retains the essential qualities that proved so popular in the first edition: it is both practical and theoretical, and highly readable. The new edition focuses on three major areas:

1. Information about health care organizations in today's dynamic environment

2. Principles of management and their application in health care settings

3. Management strategies and techniques that the nurse manager can use in daily practice

By using this approach, *Effective Management in Nursing* goes beyond leadership books and traditional management theory texts by providing practical assistance for developing important skills such as communication, recruiting, selecting and motivating staff, budgeting, risk management, managing conflict, and much more.

Multidisciplinary Authorship

The contributions of management experts often are not readily available to nurse managers. This book is unique in that the authors have drawn on the diverse expertise of management professors in schools of business and managers in private business practice, as well as that of nurse educators and nursing service administrators. This combination of theoretical knowledge and practical experience provides a rich blend of content, integrating management skills and concepts appropriate for the modern nurse manager to use in daily practice. However, each contribution has been carefully edited by the authors to conform to the goal of the book, which is to provide the best possible first course in nursing management.

New Content in this Edition

In response to suggestions from faculty and nurse managers who use the text, several new chapters and new sections have been added to this revision. Among the topics discussed in these new chapters are the following: managing change, increasing productivity, quality assurance, making ethical decisions, and managing the chemically dependent nurse. The new sections include delegation, group theory, and organizational theory.

New Five-Part Organization

This new edition has been reorganized into five parts:

1. Understanding nursing management—the basics of organization theory and management skills

2. Emerging issues in nursing management—productivity, managing change, ethics and managing chemically dependent staff, all chapters new to this edition

3. Key skills in nursing management—communication, motivation, leadership, time management, and problem solving

4. Human resource management skills—selecting, training, and appraising staff, and handling labor relations

5. Basic survival skills for the nurse manager—budgeting, using computers, managing risk, conflict, and dealing with higher management.

This five-part framework outlines the job and its environment first, then reviews emerging issues and presents basic theoretical knowledge, and, finally, examines diverse survival skills. The overall goal is to acknowledge the primacy of patient care, accountability, quality control, and productivity enhancement. This requires the right technology, the right people, creative thinking, and above all, the successful combination of all these factors into a system that runs smoothly. In achieving this, we go beyond theoretical understanding to provide suggestions for implementing practical applications, examples, and key behavior patterns.

Introductory outlines at the start of each chapter offer a convenient reference to chapter content. In addition, each chapter concludes with a summary of key points and a current bibliography.

Our society is struggling with many issues relating to sex differences. Many of these issues indirectly affect the content of this book. One affects it directly, namely the use of gender-specific pronouns when referring to nurses and nurse managers. Because more than 94% of nurses are female, the editors have resolved this issue in the interest of simplicity and clarity. The female pronoun alone is sometimes used to refer to nurses and nurse managers; this is in no way intended to diminish the contributions made by men to the profession.

Complete Teaching-Learning Package

Unique in the field of nursing management books, *Effective Management in Nursing* is only part of a complete teaching/learning package. This revised package includes an experiential skill-building workbook plus an instructors' resource manual. The workbook can be used with any nursing management text; the instructors' manual is tailored for use with *Effective Management in Nursing* and its accompanying workbook.

Acknowledgments

The authors wish to acknowledge the contributors, as well as our research assistant, Germaine Freese, our secretary, Carole Mandis, and Nancy Evans, Senior Editor at Addison-Wesley Publishing Company.

We owe a special debt of gratitude to the many reviewers who made comments and suggestions at various stages of the revision process. Their experience and insight have been essential to enhancing the quality and usefulness of this new edition. We would like to thank: JoAnn Alexander, University of Evansville; Janis Childs, University of Virginia; Mary E. Foley, St. Francis Hospital, San Francisco; Mary Geary, North Florida Regional Medical Center; June Levine-Ariff, Children's Hospital of Los Angeles; Brenda Montgomery, Dalhousie University, Halifax, Nova Scotia; Karen Mumina, The University of Oklahoma; Katy Nichols, Texas Christian University; Kitty S. Smith, George Mason University; Terrill L. Stumpf, University of San Francisco; Sharon Summers, University of Kansas; and Mary Yarborough, Mercy Hospital and Medical Center, San Diego.

Eleanor J. Sullivan and Phillip J. Decker

Contributors

Larry D. Baker, DBA
President, Time Management
  Center of St. Louis, Inc.
St. Louis, MO

Dianne Bartels, RN, MA
Associate Director
Center for Biomedical Ethics
University of Minnesota Hospital
  and Clinics
Minneapolis, MN

James A. Breaugh, PhD, MA
Associate Professor of Management
  and Psychology
School of Business Administration
University of Missouri-St. Louis
St. Louis, MO

Kenna Bridgmon, RN
President, Alternative Source
  Consulting
Shawnee Mission, KS

Phillip J. Decker, PhD
Associate Professor of Management
Department of Management
  & Marketing
College of Business Administration
Western Kentucky University
Bowling Green, KY

Dennis L. Dossett, PhD
Associate Professor of Management

Public Policy Administration
  and Psychology
School of Business Administration
University of Missouri-St. Louis
St. Louis, MO

Sandra R. Edwardson, PhD, RN
Associate Professor
School of Nursing
University of Minnesota
Minneapolis, MN

Doris A. England, RN, MSN
Associate Administrator of Patient
  Care
Children's Hospital of Michigan
Detroit, MI

Brenda Ernst, RN, MA
Vice President of Nursing
The Jewish Hospital of St. Louis
St. Louis, MO

David O. Evans, RN, MSN
Assistant Nursing Director
Ambulatory Care
Cardinal Glennon Children's
  Hospital
St. Louis, MO

David P. Gustafson, PhD
Associate Professor of Management
  and Organizational Behavior
School of Business Administration

University of Missouri-St. Louis
St. Louis, MO

Sherlyn Hailstone, RN, MSN
Vice President, Nursing
Barnes Hospital
St. Louis, MO

Marlene Hartmann, RN, MSN
Senior Vice President for Patient
 Care
Barnes Hospital
St. Louis, MO

Janalee B. Heaton, RN
% Time Management Center of St.
 Louis, Inc.
St. Louis, MO

Judith M. Hibberd, PhD, RN
Associate Professor
Faculty of Nursing
University of Alberta
Edmonton, Alberta, Canada

Ruth Launius Jenkins, RN, PhD
Associate Professor
School of Nursing
University of Missouri-St. Louis
St. Louis, MO

Linda A. Knight, BS, MEd, DA
Patient & Community Health
 Education Coordinator
Barnes Hospital Plaza
St. Louis, MO

June Levine-Ariff, RN, MSN
Assistant Director of Nursing
Children's Hospital of Los Angeles
Los Angeles, CA

Rusti C. Moore, RN, MEd
Director of Education
Hospital Division
Arabian American Oil Company
Dhahran, Saudi Arabia

Susan C. Reinhard, RN, MSN
Assistant Professor
Rutgers University
College of Nursing
Newark, NJ
            and
Lobbyist
New Jersey State Nurses' Association
Trenton, NJ

Benjamin H. Rountree, DPA
Principal
Hay Group
Atlanta, GA
            and
Assistant Professor
Health Services Management
Columbia, MO

Vicki L. Sauter, PhD
Associate Professor of Management
Science/Information Systems
University of Missouri-St. Louis
St. Louis, MO

Donna Lynn Smith, RN, BScN,
 Prof., Dip., MEd, C.H.E.
Assistant Vice President (Nursing)
University of Alberta Hospitals
Edmonton, Alberta, Canada

Marlene K. Strader, RN, MSN
Assistant Professor
School of Nursing
Southern Illinois University at
 Edwardsville
Edwardsville, IL

Eleanor J. Sullivan, PhD, RN
Associate Dean, Associate Professor
School of Nursing
University of Minnesota
Minneapolis, MN

1
Introduction to Nursing Management

NURSE MANAGERS ARE simultaneously subordinates, superiors, and customer service representatives. Think about this! As subordinates, nurse managers are held accountable by nursing administrators for the performance of their units. They are also accountable to patients and their families, and accountable for maintaining professional standards. The challenge is to fulfill the accountability to superiors, patients and their families, and professional standards, while depending on the efforts of subordinates to make this performance possible. The first edition of this book was designed to help nurse managers master that challenge. Today, there are additional challenges: increasing productivity in today's health care environment; facilitating changes brought about by internal and external forces; making ethical decisions in increasingly complex situations; and assisting a staff member who is chemically dependent. This second edition incorporates help in these areas.

Productivity is a summary measure of the quantity and quality of work performance with resource utilization considered. (See Chapter 4 for a complete discussion of productivity.) The organizational structure, work group structure, staff, and the nurse manager all have an impact on productivity. Nurse managers are in a position to directly influence the productivity of the individuals and work groups under their supervision. They may also be able to help integrate these contributions into the organization as a whole. Only when such integration occurs is high productivity possible.

Managing change is also a topic that has been of increasing importance to nurse managers. The environment of health care has seen and will continue to see a period of rapid change and evolution. The constraints of third-party reimbursement; the resulting competition among health care institutions; an increasing nursing shortage; and the increased predominance of multihospital, for profit corporations in today's health care industry ensure a changing environment. Nurse managers must be prepared for it. The status quo no longer can be the basis for decision making. Furthermore, a more worldly view is needed in order to predict and prepare for the new problems that will need to be faced tomorrow.

This changing environment and the resulting inevitable heavy emphasis on increased productivity ensures that we must reemphasize education in ethical decision making. Nurse managers will find themselves faced more and more with ethical dilemmas in making decisions, as the need for productivity, staff shortages, and the desire to provide the best possible patient care all collide.

The profession is just beginning to recognize the presence of chemical dependency in our ranks, and concern for a colleague in need challenges us to help. Legal and ethical issues emerge as the first-line manager moves to assist the nurse while ensuring patients' safety. New knowledge about chemical dependency and intervention skills must be learned and put to use. These issues and more will assuredly be among the ethical dilemmas faced by tomorrow's nurse.

Nursing isn't the safe place it used to be—especially for those who are to become nurse managers. Learning management skills is the first step. Learning to improve those skills, and to keep adding new skills in an unpredictable environment, is the second step. Learning to learn is the only real solution. Nursing and nurse managers must accept that challenge.

INTRODUCTION TO NURSING MANAGEMENT

Ever since people began forming groups to accomplish goals they could not achieve individually, the art of management has been essential to ensure coordination of individual effort. The purpose of this book is to study managers—nurse managers.

An essential factor in providing high quality nursing care is the presence of well-qualified nursing leadership. This is true throughout the hierarchy of nursing service and includes the position of nurse manager: the key leadership position directly related to the delivery of nursing care.

The nurse manager is responsible for representing the institution to the patient and the patient to the institution. The nurse manager must be proficient in clinical practice as well as able to implement on a unit the operations and goals of the institution. This is not always an easy task.

Working Within the Bureaucratic Environment

Health care institutions are unique, complex, social institutions that function as bureaucracies. They often provide a work environment in which it is very difficult for the nurse to function simultaneously as both professional practitioner and employee. Bureaucracies, by definition, subordinate the needs of individuals to the needs of the institution, and this often causes serious conflicts for professionals attempting to give individualized care. In addition, the nurse often finds that she is attempting to serve three masters: administration, physician, and patient. This contributes to the difficulties of functioning within the hospital setting.

It is the nurse manager's responsibility to assist the staff to work effectively in this environment. The manager must be advocate for both patient and staff and convince the administration of the need and value of individualized care. The staff may not always find working within a bureaucracy unpleasant; there are advantages as well as disadvantages. Employees often find that the rules and policies established by the bureaucratic institution provide more structure and a greater sense of security. The same well-defined policies and rules also give some employees a greater sense of power as well as a feeling of impartial fairness, while other employees find the rules and policies too confining and restrictive. The nurse manager must demonstrate to the staff and administration that rules and policies are necessary but that adjustments can be made when nursing care requires alterations in either. The mechanism for adjustments should be clearly defined and used whenever professional judgment indicates a need to alter a rule or policy for a specific patient or a specific incident in a patient's recovery. The nurse manager is the logical person to assume the role of patient advocate to the administration. In addition, she represents administration to the staff and patients. She is the manager closest to the direct care; her roles as patient care advocate as well as administrator help her provide the best environment for such care.

Most nurses assume administrative or management roles with the intention of contributing to patient care by ordering the environment, assigning or educating the staff, or performing some other activities that will provide an environment conducive to the patient's recovery. Too often the nurse in administration loses this orientation and begins to identify with the bureaucrats rather than the care givers. This change of orientation occurs more frequently among upper-level administrators than among nurse managers, but occurs often enough at lower levels to be disturbing.

It is essential that the nurse manager maintain a commitment to nursing care and nurses, see her role as advocate for staff and patients, and become a leader of the nursing unit.

The management skills necessary for this important and difficult position are discussed in this book, but there are other functions of management as well—these are less definitive. They include determining the character of the nursing unit, ensuring that patient care is the major priority, and establishing positive relationships with other levels of the nursing hierarchy.

Determining the Character of the Nursing Unit

Determining the character of the nursing unit is a relatively nebulous function, but probably the most important of the three listed above. The staff of the nursing unit directly reflect the beliefs and values of the nurse manager. How often have we noted differences in nursing staffs: one group is competent but "cold" and seemingly insensitive to patient-family relationships, while another is courteous, competent, and caring. What makes the difference? The nurse manager. The expectations of the first-level manager dictate the attitudes and behaviors of the staff and set the ethos of the unit.

The nurse manager also determines the character of the relationship the unit nursing staff has with other professionals and staff. If the leader interacts with physicians, housekeeping, or the other groups in a professional manner, the staff will also follow this pattern. However, if the nurse manager is not able to relate to others in a productive and agreeable manner, the staff will have similar difficulties.

Another aspect of the character of the unit is the general atmosphere. A quiet unit, with staff moving from one task to another with minimal commotion, gives a sense of competence and efficiency. This is much preferred to a nurses' station with a number of people sitting around entertaining each other while patients or families are waiting for information or assistance. Possibly the staff in the latter situation are just as competent or efficient as in the former situation, but they may not give that impression to the lay observer. Patients and families are under a great deal of stress, and they need to sense support from and confidence in the staff.

Ensuring the Primacy of Patient Care

The nurse manager must ensure that patient care is the unit's major priority. This sounds like something that does not have to be stated, but it is essential that the nursing staff understand how important care is to the patient's recovery; that's why the patient is hospitalized. Medical care without nursing care can be delivered in a variety of other settings, but in the hospital the major difference is nursing. The nurse manager must keep this distinction before the staff; nurses must take pride in the valuable contribution they are making. Too often staffs lose sight of this fact, and the morale of the unit suffers.

Establishing Relationships Within the Nursing Hierarchy

The third function of the nurse manager is establishing a positive relationship with the other levels of the nursing hierarchy. The ancillary personnel look to the nursing staff for support and direction, while the supervisory level of nursing expects the unit staff to carry out the objectives of the total nursing organization. Both levels are critical to the work of the nursing staff on a unit. The nurse manager, again, sets the relationship for all her staff. If she is able to work with both levels, then all staff will probably also fit into the nursing organization in an appropriate way.

In all three of the functions just described, it is obvious that the nurse manager is the key person on the nursing unit and that the delivery of high quality nursing care will be directly related to the quality of the leadership she provides.

ACCOUNTABILITY

Accountability is being responsible for one's actions and accepting the consequences of one's behavior. Since nursing's goal is to provide high quality care to the patient, accountability means responsibility for providing that care, and acceptance of the consequent praise or blame. The difficulty comes when one's decision about what is best for the patient conflicts with others' beliefs or goals. Traditionally, nursing has allowed others (physicians and administrators) to make patient care decisions. More recently, however, changes in women's roles and the nursing profession have encouraged many nurses to become more assertive in presenting their ideas, thereby increasing their willingness to be accountable.

Accountability can be considered within a systems framework, as shown in Figure 1–1. At the individual level, accountability is reflected in one's ethical decision-making processes, one's competence, commitment, and integrity. The American Nurses' Association code of ethics for nurses (see Chapter 6) is a guide for helping individual nurses make ethical decisions. At the institutional level, accountability is reflected in the nursing department's mission, philosophy, and objectives, and by peer review via patient audits. Professional accountability is found in standards of practice, such as those developed by the ANA (see Appendix A).

Society maintains the accountability of its members by enacting legislation that: (a) establishes rules and regulations to protect the rights, health, and safety of its members; (b) provides for an agency or group (usually a board) to monitor and enforce certain rules and regulations; and

Figure 1–1 Systems of Accountability

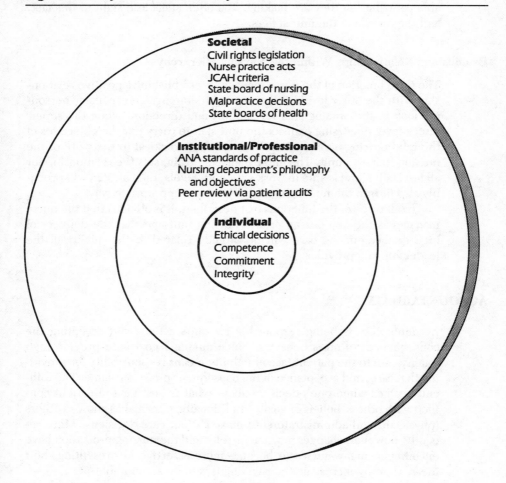

Societal
Civil rights legislation
Nurse practice acts
JCAH criteria
State board of nursing
Malpractice decisions
State boards of health

Institutional/Professional
ANA standards of practice
Nursing department's philosophy
  and objectives
Peer review via patient audits

Individual
Ethical decisions
Competence
Commitment
Integrity

(c) establishes a mechanism (usually a court of law) to protect members whose rights, health, or safety are impinged upon by other member(s) of society. Some examples of protective legislation with an impact on nursing are the state laws covering the practice of nursing as well as those governing occupational safety and health; the whole array of civil rights legislation; laws establishing state boards of nursing; and the legal precedents in court decisions involving negligence and malpractice litigation.

Society also protects its members by monitoring its allocation of resources (tax money) and by establishing requirements (standards) that both institutions and individuals must satisfy in order to qualify for certain funds. It is usually the responsibility of accrediting agencies, such as the Joint Commission on the Accreditation of Hospitals (JCAH), to set standards and check on adherence to them. Institutions must be accredited—that is, satisfy the criteria for performance—in order to receive government funds. Establishing prospective levels of reimbursement, as with the diagnostic-related groups (DRGs) utilized for medicare payments, is another way in which society attempts to maintain accountability of health care institutions.

THE NURSE MANAGER AND PATIENTS

The nurse manager interacts with patients both directly and indirectly. Although the nurse manager may only occasionally give direct patient care, she sees patients on rounds; reviews patient records; receives reports on patient status; and answers questions and requests from staff, patients, and families. The nurse manager may feel she has moved away from patient care, but her job entails far greater responsibility for the patients than she had as a staff nurse. She has an opportunity to make a substantial contribution to patient and staff well-being by ensuring that quality care is given by her staff. It is a great responsibility. A description of the nurse manager's job is outlined in Figure 1–2.

THE EDUCATION OF NURSE MANAGERS

Health care professionals have only recently recognized the need for formal preparation for those assuming supervisory and management roles within hospitals. The National Commission on Nursing has recommended that "nurse executives and nurse managers of patient care units should be qualified by education and experience to promote, develop, and maintain an organizational climate conducive to quality nursing practice and effective management of the nursing resource" (National Commission on Nursing, 1983). In recent years, graduate programs have included management courses as a functional area added to clinical specialization, and some programs offer graduate majors in nursing administration. The American Association of Colleges of Nursing and the American Organization of Nurse Executives have issued a joint position statement on graduate education in nursing administration. It is shown in Figure 1–3.

RESEARCH IN NURSING MANAGEMENT

Nursing management research is in its infancy. Those interested in this area are usually found practicing nursing administration. Because few nursing schools have offered graduate degrees in management, few mentors and senior researchers have been around to nurture the growth of

Figure 1—2 Nurse Manager Job Description

Position Purpose

Serves as the official supervisor of an assigned division and functions to plan, direct, coordinate, implement, control, evaluate, and improve the quality of patient care delivered.

Specific Responsibilities

- Interviews, selects, formally evaluates, and terminates assistant nurse manager/clinical nurses, registered professional nurses, licensed practical nurses, nurse assistants/technicians, and unit clerks in the division.

- Establishes division *standards, goals, objectives, priorities, and facilities change* based on the needs of patients and their families, physicians, staff, and on the results and recommendations of various division audits. Generally plans and executes administrative programs within the framework of the total nursing service program and follows up with a written annual report on division activities and future plans.

- Ensures competent, well-trained nursing personnel by identification of skill needs and subsequent recommendation of formal educational and developmental activities or personally instructing subordinates.

- Directs or personally engages in patient/family teaching for optimal recovery and health.

- Maintains timely documentation and anecdotal records on staff to be used in the preparation of performance appraisals.

- Holds regularly scheduled staff meetings, which provide opportunities for discussion of division problems, orientation to new projects, procedures, changes in care approaches, etc.

- Contributes to creating a work climate that encourages positive staff morale, motivation, and commitment through frequent contact with the staff (high visibility and accessibility); through the implementation of a leadership style appropriate to the demands of the situation; through consistent enforcement of division policy; through intensive evaluation of subordinates and provision for timely feedback; through interdepartmental and interpersonal mediation, troubleshooting, and problem solving; and through rendering expert service and role modeling.

- Develops the role of assistant nurse manager according to division needs and arranges for the assistant to function effectively in the absence of the nurse manager.

- Plans for future staffing, supply, and equipment requirements for maintaining or improving the quality of patient care and of the environment of the division. In conjunction with the unit manager, establishes supply standards and recommends capital expenditures.

- Supervises the allocation of division resources, remaining accountable to an established budget.

- Controls work time schedules for entire staff, makes scheduling adjustments when necessary.

- Equitably delegates patient care/division maintenance assignments and authority according to perceived strengths and limitations of subordinates, maintaining accountability.

- Directs the appropriate orientation of new staff into the division.

- Acts as a clinical resource, rendering expert service, and is prepared to assist with direct patient care when needed.

- Arranges educational inservice programs when the need and opportunity arise.

- Creates an open and accurate line of communication, upward, downward, and laterally, with particular respect to confidentiality.

- Initiates and/or delegates writing of patient care plans.

- Establishes an effective working relationship with the medical staff, admissions, dietary, housekeeping, laboratory, radiology, respiratory therapy, and other service areas related to the specialty of the division. In particular, makes daily rounds of the patients and ensures that the patient's medical plans and directives from the physicians are properly executed; surveys the environment and condition of each patient to ascertain the quality of *every* service being provided.

- Expeditiously handles staff, physicians, patient, interdepartmental complaints, and problems, providing accurate and timely follow-up.

- Responds quickly and intervenes in crises or conflicts of any nature that occur on the division.

- Remains responsible for the implementation of appropriate procedures in the event of emergencies, disaster, etc.

- Coordinates interpersonal relations among nursing staff and physicians, department heads, patients/families through problem identification and decision making.

- Attends to the various environmental cues suggestive of potential problems so as to quickly remedy: e.g., monitors physician/staff relations and patient/family perceptions of care received, interprets subtle messages conveyed by informal leaders, and so forth.

- Enforces hospital and nursing service policy and procedure.

- Counsels and provides remedial action for staff infraction of established professional guidelines.

- Supervises the documentation of pertinent and current patient information.

- Ensures that incident reports are prepared on unusual circumstances or events that occur.

- Ensures that contact is made with visiting nurses or social workers concerning post-hospital patient care.

- Reviews and responds to division mail and telephone calls/messages of a varied nature.

- Evidences involvement in the institution and its policies by providing service on committees that recommend policies, procedures, and standards of patient care delivery, such as the total head nurse group, the policy and procedure committee, the nursing audit committee, and ad hoc committees as appointed.

Used by permission of Barnes Hospital, St. Louis.

others in the field. This situation has been changing more recently, however, as schools of nursing are developing both master's and doctoral programs in management.

With the establishment (by congressional legislation) in 1985 of the National Center for Nursing Research (NCNR) in the National Institutes of Health, nursing research has moved into the mainstream of scientific efforts in the United States. The purpose of the NCNR is to support nurs-

Figure 1—3 Position Statement on Graduate Education in
Nursing Administration

The American Association of Colleges of Nursing (AACN) and the American Organization of Nurse Executives (AONE) believe that graduate education in nursing administration must be comprehensive, relevant, appropriate and responsive to present and future health care environments and nursing practice settings. AACN and AONE believe that the nurse executive is responsible for leadership and management of the nursing organization, accountable for the clinical practice of nursing, and functions as a member of the executive management team. The nurse executive is expected to facilitate effective, efficient patient care.

Educational preparation for nursing administration should take place in university schools of nursing offering specialized graduate programs in nursing administration. These programs should incorporate those appropriate academic disciplines essential to the practice of organizational management. This preparation integrates concepts from the disciplines of nursing, business, and management resulting in a unique and specialized configuration of knowledge. This knowledge provides the foundation for the theoretical base of nursing administrative practice. The synthesis and application of this knowledge is essential to the development of nurse executive leadership for professional nursing practice.

American Association of Colleges of Nursing/American Organization of Nurse Executives.

ing research and training in several areas including: health promotion and disease prevention, acute and chronic illness, and nursing systems of care delivery (where nursing management research is funded).

Increasing numbers of schools of nursing are establishing doctoral programs to help prepare the necessary cadre of nurse scientists for the future. Some of those scientists will undoubtedly focus their research efforts on nursing management. Let us consider, then, the appropriate role of the nurse manager in research.

The Role of the Nurse Manager in Research

The nurse manager's most important responsibility in research is to critically evaluate management research findings for application. However, several factors interfere with making this a reality.

First, a number of nurse managers practicing today have not had the educational preparation necessary to evaluate research. Many are graduates of associate degree or diploma programs where research evaluation is not included in the curriculum. Graduates of baccalaureate programs have received some beginning appreciation of research and have been exposed to the process of research evaluation, but it is unlikely that critical evaluation of nursing research was a priority while clinical skills were being mastered. Master's degree programs do prepare one with a basic working knowledge of the research process and with the skill to evaluate the importance of the results; however, most institutions do not require a master's degree for nurse manager positions. (This, too, is changing in the larger institutions, especially those located near a school with a master's program.)

Secondly, in order to participate in research activities, the manager must adopt a questioning frame of mind—a perspective not always congruent with the fast-paced decision making required in management. Such a frame of mind involves questioning the status quo and considering whether changes would improve the outcome of any given situation.

And, finally, most managers do not always recognize the value of research to their practice. In today's cost-containment environment, critical evaluation of research is an especially important aspect of nursing management. Research that addresses how we can provide quality services to patients in the most efficient manner must be evaluated, replicated to validate findings, and utilized appropriately. The research evaluation process will not be examined here, but many nursing research texts are available. The reader is referred especially to Castles' (1987) *Primer of Nursing Research* (Chapter 12) and Wilson's (1985) *Research in Nursing* (Chapter 4).

A changing environment demands new management skills. Effective nursing management means quality patient care, accountability to many diverse populations and associations, and productivity enhancement. It is a difficult, sometimes seemingly impossible task, but it can be done. Nurses have not been educated and nurtured in a profit-oriented, product-line, marketable product environment and, therefore, have not been exposed to the entire gamut of management skills. Yet, the 1980s are producing, and will continue to do so into the 1990s, a more traditionally industrial-type environment for health care where these skills are needed. You must acknowledge your product—quality patient care—provide the best you can, and then market it.

BIBLIOGRAPHY

Castles, M. R. (1987). *Primer of nursing research.* Philadelphia: W. B. Saunders.

National Commission on Nursing. (1983). *Summary report and recommendation.* Chicago: American Hospital Association.

Sovie, M. D. (1985). Managing nursing resources in a constrained economic environment. *Nursing Economics,* 3(2): 85–94.

Wilson, H. S. (1985). *Research in nursing.* Menlo Park, CA: Addison-Wesley.

1

UNDERSTANDING
NURSING MANAGEMENT

2

The Nature of Organization
in Health Care Settings

WE LIVE IN an organizational society, spending most of our waking hours and productive energies working toward the fulfillment of organizational goals. The justification for doing so is both rational and economic, inasmuch as we have discovered that properly organized and coordinated efforts can capture more information and knowledge, purchase more technology, and produce more goods, services, opportunity, and security than all individual efforts combined.

To achieve superior productive capability, however, an organization must depend on member behavior that is consistent with its goals. This means that individuals working in an organization must act in prescribed ways, sacrificing some of their personal freedom and autonomy. The price that people pay in loss of personal freedom must be weighed against the economic and other personal benefits they gain.

But it is a distasteful experience for most people to have little choice in the governance of their behavior, no matter how logical the reasons might be. Money alone usually provides insufficient motivation for surrendering one's autonomy. Therefore, the working relationship between organizations and their memberships must be given constant attention, and the person usually responsible for this mediating role in behalf of the organization is a manager; this activity is supervision.

This book will deal with the role and functions of a particular type of manager—the nurse manager—and the contributions he or she can make to the delivery of health services in a variety of work settings. The manager's functions are vital, complex, and frequently difficult; they must be directed toward balancing the needs of the health care organization, patients, physicians, subordinates, and self. Nurse managers need a body of knowledge and skills distinctly different from those needed for nursing practice, yet few of them have been prepared for managerial duties through education and training. Frequently they must depend on experiences with former supervisors who themselves learned supervisory techniques "in the trenches," or they must make their decisions out of some sort of instinct or common sense reasoning and with some apprehension. This book, focusing on the theory, processes, and dynamic potential of the effective nurse manager, proposes to resolve the gap in the new manager's preparation.

But the matters to be discussed must be considered within the realities of the setting in which they take place. We shall therefore first describe the role of nurse manager in terms of the most common environments in nursing, defining the organizational and environmental characteristics and constraints under which the nurse manager works. To understand the nature of nursing management, we will examine the structure of the institutions in which nursing is practiced and the environments in which the nurse manager and the institution function.

THE NATURE OF ORGANIZATIONAL THEORY

An organization is a collection of people working together under a division of labor and a hierarchy of authority to achieve a common goal. Continuously working together under authority toward a goal implies management. The activities of organized people don't just happen—they are managed.

There are many types of organizations. Organizations can be grouped, for example, by product, size, ownership, or purpose. The above definition of an organization includes division of labor and a hierarchy of authority, which are subcomponents of organizational structure (Robbins, 1983). If we wish to discuss the structure of an organization, we must consider three macro components: complexity, formalization, and centralization.

Complexity concerns the division of labor in an organization, the specialization of that labor, the number of hierarchical levels, and the geographical dispersion of organizational units. Formalization is the degree to which an organization relies on rules and procedures to direct members' behavior. It is independent of size. Centralization concerns the locus of decision-making authority.

Organizational theory is the study of organizational structure. And since all science has as its aim, the understanding, prediction, and control of an end, organizational theory is the process of creating knowledge to understand organizational structure so that we can predict and control organizational effectiveness or productivity by designing organizations. Hence, we can design organizations so that they better achieve their goals.

The most common way modern organizational theorists analyze organizations is through a systems perspective. A system is a set of interrelated parts arranged in a unified whole (Robbins, 1983). Societies, automobiles, human bodies, and hospitals are systems. Systems are either closed or open. Closed systems are self-contained and usually can only be found in the physical sciences. This perspective has little applicability to the study of organizations. The open system perspective recognizes the interaction of the system with its environment. Organizations must interact with their environments. Katz and Kahn (1978) outline ten characteristics that are common to all open systems. Understanding these characteristics will help one to conceptually understand how organizations function.

The first characteristic is *input*, or *importation of energy*. See Figure 2–1. Open systems import forms of energy from the external environment. Thus, the human cell receives oxygen and nourishment from the bloodstream, and an organization receives capital, human resources, materials, or energy (e.g., electricity) from its environment.

The second characteristic is *throughput*, whereby open systems transform the energy and materials available to them. Just as the human cell transforms nourishment into structure, an organization can create a new product, process materials, train people, or provide a service in the transformation process.

The third characteristic is *output*. Open systems export some product—a manufactured substance, an inquiring mind, or a well body, for instance—into the environment.

Fourth, an organization's throughput will work as a *system of cyclic events*. Organizational activities occur over and over again in a self-closing cycle, as the material that is input is transformed by throughput and results in output.

The fifth open system characteristic is called *negative entropy*; that is, the system reserves some of the input material so that it will be available for future use. For example, the human body stores fat that can be used for energy in lean times. Similarly, an organization can put extra money in the bank or employ extra manpower for availability in times of need.

The sixth characteristic of an open system is *information input*: the feedback and coding process. Every organization must take in information

Figure 2–1   The Hospital as an Open System

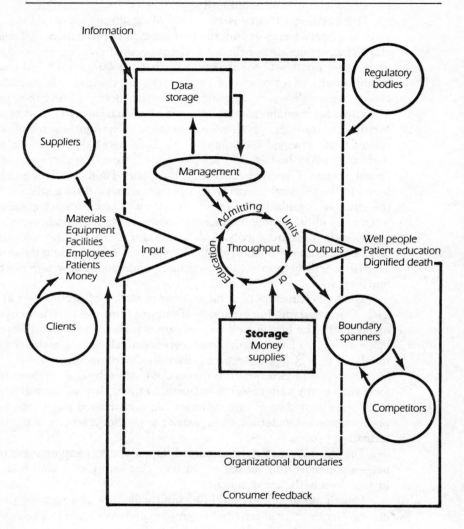

and feedback from the environment, code that information, and then store it so it can be used to predict the environment. This enables the organization to maintain a *steady state*, the seventh characteristic of an open system.

Sometimes called homeostasis, a *steady state* refers to the ability and desire of an organization to maintain some constancy in energy exchange. Just as the human body stays in a steady state, with no significant variation in its size and mass over time, so an organization attempts to stay in a steady state by predicting the environment and increasing and decreasing the input as information about output (market analysis) is generated. The basic principle is preservation of the character of the system.

The eighth characteristic is *differentiation*; organizational patterns tend to develop into specialized subsystems for specialized tasks (e.g., the nervous system in the body). Mechanization and computerization would be considered differentiation in an organization.

Two processes combine to form the ninth characteristic: *integration/ coordination*. As differentiation proceeds, it is countered by processes that bring the system together. Thus, management is an integration/ coordination subsystem in an organization, just as the cerebral cortex is the integration/coordination subsystem within the human body.

The last characteristic of an open system is *equifinality*: the principle that any final goal or end can be reached by a variety of means. As open systems move and develop within their environment, they may set different goals at different times and choose different methods to attain them, but the ultimate goal of any open system is to survive. The adaptability of humans for survival, for instance, represents equifinality. So does the behavior of organizations like the National Foundation for Infantile Paralysis; when its original purpose was achieved, it found another cause in order to survive.

As just one example of using the Katz and Kahn open systems perspective, we can look at nursing as a product line. This approach has recently been advocated in nursing (see Stanton, 1986, and Anderson, 1985). Product-line management is a technique developed in the late 1920s by Procter & Gamble. It evolved from the need to decentralize production and marketing decisions in order to maximize efficiency and profits. One person (the product-line manager) close to the product is given authority over it. The product-line manager can respond quickly to the changing environmental pressures impacting this one product. Thus, he is responsible for all forecasting, planning, production, and marketing—for that product. In open system perspective, the product-line manager is in charge of all functions—input, throughput, and output—related to one product. In contrast are the specialists, each of whom is in charge of a particular function (input, throughput, or output) for all products. For example, nursing, records staff, physicians, and purchasing staff are in charge of all respective inputs; nursing, dietetics, and other specialty departments are responsible for throughput; nursing and DOT (Department of Education and Training) are in charge of output.

Hospitals have traditionally neither defined their product nor managed it in a product-line manner. From a marketing perspective, a product is defined in relation to customer need. Hope for a better appearance or more sex appeal are customer needs that many companies produce products to satisfy. A hospital's product is improved health, a better quality of life, health education, or wellness. These are not always easily definable or packageable, and this is the dilemma for health care. But a product can be defined, and input, throughput, and output for that product can be managed. The major question is: Will nursing manage one or more of these products itself, or allow others to do it? One or the other will happen because product-line management makes sense in tighter economic times.

A business must develop a method of accounting for the revenue (input) it makes for producing a product (output) so that it can determine the efficiency of production (throughput). Nursing is a production process. The hospital thus can determine profit or loss and tie it to product line. Traditionally, health care has been able to freely pass increased costs to the customer, but this has changed with the introduction of the government's prospective payment system utilizing diagnostic-related groups (DRGs) to pay for health care and the corresponding responses by cost-conscious insurers. The government (which pays almost 40% of U.S. health expenditures) and the business community (which pays another 30%) have tired of the relentless escalation of health care costs. Consequently, the need to determine costs and generate revenue by product or service has become crucial in health care. Product-line management, therefore, will get increased attention from nursing. Nursing is an expense center (a big one) for a product line. The product may not yet be defined well by the institution, but that will also change as marketing departments are springing up in hospitals. One cannot market without defining the product and the customer need for which it is produced. Furthermore, the price given to a product and the quality of that product are directly affected by the producing department—in this case, nursing. Power and influence can be gained from this role. But tremendous responsibility for the viability and survival of the institution also goes with it. Thus, the efficiency of throughput (largely nursing, but also medical and other staff) is related to the quality of output, which, to a large extent, determines critical inputs.

As a final aside to this example, let us examine the possible products of nursing. Education and wellness are examples that have received attention to date. Health care is an obvious one and can now be organized by DRG—467 product lines in their own right. The future will show that some hospitals are more efficient than others for a given product line (DRG), and each will begin to specialize in those particular lines in order to maximize input (or profit). Nursing's largest role in the throughput of a product line is the management of production. Industrial wellness, physical fitness, and health education are other examples of products. Overall, we believe that the value of an open systems perspective and of putting product-line management within that rubric is not developing new products but realizing that nurse managers manage an expense center that has great control over the throughput of a product line. They thus control, to a large extent, the viability of the organization in which they exist.

HEALTH SERVICE ORGANIZATIONS

Health service organizations transform such inputs as money, people, supplies, and technology into health care services; as outputs, they produce clients with improved physical, mental, or emotional health. This transformation can take place only when there are adequate inputs to allow the process to occur. Hence, anything affecting inputs becomes a real concern for those charged with looking out for the general health and well-being of the institution.

Consider, for example, the influence of physicians on a hospital's purpose. Controlling to a significant extent the admission of patients to a hospital (input), physicians can thus also control the input of money necessary to operate the facility. The organization can therefore be expected to be sensitive to physicians' wants, needs, and expectations.

However, physicians are by no means the only influence on the purpose or mission of a health care institution. Hospital social workers, as well as the patient and patient's family, can influence the selections of the long-term care facility to which a patient is discharged. Which community mental health center is selected may be influenced by personnel in other social service agencies. A resultant reduction in client flow to any institution can in turn affect the funding decisions made by governmental and voluntary agencies, such as United Way.

Insurance companies or governmental agencies (Medicare, for instance) acting as third-party payers can also alter the mission of an institution through restriction of payments for certain services. In fact, the federal government did just that with the enactment of Public Law 98-21 utilizing DRGs for payment of Medicare benefits through a system of prospective rather than retrospective reimbursement.

Many other factors are also having a dramatic impact on health care institutions—among them, nurse supply, competition, and marketing. The current (and increasing) shortage of professional nurses has forced hospitals to adopt drastic measures, such as closing units, mandating overtime, or risking patient care with a low staff-to-patient ratio.

Competition has become the reality in health care delivery systems. Free-standing clinics and health services advertising are but two of the ways organizations are attempting to capture the health care market. To add to the confusion is the problem of increasing patient use while dealing with a nursing shortage.

The implications of competition are being much debated, but there seems little doubt but that the extraordinary changes taking place in the health care field will result in the demise of many institutions. The hospitals that succeed in filling their beds to or near capacity are quite likely to put others out of business. But hospitals are now developing new marketing strategies as a defense against competitors. Those strategies have a very definite bearing on the purpose of the institution, for organizations, like their human memberships, tend to fight to survive. In so doing, the institution must adapt itself to a constantly changing environment, one in which relationships between the organization and its environment play a significant role in shaping the organization's purpose.

In brief, an organization's purposes are the products of the environments in which the organization functions and, in the long run, it is society as a whole which creates an environment. James Thompson (1967) has suggested that certain identifiable persons and groups within that society determine or shape an organization's purpose and influence its structure and operations. He calls these persons and groups the "task environment" and identifies four elements or clusters, shown in Figure 2–1. They include (a) clients who use the services of the organization; (b) suppliers who provide essential labor, capital, supplies, equipment, and property; (c) competitors who challenge the organization for clients or supplies; and (d) regulatory bodies such as governmental agencies, standard-setting professional organizations, collective bargaining units, and all others who might act to restructure or restrain the operation of the organization.

The relationship between the organization and its task environment becomes one of exchange, one earning resources that it may export in order to acquire the needed inputs from the others. The greater the need of one organization for the exports of another, the greater the control, presuming the entity has the ability to produce at the desired level.

Nested in the innermost core of the organization are the central activities or functions of the health service organization as supplied by the deliverers of health care. This core, which depends totally on a steady and predictable stream of inputs from the task environment, operates most effectively and efficiently when the traumas and uncertainties of the task environment are absent. In other words, the central activities of the health service organization must somehow be buffered from the uncertainty and instability of the environment.

In an optimal environment for the delivery of hands-on care, patients/clients arrive in a steady and predictable stream, and needed supplies are always available. Playing a role Thompson calls "boundary spanning," these individuals (elements) serve to protect the central activities (technical core) of the organization from the uncertainties of the task environment. Boundary spanners in a hospital include personnel in purchasing or medical records, those responsible for Joint Commission on the Accreditation of Hospitals (JCAH) liaison, and nurse managers—all of whom buffer the direct-care givers from the environment, assuring to the fullest possible degree the availability of inputs.

The closer we move to the actual level at which care is rendered, the more focused the individual roles become, the more specific the information used. To coordinate and control the care delivery process, anticipate problems, and provide needed supplies, the persons at the top of the hierarchy must depend upon information from their subordinates.

THEORIES OF ORGANIZATION

The earliest recorded systematic organizational thinking was done by the ancient Sumerian civilization around 5000 B.C. The early Egyptians also dealt with this topic as did the Babylonians, Greeks, and Romans. However, organizational theory remained largely unexplored from ancient times until the Industrial Revolution (a few people did examine it—for example, Machiavelli in the 1500s). In 1776, Adam Smith (see Cannon, 1925) first established the management principles we know as specialization and division of labor.

In the late 1800s and early 1900s, other persons started to systematically think about the organization of organizations. The result today is a number of schools of thought or approaches to the organization and management of organizations. These approaches are traditionally labeled the classical, neoclassical, technological, and modern systems theories.

Classical Theory

The classical approach to organizations deals almost exclusively with the anatomy of formal organization. The main thrust is efficiency through design. People are seen as operating most productively within a rational and unambiguous task/organizational design. Therefore, one designs an organization by subdividing work, specifying tasks to be done, and only then fitting people into the plan. Classical theory is built around four elements: division and specialization of labor, chain of command, structure of the organization, and span of control.

Several theorists have contributed to classical organizational thought. In 1911, Frederick Taylor wrote *The Principles of Scientific Management*. This book became an early cornerstone of management theory. In it, Taylor offers four principles of scientific management:

1. Develop a "science" for every job by studying motion, standardizing the work, and improving working conditions.

2. Carefully select workers with the correct abilities for the job.

3. Carefully train these workers to do the job and offer them incentives to produce.

4. Support the workers by planning their work and by removing obstacles (Schermerhorn, 1984).

These principles were given to maximize individual productivity.

Frank and Gillian Gilbreth added to scientific management by proposing time and motion study, the science of reducing a job to its basic physical motions. Thus, wasted movements are eliminated and incentives are based upon the newly designed job. Scientific management is the basis of job simplification, work standards, and incentive wage plans as used today.

Henri Fayol, in 1916, published *Administration Industrielle et Generale* in which he proposed five rules of management:

1. Foresight—to plan for the future, specify goals

2. Organization—to provide resources for the plan

3. Command—to select and lead people in implementing the plan

4. Coordination—to ensure all employees' efforts fit together to achieve the goal

5. Control—to verify progress toward the goal

These rules were the basis for classical management functions: planning, organizing, controlling and decision making. Fayol also specified 14 principles of management (see Figure 2–2), which would be used to implement the five rules. These rules and principles are the subject of Chapter 3.

Max Weber (1958) proposed the term *bureaucracy* (which to most of us today is a dirty word connotating long waits, inefficiency, etc.) to define the ideal, intentionally rational, most efficient form of organization. Much of Weber's suggestions for the most rational, fair, and efficient organization parallel the work of Fayol and his contemporaries.

Although the work of the scientific management theorists has been the core of industrial engineering, much of classical organizational theory has been criticized. Without considering factors such as technology, labor pool, and organizational climate and environment, there is no one best way to design an organization. Howell and Dipboye (1982) suggest that many of the classical prescriptions are not as explicit as they seem. How far, for example, should specialization be carried? At the extreme, it becomes ridiculous: thousands of very bored people doing one-minute tasks each. Thus, how far specialization should be taken is a matter of human judgment—and our "objective" principle turns out to be highly subjective. Many other criticisms have been given. Most of these concern lack of correspondence between the formal or planned organization/task and the actual organization, dehumanization of the worker, and rigidity of operation.

Neoclassical Theory

The criticisms of classical theory led to neoclassical theory. Neoclassical theory takes the postulates of the classical school as given, but these postulates are seen as being modified by people. This approach is often identified with the human relations movement of the 1930s. A major assumption of this school of organizational thought is that people desire social

Figure 2–2 Fayol's General Principles of Management

1. *Division of work* The object of division of work is to produce more and better work with the same effort. It is accomplished through reduction in the number of tasks to which attention and effort must be directed.

2. *Authority and responsibility* Authority is the right to give orders, and responsibility is its essential counterpart. Whenever authority is exercised responsibility arises.

3. *Discipline* Discipline implies obedience and respect for the agreements between the firm and its employees. Establishment of these agreements binding a firm and its employees from which disciplinary formalities emanate should remain one of the chief preoccupations of industrial heads. Discipline also involves sanctions judiciously applied.

4. *Unity of command* An employee should receive orders from one superior only.

5. *Unity of direction* Each group of activities having one objective should be unified by having one plan and one head.

6. *Subordination of individual interest to general interest* The interest of one employee or group of employees should not prevail over that of the company or broader organization.

7. *Remuneration of personnel* To maintain the loyalty and support of workers, they must receive a fair wage for services rendered.

8. *Centralization* Like division of work, centralization belongs to the natural order of things. However, the appropriate degree of centralization will vary with a particular concern, so it becomes a question of the proper proportion. It is a problem of finding the measure that will give the best overall yield.

9. *Scalar chain* The scalar chain is the chain of superiors ranging from the ultimate authority to the lowest ranks. It is an error to depart needlessly from the line of authority, but it is an even greater one to keep it when detriment to the business ensues.

10. *Order* A place for everything and everything in its place.

11. *Equity* Equity is a combination of kindliness and justice.

12. *Stability of tenure of personnel* High turnover increases inefficiency. A mediocre manager who stays is infinitely preferable to an outstanding manager who comes and goes.

13. *Initiative* Initiative involves thinking out a plan and ensuring its success. This gives zeal and energy to an organization.

14. *Esprit de corps* Union is strength, and it comes from the harmony of the personnel.

Abridged from Fayol, Henri. *General and Industrial Administration* (New York: Pitman, 1949), pp. 20–41. Used by permission.

relationships, respond to group pressures, and search for personal fulfillment. Mary Parker Follet was an early advocate for the social aspects of organizations and in fact proposed the coordination of effort through mutual agreement (participative management) long before the human relations movement (see Metcalfe & Urwick, 1940).

Between 1924 and 1929, the Western Electric Company instituted a series of studies at their Hawthorne plant in Chicago. The Hawthorne studies were originally designed to study scientific management principles. The first study was an examination of the effect of illumination on productivity. This study failed to find any relationship between level of illumination and production. Productivity in some groups varied at random, while in one it actually went up as illumination went down. The researchers concluded that unforeseen "psychological factors" were responsible. Further studies examined physical working conditions such as rest breaks and length of workweek. Again no relationship to productivity was found. The researchers concluded that the social setting created by the research itself accounted for the increased productivity. Workers felt special because of the attention given them as part of the research and thus worked harder. These studies led to identification of what is known as the *Hawthorne effect*—the tendency for persons to perform as expected because of special attention. They also led to a focus by organizational theorists on the social aspects of work and organizational design.

In 1938, Chester Barnard wrote *The Functions of the Executive,* in which he asserted that individuals cannot be coerced or bribed to do things considered unreasonable. Barnard recognized that formal authority does not work without willing participants. Later theorists, such as Maslow and McGregor, were also influenced by the Hawthorne studies and the human relations movement. These researchers proposed motivational theories to explain the link between organizational design and productivity. The work of these individuals is examined in Chapters 4 and 9.

The neoclassic theorists had in common a desire to humanize classical theory without total rejection of the structural view. All recognized the need to design a rational organizational structure, but proposed that it be done through cooperation, participation, and a view to the motivation of the individual. In a sense, these researchers bridge the gap between classical theory and systems theory. They took structure and added the individual. The systems theorists view productivity as a function of structure, people, technology, and environment.

Technological Theory

During the 1960s a number of researchers focused their attention on the connection between technology and organizational processes. Woodward (1965), for example, surveyed 100 British manufacturing firms in an effort to find what management practices contribute to business success. She concluded that the demands of different technologies tend to shape the kind of organization that develops. Woodward categorized firms into three types of technology: unit (custom-made products), mass (large-batch manufacturing), and process production (continuous-process manufacturing). The most successful firms in her survey tended to cluster around the typical pattern in each production type.

The work of Woodward and others in this area helped make the final leap to modern systems theory, in which the organizational structure, the individual, technology, and the organization's environment all combine to determine organizational effectiveness.

Modern Systems Theory

An organization is a complex sociotechnical system. This concept is what integrates modern systems theory. The organization is viewed as a system that operates on certain inputs to produce certain outputs in a certain kind of environment (open systems). Modern organization theory also often relies on a conceptual analytical base, empirical research, and its integrating nature. Yet it is diverse. Examples are the open systems approach of Katz and Kahn (1978) described earlier, the decision system approach of March and Simon (1958), and the information-processing approach of Galbraith (1977).

Modern theorists ask a number of related questions. Key among them are: (1) What are the strategic parts of the system? (2) What is the nature of their mutual dependency? (3) What are the main processes in the system that link the parts together and facilitate their adjustment to each other? (4) What are the goals sought by systems? (See Scott, 1961.)

The basic part of an organizational system is the individual and the role he or she occupies. Next is the formal arrangement of functions and subparts of the organization. These are arranged in an interrelated pattern called the formal organization. Also important is the informal organization. Thus, both formal role demands from the organization and informal demands from the work group are taken into account. The physical setting is also studied.

Linking processes that are studied include role taking, communication, group processes, balance between organizational subparts, control and regulatory processes, feedback mechanisms, decision making, motivation, and leadership. Finally, goals such as organizational effectiveness, productivity, stability, and survival are studied.

Modern systems theorists view their approach as a framework for analyzing organizational behavior and effectiveness. Systems theory is an excellent method to account for general concepts of organizational functioning, but these concepts don't always lead to specific testable hypotheses. It is best to think of the systems approach as a general way of looking at organizations while we examine the specifics of organizational behavior. It is a "big picture."

Katz and Kahn (1978) view organizations as a recurrent cycle of input, transformation, and output. Organizations lack physical structure such as that of the human body. One can destroy the physical plant, but unless the articles of incorporation, charter, people (who may come and go), and job descriptions (definition of roles and authority structure) are destroyed, the organization survives. Even the goal can disappear and the organization will survive by developing new inputs, throughput, outputs, and goals. The March of Dimes is a good example. The goal of the March of Dimes was to provide care for polio victims. When polio was eliminated, the goal was irrelevant. Thus, the organization established new goals based on needs of the handicapped. The patterns of the events of organizational life are what is important. Katz and Kahn rely on role-taking and role-maintaining processes for their analysis.

March and Simon (1958) view an organization as an information-processing network with many decision points for both individual members and the organization. If we can understand those decision points and the variables or forces acting on the decision maker, we understand the most critical behavior of the system. March and Simon suggest that the classical concept of rational decision making is limited in organizations. The problem solver does not always know all the alternatives and may not have the criteria to evaluate them. These are the basic premises of rational decision making. However, decision making is rational within certain limits—"bounded rationality."

Rather than use rational decision making to optimize economic return, organizations and their members often satisfice—that is, decision makers set some minimum acceptable level of return and pick the first alternative that promises to exceed this level.

Furthermore, March and Simon suggest, instead of continually making decisions, organization members develop programs—sets of complex, organized behaviors used to respond to common environmental stimuli. These programs are why much human behavior is so predictable. Thus, March and Simon view organizational change as a process of changing the basic behavioral programs of organizational members or of changing the stimuli that affect decisions.

Galbraith (1977) views an organization as a large communication system. He suggests that as uncertainty in organizations increases, the amount of communication required (or information to be processed) to keep the organization stable goes up. Thus, the organization is a system in which the goal is the reduction of uncertainty. Since all communication channels have some limit as to what they can carry, and increased uncertainty (from an unpredictable environment such as that now faced by nursing with DRGs, increased health care competition, etc.) will eventually exceed the capacity of existing channels to reduce it. When this happens, it becomes necessary to (a) increase capacity or (b) reduce the quality of communication. Galbraith not only discusses strategies for increasing capacity and other methods of decreasing uncertainty, he also outlines different system types that deal with uncertainty to various degrees. One of these is the matrix organization, in which two distinct management systems—a departmental structure and a project or product structure—overlap. With this approach, an organizational member reports to two bosses, which is a direct violation of classical rules. Yet, the matrix organization is often used in engineering and research firms because of its high information-processing capacity.

Overall, modern systems theory is a useful tool for understanding organizations. Often, it is difficult to test empirically many of the hypotheses generated by the theory, but the aim is not to present the ideal organizational plan. The theory does recognize the vast complexity of organizations and the interactive effects of many variables. Great progress has been made in this theoretical school in specifying what the important organizational variables are and in considering the human variables as well.

ORGANIZATIONAL STRUCTURE IN HEALTH CARE

A bureaucratic structure, as depicted in Figure 2–3, characterizes the majority of today's health service organizations. Such a structure maintains command and reinforces authority; provides for a formal system of communication up, down, and across the facility; and buffers the caregivers from the task environment. But a bureaucratic structure is also impersonal and not always comfortable for the individuals working within the system. Formal communication often takes on an autocratic, downward orientation. Even more detrimental, however, is the fact that the inflexibility of the structure renders individuals unable to respond to their changing environments.

Administrators structure or design health service organizations in ways designed to increase the probability of their organizations' survival and success. But they do so within differing social, political, economic, and resource climates, and they impose their own perspectives. Naturally, then, the formal structure of hospitals tends to vary.

Characteristically, however, these structures take the form of a set of differentiated but interrelated functions. These broad functions are, in turn, broken down into tasks to be performed by persons in formal work groups. The decision as to how the pieces should be fitted together is usually based on the basic assumptions of bureaucracy.

The vertical dimension of Figure 2–3 deals with the organization's hierarchy—that is, the lines of authority and responsibility. The organization must be able to exercise control over the behavior of its membership, and hierarchy provides the authority for such control. On the other hand, the horizontal dimension of the chart relates to the division and specialization

Figure 2–3   Typical Bureaucratic Structure, with Special Focus on the Nursing Department

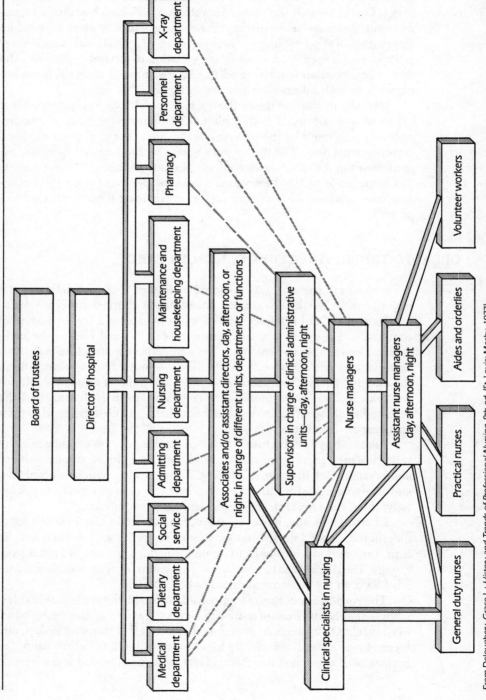

From Deloughery, Grace L.: *History and Trends of Professional Nursing,* 8th ed. (St. Louis: Mosby, 1977).

of labor—functions attended by specialists. A look at the vertical dimension will provide some understanding of how hospital organizations use differentiation in pursuit of their goals and how differentiation results in an organizational prescription for the nurse manager.

The Vertical Dimension

The pyramid is differentiated into several vertical levels based on the administrative need to dispense authority and responsibility in the interest of control. Authority exists most substantially at the top, decreasing as one descends the bureaucracy. Individuals occupying positions at the top of bureaucratic structures are usually referred to as executives. Responsibility at this highest level is very broad, embracing the general well-being and direction of the organization.

To those lower in the hierarchy—and this includes many nurses—executives may appear aloof from the real purposes of the hospital; they often appear to focus on issues less directly associated with patient care than clinical staff believe necessary and appropriate. Yet today's economic system is built upon competition, and health service organizations are beginning to operate within that system on more nearly the same basis as other "people-serving" institutions. Hence, executives tend to perceive and evaluate their organizations with an eye on the task environment.

For example, should the hospital open an outpatient clinic in a shopping mall in order to maintain its share of the health care market, keep beds filled through resulting referrals, and provide additional income? The survival of the organization may well depend on decisions of this kind and the coordination of highly disparate activities to accomplish them. Moreover, the administrative attention devoted to the actual operation of the facility focuses, generally, on the total institution. Small wonder, then, that executives may seem "aloof" to the staff nurse who attends, principally, to the specific internal tasks of the organization.

The level below executives in hospital structure is called middle management. These individuals attempt to coordinate and control the activity of functional work groups in order to accomplish directives from executives. The nursing director, for example, heads a department composed of a significant number of individuals working on different units. This role also includes representing the profession, a responsibility that will be discussed later in more detail.

The perspective of the nurse manager, although lower in the managerial hierarchy and more internally focused than that of her superior, usually responds indirectly to patient-staff interaction. Managers tend to be more concerned with what work has to be done rather than how the work is to be done, mustering often diminishing nursing resources and planning for the future. In short, their efforts are boundary spanning, coordinating, and controlling.

The Horizontal Dimension

The horizontal dimension in Figure 2–3 relates to specialization of labor. In hospitals this usually results in an array of departments similar to those depicted in the figure. Each department, service, or program represents a particular portion and type of human input necessary to the total care-giving process. The task at hand is to fit those pieces together to produce quality, as well as quantity, of care.

Conflict is inevitable among the horizontal units in health service organizations, since many of these units are derived from specific disciplines (nursing, medicine, or social work), and each group of professionals has its own set of values, attitudes, and perspectives. Since each one is likely to consider its contribution to be more important than the whole, and since each must compete for limited resources, conflict often results. Moreover, professionals communicate most frequently and comfortably within their own peer groups, which tends to reinforce peer decisions and control and thus compounds the difficulty in interaction with other unit groups.

Yet the intensive technology associated with health services makes it imperative that unit groups coordinate their efforts. Health services are administered on the basis of client need, and significant numbers of individuals, each with their own expertise, must work together in delivering care. In a hospital, for example, the degree to which services are provided in a smooth and appropriate flow conditions the institution's "continuity of care," a primary concern and function of the system.

TYPES OF HEALTH CARE ORGANIZATIONS

Health care organizations can be categorized as: (a) acute care institutions; (b) long-term care institutions; (c) ambulatory care organizations; (d) home health care agencies; and (e) temporary health care services. In addition, they may be private or public and proprietary or nonprofit. Most health care institutions and agencies are not for profit, but this picture may be changing with the recent development of proprietary, or for profit, hospitals or chains of hospitals. Some of these institutions specialize in one area of health care, such as alcohol treatment, but most function as general hospitals.

The largest number of health care organizations in this country today are acute care hospitals. Some hospitals are private, of which most have been founded by religious organizations, while others are public and are owned and operated by local, state, or federal governmental agencies—for instance, Veterans' Administration hospitals or state mental hospitals.

Many hospitals, regardless of other characteristics, also serve as teaching institutions for physicians, nurses, and other health care professionals, but the term "teaching hospitals" commonly designates those hospitals with a house staff of residents on call 24 hours a day. This is in comparison to a community hospital, with only physicians in private practice on the staff. These private physicians tend to be less accessible than a house staff, so the medical supervision of patient care differs. For the staff and supervisory nurses, patient care also will differ in the two types of institutions.

The growth of long-term care institutions has paralleled the increase in the elderly population. Today more people are living longer and living with poorer health, thus increasing the demand for long-term care.

Health care is also provided in ambulatory care settings, the home, and by agencies that provide personnel for temporary service. Ambulatory care providers are similar to hospitals in that they may be private (emergency aid facility) or public (county health department clinic), and proprietary (physician's office) or not for profit (church-operated screening clinics).

The trend toward home health care has also grown in recent years. Inflation and cost containment, for one thing, have forced hospitals and third-party payers to examine critically the length of patient stay. The result has been earlier discharge of patients and a more acutely ill patient population returning home. Further, more people are surviving life-threatening illness or trauma and thereby needing care. Visiting nurse associations (nonprofit, private), local health departments (nonprofit, public), temporary service agencies (proprietary, private), as well as departments of acute care hospitals all provide home health care. The largest growth, however, has occurred in private (for profit and not for profit) home care agencies. Services provided by home care agencies are primarily nursing, but some larger agencies also offer other professional services such as physical therapy or social work.

The temporary service agencies have grown in response to nursing shortages. These agencies provide nurses and other health care workers to hospitals who are temporarily short-staffed as well as providing private duty nurses to individual patients. Some hospitals rely a great deal on these agencies to provide staffing when staff shortages and variations in the patient census make scheduling difficult and inefficient.

Multihospital systems are becoming increasingly more common. Nursing homes, psychiatric facilities, HMOs, and home care agencies are also often part of the multiunit systems.

Multi-institutional arrangements take many forms (Freund & Mitchell, 1985): (a) *formal agreement,* where two or more institutions engage in a joint program while maintaining responsibility for separate actions or services; (b) *shared services,* where clinical or administrative functions common to two or more institutions are carried out cooperatively; (c) *consortia on planning or education,* where groups of institutions meet together and with health systems agencies to determine which institutions will provide specific services to the community; (d) *contract management,* in which an outside management firm contracts to take over day-to-day responsibility for managing an organization (no change of ownership occurs); (e) *leasing,* similar to contract management but the management

Figure 2—4 Multi-Institutional Benefits/Constraints for Nursing

BENEFITS

Economic:
- access to capital to finance new programs, services, and continuing education
- support for otherwise failing institutions
- program start-up costs spread over larger base

Improved Technology:
- corporate production of patient education and training aids
- corporate-wide computerized cost accounting, patient care information, and patient classification systems
- availability of new sophisticated patient care equipment

Diversification:
- market analysis for special projects
- new programs/services involving nursing (surgical centers, home health programs, wellness centers, child day care, hospice programs) bringing enhanced career mobility within the same corporate structure
- nonhealth lines of business, such as uniform companies for staff purchase at lower than market prices

Fringe Benefits:
- stock option purchases at reduced rates
- end-of-year stock bonuses
- vested retirement system through corporation that is transferable with relocation
- continuing education for nursing staff and management
- educational leave program
- financial rewards for writing and publication
- awards (with monetary value) for community services and excellence
- attractive insurance and tax deferral benefits
- benefits transferable if relocate within the system

Professional:
- improved registered nurse ratio
- increased number of clinical specialists and nurse researchers
- decentralized nursing organizations
- specialists attracted to rural areas
- upward mobility for nursing staff
- systemwide mobility

CONSTRAINTS

Reduced Autonomy:
- nurse executive autonomy reduced, especially in regard to institutional governance and diversification
- nurse executives have not recognized their corporate responsibility; tend to be myopic toward their own insitution

Quality:
- rapid expansion without the necessary resources and personnel results in current staff overload and reductions in quality initially
- reduced registered nurse mix due to regional determination of standard registered nurse mix
- consultants have no ongoing influence in a given institution

Reprinted with permission of Anthony J. Janetti, Inc., publisher, *Nursing Economics*, 3 (Jan/Feb), p. 30, 1985.

firm regulates not only day-to-day operations but policy as well; (f) *corporate ownership with separate management,* where a corporation owns several institutions and contracts for their administration with independent firms; and (g) *complete corporate ownership,* where a corporation owns and manages several institutions.

Multiunit systems can integrate horizontally or vertically. A horizontally integrated system is one in which the units provide the same or similar services. A vertically integrated system is one in which the units provide different services. An example of the latter would be a system with an HMO, psychiatric hospital, acute care hospital, and nursing home.

Freund and Mitchell (1985) suggest that although these arrangements have been highly touted, the final verdict on performance/efficiency will have to await the test of time and empirical studies. The authors have delineated the possible benefits and constraints of such organizations; these are displayed in Figure 2–4.

The nurse manager may be responsible for supervising patient care in all of the various types of health care organizations described. The knowledge of organizations and management principles presented here are applicable in all health care settings. Because most nurses are employed in hospitals, however, the examples focus primarily on nursing management in hospitals. When appropriate, other health care settings are also discussed.

THE DEPARTMENT OF NURSING

Nursing is the largest department in any hospital. At its head is the nursing service administrator, who is called the nursing administrator, director of nursing, vice-president for nursing, or one of many other titles. The nursing director will have at least one assistant for every period of the day, since the nursing department is staffed around the clock. Each nursing department will have clinical specialists in such areas as maternity, pediatrics, and the operating room, and every clinical service will usually have more than one division with a nurse manager in charge. There may also be staff positions in such areas as inservice education and recruiting. Special nursing units include medical, surgical, pediatric, obstetric, psychiatric, operating room, recovery room, emergency room, and intensive care.

Figure 2–5a illustrates an organizational chart for the typical centralized department of nursing, formed in a hierarchical authority pattern. Figure 2–5b illustrates a decentralized nursing service.

A recent phenomenon in the structuring of nursing departments has come from the desire to democratize decision making in hospitals, especially decision making among the nursing staff. These innovations may simply take the form of participative decision making (which is discussed

Figure 2–5a Traditional Centralized Nursing Service

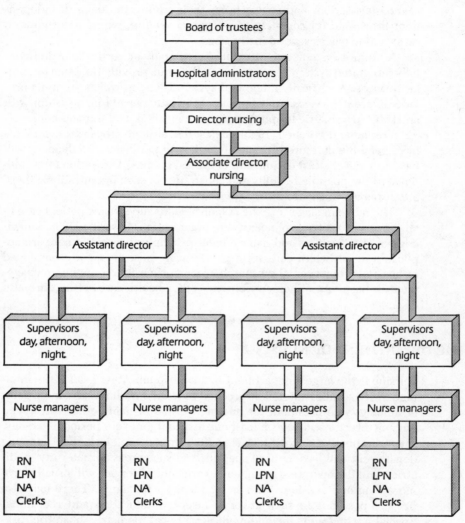

H. S. Rowland, B. L. Rowland: *Nursing Administration Handbook* (Germantown, MD) Aspen, 1980. Used with permission.

Figure 2–5b Decentralized Nursing Service

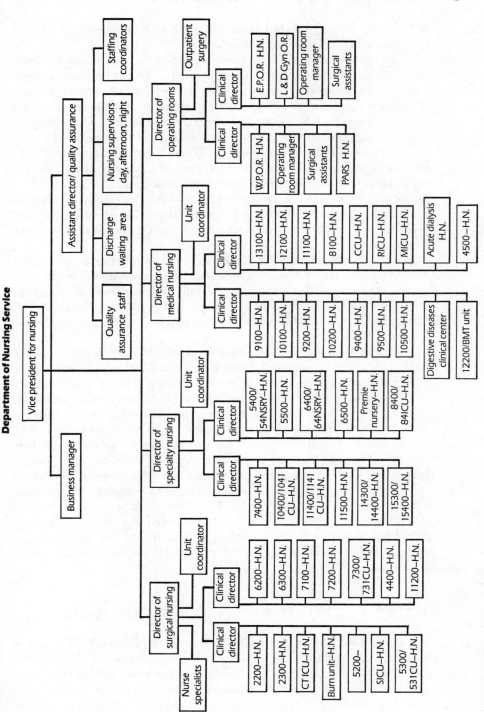

Used by permission of Barnes Hospital, St. Louis.

in Chapters 10 and 12), but more elaborate systems known as "shared governance" have begun to be developed.

Shared governance is a system that allows the staff nurse an equal vote in major decisions about nursing practice. These systems are usually built on a foundation of primary nursing, peer review, and some provision for clinical advancement. Most shared governance systems are designed along the lines of academic or medical governance models. That is, nurses elect a "congress" that represents all nurses. Operating under the congress may be a council (human resources) in charge of staffing levels, recruitment, and retention; and a council (nursing care) in charge of care standards, audit criteria, research, and staff education.

Some shared governance systems incorporate elected advisory boards for each service and/or clinical department. From these boards is elected a senate or congress that will meet several times a year to decide larger issues.

The ultimate outcome of shared governance is that nurses participate in a democratic forum to control their own practice within the health care system. The assumption is that nursing staffs, like medical staffs, will predetermine the clinical skills of staff nurses and monitor the work of each through peer review, while deciding other practice issues through elected forums.

Such systems should increase job satisfaction and lower turnover among those nurses who wish to participate in deciding the direction of their practice in an institution. However, it may also lower satisfaction for the inevitable minority who do not wish to participate in democratic forums or spend the time in the meetings and the other group work required of a democratic shared governance system. Nevertheless, efficiency may be improved by such systems as nurses take charge of their units/divisions/practice and move away from reliance on float pool or agency nurses to fill the gaps. Patient care should improve when nurses control their own practice. Many hospitals are examining such systems and weighing the costs and benefits. Only time will give us the answers to the economic questions. We feel, however, that regardless of the economic outcomes, such systems are good for nursing. Through such systems nurses can gain an equal voice not only in nursing practice but in health care.

ORGANIZATIONAL EFFECTIVENESS IN HEALTH CARE TODAY

It is difficult to define organizational effectiveness, especially in a service industry such as health care. Do we look at the number of patients processed or the outcomes? In teaching hospitals, do we look at curing patients or providing learning for interns and nurses? We must recognize that open systems have multiple functions and exist within environments that provide uncertainty, and that their effectiveness may be measured by their ability to survive, adapt, maintain themselves, and grow. Viewed through a systems perspective, effectiveness comes to be defined by how well an organization copes with its environment. Nothing could be more meaningful for health care today.

Many factors today make it difficult for bureaucratically structured organizations to be effective. A bureaucracy's strength is its capacity to manage routine and predictable activities in a stable and predictable environment with its well-defined chain of command and rules. But many organizations, especially in health care, are not well equipped to deal with today's rapid and continuous environmental change. In addition, growth is a factor that introduces complexity in a bureaucratic pyramid. Increased administrative overhead, tighter controls, rigid rules, and greater impersonality all result from increased organization size. Increased diversity also results from growth. Today's environment demands diverse, highly specialized competence that is often incompatible with a bureaucracy's hierarchy and rigidity. Also needed today is a change in managerial philosophy. New concepts of people, their values, needs, and reaction to uses of power are needed. Finally, the need to integrate innovative, non-status quo thinking into organizational decision making is needed. Any organization designed to deal with a stable environment where organizational processes are rigid or based on past history will not react to environmental pressures in such a way as to be effective. In fact, many have not survived.

Bureaucracies do abound, however, and many are successful. But some organizations exist in stable environments and are not growing rapidly. Furthermore, many are run by centralized control and rigid sets of regulations, which is the management style usually desired by the dominant organizational coalition. Where technology is stable, such power maintenance may not inhibit an organization.

It is difficult, though, to view health care today in a stable, predictable environment. Organizational effectiveness for health care institutions in today's environment entails, therefore:

1. *Adaptability*—the ability to solve unique problems quickly in reaction to a changing environment

2. A *sense of organizational purpose*—knowledge and insight as to where an organization is headed and why. This is shared by all members of the organization.

3. *Ability to test reality*—the ability to search out, accurately perceive, and correctly interpret the environment and its implications for the organization.

4. *Integration*—the ability to ensure that all organizational subparts are integrated and not working at cross purposes (see Schein, 1980)

From an open systems viewpoint, such organizational effectiveness means sensing a change in the environment, inputting relevant information and digesting that information, using that information rather than organizational past history to make creative decisions, changing the throughput according to those decisions while managing undesired side effects, outputting new products or services in line with perceived environmental demands, and obtaining feedback on the change.

If we examine these processes from another perspective, we note that there are many points at which these processes could fail, thus reducing effectiveness:

1. Failure to sense environmental changes in a timely manner

2. Misperception of environmental changes

3. Failure to attempt to gain a market share in innovations until all or almost all the competition has done so

4. Failure to transmit relevant information to organization decision makers

5. Failure to foster creative decision making

6. Failure to recognize assumptions inherent in decisions made internally or by external change agents/consultants

7. Failure to convert the production system completely to the change

8. Failure to realize that simply announcing change doesn't make it happen

9. Failure to allow participation in change by organizational members responsible for implementation

10. Failure to recognize and deal with the inevitable resistance to change

11. Failure to ensure that all subsystems change as needed

12. Failure to communicate to the environment that change is taking place so that the product or service can be exported in a timely manner

13. Failure to obtain feedback

14. Failure to use the feedback to modify the change

All these do's and don'ts are subparts of an overall coping strategy to be used in a changing environment and they are integrated. It does little good to have the best market research department if the organization fails to influence its production system to change nor does it help to have a flexible production system if the organization cannot perceive environmental change.

Furthermore, to be innovative in today's environment, organizations must have three kinds of people (see Galbraith, 1982): *creative idea generators* (entrepreneurial risk-takers who champion innovative solutions); *sponsors* (middle managers who recognize the business significance of new ideas, can carry ideas to implementation, and can balance the operating and innovating needs of the organization); and *orchestrators* (those with the political skills to ensure that innovation, which causes massive change, survives).

There are many ways to accomplish the ends advocated here for a coping strategy. One way is to ensure that new ideas are kept apart from the operations section of the organization—especially, staff controls—until they are proven. Innovation and operation are inherent opposites, much as creative and status quo decision making are.

Another method is to create research and development (R & D) departments whose entire function is to create and rigorously test new ideas. Project management and matrix organizations are, on a larger scale, also useful.

In designing and operating their organizations, nurse managers are by no means restricted to a bureaucratic model. Productivity, survival, and continued growth in today's health care environment require innovative organizational design and management. Since this book is designed for the nurse manager rather than the administrator, we will focus upon management. The concepts of productivity enhancement and innovation are themes that run throughout. They are requirements in today's health care industry.

SUMMARY

- We live in an organized society where individuals balance lack of personal freedom in furthering organizational goals with the economic and personal benefits of increased productivity. Managers mediate the process in which individuals surrender autonomy for other benefits.

- Organizations are open systems that operate much like the human body. Their ultimate goal is to survive and they change various resources (people, capital, supplies) into services.

- Organizations produce goods and services that are exchanged for the resources required to survive. Many factors influence the organization's performance (e.g., patients, suppliers, competitors, governmental regulatory bodies, physicians, third-party payers, and the labor market).

- Organizations can be viewed as social systems consisting of people working in a predetermined pattern of relationships toward a goal. The goal of health care organizations is to provide a particular mix of health services.

- There are four differing schools of organizational theory: classical, neoclassical, technological, and modern systems.

- Within the organization, an authority structure is created that determines the formal communication system and guides the organizational activities. This structure can be examined on two dimensions: horizontal and vertical.

- There are five types of health care institutions: acute care, long-term, ambulatory care, home health care, and temporary health care. They may be private or public, proprietary or nonprofit.

- Nursing is the largest department of a hospital, includes many units, and can be organized in a centralized or decentralized manner.

- The nurse manager interacts with patients and staff to manage a nursing unit. Accountability in nursing means responsibility for providing high quality patient care and acceptance of the consequent praise or blame. There is a difficulty when one's decision about what is best for the patient conflicts with others' (physicians' and administration's) beliefs.

- Organizational effectiveness is a difficult concept in health care today. Innovation and creative problem solving are needed and must be fostered.

BIBLIOGRAPHY

Anderson, R. A. (1985). Product and product-line management in nursing. *Nurs Adm Quart*, 10(1): 65–72.

Barnard, C. I. (1938). *The functions of the executive*. Cambridge: Harvard University Press.

Cannon, E. (Editor). (1925). *Adam Smith, An inquiry into the nature and causes of the wealth of nations*. 4th ed. London, Methuen. Originally published in 1776.

Fayol, H. (1949, English version). *General and industrial administration*. London: Pitman.

Freund, C. M., and Mitchell, J. (1985). Multi-institutional systems: The new arrangement. *Nurs Econ*, 3(Jan.–Feb.): 24–31.

Galbraith, J. R. (1977). *Organizational design*. Reading, MA: Addison-Wesley.

Galbraith, J. R. (1982). Designing the innovating institution. *Organizational Dynamics*, (Winter): 5–15.

Howell, W. C., and Dipboye, R. L. (1982). *Essentials of industrial and organizational psychology*. Homewood, IL: Dorsey.

Katz, D., and Kahn, R. (1978). *The social psychology of organizations*. New York: Wiley.

March, J. G., and Simon, H. (1958). *Organizations*. New York: Wiley.

Metcalfe, H. C., and Urwick, L. (Editors). (1940). *The collected papers of Mary Parker Follet*. New York: Harper.

Robbins, S. P. (1983). *Organizational theory*. Englewood Cliffs, NJ: Prentice-Hall.

Schein, E. H. (1980). *Organizational psychology*. Englewood Cliffs, NJ: Prentice-Hall. Chapter 13.

Schermerhorn, J. R., Jr. (1984). *Management for productivity*. New York: Wiley.

Scott, W. G. (1961). Organization theory. *J Acad Mngmt*, 4(1): 7–26.

Stanton, L. J. (1986). Nursing care and nursing products: Revenue or expenses? *J Nurs Adm*, 16(9): 29–32.

Taylor, F. W. (1911). *The principles of scientific management*. New York: Harper & Brothers.

Thompson, J. D. (1967). *Organizations in action*. New York: McGraw-Hill.

Weber, M. (1958). In: *From Max Weber: Essays in sociology*. Gerth, H., and Mills, C. W. (editors). New York: Oxford University Press.

Woodward, J. (1965). *Industrial organization: Theory and practice*. London: Oxford University Press.

The Functions of a Nurse Manager in a Health Care Setting

Management Functions
Planning
Organizing
Controlling
Decision Making

Management Functions for the First-Level Manager
Planning
Organizing
Controlling

THIS CHAPTER WILL discuss the functions of a supervisor (nurse manager) in a health care setting with particular attention to the traditional functions of management. In addition, it will provide an introduction to some of the more current functions of human resource management and review some of the functions that are especially characteristic of health care settings, such as multiple bosses, role conflict, and patient care management. Figure 3–1 illustrates many of the environmental, institutional, and human factors that converge on the nurse manager.

MANAGEMENT FUNCTIONS

Supervision can be defined as the process of getting work done through others—done properly, on time, and within budget. Throughout this book the terms *supervision* and *management* will be used almost interchangeably although, conceptually, management can be viewed as a broader role that goes beyond direct supervision of people to include also the deployment of resources to accomplish organizational ends. Management functions can be defined as follows:

Figure 3–1   Factors Affecting the Nurse Manager

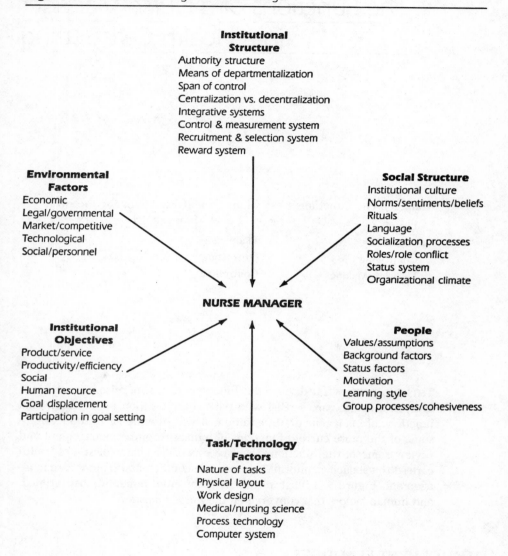

**Institutional
Structure**
Authority structure
Means of departmentalization
Span of control
Centralization vs. decentralization
Integrative systems
Control & measurement system
Recruitment & selection system
Reward system

**Environmental
Factors**
Economic
Legal/governmental
Market/competitive
Technological
Social/personnel

Social Structure
Institutional culture
Norms/sentiments/beliefs
Rituals
Language
Socialization processes
Roles/role conflict
Status system
Organizational climate

NURSE MANAGER

**Institutional
Objectives**
Product/service
Productivity/efficiency
Social
Human resource
Goal displacement
Participation in goal setting

People
Values/assumptions
Background factors
Status factors
Motivation
Learning style
Group processes/cohesiveness

**Task/Technology
Factors**
Nature of tasks
Physical layout
Work design
Medical/nursing science
Process technology
Computer system

1. *Planning*: Determining the long- and short-term objectives (ends) of the institution or unit and the actions (means) that must be taken to achieve these objectives.

2. *Staffing*: Selecting the personnel who will be involved in carrying out these actions and placing them in positions appropriate to their knowledge and skills.

3. *Organizing*: Mobilizing the human and material resources of the institution so that the latter's objectives can be achieved.

4. *Directing*: Motivating and leading the personnel to carry out the actions needed to achieve the institution's objectives.

5. *Controlling*: Comparing results with predetermined standards of performance and taking corrective action when performance deviates from these standards.

6. *Decision making*: Identifying a problem, searching for alternative solutions, and selecting the alternative that best achieves the decision maker's objectives.

This chapter will give special attention to planning, organizing, and controlling for the nurse manager, with less attention to staffing, directing, and decision making, as these are covered elsewhere.

Planning

Planning is always important since the future is uncertain, especially in such areas as the health care field, where environmental factors are rapidly changing. Planning is a four-stage process: (a) establish objectives (ends); (b) evaluate the present situation and predict future trends and events; (c) formulate a planning statement (means); and (d) convert this into an action statement.

One can usually differentiate between strategic planning and contingency planning, although in both cases a similar process is used. *Strategic planning* refers to determining the long-term objectives of the institution and the policies that will be used to achieve these objectives; such planning is carried out primarily by the chief administrative head and/or the board of directors in a health care institution. Although lower-level managers are not directly involved in strategic planning, they are affected by the strategic plan since it will determine both the objectives they must achieve and the means by which they can do so. A manager's effectiveness is directly related to her or his knowledge of the institution's strategy and its application to the unit for which the manager is responsible.

Contingency planning refers to identifying and dealing with the many problems that interfere with getting the work done. This requires advance identification of the department's or unit's objectives, the contingencies that may prevent the achievement of these objectives, and how the work can be organized or assigned to prevent these contingencies from getting out of hand.

Setting objectives. Contingency planning essentially flows from strategic planning. Since the latter involves establishing objectives as well as policies to achieve them, a discussion of institutional objectives is in order. These can be categorized into four general areas: product/service objectives, efficiency objectives, social objectives, and human resource objectives.

Product/services. For health care facilities this is the most important area because of its relationship to patient care. What patient care needs will be directly satisfied by the institution? What types of patients are to be served? What types of services will be offered? Some health care facilities also set goals (objectives) in the areas of teaching and/or research. The relative importance of each of the above will depend on such factors as whether the institution is a private or public facility, whether it is affiliated with a university or some other type of institution, and its size and geographical location.

Efficiency. This refers, of course, to efficiency in the performance of the institution's work. How many resources are required per unit of care—for instance, the number of nurses per patient day? How much time is expended per procedure? How many square feet are allocated per service? How will the efficiency of the unit be measured (e.g., average hospital stay, occupancy rates, within budget, hours of nursing care required for a given mix of patients)? Outside agencies such as third-party payers and governmental agencies are particularly concerned with these matters, in view of the rapid growth in health care costs over the last ten years.

Social. Objectives in this area relate to meeting the obligations that have been established by the community or society in which the institution resides. Will the institution actively seek to be a good citizen or will it merely meet its minimal obligations by obeying the letter of the laws governing its behavior? It should be noted that hospitals themselves possess considerable political power through such lobbying organizations as the American Hospital Association and the American Medical Association and may therefore influence the laws under which they are regulated.

Human resources. This has to do with the efforts that will be made to satisfy employee needs in order to maintain their commitment to the objectives of the institution. Will specific objectives be set in the areas of nurse manager/supervisor development and employee attitude and satisfaction?

Figure 3–2a shows the mission statement of one university-affiliated private hospital, which presents the nature of the institution and the direction in which it plans to go in the future. It is followed by the philosophy statement and an annual corporate goals and nursing service objectives statement (see Figure 3–2b, c). It also includes some specific objectives needed to achieve these overall goals. Obviously, goal statements for non–university-affiliated hospitals or community hospitals that focus on secondary care might be very different. Goal statements need to be reviewed periodically to keep them realistic and consistent with environmental trends.

Figure 3—2a Midwest Teaching Hospital Mission Statement

- To be dedicated to excellence and international health care leadership in affiliation with an out-standing medical school.

- To serve as one of the world's pre-eminent providers of health care, engaging in a full range of services, including primary, secondary, and tertiary acute patient care.

- To provide resources necessary to serve as a national and international institution for medical education at all levels and for applied research in the biosciences.

- To strive towards ensuring the availability of compassionate, cost effective, quality health care services throughout the metropolitan region.

- To provide an environment which is conducive for the medical staff members to practice to the extent of their qualifications in accordance with by-laws, rules and regulations approved by the Hospital Board of Directors.

- To provide employees with a high quality of working life, including equitable compensation and benefits, and opportunities to achieve their full potential as individuals and as members of the health care team.

- To meet the financial requirements of the institution necessary to remain fiscally viable.

Used by permission of Barnes Hospital, St. Louis.

Figure 3—2b Hospital Nursing Service Philosophy

Nursing is the individualized process of caring for and supporting patients as they progress through the changing levels of health.

We are committed to the development of patient-centered nursing care and the accountability of individual professional nurses for specific patient care through the nursing process. This process includes assessment of patients' health care problems, establishing nursing diagnosis, planning for and instituting goal-directed nursing activities, and critically evaluating the effectiveness of that care on a continual basis.

We support the dignity of the individual and believe that patients have the right to respectful care. We believe that nurses are patients' advocates, who participate in communications relative to the various aspects of patient care and the coordination of that care. Collaboration with other health care professionals and support of therapeutic medical treatment is recognized as essential throughout the process of care. We believe that patients and/or their important others should be included in the development and evaluation of their care.

We are committed to health teaching which promotes an optimum level of functioning. We believe that discharge planning, which provides for the transition from hospital to community, is an integral part of the patient's plan of care.

We believe that professional growth of nurses is related to the development of competency in nursing practice and the acceptance of responsibility for one's own actions and judgements. We provide experiential and educational opportunities which support professional growth and recognize that research activities are necessary to the continued development of nursing practice.

In response to expressed health needs of the community, we accept the responsibility to share relevant knowledge and information. We recognize the community has the right to expect that care be provided in a manner which demonstrates concern for cost effectiveness.

Used by permission of Barnes Hospital, St. Louis.

Figure 3—2c Corporate Goals and Nursing Service Objectives 1987

I. Patient Care Delivery

Goal A. To develop a coordinated continuum of care:

* Objective 1. To expand the heart transplant program by implementation of Mechanical Assist Program.
* Objective 2. To explore the feasibility of developing a Comprehensive Critical Cardiology Service (CCCS).
* Objective 3. To develop a geriatric psychiatric program.
* Objective 4. To develop systematic process for organ retrieval in support of the organ transplant program.
* Objective 5. To further develop the Epilepsy program on Neurosurgery.
* Objective 6. To explore the development of a Cooperative Care Unit.
* Objective 7. To assist in the development of a plan to create a center of excellence in pulmonary medicine.
* Objective 8. To develop an outpatient Psychiatric Day Hospital.
* Objective 9. To develop an outpatient center for cardiac assessment and screening.
* Objective 10. To develop an outpatient diabetic center.
* Objective 11. To develop a plan for centralized outpatient facility for medical therapies or diagnostic procedures.
* Objective 12. To investigate the feasibility of developing a comprehensive outpatient treatment facility for dermatology patients.
* Objective 13. To assist in the development of a sports medicine rehabilitation program.
* Objective 14. To develop a business plan for Obstetrics following the movement of patients to Regional.

Goal B. To improve the efficiencies and effectiveness of operations.

* Objective 1. To develop, where appropriate, intermediate care units for patients who do not need intensive care but need more than general ward care and evaluate effectiveness.
* Objective 2. To design cost-effective nursing care delivery practices and systems.
* Objective 3. To determine nursing care cost information per DRG.
* Objective 4. To implement nursing portion of computerized pharmacy information system.
* Objective 5. To ensure quality patient care through the establishment of standards and revision of documentation and quality monitoring systems.

Goal C. To identify new markets and improve the awareness, utilization and value exchange of services.

* Objective 1. To promote Cardiology services.

II. Personnel

Goal A. To bring about increased sensitivity to consumers.

* Objective 1. To participate in revising the consumer relations program and implement changes applicable to Nursing.

Goal B. To implement career development programming.

* Objective 1. To continue development of an RN career ladder program during 1987.

Goal C. To manage compensation systems.

Goal D. To ensure recruitment and retention.

Goal E. To improve benefit systems.

Goal F. To improve communications.

* Objective 1. To establish a framework for communication which ensures staff involvement in problem identification and resolution.

III. Financial Viability

Goal A. To achieve targets for operating and non-operating net excesses of revenues over
 expenses.

* Objective 1. To review pricing structure for all areas, recommending changes where
 indicated.

Goal B. To increase donor contributions.

Goal C. To maintain an AA rating for capital access.

Goal D. To provide the financial support necessary to meet community responsibility for
 indigent care.

Goal E. To maximize participation in viable alternate delivery systems.

Goal F. To develop finanical systems which are responsive to the changing environment.

IV. External Environment

Goal A. To influence the development of clinical service management and medical staff
 relations.

Goal B. To participate in medical, nursing and allied health education and research
 programs.

Goal C. To pursue opportunities in the hospital's relationships in the medical center.

Goal D. To develop an ongoing rapport with political and health care leaders.

Goal E. To establish a long-range strategy in relation to competition and new business
 opportunities.

Used by permission of Barnes Hospital, St. Louis.

Statements of goals, as in Figure 3–2c, focus thinking on the future, on what might happen in the future, and on how present activities help to move the institution towards these goals. Institutions with such specific goals are called proactive institutions; their administrators spend much of their time on future events and on preparing the institution to deal with them. Institutions without clear goals are reactive institutions—ones that tend to operate on a day-to-day basis and spend much of their time and attention on "fire-fighting" instead of "fire prevention."

These same principles can be utilized by first-level managers also. For example, Barnes Hospital in St. Louis recently developed a nursing service strategic planning model that fits with the current hospital process. The process incorporates the corporate strategy, assessment of the Nursing Service Department, planning sessions with the clinical service division chiefs, and any assessments of new business lines that may have been completed during the previous year. The key groups assessed in the environment assessment include patients, families, physicians, staff, internal hospital departments, and the local and national nursing issues. In assessing the external environment, the nursing service focus was mainly on corporate directions and evaluation of corporate issues to determine department applicability. Examples of issues assessed would be the aging population, clinical service strengths, physician relations, etc. The second component of the environment assessment is the market assessment. Future directions for consumer relations were examined, patient satisfaction surveys were summarized, and public expectations of nursing care were reviewed. Manpower availability for nursing was included in the market assessment. Both national trends and Barnes Hospital nursing service recruitment data for the past four years were examined. The entry-into-practice issue was also addressed, as were the quality directions for the hospital as a whole. A physician evaluation of the nursing services provided would also be important to include in a market assessment.

In assessing the nursing department as a whole, the nursing service reviewed several issues. The current employee attitude survey and actions taken to correct deficiencies were reviewed. Area salary and benefit surveys were examined to determine the nursing service position. The latest Joint Commission recommendations and their progress in meeting the deficiencies were reviewed. Other active nursing service committees such as Career Ladder and Nurse Practice Committee efforts were incorporated. During the organizational assessment component, the nursing department's relationships with other hospital departments and with the local and national nursing community in the areas of education, research, and publishing were explored. The expectation was to develop a three-year departmental plan. An objective for nurse managers was set up on their divisions to identify issues to be addressed for the next three years. The nurse managers would have to be knowledgeable of the corporate strategy, the nursing department goals and objectives, and any clinical service activities that affect their area.

When doing a division assessment, the following items were thought to be important: patient care delivery systems, quality scores, staff development, patient/physician satisfaction, staff satisfaction, support department evaluation, physical plant assessment, equipment needs identification, and clinical practice changes that would be impacting the area. It is expected that division planning will be a participative process where unit goals and objectives would be set and prioritized, and action plans developed. It is clear that division planning fits in with both the departmental and hospital planning. And nurse managers will be expected to do such planning in the future (Hailstone, 1987).

One common problem that has been found in many institutions, especially those without clear-cut operational goals, is goal displacement. Goal displacement means that a hospital unit pursues its own narrowly defined goals rather than the overall goals of the institution. Sometimes goal displacement manifests itself as excessive enforcement of rules (or excessive concern over the means of the unit) rather than the ends of the institution; this is especially likely to occur in bureaucratically organized institutions, or when the official goals of the institution are general and ambiguous. Such ambiguity often results when there is difficulty in achieving agreement among units as to the institution's overall goals, so that each unit pursues its own goals.

It is not only important for an institution to establish objectives, but each individual in the institution should be involved in the process. One popular technique for doing this is what is known as management by objectives (MBO) (De Fee, 1977). MBO involves several stages. Ideally, the first stage is the determination of the overall objectives of the institution. These objectives are shared with subordinates, who then formulate objectives for their particular units. These latter objectives are discussed by the subordinates and their managers to be sure that overall and unit objectives are in congruence.

Once the objectives are formulated, the subordinate works on developing a plan (means) to achieve them. Measures of achievement are predetermined, and feedback as to whether or to what degree the objectives are achieved is given to the subordinate at specified intervals. Periodic subordinate/supervisor review of the MBO plan is useful so that corrective action may be taken. In some cases adjustment of the objectives (up or down) may be necessary; in other cases changes will be made in the means used to achieve them.

Both academicians and management practitioners have raised questions as to the effectiveness of this technique. The literature shows that MBO is usually more effective in improving employee satisfaction and morale than in improving employee productivity, but MBO can nevertheless serve as both a planning and a control technique. It tends to work best in situations where there are clear-cut institutional objectives; top administrators are committed to lower-level participation in goal setting; individual and measurable tasks are involved; performance feedback can be given; there is considerable trust between the supervisor and the subordinate; true participation in objective setting is afforded; and where the subordinate is highly motivated toward achievement. Some would argue that the above situation represents a very favorable work environment and that MBO is likely to work best where it is needed the least. Nevertheless, objective setting (see Chapter 11) is an important supervisory function.

Evaluating and predicting. The second stage in the planning process is evaluation of the present situation and prediction of future events. From a strategic planning point of view, this stage requires an evaluation of the internal and external environment of the institution. The former calls for evaluating the present strengths and weaknesses of the institution. What activities does the institution perform well or poorly? Present activities and the policies relating to them might be grouped into the following categories: patient care/teaching/research; physical facilities; human resources; budgets (financial development); organizational system; technological capabilities; auxiliary services; finance/accounting; and management/administrator reputation.

The factors in the external environment that must be evaluated, along with some examples of their effects on health care institutions, are shown in Figure 3–3.

After both the internal and external environments of the institution have been evaluated, specific policies can then be formulated. These can best be expressed in the double-column format below, with questions on the left and possible answers, choices, or observations on the right.

POLICY QUESTIONS	HEALTH CARE EXAMPLES
What services will be offered by the organization?	Types of patient care Teaching Research
What kinds of patients will be served?	Children, the aged, special conditions
How will these services be delivered?	Free-standing treatment facilities such as emergency aid clinics, surgical centers, and outreach programs
How will these potential patients be informed about the services offered?	Note the recent advertising by organizations providing alcoholism treatment, billboards advertising emergency aid facilities
How will these services be priced?	Percentage of indigent patients served, relationship with Blue Cross, Medicare, Medicaid, etc.
How will the institution be financed?	Sources of funds for new building/wing/special care facilities
On what basis will the institution choose to compete? What will be emphasized? What kind of care? What patient mix of acuity levels?	General, specialties, trauma, referral, pediatrics

Figure 3—3 External Environmental Factors and Effects

External Environment Factors	Some Effects on Health Care Institutions
Economic	
Inflation	Increased costs of equipment
State of the economy/business cycle	Decreased elective surgery/fewer beds filled during recessions
Fiscal/monetary policies	Availability of government funds to support health care
Legal/Governmental	
Health care regulation	Professional standards review Organization law State review of rates State certificate of need for opening new facilities Reimbursement mechanisms
Health care support	Related to fiscal policies-support for research, teaching in health care
Legal liabilities	Increased malpractice suits
Accreditation agencies	Must meet JCAH or state division of health criteria or lose governmental support
Market/Competitive	
Non-health care competitors	Emergence of new services or elimination of unneeded services
Changes in patient needs	
Changes in population—eg, aging	Increased demand for long-term health care facilities
Substitute products	Emergency aid facilities
Technological	
Changes in technology	Need for retraining
Cost of new technology	Increased cost of hospitalization
Social/Personnel	
Availability and cost of personnel	Nursing shortage/surplus
New opportunities for women	Nurses demand more participation in decision making
Changing attitudes towards health care, death, physical fitness	Increased number of sports injuries Holistic health care "Right to life" movement

From these general policies then come specific allocations of resources to achieve the institutional goals. Procedures, rules and regulations, schedules, and budgets are established as part of the overall institutional plan.

Organizing

Once a strategic plan is established, the organizational structure to carry out that plan must be established. (Figure 3–1 shows some of the factors that influence the institution's structure.) The plan determines what tasks need to be performed in order to achieve the goals. •

These tasks are then subdivided into subtasks. It is from such division of labor/specialization—e.g., one person to give the medications, another to transport patients off the unit—that the efficiency of an institution comes.

These tasks, however, need to be coordinated. One way to do this is by grouping them into departments, as in, say, nursing and housekeeping. Departmentalization can be based on: product or service (maternity, psychiatric); type of client (elderly, children); functions (accounting, finance, housekeeping); process (operating room, radiology); time (evening/night nurse); or geography (emergency).

Authority and power. The most important means of coordination is the authority structure of institutions. According to Scott and others (1967) (Scott et al., 1967), authority involves certain kinds of rights that are possessed by members of the institution. There are two general types of authority rights: the right to allocate institutional tasks, and the right to evaluate the performance of these tasks. These evaluations affect the rewards and sanctions received by employees from the institution.

A variety of individuals may possess these rights. Whether a person has these rights can be determined by the answers to two questions: Would the person A allocating institutional tasks or evaluating the performance of these tasks be negatively evaluated by their supervisors for doing so? Would the person B to whom the tasks have been assigned be negatively evaluated for noncompliance with these orders? If the answer to the first question is no and the answer to the second question is yes, then we can say that A has authority rights over B.

Allocation rights can be exercised either by direction or by delegation. The first would include specifying how a task is to be performed, and the second would leave to the subordinate how the task is to be performed. The latter type of allocation is most commonly found in institutions employing professionals.

Evaluation rights are broken down into three stages: criteria setting, sampling, and evaluating. In institutions employing professionals, such as health care facilities, the profession itself frequently establishes the criteria by which an individual should be evaluated, but it is usually the manager's right to sample work behavior and then compare this behavior with the established standard.

A second theory of authority is the "zone of indifference" theory developed by Barnard and elaborated on by Simon (Simon, 1976). This theory places less emphasis on the institution as a source of authority and focuses more on the relationship between the supervisor and subordinate and on the sources of power that the former has over the latter.

French and Raven have classified sources of power into five main categories: reward, coercive, legitimate, expert, and referent (French & Raven, 1959). *Reward* and *coercive* power have to do with the ability of the supervisor to mediate positive or negative rewards for the subordinate, including such items as pay, recognition, work schedule, duties, continued employment, and so forth. *Legitimate* power relates to the belief that the supervisor has the right to give commands; it is frequently based on acceptance of the social system. *Expert* power refers to the belief by the subordinate that the supervisor has superior knowledge in this particular area. *Referent* power refers to the degree to which the subordinate identifies with the superior and therefore patterns his or her behavior accordingly.

Nurse managers have reward and coercive power over their subordinates. Many newer staff nurses tend to believe that the nurse manager also has legitimate power over them. Expert and referent power would more likely come after nurse manager and staff nurse have worked together for some time. More experienced nurses might also share expert and referent power with the nurse manager over the newer staff nurses. The more types of power a supervisor has over a subordinate, the greater the control that supervisor has. This makes it extremely important for nurse managers to be selected on the basis of their technical expertise and personal leadership qualities, including their ability to serve as a role model.

Bureaucracies. Although authority is the most common means used to link the tasks, people, and technology of the organization, other integration techniques are also used. Rules and regulations, for instance, are especially important within the bureaucratic type of organization. The bureaucratic organization consists of a set of positions arranged in a hierarchical manner, wherein each position holder has formal duties with a high degree of specialization and a formally established system of rules and regulations that governs his or her decisions and actions. Individuals are employed on the basis of professional or other qualifications rather than political, family, or other connections, and the person seeks this particular position as a career. In this "ideal" type of organization, bureaucratic officers hold their positions because of their expertise; they apply the rules and regulations in an impersonal manner, without favoritism, to make rational decisions and achieve administrative efficiency.

"Bureaucracy" is often used pejoratively to connote an institution where excessive enforcement of rules leads to inefficiency. The major problem that most bureaucratic institutions face is a form of goal displacement, where the energies of the participant in the unit are focused more on enforcing the rules than providing service to the clients; this is a not unusual situation within public health care institutions. Nevertheless, the bureaucratic model is still followed in parts of most health care institutions, especially in support and administrative departments.

Other commonly used means of integration, especially between different units within the institution, according to Jay Galbraith, include direct contact, liaison roles, task forces (temporary committees), teams (permanent committees), integrating personnel, integrating departments, and, finally, matrix organizations (Galbraith, 1977). For example, nursing committees can be viewed as an integrating force. Galbraith, as well as Jelinek and colleagues, discuss these means of organizing in some depth (Galbraith, 1977; Jelinek, Litterer & Miles, 1981).

Controlling

Control involves establishment of standards of performance, determination of the means to be used in measuring performance, evaluation of the performance, and feedback of performance data to the individual so behavior can be changed.

MBO, presented earlier as a planning device, can also be considered as a control mechanism. First, it entails the determination of objectives (standards) against which performance can be measured. Second, specific measures have to be established to determine whether these objectives are met. Third, the actual accomplishment of the objectives would be measured in relation to the standard and this information would be fed back to the individual. Then corrective action could be taken as indicated.

The MBO process is a rather mechanistic system that is applicable to only a limited range of tasks and situations. It involves a lot of self-control, and many health care organizations rely heavily on internalized "self-control." This type of control depends heavily on proper selection and training of individuals to insure that they have the capability and desire to behave in the manner required by the organization to accomplish its tasks. Especially important to self-control are the socialization processes that cause persons to internalize the values of their profession and accept a code of behavior. Socialization as a means of control is useful in health care organizations because continuous monitoring of behavior is difficult.

Socialization. There are five important stages in the socialization process (Klein & Ritti, 1980). The first stage is *anticipatory socialization*, during which individuals acquire what they believe to be the attitudes, values, and beliefs of the group to which they hope to belong. Some of this learning, unfortunately, comes from the myths that are presented in the media and from contacts with individuals in these occupations. Consider, for instance, how the numerous television series on hospitals have often encouraged would-be nurses to develop erroneous conceptions (e.g., subservience) about nursing as a profession.

The second stage involves learning in a presocializing institution such as a school of nursing. During this period, which culminates for most nursing professionals in graduation and passing of the licensure examination, an individual becomes more aware of the real norms of the profession. The third stage comes with recruitment, when the institution seeks to select individuals who already possess the skills and values desired by the institution. Proper selection makes the job of the nurse manager in the health care facility easier.

The next stage, institutional socialization, introduces individuals to the norms and values of the particular institution in which they are employed. "Reality shock" occurs when individuals find that the norms and values of the "aspired-to" group are different from those learned in the first two stages and anticipated for the third stage. This results in feelings of helplessness, powerlessness, frustration, and dissatisfaction (Schmalenberg & Kramer, 1979).

The final stage of socialization is sometimes referred to as "the rite of passage." It occurs when a person is accepted into full membership status and is committed to the actual norms and values of the institution.

Schmalenberg and Kramer perceive four phases in the role transformation from student to staff nurse: honeymoon phase, followed by shock, recovery, and resolution stages. They argue that the subcultures of school and work have different values and norms. In nursing schools, "the dominant values transmitted are comprehensive, total patient care with individualization and family involvement. Use of judgment, autonomy, cognitive skills, and decision making are strongly promulgated in this system. In the work subculture, the emphasis is on the value of providing safe care for all the patients. Organization, efficiency, cooperation, and responsibility are highly valued" (Schmalenberg & Kramer, 1979:1).

During the honeymoon phase the new graduate is pleased with her first job as a "real nurse" and focuses on learning the routines of the hospital, perfecting her skills, and becoming accepted by other staff. The second stage begins when she finds that some of the values taught in school are not as highly valued in the work setting. In the recovery stage the nurse begins to tolerate some of the aspects of the situation that before seemed intolerable. The final phase involves constructive resolution of the conflict between work and school values.

An effective and understanding nurse manager can help new nurses deal with this socialization process and facilitate the sharing of experiences in resolving the conflict. Newly graduated nurses need to understand the universal nature of the process they experience and be allowed to express and explore their feelings with others during the process.

Managerial surveillance. A second type of control system is managerial surveillance, which involves both direct observation of subordinate behavior and indirect observation through records. The amount of control from this source is related to the authority structure of the organization. For some types of managerial situations in a health care facility, control through direct observation may be very important: in emergency rooms; units with a large number of beginning nurses; highly technical areas that lack experienced personnel; or units with a number of non-professional staff such as nursing assistants. In units staffed by highly qualified and experienced professionals, managerial surveillance through direct observation may be less important.

Related to managerial surveillance is the "span of control" of the supervisor, or the number of individuals for whom the supervisor is directly responsible. Narrow spans of control, with only three to five subordinates, allow for a great degree of control, while spans of control for over ten employees make it difficult to control each subordinate by direct observation. Some of the factors that allow for wider spans of control include very routine work, well-trained subordinates, a highly capable manager, personal assistants, stable operations, similar functions among subordinates, highly formalized tasks, and spatially dispersed subordinates (Van Fleet & Bedeian, 1977). When the individuals being monitored are physically isolated or dispersed, indirect observation is obviously difficult.

A number of sources of information are frequently used for indirect observation—among them, budgets, schedules, time sheets, activity reports, statistical reports, patient surveys, narcotic reports, and patient charts. The types of information available are specific to each institution as are the standards used to evaluate that information.

The more sources of power that a supervisor has over a subordinate, such as reward, coercive, legitimate, referent, and expert, the more likely it is that the supervisor will be able to control the subordinate's behavior and direct it toward the accomplishment of institutional objectives. Rules and regulations also serve as a source of control, especially in situations where these rules and regulations have been internalized. Reliance on this means of control is most common in those parts of the institution that have a bureaucratic structure.

Principles of control. Whatever method is used to control the performance of others, the manager should be aware of several principles of control. The first one has been referred to by Klein and Ritti as "setting the fox to watch the henhouse" (Klein & Ritti, 1980). In this situation, individuals themselves provide their supervisors with the information that will be used to evaluate their performance. It is relatively easy for them to modify or in some other way manipulate the information, because it is subjective or judgmental and therefore not easily detectable. When such self-reported data are used for evaluation, caution is advised.

Another important principle is the notion that "measured behavior" drives out "unmeasured behavior." If a supervisor focuses on specific, measurable aspects of the job in giving feedback to an individual, it may drive out unmeasured (and unrewarded) behavior.

Finally, there is what has been referred to as the "paradox of control" (Dalton, 1971). In attempting to control others, an individual may impose new requirements on them. This leads to countermeasures by the controllee, either to avoid this control, to modify the information, or even to seek substitutes for the desired action. This leads to countermeasures by the controller, and the whole process can become a vicious cycle. Frequently greater control over the behavior of others can be gained by giving up control—giving people greater freedom and trusting that they will do what is right.

Decision Making

Decision making permeates all aspects of the manager's job (Chapter 12). It includes: (a) the identification of a problem; (b) the establishment of the criteria that will be used to evaluate potential solutions to the problem; (c) a search for alternative solutions/actions (recognizing that no action is always an alternative choice); (d) evaluation of the alternatives; and (e) selection of a particular alternative. This process can take place in a second (e.g., deciding to whom you will give a certain task) or may take place over months or even years (e.g., choosing a career, spouse, or a new job).

March and Simon have pointed out that in using this approach to decision making, real decision makers tend to use a simplified model of the real situation and tend to seek satisfactory rather than "optimal" solutions (March & Simon, 1964). Most decision makers establish some minimum criteria as to the acceptability of a decision and then search until a solution is found that meets this minimum acceptability.

MANAGEMENT FUNCTIONS FOR THE FIRST-LEVEL MANAGER

Particularly relevant to the first-level manager's position are the functions of planning, organizing, and controlling; most of the time, for the person in this position, these involve dealing with contingencies. Since the nurse manager's job is to maintain the highest possible level of patient care while at the same time meeting other conflicting goals such as staying within budget, keeping staff satisfied, and so on, it is important to consider those factors referred to as contingencies, which prevent these goals from being achieved. Gellerman (1975) defines contingencies as those unplanned interruptions, unanticipated events, and inconvenient or awkward circumstances that prevent the work from being accomplished. Much of the content here on planning, organizing, and controlling for the nurse manager stems from Gellerman's ideas. He states:

Planning, for a supervisor, means identifying the most probable sources of contingencies in advance. . . . Organizing, for a supervisor, means making sure that when contingencies occur . . . his/her subordinates are ready for them. This means that they are properly equipped and in the right places at the right times; and above all that they are properly trained. Controlling means making sure that contingencies are properly dealt with, and—when necessary—intervening in the subordinate's work to prevent a contingency from getting out of hand (Gellerman, 1975).

The fundamental principles of the nursing process—assessing, planning, implementing, and evaluating—are very similar to the management concepts of planning, organizing, and controlling, as shown in Figure 3–4.

Planning

Contingency planning is very difficult because of the crisis nature of hospital work and the unknowns involved in patient care. Nevertheless, the nurse manager must try to be aware of the contingencies that may prevent the work from being accomplished. For instance: new, inexperienced, part-time or temporary staff, who do not know the policies and procedures of the institution well and may not be very committed to it; tardiness or unexpected absenteeism, which leaves the unit short of personnel (holidays, weekends, or vacations); staff tardiness from lunch or

---

Figure 3–4   Comparison of Tasks of Clinical Nurse and Nurse Manager

ASSESSMENT

Clinical nurse	**Nurse manager**
Observation of the patient/client and his environment.	Observation of staff reactions to policies and objectives.
	Observation of needs of community—priorities in health care—manpower trends and availability of resources.
Communication skills. Art of listening and interviewing.	Communication skills—art of listening and interviewing.
Collection of facts, identifying priorities.	Collection of facts. Identifying priorities.

PLANNING

Interpretation in the light of clinical knowledge and the facts.	Interpretation in the light of "managerial" knowledge and the facts.

Setting short- and long-term goals for the patient and his family.

Deciding what to do to solve the problems, keeping in mind quality of care, safe care, and the nursing policies laid down.

Involving the patient and his family in the plan of care, and other disciplines as required, in order that there is co-ordination and progress toward similar goals.

Setting short- and long-term goals for service.

Deciding what to do to solve problems, keeping in mind quality of care, safe care, and revising policies if necessary.

Involving the staff and other disciplines in order that there is co-ordination of planning, and progress toward similar goals.

Innovating/using creativity.

IMPLEMENTATION
(Organization)

Setting the plan into action, taking into account:
   The patient's ability to help himself.
   Professional resources.
   Equipment available.

Teaching needs—of patient, family, nursing and other students.

Organizing for continuity of care.

Providing team leadership and an environment in which good work can be done.

Setting the plan into action, taking into account:
   The amount of delegation which can be safely undertaken.
   Professional resources.
   Time available.

Teaching needs—development of staff—orientation of new staff to fulfill their respective roles.

Organizing for continuity in providing a service.

Providing leadership in the area of responsibility and an environment in which good work can be done.

Organizing the budget.

Consumer relations.

EVALUATION
(Control)

Analyzing results of implementation of plan for patient and family.

Considering changes which have taken place which necessitate reassessment.

Considering quality of care provided, alongside the standards and policies which have been agreed.

Identifying areas of nursing practice which require revision of research. Communicating the need together with a suggestion for action to appropriate level.

Communicating changes in planning which may be required to keep patient/client, colleagues, and other professionals informed.

Analyzing results of implementation of plan in consultation with those delivering nursing care.

Considering changes which are necessary and the case for re-planning or adjustment of the plan.

Considering quality of care provided alongside the standards and policies which have been agreed. Taking action where needed.

Facilitating clinical nurses and managers to undertake research projects and critiquing practice.

Communication changes in planning which may be required to keep staff and other professionals informed.

Schurr, M. Getting It Together. *Nursing Times,* Vol. 75, August 30, 1979. Used with permission.

breaks; excessive demand for space when the division is at full capacity; new residents who need to be oriented; unexpected number of critical care patients; physician requests for special services; patients scheduled to be in two or more places at the same time; unavailability of staff, especially for evenings and nights; unavailability of medications, supplies, or equipment at the right time; staff quitting without giving notice.

Once the nurse manager is aware of the contingencies, she or he must be alert to detect their occurrence before they are out of control. This involves nursing rounds at the beginning of each shift and thereafter as needed. A good nurse manager attempts to make frequent but brief contacts with her subordinates to determine whether the work of the unit is progressing satisfactorily. It is important to remember the word "brief." Personal interchanges can best be left to breaks, lunch hours, or other social occasions. Also one can be seduced into spending extra time with subordinates if they are working on an interesting task. If the subordinate is adequately handling a particular situation, then the nurse manager should be elsewhere, making sure that a problem is not starting up at another location.

Making rounds also enables the nurse manager to assess patient care and staff performance on the unit. She or he can assess the quality of care being provided, a staff member's organizing abilities and interpersonal skills, team cohesion, and individual patient status. "Paper patrolling," such as reviewing records, budgets, and performance data, can also ensure that work is being performed satisfactorily. A nurse manager should develop a system of "red flags," things to look for that show that work is not being done correctly, on time, and within budget. Here one would look for such things as patterns of absenteeism or lateness, direct nursing care hours versus overhead, patient days volume, use of medical-surgical supplies or pharmacy items, or failure to fill out reports (including patient charts) adequately that indicate a potential problem. This review should be done periodically to enable early correction of problem situations.

Finally, what activities will be necessary to prevent problems from happening and what are the plans for dealing with problems once they have occurred? For example, does the unit have plans on dealing with certain kinds of disasters—external disasters, for instance, that increase demand for unit space, or snow or floods that prevent employees from getting to work, or internal disasters such as fire or loss of power?

Organizing

Organizing means having qualified people and the right materials, information, and equipment needed to deal with contingencies. The latter three items are specific to an organization and the type of services it provides. It is important for the nurse manager to identify these needs and make sure that her subordinates have the resources available. Backup materials and equipment are especially important. It is also critical for the nurse manager to be aware of the state of the unit's equipment.

Having qualified personnel at the right time and place to take care of the division's work is one of the most important responsibilities of the nurse manager. He or she needs not only to be sure that the unit personnel have the knowledge and ability to do the job, but also that they are familiar with the policies and procedures of the specific unit. This is frequently achieved through training, which must be an ongoing, almost continuous process to ensure adequate patient care. Refresher (or developmental) training may also be indicated so that seldom used but important skills such as cardiopulmonary resuscitation are retained. Just as ball players have spring training and firefighters hold fire drills, so must nurses and nursing support staff engage in periodic rehearsals of appropriate behavior in specialized situations; they should also understand the reasons behind the policies, procedures, rules, and regulations in the organization. Sometimes these do not make sense to new or inexperienced personnel. Helping staff nurses to understand the "why" behind them will frequently lead to greater compliance with these institutional requirements.

Another important aspect of organizing is scheduling—making sure that persons with the appropriate skills are available on each shift. Obviously, scheduling is very much affected by the institution's policies. In some institutions scheduling is centralized, while in others the nurse manager is responsible. In the former the nurse manager would have to work closely with the centralized scheduler to make sure that adequate personnel were available. In the latter situation, the nurse manager would need to develop scheduling skills.

Proper scheduling includes knowing in advance the capabilities, availability, needs, and desires of the unit personnel. A nurse manager must anticipate needs, estimate when additional personnel will be needed, and have backup personnel plans. Knowing about each person's knowledge, skill, home situation, and even his or her "biological clock" can help insure the availability of adequate personnel to meet contingencies. Working out potential substitutions in advance can help to reduce conflicts in crises. Scheduling is discussed in Chapter 14.

In addition to the above, the nurse manager must help each staff nurse to organize his or her time and activities. Time management (see Chapter 11) is an important aspect of this. Techniques for improving time management are as important to the staff nurse as they are to the nurse manager. Nurse managers can demonstrate effective time management by example.

Patient care is organized according to the type of delivery system used in the unit. Generally, there are three means of organizing the tasks of nursing: functional, team, and primary nursing. These three methods, as described below by Kron (1981), lead to different problems for the nurse manager.

1. *Functional Nursing.* In this method, nursing care is divided into separate tasks. These are performed by varying levels of nursing personnel, depending upon the complexity of each task in terms of judgment and technical knowledge, and the preparation of the individual staff members. Each staff member is responsible for only the tasks done during a given tour of duty.

2. *Team Nursing.* This method utilizes a heterogeneous team of nursing personnel to deliver nursing care to a group of patients. The leader of the team is a registered nurse. The team leader is given the responsibility for the planning, continuity, and evaluation of the nursing care regimens of all patients cared for by the team, for supervising the team members in the implementation of nursing actions, and for evaluating the results.

3. *Primary Nursing* (in a hospital setting). Developed by Marie Manthey (1980), in this method of delivering nursing care, registered professional nurses are given total responsibility and authority for assessing, planning, implementing, and evaluating the nursing care regimens of a specified number of patients within the health care facility. The primary nurse is responsible for the care of a patient 24 hours a day, from the time the patient is admitted to the nursing unit until the patient leaves it. An associate professional nurse carries out the nursing orders when the primary nurse is not on duty (Kron, 1981).

In functional nursing, the nurse manager is actively involved in planning patient care. She or he makes specific assignments, is personally responsible for coordination between staff and shifts, and is the person to whom the staff go for questions and answers. The nurse manager has total responsibility for the unit and must act as a first-level supervisor. In team nursing some of the supervisory functions, especially planning the patient care, assigning tasks, and coordinating these tasks, are taken over by the team leader. In primary nursing the primary nurse is also responsible for planning the nursing care and is usually responsible for care of the patient over 24 hours, even when not on duty.

In team nursing, the nurse manager becomes a manager in that she is really responsible for managing other managers—i.e., the team leaders. The nurse manager must be an effective delegator if team nursing is to be effective, must work cooperatively with these team leaders, and be a resource person for them.

In primary nursing, the nurse manager is often responsible for assigning primary nurses to patients, coordinating the activities of the primary nurses on all shifts, and scheduling so that associates are available when the primary nurse is off duty.

Controlling

Controlling means that the nurse manager must monitor the performance of her subordinates and take corrective action when performance deviates from the established standards. Thus nurse managers would take corrective action when contingencies are about to or have gotten out of control.

One specific concern is when to take corrective action or intervene and how to intervene. An effective nurse manager will intervene when a specific policy, procedure, rule, or regulation has been or is likely to be violated, when there is danger to the patient or personnel, when the subordinate is overloaded or does not possess the necessary skill, information, or authority to act properly, or when there is threat to the property of the institution. For example, the nurse manager would intervene upon observing a staff nurse using incorrect procedures that might affect the patient's health and safety. The nurse manager would also help in emergency situations where the staff nurse was overloaded. On the other hand, the nurse manager may delegate handling of certain contingencies by assigning specific duties to other individuals. Effective delegation is important.

The act of controlling, intervening, or correcting the behavior of a subordinate can be a frustrating experience for both controller and controllee. Too frequent intervention may lead subordinates to lose confidence in themselves or lead to less risk-taking behavior in the future. But failure to intervene can lead to serious problems.

Both nurse managers and subordinates should know in advance the situations or "trigger points" that call for nurse manager intervention. Subordinates should also know under which conditions the nurse manager is willing to provide assistance to ensure that a situation remains under control. It is necessary to stress the importance of frequent patrolling whether it be nursing rounds or "paperwork patrolling." The nurse manager should spend as much time as possible on prevention of problems rather than on later corrective action.

This chapter has focused on the traditional functions of management, namely, planning, organizing, and controlling. Frequent references have been made to other chapters in the book that focus on some of the other functions of management, especially the modern functions of motivation, leadership, and human resource management. The rest of the book will present: emerging issues in nursing management (productivity, change, ethics, and chemical dependency); the modern functions of management (communication theory, decision making, leadership, and motivation); human resource management (recruitment, selection, training, and performance appraisal), and other aspects of management appropriate for nursing (budgeting, risk management, conflict management, and labor unions).

SUMMARY

- Management is the process of getting work done through others, done properly, on time, and within budget. Traditionally, management functions have included planning, staffing, organizing, directing, controlling, and decision making.

- Planning is a four-stage process: establish objectives, evaluate the present situation and predict future trends, formulate a plan, and convert this into action.

- Objectives can be categorized into four general areas: product/service, efficiency, social, and human resource objectives. Predicting trends must be done inside and outside the organization. These objectives can be used in MBO systems to guide action.

- Once a plan is established, an organizational structure must be established to carry out the plan. This is organizing. Organizations are organized by task, department, client, time, and/or geography.

- The most important means of coordination is the authority structure. Authority involves two general types of rights: allocation of tasks and evaluation of performance. Furthermore, direction can be exerted from other sources besides legitimate power: reward, coercion, expert, and referent power.

- Roles and role definitions help define the authority structure of an organization.

- Socialization is the process of fitting people into the roles and informing them of the rules inherent in any authority structure. Socialization includes five stages: anticipatory socialization (beliefs), learning in a presocialization institution (school), recruitment, institutional socialization, and the final "rite of passage." Nurse managers can facilitate the socialization process.

- Managerial surveillance (through observation of behavior or records) is a key to control. The manager's span of control may determine the amount of time available for surveillance.

- Measured behavior tends to drive out unmeasured behavior. Staff will do what is focused on by the manager and/or what is rewarded.

- Nurse managers plan, organize, direct, and control as do all managers.

BIBLIOGRAPHY

Christen, J. W. (1987). The changing nature of first-line supervision. *Health Care Supervisor,* 5(2): 65–70.

Dalton, G. W. (1971). Motivation and control in organizations. In: *Motivation and control in organizations.* Dalton, G. W., and Lawrence, P. R. (editors). Homewood, IL: Irwin-Dorsey. P. 4.

De Fee, D. T. (1977). Management by objectives: When and how does it work? *Personnel Journal.*

Douglass, I. M. (1984). *The effective nurse: Leader and manager.* 2nd ed. St. Louis: Mosby.

French, J. R. P., and Raven, B. (1959). The bases of social power. In: *Studies in social power.* Cartwright, D. (editor). Ann Arbor: University of Michigan Institute for Social Research. Pp. 150–167.

Galbraith, J. R. (1977). *Organization design.* Reading, MA: Addison-Wesley.

Gellerman, S. (1975). *Leader's guide to accompany . . . "Effective supervision: Planning, organizing and controlling."* Rockville, MD: BNA Communications. P. 1.

Gillies, D. A. (1982). *Nursing management: A systems approach.* Philadelphia: Saunders.

Hailstone, S. (1987). Interview with Sherlyn Hailstone, Associate Vice President, Nursing Service, Barnes Hospital, St. Louis, MO (May).

Jelinek, M., Litterer, J. A., and Miles, R. E. (editors). (1981). *Organizations by design: Theory and practice.* Plano, TX: Business Publications.

Klein, S. M., and Ritti, R. R. (1980). *Understanding organizational behavior.* Boston: Kent. P. 124.

Kron, T. (1981). *The management of patient care: Putting leadership skills to work.* 5th ed. Philadelphia: Saunders. Pp. 210–211.

Manthey, M. (1980). *The practice of primary nursing.* Boston: Blackwell.

March, J. G., and Simon, H. A. (1964). *Organizations.* New York: Wiley.

Marriner, A. (1984). *Guide to nursing management.* 2nd ed. St. Louis: Mosby.

McClure, M. L. (1984). Managing the professional nurse. Part II. Applying management theory to the challenges. *J Nurs Adm, 14*(3):11–17.

Rowland, H. S., and Rowland, B. L. (1985). *Nursing administration handbook.* 2nd ed. Germantown, MD: Aspen Systems Corporation.

Schmalenberg, C., and Kramer, M. (1979). *Coping with reality shock.* Wakefield, MA: Nursing Resources. P. 1.

Scott, W. R., et al. (1967). Organizational evaluation and authority. *Adm Sci Quart, 12*:93.

Simon, H. A. (1976). *Adm Behav.* 3rd ed. New York: The Free Press. P. 126.

Van Fleet, D. D., and Bedeian, A. G. (1977). A history of the span of management. *Academy of Management Review, 2*:364.

van Servellen, G. M., and Mowry, M. M. (1985). DRGs and primary nursing: Are they compatible? *J Nurs Adm, 15*(4): 32–36.

2
EMERGING ISSUES IN NURSING MANAGEMENT

What Is Productivity?

Economics/Industrial Definitions

Attempts to Define Productivity
in Health Care

What Is Nursing Productivity?

**Current Methods for Measuring
Nursing Productivity**

Resources per Patient Day

Degree of Occupation

Utilization Rates

Improving Nursing Productivity

Changes in the Use of Inputs

Changes in the Care Process

Summary

AMERICANS INVEST BILLIONS of dollars in health care each year. In return for that investment they expect health care providers to give an accounting of how the money was spent and with what result. As health care costs continue to rise faster than the overall rate of inflation, consumers and policymakers demand decreased health care costs and waste, more careful allocation of scarce resources, and evidence that the care given is of adequate quality.

These externally imposed financial constraints have led health care facilities to become much more attentive to productivity in recent years. Nursing is one health care service that is very likely to be subjected to productivity evaluation. Nursing not only comprises the largest single group of health care providers, but can account for 50% or more of the operating budgets of institutions such as hospitals and nursing homes. Because of their size, and because reductions in the number of nurses hired can appear small in relation to reductions in other smaller departments, nursing services are likely to be reduced in an attempt to cut budgets. Consequently, the definition and measurement of nursing productivity has become a high priority for most nursing managers.

Unfortunately, nursing productivity is a concept that is ill defined. In this chapter, the concept of productivity is reviewed, and then ways of defining and measuring nursing productivity will be discussed. The chapter concludes with specific strategies a nursing manager might use to improve productivity.

WHAT IS PRODUCTIVITY?

Economic/Industrial Definitions

As an economic concept, productivity describes the relationship between the output of an industry and the resources required to produce that output (output per input). It is measured by a number of different methods, the most common of which is the labor productivity statistic. Labor productivity measures the dollar value of output per worker-hour used to produce the output; this gives a simple estimate of whether industries are becoming more or less efficient in their production methods. But this single factor output-input ratio fails to take into account possible reasons for increases or declines in efficiency other than the cost of labor or how hard employees work. To account for the contribution of inputs other than labor, a total factor productivity measure must be used. These other relevant inputs include the introduction of new technology, increases in the cost of raw materials, substitution of equipment or supplies, etc.

Attempts to Define Productivity in Health Care

Finding a definition of productivity for health care is more complex than determining whether only labor or all relevant factors should be used to measure input. Fundamental questions remain about what should be considered an input. Moreover, there is considerable debate about how output should be measured.

The nature of health care inputs. Inputs present fewer measurement problems than outputs. Inputs include the labor, materials, and equipment used in the production of services. These inputs usually can be measured in physical units such as hours of labor; dollars spent on equipment, remodeling, or building expense; and number of supplies used. But the measurement of some inputs is not as simple as it seems. Nursing personnel, for example, is not a homogeneous group, since nurses vary in their level of education, experience, and skill. Some of the differences in educational level and experience may be reflected in differences in pay rates. Yet any two nurses with equivalent education and years of experience are likely to differ considerably in their efficiency and ability to perform a quantity of work. Methods for quantifying differences in skill level are rudimentary.

The nature of the hospital's product. As difficult as it may be to find an adequate definition of input, defining the output of health care is even more problematic. There are, for example, several definitions of hospital output. Until recently, hospital output was most frequently defined as patient days, i.e., the total number of days all patients were hospitalized in a facility over a period of time (Feldstein, 1971). Then it was realized that some patient days require the use of many more resources than others. A day of care for a transplant patient is much more costly than a day of postpartum care, for example. As a result, it has become necessary to consider some new definitions of output.

Most of the new concepts of hospital output assume that the hospital has more than one product (patient days)—that it is instead a multiproduct firm. Currently, most attention is focused on refining the meaning of "patient days" by using the concept of case mix, a set of methods for clustering patients into groupings that are homogeneous with respect to the use of resources. Factors used to cluster patients have included diagnosis, prognosis, utilization, organ system, hospital department, and patient demographic characteristics (Hornbrook, 1982). The best known of these case-mix measures is the diagnosis-related groups (DRGs) system, which groups patients into 468 resource-use groups based on information about their diagnosis and age, and on the use of certain procedures. Using the DRG case-mix measure, the hospital could potentially produce 468 distinct products that vary from one another in the cost of production. Each DRG is weighted to represent the average cost of providing care to patients in that category. While there are many arguments about the validity of the resource clusters produced by the DRG system, it or a case-mix method similar to it is likely to remain in use since it provides greater precision in measuring hospital output.

Output or outcome? Case-mix measures have refined how hospital output quantity is measured, but they do not address the question of output quality. Estimating the quality of health care services output is a particularly vexing problem. In purchasing goods such as household appliances and automobiles, the consumer is usually able to judge the quality of a product by inspection or referring to a consumers' guide to that product. If a manufacturer consistently puts out inferior goods, consumers can express their quality preferences by not purchasing the product.

The purchase of health care services, however, is fundamentally different. Because health care is a service, its production and consumption are simultaneous events. The consumer cannot return a defective product and often cannot reverse the effects of poor service. Furthermore, there is no consumers' guide to health care services and most consumers cannot or do not have time to learn how to evaluate the quality of health care services. Instead, the health care consumer must rely on the ethical obligation of the professional to exercise sound judgment in making decisions about the type and quantity of health care required.

To protect further the interests of the consumer, therefore, health care output is increasingly being defined in terms of quality as well as quantity of services. The goal is to describe output as a quality-adjusted output, or as an outcome.

Quality adjustments of outputs can be made in one of two ways—in terms of the soundness of the care process used to produce the output or in terms of the quality of the output itself. The soundness of the care process is generally the most convenient to measure, but it is based on the assumption that a demonstrable link exists between the care activities performed and the outcome achieved by the patient. Is there, for example, a verifiable cause and effect relationship between preoperative teaching and improved recovery following surgery? If the link between process and outcome is demonstrated, evidence that the best process was used constitutes evidence of the quality of the service. While researchers have made much progress in demonstrating these links in nursing care, the work proceeds at a relatively slow pace.

The alternative to measuring the care process is to assess the quality of the output (i.e., the outcome of care) directly. Measuring outcome is both difficult and expensive. It is difficult because the ultimate outcome of many episodes of illness or care and treatment encounters is not known for some time after the care ceases. It is expensive since it may entail locating the patient after the care and treatment ends in order to perform special, nonroutine evaluations. Finding a meaningful indicator of quality that is also easy to measure is likely to be a key task for the next decade.

WHAT IS NURSING PRODUCTIVITY?

As the prior discussion indicated, there are two basic approaches to measuring productivity. The economic/industrial concept tells us that productivity is the ratio of work output to work input: units of output/units of input. This approach comes out of the scientific management tradition of the 1920s, where the question asked was: How can we design processes and procedures to produce the product most efficiently? An example of the use of scientific management principles in nursing is found in the development of patient classification systems for measuring nursing work load.

Although the principles of scientific management have been applied to the area of nursing productivity, a second, more comprehensive model for evaluating productivity is currently being advocated in the health care and nursing literature. This model attempts to place productivity within a systems framework and incorporates the concept of effectiveness as well as efficiency. Jelinek and Dennis (1976) were among the first to articulate this concept in nursing, when they used an open systems model (see Figure 4–1) showing the relationship between inputs, processes, and outputs and suggested that it is also necessary to consider the influence of the environment in which these three elements exist.

Input includes the number and type of nursing personnel, equipment

Figure 4—1 Nursing Productivity Framework

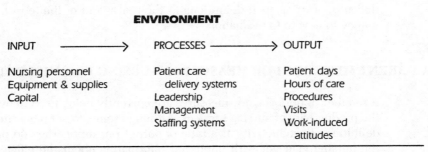

ENVIRONMENT

INPUT ————————> PROCESSES ————————> OUTPUT

Nursing personnel	Patient care	Patient days
Equipment & supplies	delivery systems	Hours of care
Capital	Leadership	Procedures
	Management	Visits
	Staffing systems	Work-induced attitudes

Adapted from Jelinek & Dennis, 1976.

and supplies used, and the capital costs incurred in providing care. Processes include all of the activities and resources required to convert inputs into outputs. Output represents the "product" resulting from the application of processes and inputs. The environment is everything external to the organization over which the nursing manager has little control, including labor laws, health care financing policies, and personnel licensing laws.

In addition to developing a framework for understanding nursing productivity, Jelinek and Dennis proposed that in defining nursing productivity, we must be as concerned about the quality as the quantity of output:

The concept of productivity encompasses both the effectiveness of nursing care, which relates to its quality and appropriateness, and the efficiency of care, which is production of nursing output with minimal resource waste. (1976, p. 3).

This definition is consistent with standard economic definitions of productivity and also takes into account some of the special characteristics of nursing services (Edwardson, 1986). There is an increasing tendency to incorporate both efficiency and effectiveness into the operational definition of the output of health care organizations (AMSI, 1980).

Effectiveness of a hospital's output refers to the safety, appropriateness, and excellence of its care, and encompasses the issues of health status changes, patient outcomes, and patient satisfaction (AMSI, 1980). Efficiency refers to a state in which the inputs and methods used to produce a product or service result in the maximum feasible output (Pauly, 1970).

These two approaches to defining productivity offer practicing nurses a difficult choice. On the one hand, nurses are drawn to the simplicity and easy measurement of industrial definitions of the concept, but are repulsed by the way industrial models reduce the complicated process of care to crude output-input ratios. On the other hand, nurses' professional instincts draw them to the comprehensive definitions of productivity that incorporate estimates of effectiveness. But they are fully aware of the difficulty of using such definitions in the real world of limited time and money to devote to evaluation.

CURRENT METHODS FOR MEASURING NURSING PRODUCTIVITY

A number of performance measures are currently being used to evaluate the productivity of nursing services. Although some do not meet the strict definition of productivity as a ratio of output per input, they do provide the nursing manager with important information about the efficiency of nursing care delivery.

Resources per Patient Day

Nursing hours per patient day is a commonly used indicator of labor productivity that is simple and easily understood. As shown in Figure 4–2, it is calculated by totaling the paid hours for nursing personnel for a period of time and dividing that total by the total number of patient days for the same time period. To accurately reflect the true cost of nursing care, the

Figure 4–2 Calculating Resources Used per Patient Day

I. Nursing Hours per Patient Day

$$\frac{\text{Total paid hours for nursing personnel for time } X}{\text{Total number of patient days in time } X}$$

Direct Nursing Hours per Patient Day

$$\frac{\text{Total paid hours for nursing personnel}}{\text{providing direct care in time } X}{\text{Total number of patient days in time } X}$$

II. Nursing Salary Costs per Patient Day

$$\frac{\text{Total payroll expenses for nursing personnel in time } X}{\text{Total number of patient days in time } X}$$

Direct Nursing Care Salary Costs per Patient Day

$$\frac{\text{Total payroll expenses for providing}}{\text{direct nursing care in time } X}{\text{Total number of patient days in time } X}$$

total paid hours should include the fringe benefit hours (e.g., vacation, holiday, and sick hours used) and the paid hours for nursing administrators as well as the hours required for direct patient care.

While nursing hours per patient day is one of the oldest and most frequently used performance measures, it attributes productivity and all changes in productivity from one time period to another to a single input: the number of hours of nursing care. It fails to consider any changes that may have been made in the care process or in the supplies and equipment used—changes that may have increased or decreased the efficiency or effectiveness of the care given. It also fails to consider changes that may have been made in the skill level of the staff providing the care, the type and intensity of patient days being considered, or the quality of the patient days being produced.

Another, very similar performance measure used is nursing salary costs per patient day. It is a slightly more refined measure, however, in that the use of salary costs provides some information about the skill mix of the staff. Nursing salary costs per patient is calculated by totaling the actual salary costs for nursing personnel and dividing by the total patient days for the same time period.

Standardizing patient days.   Both nursing hours per patient day and salary costs per patient day are useful as measures of labor productivity (i.e., personnel costs per unit of output), but only if the nature of the patient day is held constant. If the nature of the patients cared for on a nursing unit changes, it is difficult to know whether productivity also changes unless an adjustment is made. As an example, consider a nursing unit that provides the same number of hours of care during two time periods. If the level of patient acuity or dependence remains the same during the two time periods, labor productivity will remain unchanged. But if the overall level of patient dependency on nursing care increases during the second time period, labor productivity will increase.

One way to factor in patient dependency levels is to standardize patient days using information from the patient classification system designed to measure nursing work load. Patient days can be standardized by substituting the required hours of care as calculated by the patient classification system for patient days. Productivity ratios can then be calculated as shown in Figure 4–3. If desired, the required hours of care can be divided by 24 hours to produce required days of care. Such standardization of the nature of the patient days produced improves the validity of comparisons of nursing hours and nursing salary costs per patient day in two or more monitoring periods.

Degree of Occupation

Another productivity indicator in common use is the degree to which the nursing staff is occupied. Degree of occupation is regularly measured by nursing managers on a very informal basis using a "busyness scale."

Figure 4-3   Resource Use per Standardized Patient Day

I. Nursing Hours per Standardized Patient Day

$$\frac{\text{Total paid hours for nursing personnel for time } X}{\text{Total required hours (or days) of care in time } X}$$

II. Nursing Salary Costs per Standardized Patient Day

$$\frac{\text{Total payroll expenses for nursing personnel in time } X}{\text{Total required hours (or days) of care in time } X}$$

The nursing manager observes the unit staff and makes a judgment as to whether the number of staff members available is sufficient to handle the work load.

While this procedure may appear to be too informal to be valid, many observers strongly believe that a skilled and experienced charge nurse or head nurse can, in fact, be a very finely tuned measurement instrument of staffing adequacy. This assumption has led to the development of at least one method for helping charge nurses assess degree of occupation—i.e., staffing adequacy—more systematically. The method, developed by Williams and Murphy (1979), requires the charge nurse to answer a series of questions about the activity level on the unit that day (e.g., number of admissions and surgeries) and to judge the adequacy of the number of staff assigned and of the care given.

Some researchers question, however, whether degree of occupation is a valid productivity measure. It could be argued, for example, that a fully occupied staff is not necessarily a productive staff if the work is poorly organized and sequenced or if the support services and equipment available are inadequate for allowing the staff to perform efficiently. The staff may be exceedingly busy and understaffed using current practice models, but that does not preclude the possibility that the quantity and quality of care given can be improved considerably without increasing costs (Edwardson, 1986).

Utilization Rates

One of the best known performance measures used in nursing is the ratio of required to actual staffing levels. This performance measure is produced by most nurse staffing systems based on patient classification.

To obtain information for calculating utilization rates, the patient classification system used for nurse staffing is used to predict the amount of care each patient will require in the near future (usually one or two

Figure 4—4   Example of a Productivity Monitoring System

Cost Center	Hours (or FTEs)			Percent Productivity
	REQUIRED	ACTUAL	VARIANCE	
432	45	45	0	100%
433	45	42	3	107%
434	45	48	−3	94%

shifts hence). The time required by all patients on a unit is summed and then labeled "required hours of care." Additional time is factored in for indirect care activities (e.g., charting, making referrals), unit maintenance activities, and the nurses' break time. At the end of the shift for which the prediction was made, the actual hours of nursing time paid is calculated. The utilization rate is then calculated as:

$$\frac{\text{Required hours of care}}{\text{Nursing hours paid}}$$

Figure 4–4 shows an example of how utilization rates ("productivity") are frequently reported in nursing management information systems. The actual hours of care provided are subtracted from the required (or predicted) hours of care to give a variance. The percentage of productivity is then calculated by dividing the required hours of care by the actual hours provided and then multiplying the quotient by 100. A productivity rate of 100% indicates that the actual hours of care matched the required hours. A rate greater than 100% indicates that actual hours were less than required, while a rate less than 100% shows that more hours of care were provided than were required. Most institutions set acceptable productivity ranges of 85% to 115%.

While these rates are perhaps the single best day-to-day control monitor available to nursing managers, they are more appropriately called a utilization rather than a productivity indicator unless certain assumptions are made about required hours of care. When compared to standard economic definitions of productivity, the ratio of required to actual hours of care has an input measurement (actual hours) but does not have a commonly used output measurement.

Required hours of care as an output.   The required-actual ratio is useful as a productivity measure only if the nursing service assumes or has demonstrated that the required number of nursing hours can provide the quantity and quality of care the hospital wishes to provide. In other words, the use of staff utilization ratios to judge productivity is based on one very important, but frequently unacknowledged, assumption: the standard hours of care used by the patient classification system to calculate required nurse hours provide the'desired level of service.

To be used as an output indicator, the required hours of care should be thought of as targeted hours of care—i.e., the hours of care required to produce the desired level of care quality. To affirm the validity of targeted hours as a substitute measure of desired output, the nursing department either needs to use the research findings of others to show that a certain amount of care produces the desired results or must do its own evaluation studies to demonstrate that a given level of care quantity and quality can be produced by a given number of nursing care hours.

An example from a maternity service will illustrate the point. Assume that a maternity service has determined that five hours of professional and two hours of nonprofessional nursing care during the postpartum period meet the outcome standards set by the service (see Figure 4–5). By a careful evaluation of outcomes, the providers of this maternity service have determined that patients are discharged in a reasonable number of days and that the mothers are satisfied with their care and are able to care

Figure 4–5 Example of the Use of Targeted Hours of Care as an Output Indicator

---

I. Outcome Standard

Average length of stay = 2.9 Days
Knowledge & Skill
 90% score above 90% on a post-teaching test of knowledge
 98% give satisfactory return baby bath demonstration
Satisfaction
 90% satisfied or very satisfied on satisfaction questionnaire
Complications
 2% postpartal and newborn infection rate
 50% of mothers continue breast feeding for at least one month

II. Calculating Productivity

These standards can be met at 7 hours of care per patient day. Therefore, productivity can be calculated as follows, using hypothetical actual hours of care provided.

a. $\dfrac{\text{Target}}{\text{Actual}} = \dfrac{7}{7} = 100\%$

b. $\dfrac{\text{Target}}{\text{Actual}} = \dfrac{7}{7.9} = 89\%$

c. $\dfrac{\text{Target}}{\text{Actual}} = \dfrac{7}{6.5} = ?$

---

for themselves and their infants. The complication rate is also judged to be adequate. If a nursing service provides this type of evidence that it is able to meet the institution's own standards of care, then targeted hours of care could quite legitimately be substituted as an indicator of output— the appropriate quantity and quality of care (Edwardson, 1986).

The process for calculating the productivity of the unit is shown in part II of Figure 4–5. When the actual hours of care provided match the target, productivity is 100%, but when actual hours exceed the target, productivity falls below 100%. A problem arises in calculating productivity when the actual hours provided are fewer than the target. Although most institutions would calculate productivity as 108% in this case, there is a question as to whether this is a legitimate calculation. When the actual use of staff is less than the targeted level, it suggests that the standards used to establish the target are too high or that the organization is willing to compromise its standards with unknown consequences. For these reasons, some have suggested that productivity levels should never exceed 100% unless the clinical service can show that the care process has been made more efficient by using new methods or new equipment and that the quality of the outcome has not suffered.

IMPROVING NURSING PRODUCTIVITY

Having reviewed and critiqued some of the common indicators of nursing performance and suggested ways to improve them, we now consider how the manager can improve nursing productivity. As the model in Figure 4–1 suggests, there are two possible points at which productivity gains may be made: through changes in the use of inputs and through changes in the care process. Changes to elements of the environment are largely beyond the control of the nursing manager, at least in the short run.

Changes in the Use of Inputs

Inputs include the raw materials, manpower, supplies, and equipment used to provide a service or produce a product. Little attention has been given to the "raw material" of nursing services since it is a little disconcerting to think of patients and clients as raw material. Nurses have traditionally had little control over the type of patients presented to them. Recent activities among hospitals to identify areas of excellence and market those selected services to potential consumers may change all that. Increasingly, nursing departments and individual nursing practitioners are marketing their services as well, thereby exerting some influence themselves over the type of patients for whom they care.

Matching supply with demand. The most costly input in the provision of nursing care is labor input. Therefore, the greatest productivity gains can be achieved by careful selection and use of personnel. The easiest method for controlling labor input is to measure requirements for care based on patient classification data and then schedule nursing personnel to meet the expected demand.

Before patient classification systems (PCSs) were developed, the number of nursing staff members scheduled was determined by global staff-patient ratios (often one nurse to three or four patients). These global standards were insensitive to differences in care requirements among patients; some patients, for example, required more care than was available with fixed staff-patient ratios and some required less (Giovannetti, 1978).

PCSs were designed to recognize this variation by grouping patients into categories with similar nursing care requirements. Using concepts that derive from the scientific management theoretical framework, PCSs assume first that work can be subdivided into specific functions that vary as to length of time and skill required to perform them.

After specific functions have been identified, it is necessary to measure the time required to care for patients needing different combinations of tasks. Two basic approaches to work measurement are taken. PCSs of the factor type use a long and comprehensive list of tasks, each with an associated time requirement. With this approach, patients are categorized into groups (usually four or five) based on the time required for staff to complete all of the tasks identified for them.

Prototype PCSs, on the other hand, use only a few tasks (e.g., bathing, feeding, ambulation) that have been shown to be critical indicators or predictors of the amount of care required (Giovannetti, 1979). Patients are categorized into groups (usually four or five) based on whether they demonstrate one or more of these critical indicators. Then the average amount of time required to care for patients in each of the categories is measured.

Regardless of the type of PCS in use, the most important characteristic is that it be valid and reliable. Invalid or unreliable PCSs will not only lead to inappropriate use of nursing personnel, but can lead to dissatisfaction among the staff. Staff members may attempt to undermine systems that are perceived to be inaccurate. The validity and reliability of a PCS can be maintained only through regular monitoring and adjustments to changing conditions.

Once the nurse manager is convinced that the PCS produces valid and reliable data, the system can be used from one to three times a day. Classification tools consist of descriptions or checklists of variables. The decision as to how often patients are classified is made by the nursing division based on a number of considerations including the degree of change in patients' conditions from shift to shift and the ability of the staffing system to make changes in staff allocation.

After the nursing care requirements of each patient have been measured, the total time required by all patients on the unit is calculated according to the methods specified by the PCS. This total time then predicts the amount of care time that will be required for that set of patients one or two shifts hence.

To determine the number of staff members needed to care for these patients in those future shifts, divide by 8 (the number of hours worked by each nurse per shift) the total time required. The number of staff members required is then compared to the number who have been scheduled to work that shift minus any known absences.

The key to efficient resource use is to match the required and available staff. If more nurses are needed than are scheduled, the nurse manager will need to identify other nurses who can work that shift by calling upon a float pool, unscheduled employees, or a substitute nurse service. If more nurses are scheduled than are needed, the nursing manager may need to ask some of the staff to float to other units with greater need or not come to work that day.

Making staff substitutions. As noted earlier, because of differences in education, skill, and experience among individual nurses, the nursing labor input usually does not exist in homogeneous units. Some differences are reflected in salary differences. Many would argue that it is logical to take advantage of these differences in payment rates. To the casual observer, it would seem that employing more nonprofessional staff who receive lower salaries should reduce personnel costs; increasing the number of LPNs and nursing assistants in relation to the number of RNs, for example, would result in more available hours of personnel time per patient day with no increase in cost.

There are, however, theoretical arguments for and against staff substitution as a method of improving nursing productivity. Adherents of the scientific management tradition feel that productivity is greatest when the work of providing care to individual patients is divided into its component parts and the tasks assigned to staff members according to their ability. Tasks are assigned to the least costly personnel category capable of doing the tasks; the most qualified individuals are assigned only those tasks requiring their special expertise. Supporters of the human relations theoretical framework, on the other hand, argue that knowledgeable workers such as nurses are most satisfied, and therefore most productive, when they are allowed to perform "whole tasks," i.e., provide total patient care for a caseload of patients. They argue against dividing the work into component parts and assigning isolated tasks to individuals.

If there are conflicting theoretical predictions as to what division of labor will be most productive, the empirical evidence is also inconclusive. Unfortunately, some experiments with increasing the proportion of professional to nonprofessional staff were done in conjunction with the introduction of primary nursing (Dahlen, 1978; Marram, Barret & Bevis, 1979; Osinski & Powals, 1980; Nenner, Curtis & Eckhoff, 1977). The use of two experimental treatments simultaneously makes it impossible to sort out which of the reported changes are attributable to alterations in skill mix, which to the change in the mode of care, and which to a combination of the two. Other studies of all-RN or predominantly all-RN staffing have been uncontrolled case studies rather than experiments (e.g., Burt, 1980; Hinshaw, Scofield & Atwood, 1981; Miller, 1980).

Although there are acknowledged methodological problems in the study of skill mix in providing nursing care, a situation with a high proportion of professional staff has several reputed advantages. First, it has been reported that such a situation leads to greater patient satisfaction (Abdellah & Levine, 1958) and better coordination and quality of care (Georgopoulous & Mann, 1962; Miller & Bryant, 1965). Two other studies suggest that it may be relatively costly to use nursing assistants because nursing assistants require greater supervision and more instruction as to what they should do next. It has been found that nursing assistants are occupied only 65% to 73% of their scheduled work time as opposed to RNs, who were occupied 92% to 100% of the time (Clark, 1977; Christman, 1978).

These findings suggest that nursing services in a hospital are too variable and unpredictable to take full advantage of the theoretical economies to be achieved by assigning tasks to the least qualified individual capable of performing them. Although there is tentative evidence that high professional to nonprofessional ratios may be no more costly, and frequently are less costly, in terms of salary costs and turnover rates (Dahlen, 1978; Burt, 1980; Marram, et al., 1976; Marram, Barret & Bevis, 1974; Osinski & Powals, 1980; Hinshaw, Scofield & Atwood, 1981; Nenner, Curtis & Eckhoff, 1977; Miller, 1980; Forseth, 1980; Corpuz & Anderson, 1977), methodological problems in some of the available literature make it essential that investigation continue.

Controlling the use of supplies and equipment. The nurse manager can also control input costs by the wise use of supplies and equipment. One method for doing this is to compare the cost and features of roughly equivalent supplies and equipment, selecting products that have the desired qualities at the lowest cost. At times, the individual manager or the institution's purchasing department may be able to use competitive bidding procedures in which vendors submit bids as a method for obtaining the lowest cost.

Once supplies and equipment have been purchased, cost can be controlled by using them wisely. For example, the nurse manager can implement systems that carefully monitor the use of supplies in order to reduce waste and prevent theft. Increasing cost sensitivity among nursing personnel is another method. One nurse manager was able to produce large savings by simply placing price tags on chargeable supplies. Nurses in the study hospital discovered that they could substitute less costly items with no untoward effects and avoid using some items altogether (McVay, 1983).

Changes in the Care Process

Finding ways to improve productivity by making changes in the care process allows the nursing manager to use his or her creativity to the fullest. Jelinek and Dennis (1976), in their comprehensive review of the literature on nursing productivity, called the care process the "technology of nursing." According to their definition, technology "comprises all methodologies employed in converting inputs into outputs" (1976:12). In this concept of productivity, technology includes the physical and managerial organization of nursing services, leadership and supervision, patient care delivery systems, staffing and scheduling practices, care planning and documentation procedures, and the performance of nursing activities themselves. Clearly, there are many opportunities here to experiment with methods for improving the quantity and quality of nursing care given.

Selected examples. It would be impossible to give examples of all the ways the process of care may be changed. The following few, however, are representative.

One of the most frequently used methods for improving the process of care is to alter the work schedules of nurses. Use of restructured workweeks—such as four 10-hour shifts, three 12-hour shifts, or special weekend schedules—has been reported to improve staffing efficiency while also meeting some nurses' needs for leisure time (Huey, 1981; Hutchins & Cleveland, 1978; Kent, 1972; Mills, Arnold & Wood, 1983). Job sharing or job pairing, in which two individuals divide one full-time position, is another possible scheduling modification.

Some have suggested that nursing might become more productive if nurses were to give up some of the rituals of nursing care. "Rituals" include those routine activities such as linen changes and vital signs monitoring that are sometimes completed out of habit and without regard for the individual patient's need for them. Of course, some activities that may appear to be unnecessary, habitual behavior may be required to protect the institution from liability. But a careful needs evaluation may enable a nursing unit to free up time for more important work.

Other changes in the direct care process may lead to improvements in the quantity and quality of care delivered. Experiments with new approaches to common clinical problems such as incontinence and situational confusion may be fruitful. Investigating alternative modes of nursing care delivery such as primary nursing (as described in Chapter 3) or a modular delivery system (a combination of primary and team nursing in which teams of primary and associate nurses care for a group of patients) might also improve productivity. Using new or improved products or equipment can have positive results in some cases.

Documenting changes. Regardless of the nature of the changes made in the care process, it is essential that they and their consequences be measured and evaluated. Without careful documentation, it may be impossible to convince others that the innovations introduced are safe, effective, and efficient.

Consider the example of one nurse midwifery clinic. Several years ago the staff of the clinic decided they could be more efficient if they replaced an individual approach to early prenatal teaching and orientation to the clinic with a group approach. After some time it became apparent that the clientele, which represented several ethnic groups, some with limited command of English and little formal education, was too diverse to make group teaching practical. Class members frequently were forced to wait while the instructor attended to language or other unique individual needs. Original estimates of a one-hour class turned into several actual hours, attendance dropped, and concerns grew about the women's ability to care for themselves in early pregnancy.

The staff of the clinic decided an evaluation of the patient teaching program was in order. By totalling the cost of staff time (including the time of staff members who were largely unoccupied during the class) and the cost of the unused clinic rooms and comparing them with the attendance rate and knowledge outcomes, it became clear that the group approach for this set of patients was inappropriate and at least as costly. The clinic reverted to the one-on-one teaching strategy.

To evaluate the effects of changes in process, therefore, the nurse manager should collect cost and outcome data as a part of all clinical studies. This is a less formidable task than it may appear on the surface. Cost accounting methods are well understood and relatively easy to apply. Most financial officers are eager to· assist managers in performing cost analyses. While outcome evaluation can be difficult, studies of outcome, when they are used for managerial purposes, need not meet all the rigorous criteria applied to research studies.

Calculating costs. Costs can be calculated using one of two approaches. In some cases it is necessary to estimate only the direct costs of the change—for example, costs associated with changes in the brand of a product used or with the introduction of a new record-keeping system.

In other cases the relevant unit of analysis is an episode of care or a patient stay. The manager must estimate the total cost of nursing care for patients affected by the change in practices. Fortunately, data available from the PCS can also be used to compute the nursing care costs for individual patients and groups of patients.

Figure 4–6 presents an example of how this is accomplished. First, patients are classified in the usual manner. It is important that the classification for each patient be recorded in a retrievable fashion such as on the patient record or on a computer file. After discharge, the total hours of care are totalled and multiplied by the hourly nursing care salary cost (Total salary costs/Total number of paid hours). Then all indirect nursing costs are added in. Indirect nursing costs include the unit's share of the

Figure 4–6 Cost Estimation Example

	Day of Stay	A	B	C	D	E	F
		Hours for Each Patient Served					
I. Apply workload measurement system	1	3	5	4			
	2	2.8	5	4	5	3	
	3	2.5	4.8	4	4.9	3	2.8
	4	2.5	4.6	3	4.9	2	2.8
	5	2.3	4.6	3	4.6	2.3	2
II. Add hours of care for length of stay		13.1	24.0	18	19.4	10.3	7.6
III. Assign hourly cost of nursing care to individual patients (e.g., \$12/hour)		× \$12	× \$12	× \$12	× \$12	× \$12	× \$12
		\$157.2	288.0	216.0	232.8	123.6	91.2
IV. Add indirect costs (e.g., \$20/patient day)		\$257.2	388.0	316.0	312.8	203.6	151.2

V. Calculate average cost per case

A. Add total cost for all relevant patients

$$
\begin{array}{r}
\$\ 257.20 \\
388.00 \\
316.00 \\
312.80 \\
203.60 \\
151.20 \\
\hline
\$1628.80
\end{array}
$$

B. Divide sum by number of patients $\dfrac{\$1628.80}{6} = \$271.47$

expenses of nursing administration, staff development, the cost of operating the physical plant, and similar non–patient-specific expenses. These costs are generally prorated on a per-patient day cost basis (Total indirect costs/Number of patient days). To obtain an average cost for all patients being studied, the total costs of each patient's care is totaled and divided by the number of patients in the sample. The average costs before introduction of the innovation can then be compared to costs after its introduction to identify cost savings.

Measuring outcome.   Measuring the effects of a change in practice can be more difficult. In a few cases, a change in the care process may have been evaluated in a research study reported in the literature. If that is true, the nursing unit may be able to replicate the outcome measurement made in the original study.

In most instances, however, the nursing staff will need to design its own outcome evaluation method. The first question to be asked in developing an evaluation strategy is: What is the outcome that should be measured? The answer lies in what the innovation is intended to do, what the possible untoward consequences could be, and what the institution can afford to measure. In evaluating a new method for caring for incontinent patients, for example, intended outcome could be to reduce the number of times the patients are incontinent and reduce skin breakdown. Outcome criteria would then include the number of incontinent episodes per day and the degree of skin excoriation. Untoward consequences might include unsightly garments or decreased patient autonomy. Procedures for evaluating patients' emotional responses could be used to evaluate such potential untoward results. Each of the proposed outcomes could be measured during the hospitalization at a relatively modest cost.

But the nursing staff may also want to know the long-term outcome of their new care strategy. This implies that patients will need to be located after hospital discharge, and outcome measurements made at that time—a potentially costly procedure. There are several ways to complete this type of evaluation with little cost to the unit. One approach might be to enlist a nurse researcher interested in the problem. Another would be for the unit staff to apply for external grant funding to perform their own evaluation. Finally, it may be possible to get information about patient outcome from colleagues working in other settings. Sending evaluation forms or conducting telephone interviews with nurses working in home care or in long-term care settings can provide the needed outcome data.

Using the cost and outcome data.   Once cost and outcome data are gathered, the nursing manager must relate one to the other to decide if the innovation was beneficial. One method for doing this is to use a decision model proposed by Fishman (1975) for applying cost-effectiveness analysis to evaluation studies in a service setting.

As shown in Figure 4–7, the decision-making strategy relies on comparisons of the cost and results of two methods for accomplishing a goal. Any option that produces equal or superior results and costs less, or any option that produces superior results for equal cost should be chosen. Similarly, any option that produces inferior results for equal or greater cost should be rejected. Ambiguity arises when a superior result costs more or when the costs and results are equal for the two options. In these cases, the decision about which option to choose would depend on whether the goals to be achieved by the options in question were more or less valuable than other organizational objectives. An ambiguous choice situation may also inspire the staff to identify third and fourth options for achieving the same objective at a lower cost.

Figure 4–7 Cost Effectiveness Matrix

	Cost of New Program Relative to Old Program		
Effectiveness of New Program Relative to Old Program	New Less Costly	New As Costly	New More Costly
New Less Effective	?	Choose Old	Choose Old
New As Effective	Choose New	Choose Either	Choose Old
New More Effective	Choose New	Choose New	?

The evaluation strategy described here for assessing the effects of changes in the care process is but one of several that could be used. Whichever evaluation method is selected, it is important that it be selected before an innovation or change is made. Unless an evaluation method is planned in advance, the manager will lack the data to determine whether the change did or did not enhance the productivity of the nursing unit.

Sovie (1985) has developed a list of strategies that can be used to manage nursing resources in hospitals more productively. Sovie suggests:

1. Do more with no more. Reduce specialized staff and return some activities assigned to other departments to nurses. For example, many institutions support IV teams at considerable cost yet there is no evidence to indicate patient welfare is thus enhanced. This may require an all-RN staff, however, if done by staff.

2. Use generic care plans. If one to two hours of nursing hours are required for each patient care plan, and an institution uses generic care plans judiciously, several nurse full-time equivalents (FTEs) could be saved.

3. Develop new flow sheets to streamline documentation. Since nurses may spend up to 40% of their time documenting patient care, bedside flow sheets with appropriately labeled sections may contribute to efficient use of nursing time.

4. Use group counseling and teaching methods to meet patient and family needs. In selected circumstances, group methods may be much more effective than the traditional one-on-one approach. For example, group

methods could be used for discharge instructions for patients in the same DRG, or to provide baby care instruction for new mothers.

5. Package nursing programs and information. Any common presentation, such as orientation to the unit or preparing a family to take a patient home, could be put on video or print media. Medication fact sheets can be prepared.

6. Separate nursing charges from room charges. Patient classification systems allow average hours of nursing care per category to be developed. This will allow nursing to become a unit cost center where costs can be compared across hospital or unit per DRG. Furthermore, nursing costs per DRG could be used in incentive programs.

7. Increase use of ambulatory surgery facilities and day of surgery admissions programs. This has happened already. For these programs to function effectively, nursing must work closely with medical staff.

8. Effectively manage materials and shared services. Every entrepreneur knows the importance of inventory control and lower price/same quality substitution. Nursing has not yet learned this.

9. Think "competitive marketing" and "consumer choice." Nurses have never viewed their services as a consumer choice, but it is. Nurses represent the institution and form its image to the patients and family who go back to the community and share their experiences.

10. Develop new products. By taking on the philosophy of wellness rather than acute care, one can think of all kinds of new marketable programs/ services in the health promotion business.

11. Create a learning culture with staff. Economics, accountability, marketing, change management, productivity, cost containment, networking and, especially, human resource management are only a few of the many topics on a potential learning agenda.

12. Maximize the contributions of professional nursing through participative management, effective staff organization, professional recognition, and shared governance programs.

13. Consider matrix staffing. Unit-based nurses have traditionally accepted that floating within their own service may be required to meet nursing care requirements. However, in matrix staffing, nurses develop or are hired for competencies in at least two services and can float between services.

14. Develop and use nursing productivity standards and implement control systems. Productivity standards per DRG are essential to efficient use of staff and control of overtime.

Overall, these are just a sampling of the kinds of things nurse managers can do in concert with administrative staff and physicians to find ways to deliver quality care while meeting an institution's financial objectives.

The American public demands and is entitled to information about the efficiency and effectiveness of the health care services provided to them. The nursing profession can do one of two things: (a) develop methods to demonstrate its own value as a health care discipline, or (b) wait for others to do that evaluation. The choice seems clear. The profession must move to define the product of nursing services, provide scientific evidence of the links between nursing intervention and patient outcome, and then use professional and scientific knowledge about productivity to affect health care policy.

SUMMARY

- Productivity is a concept that describes the relationship between inputs and outputs.

- Productivity refers to the resources used to produce a product or provide a service and to the quantity and quality of that product or service.

- It has been difficult to measure productivity in health care in general and nursing in particular because of the unique nature of the service provided and a lack of consensus about how best to measure output.

- Standardizing the nature of patient days (output) and estimating the validity of measurements made by patient classification systems are just two of the simple modifications that can improve the validity of current methods for evaluating productivity.

- Nursing productivity can be enhanced by making changes in the use of inputs and in the processes used to deliver care.

- Nurse managers can improve the use of inputs by matching the supply of staff with the demand for care, by carefully evaluating the consequences of staff substitutions and by controlling the use of supplies and equipment.

- Demonstrating the relative productivity of nursing services is the responsibility of every nurse manager.

BIBLIOGRAPHY

Abdellah, F., and Levine, E. (1958). Developing a measure of patient and personnel satisfaction with nursing care. *Nursing Research*, 5:100–108.

American Management Sciences, Inc. (AMSI). (1980). *Productivity and health*. (DHHS No. (HRA) 80-14028). Bethesda, MD: Office of the Assistant Secretary of Health.

Burt, M. L. (1980). The cost of all-RN staffing. In: *All-RN nursing staff*. (Pp. 87–90). Alfano, G. (editor). Wakefield, MA: Nursing Resources.

Christman, L. (1978). A micro-analysis of the nursing division of one medical center. *Nursing Digest*, 6(2): 83–87.

Clark, E. L. (1977). A model of nursing staffing for effective patient care. *J Nurs Adm*, 7(2): 22–27.

Corpuz, T., and Anderson, R. (1977). The Evanston story: Primary nursing comes alive. *Nursing Administration Quarterly*, 1(2): 9–50.

Dahlen, A. (1978). With primary nursing, we have it all together. *American Journal of Nursing*, 78:426–428.

Edwardson, S. R. (1986). The cost-quality tradeoff in productivity management. In: *Patients and purse strings—Patient classification and cost management.* (Pp. 259–271). Shaffer, F. A. (editor). New York: National League for Nursing.

Feldstein, M. S. (1971). *The rising cost of hospital care.* Washington, DC: Information Resources Press.

Fishman, D. (1975). *Development and testing of a cost-effectiveness methodology for CMHC's.* Springfield, VA: NTIS. (NTIS Nos. PB 246-676 and PB 246-677).

Forseth, J. (1980). Does RN staffing escalate medical care costs? In: *All-RN nursing staff.* (Pp. 103–110). Alfano, G. (editor). Wakefield, MA: Nursing Resources.

Georgopoulous, B. S., and Mann, F. C. (1962). *The community hospital.* New York: Macmillan.

Giovannetti, P. (1978). *Patient classification systems in nursing: A description and analysis.* (DHEW Publication No. HRA 78-22). Washington, DC: U.S. Government Printing Office.

Giovannetti, P. (1979). Understanding patient classification systems. *J Nurs Adm*, 8(2): 4–9.

Hinshaw, A. S., Scofield, R., and Atwood, J. R. (1981). Staff, patient, and cost outcomes of all-registered nurse staffing. *J Nurs Adm*, 11(11 and 12): 30–36.

Hornbrook, M. C. (1982). Hospital case mix: Its definition, measurement and use: Part I. The conceptual framework. *Medical Care Review*, 39(1): 1–43.

Huey, F. (1981). The demise of the traditional 5-40 workweek? *American Journal of Nursing*, 81:1138–1141.

Hutchins, C., and Cleveland, R. (1978). For staff nurses and patients—The 7-70 plan. *American Journal of Nursing*, 78:230–231.

Jelinek, R. C., and Dennis, L. C. (1976). *A review and evaluation of nursing productivity.* (DHEW No. (HRA) 77-15). Bethesda, MD: Health Resources Administration.

Kent, L. A. (1972). The 4-40 workweek on trial. *American Journal of Nursing*, 72:683–686.

Marram, G., Barret, M. W., and Bevis, E. M. (1974). *Primary nursing: A model for individualized care.* St. Louis: C. V. Mosby.

Marram, G., Flynn, K., Abaravich, W., and Carey, S. (1976). *Cost-effectiveness of primary and team nursing.* Wakefield, MA: Contemporary Publishing.

McVay, E. (1983). Lost supply charges: Would visible price tags reduce their number? Master's thesis. University of Minnesota, Minneapolis, Minnesota.

Miller, P. W. (1980). Staffing with RNs. In: *All-RN nursing staff.* (Pp. 91–95). Alfano, G. (editor). Wakefield, MA: Nursing Resources.

Miller, S. J., and Bryant, W. D. (1965). *A division of nursing labor: Experiment in staffing a municipal hospital.* Kansas City: Community Studies Inc.

Mills, M. E., Arnold, B., and Wood, C. M. (1983). Core-12: A controlled study of the impact of 12-hour scheduling. *Nursing Research*, 32:356–361.

Nenner, V. C., Curtis, E. M., and Eckhoff, C. M. (1977). Primary nursing. *Supervisor Nurse*, 8(5): 14–16.

Osinski, E. G., and Powals, J. G. (1980). The cost of all RN staffed primary nursing. *Supervisor Nurse*, 11(1): 16–21.

Pauly, M. V. (1970). Efficiency, incentives and reimbursement for health care. *Inquiry*, 7:114–131.

Sovie, M. D. (1985). Managing nursing resources in a constrained environment. *Nurs Econ*, 3(3): 85–94.

Williams, M. A., and Murphy, L. N. (1979). Subjective and objective measures of staffing adequacy. *J Nurs Adm*, 9(11): 21–29.

Managing and Initiating Change

CHANGE IS INEVITABLE, if not always welcome. Change is necessary for growth, though it often produces anxiety and fear. Even when it is planned it can be threatening, because change is the process of making something different from what it was. There is a sense of loss of the familiar, the status quo. This is particularly true when change is unplanned or beyond human control. And even when the change is expected and valued, a grief reaction, for example, may occur. Those who manage and initiate change often encounter resistance from those experiencing symptoms of anxiety and grief.

Though nurse managers should understand and anticipate these reactions to change, they need to develop and exude a different approach, a positive aura for change. They can view change as a challenge and encourage their colleagues to participate. They can become uncomfortable with the status quo and find comfort in taking risks. The health care system is changing, with or without nurses' contributions. Leaders initiate change—followers survive it. Nurse managers must become skilled in implementing change introduced by the board of directors. But they should work to get nurses on that board—nurses who are as comfortable in the boardroom as they are at the bedside. Nurse leaders must initiate the changes they believe are necessary to strengthen nursing practice, provide quality care, and create a better system.

CLIMATE FOR CHANGE

The health care system is in the midst of unprecedented change. Much of this change is economically driven, with the emphasis on reducing health care costs. The government, insurance companies, and employers are exerting external pressure to alter past reimbursement policies, which reinforced a "blank check mentality." Incentives are in place to curb spending or absorb the difference between what providers charge and reimbursers are willing to pay.

Federal regulations establishing DRGs have produced a shock wave of change throughout the system. There are restrictions for admission to the hospital, the most expensive part of the system. Charges are set in advance for specific diagnoses, and limits are placed on the length of stay clients are expected to remain. The external pressure is to admit only the sickest and for the shortest time possible, and to use alternative, less expensive settings where possible. Many employee benefit programs require second opinions for surgery and approval for hospital admission. In some cases, employees are encouraged to use free-standing "emergicenters" instead of hospital emergency rooms.

Such changes have a rippling effect. Health care organizations must change internally if they are to survive—and most are changing. Hospitals are reorganizing into multihospital systems. They are diversifying to provide for profit services such as durable medical equipment and home care. Some are specializing to increase the volume of sophisticated, high-priced problems—they are developing particular expertise in these areas and learning to handle cases expeditiously. These changes require modifications in technology, personnel, and structure. In today's economic environment, organizational change is essential for adaptation. Creative change is mandatory for growth.

This climate for change produces new opportunities for nurses. Those working in hospitals find top-level management is listening to what they have to say. Innovation is "in." The participatory approach is popular because status quo management will not work when a whole system is in transition. Transitional times demand new ways of thinking, creative strategies, fresh options. The door is open for those who dare to think beyond "the way we were."

Nurses outside hospitals are forging new roles. Some are opening their own businesses in home health care and preventive health programs. As third-party payers of health care push for options to expensive disease-oriented institutional care, opportunities arise for innovative nurses. Whether they practice independently, work in bureaucracies, or form their own organizations, today's nurses need to understand, manage, and produce change.

NURSE AS CHANGE AGENT

The notion of the "nurse as change agent" is not new. A "change agent" is one who works to bring about a change. The nurse often acts as an "insider," a change agent who is part of the system being altered (usually the unit she or he manages). But nurses can also be "outsiders" or consultants for change in other systems. Nurses have been prepared for the former more than the latter. In either case, though, there has never been a better time for the nursing profession to take the initiative. As the largest health profession, nurses make the health care system run. They have concrete ideas about how to make it run better.

Although many patients are admitted to hospitals for technological intervention, they remain for 24-hour nursing care. To a large extent, nurses control length of stay. Their expertise and organization can determine the cost and quality of care a hospital offers. On the one hand, nursing represents the biggest slice of the hospital budget. On the other hand, the quality of nursing care is a "differential advantage" for the organization. A hospital known for its excellent nursing care has a competitive edge. Nurses who can suggest changes to control costs, improve quality, or offer new services will be change agents in great demand in hospitals.

Outside hospitals, nurse change agents can move the health care system from a medical to a nursing model. Fueled by businesses' interest in holding down the cost of illness care by encouraging employees to promote healthy living, nurses can create new niches in the business world. They can develop and manage prevention programs. They can case manage employees' health problems by linking them to existing services. They can create the gap-filling services consumers will require as they are left to care for themselves, outside of hospitals. In addition, nurses are the most logical problem solvers for creating cost-effective ways to care for the elderly.

Changes will continue at a rapid pace with or without nursing's expert guidance. However, nurses, like organizations, cannot afford to merely "survive" changes. If they are to exist as a distinct profession that has expertise in solving "human responses to actual or potential health problems" (ANA, 1980), they must be proactive in shaping the future. The opportunities exist now for nurses, especially those in management positions, to change the system about which they so often complain.

CHANGE WITHIN A SYSTEMS FRAMEWORK

Most nurses work in organizations. As described in Chapter 2, modern organization theory conceptualizes the organization as a complex social system within the suprasystem of society (Kast & Rosenzweig, 1970). It is an integrated whole of mutually dependent parts that exchange information and energy through semipermeable boundaries (Chinn, 1969). There is also constant interaction with the environment. Because this dynamic interaction change is inevitable, a change in one part of the system produces change throughout the system. Though change is considered necessary for growth, integrative processes are required to achieve system viability and goal achievement.

Successful organizations achieve organization equilibrium, or a balance among the forces operating on it and within it. Dynamic equilibrium occurs when an organization responds to change by shifting to a new balance or by modifying its goals (Chinn, 1969). Every system experiences stresses, strains, and conflicts, produced in part by the opposing forces of the system's maintenance and adaptive mechanisms. Maintenance mechanisms prevent change from occurring too rapidly while adaptive mechanisms work to keep the system changing over time. The significance of these forces cannot be overemphasized, for the scope and pace of organizational change depend on how they are managed. While managers work to reduce tensions, relieve stress (see Chapter 23), and resolve conflict (see Chapter 22), they must do so cautiously or pay "the price of overlooking the possibility of increasing tensions and conflict to facilitate creativity, innovation and social change" (Chinn, 1969:301).

There are several advantages in using the systems frame of reference to understand and manage change. First, it mandates integrative thinking. The change agent must analyze the system and system-environment boundaries, mechanisms, and flow of information and energy. At the same time, she or he must always recognize that the whole is greater than the sum of its parts. This complex and comprehensive approach precludes the search for simple causal relationships. Instead, the manager searches for the multiple, interacting variables that facilitate and restrict system changes. The importance of external (environmental) variables is examined in relation to internal variables.

The systems framework also directs attention to the hierarchical arrangement of the system's subsystems. Understanding this hierarchy facilitates coordination of communication and activities (see Chapter 8), and thus the change agent can assess the transactions taking place at all levels of the system. This assessment begins with the suprasystem—that is, management of change begins with those who have an overall view, because effective managers know external forces have a pervasive effect on the whole system. They know the search for organizational problems and solutions does not begin and end on the unit, in the department, or even within the organization itself. Often, change *outside* the system holds the greatest promise, if not the greatest challenge. For example, nurse staffing and recruitment problems include such suprasystem variables as: state regulatory ceilings on hospital expense budgets, which restrain substantive professional nurse salary increases; reductions in federal financial support for professional nurse education; and Medicare's hospital payment scheme based on medical diagnostic categories that do not factor in the *intensity of nursing care required*. These variables are only a few of the environmental factors influencing the education and recruitment of nurses whose job is to give intensive care to large caseloads of "general medical patients" in hospitals. They point out the need to make changes in the suprasystem known as the health care delivery system.

These issues are serious and demand attention from nurse managers who have a macroperspective and change agent skills. Reshaping the health care delivery system necessitates political action. Governmental policies influence the financing, structure, content, and process of delivering health care. Nurses *must* become comfortable with and sophisticated in formulating policy beyond their unit or hospital. What nurses can legally do, what kind of care third-party payers will pay for, and even how nurses dispose of syringes are policy issues decided in the political arena. Though nuances vary according to the political body (legislature, regulatory boards, departments, etc.), the political process is the change process.

At the organizational, departmental, and unit levels, creative change also begins with this macroperspective. The nurse change agent starts by thinking broadly. Looking at the sociopolitical and economic picture, she or he checks the pulse of the external environment, competing organizations, the board of directors, the professions. What is the climate? What are the trends? What does the consumer want and need? What does the nursing profession propose? Combining ideas from unconnected sources (Kanter, 1983), innovative thinking "percolates." The more "fluid" the vertical and horizontal organizational boundaries, the better the communication is from top-down, bottom-up, and lateral directions. Creative ideas flow best from managers who think big, brainstorm ideas, and stimulate "grassroots" staff talents.

THE PROCESS OF CHANGE

Whether it is environmental, systemwide, or unit-based, change is a process that involves strategies. It is a process that can and should be learned by all nurses, especially managers. The nurse manager needs to develop a system of integrative thinking that demands that problems be looked at as a whole. Skill in applying change theory is a most valuable management tool—inside or outside the hospital setting. The change process based on this theory is a problem-solving process, much like the nursing process. Different experts identify different numbers of steps or stages in the change process. The number of steps is unimportant. What is important is understanding what the change agent needs to do and why. The process is dynamic and fluid. As one becomes experienced with change, the sense of that "flow" becomes incorporated into the nurse's repertoire of nursing skills. Those who can master the nuances of communication skills can become "Change Masters" (Kanter, 1983).

The problem-solving change process described in this chapter synthesizes classical change theory and current nursing, sociological, psychological, and organizational thought. However, the nurse educated to manage and initiate change should know the theoretical foundation for the change process she or he implements. Therefore, key aspects of selected change theories are summarized in the following section; then a seven-step process is delineated with examples. Readers are encouraged to consult primary references for a fuller understanding of each. There are many similarities among these theoretical views, but the unique insights of each are also rich sources of contemporary approaches to change.

SELECTED CHANGE THEORIES

Lewin's Force-Field Model

Lewin (1951) provided a social-psychological view of the change process. He saw behavior as a dynamic balance of forces working in opposite directions within a field (such as an organization). "Driving forces" facilitate change because they are pushing participants in the desired direction. "Restraining forces" impede change because they are leading participants in the other direction. To plan change, one must analyze these forces and shift the balance in the direction of change through a three-step process: unfreezing, moving, and refreezing. Change occurs by adding a new force, changing the direction of a force, or changing the magnitude of any one force. Basically, strategies for change are aimed at increasing driving forces, decreasing restraining forces, or both.

Lewin's force-field model and an example are diagrammed in Figure 5–1. This scheme shows a system's opposing driving and restraining forces of change. These forces, part of the system's maintenance and adaptive mechanisms, are balanced at the present, or status quo, level. To achieve change, there must first be an imbalance between these driving and restraining forces (as seen in the example). This imbalance *unfreezes* the present patterned behavior. Behavior *moves* to a "new level," at which the opposing forces are brought into a new state of equilibrium. Once par-

Figure 5—1 Lewin's Force-Field Model of Change

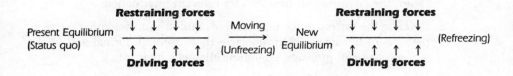

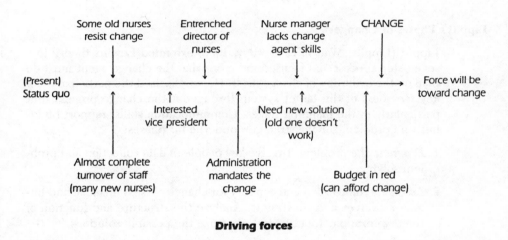

Lewin, K., 1951.

ticipants integrate the new patterns of behavior into their personalities and relationships with others, a *refreezing* takes place. The "new level" becomes institutionalized into formal and informal behavioral patterns.

Lewin's change strategies fall within his three-step process. Briefly stated, they are:

1. *Unfreeze* the existing equilibrium. Motivate participants by getting them ready for change. Build trust and the recognition for the need to change. Active participation in problem identification and generation of alternate solutions helps to "thaw" attitudes.

2. *Move* the target system to a new level of equilibrium. Get participants to agree that the status quo is not beneficial to them. Encourage "cognitive redefinition" by helping them view the problem from a new per-

spective. Stimulate "identification" by linking their views to those of a respected or powerful leader who supports the change. Help them "scan" the environment to search for relevant information.

3. *Refreeze* the system at the new level of equilibrium. Reinforce the new patterns of behavior. Institutionalize them through formal and informal mechanisms (policies, communication channels, etc.).

Lewinian thinking is fundamental to the views of later theorists. Clearly, it is a behavioral approach that nurses find consistent with their theoretical understanding of humans. The image of people's attitudes thawing, becoming more fluid, shifting to a desired state, and then refreezing is conceptually useful. This symbolism helps to keep theory and reality in mind simultaneously.

Lippitt's Phases of Change

Lippitt (Lippitt, Watson & Westley, 1958) extended Lewin's theory to a seven-step process and focused more on what the change agent must do than on the evolution of change itself. He emphasized the participation of key members of the target system throughout the change process, but particularly in the planning stages. Communication skills, rapport building, and problem-solving strategies underlie his phases:

1. *Diagnose* the problem. Involve key people in data collection and problem solving.

2. *Assess* the motivation and capacity for change. Assess financial and human resources and constraints. Analyze the structure and function of the organization. Identify and prioritize the possible solutions.

3. *Assess* the change agent's motivation and resources. Identifying this self-assessment phase is an important contribution. One's own commitment to change, energy level, future ambitions, and power bases must be considered. Starting a change and dropping it midstream can waste valuable personal energy and undermine the confidence of colleagues and subordinates.

4. *Select* progressive change objects. Develop the action plan, evaluation criteria, and specific strategies.

5. *Choose* a change agent role. The change agent can act as cheerleader, expert, consultant, or group facilitator. Whichever role is selected, all participants should identify it so that expectations are clear.

6. *Maintain* the change. Communication, feedback, revision making, and coordination are essential components of this phase.

7. *Terminate* the helping relationship. The change agent withdraws from the selected role gradually as the change becomes institutionalized.

Those who must continually implement the innovation need to have authority and accountability to do so.

Havelock's Model

Havelock (1973) developed a six-step process, also a modification of Lewin's model. It is included here only briefly. Havelock emphasized the unfreezing or planning stage, which he defined as: (a) building a relationship; (b) diagnosing the problem; and (c) acquiring resources. This planning is followed by the moving stage of: (d) choosing the solution and (e) gaining acceptance. Refreezing is referred to as (f) stabilization and self-renewal. Havelock described an active change agent who prefers a participative approach.

Rogers's Diffusion of Innovations

Rogers (1983) took a broader approach than Lewin, Lippitt, or Havelock. His five-step "innovation-decision process" details how an individual or "decision-making unit" passes from "first knowledge of an innovation" to confirmation of the decision to adopt *or reject* a new idea (1983:20). His framework emphasizes the *reversible* nature of change because participants may initially adopt a proposal but later "discontinue" it, or the reverse—initially reject it but adopt it at a later time. This is a useful distinction. If the change agent is unsuccessful in achieving full implementation of a proposal, she or he should not assume the issue is dead. It can be "resurrected," perhaps in an altered form, or at a more opportune time. However, if it is accepted, one cannot assume permanence.

Briefly, Rogers's five steps to the diffusion of innovation are:

1. *Knowledge.* The decision-making unit is introduced to the innovation and begins to understand it.

2. *Persuasion.* A favorable (or unfavorable) attitude toward the innovation forms.

3. *Decision.* Activities lead to a decision to adopt or reject the innovation.

4. *Implementation.* The innovation is put to use and reinvention or alterations may occur.

5. *Confirmation.* The individual or decision-making unit seeks reinforcement that the decision was correct. If there are conflicting messages or experiences, the original decision may be *reversed.*

Finally, Rogers stressed two important aspects to successful planned change: key people and policymakers must be *interested* in the innovation and *committed* to making it happen.

Figure 5–2   Comparison of Change Models

Levin	Lippit	Havelock	Rogers
1. Unfreezing	1. Diagnose problem 2. Assess motivation 3. Assess change agent's motivations and resources	1. Building a relationship 2. Diagnosing the problem 3. Acquiring resources	1. Knowledge 2. Persuasion 3. Decision
2. Moving	4. Select progressive change objects 5. Choose change agent role	4. Choosing the solution 5. Gaining acceptance	4. Implementation
3. Refreezing	6. Maintain change 7. Terminate helping relationship	6. Stabilization	5. Confirmation

Summary of Selected Theoretical Perspectives

These models of change are not the only ones that exist. They are classic perspectives that demonstrate overlap despite differences in perspective (see Figure 5–2). A seven-step eclectic approach based on the nursing process can abstract the common points and flesh out those significant for the nurse change agent. Insights from current experts of innovation are integrated into this model.

THE SEVEN STEPS TO PLANNED CHANGE: AN ECLECTIC APPROACH

The "nursing process" arose in the 1950s when nurses sought a framework for problem-solving patient care. The process of assessment, planning, implementation, and evaluation now structures nurses' thinking and care delivery—it is "second nature" to the professional nurse. Essentially, managing change follows the same path as the nursing process: assessment, planning, implementation, and evaluation (see Figure 5–3). However, since many nurses are less comfortable with change than with patient care, these steps are subdivided and extended into seven steps. Much emphasis is placed on the assessment phase of change for two reasons. First, without thorough data collection and analysis, planned change will not proceed past the "wouldn't it be a good idea if we . . ." stage. Second, nurses are often not familiar with the kind of data they need to collect and/or with the methods by which to analyze them in order to manage and initiate change.

Two situations will be presented to illustrate the steps in the change process. Each is intended to stimulate application of the change process regardless of setting or specific problem addressed. *Situation one* involves a hospital *staffing* problem while *Situation two* describes a *communication* problem within a community health organization. Readers are also encouraged to identify a situation relevant to their own practice or management role. For example, nurses in private practice might consider how to obtain hospital admitting privileges. Nurse managers could substitute the initiation of an improved patient classification system (see Chapter 19) to link patient acuity levels to staffing patterns.

Assessment

1. Identify the problem of opportunity.

Opportunities demand change as much (or more than) problems do. They are often overlooked by managers who manage but do not lead. That is, change is often planned to close a performance gap, a discrepancy between the desired and actual state of affairs. Performance gaps may arise because of problems in reaching performance goals or because new goals have been created. Be it a problem or opportunity, it must be identified clearly. If perceived differently by key persons, the search for solutions becomes confused. Start by asking the right questions, such as:

1. Where are we now? What is unique about us? What *should* our business be?

2. What can we do that is different and better than what our competitors do?

3. What is the driving stimulus in our organization—what determines how we make our final decisions?

Figure 5–3   Seven Steps of Planned Change: An Extension of the Nursing Process

Nursing Process	Change Process
Assessment	1. Identify the problem or opportunity 2. Collect data 3. Analyze data
Planning	4. Plan the change strategies
Implementation	5. Implement the change
Evaluation	6. Evaluate effectiveness 7. Stabilize the change

4. What prevents us from moving in the direction we wish to go? What is the problem?

5. What *kind* of change is required?

This last question generates integrative thinking on the potential effect of change on the system. Organizational change involves modifications in the system's interacting components, that is, in technology, structure, and people. For example, the introduction of new *technology* may necessitate changes in the *structure* of the organization. The physical plant will be altered if open-heart surgery is added as a new service. Relationships among the *people* who work in the system change when the structure is changed. New units are opened, others close. New rules and regulations, new authority structures, and new budgeting methods are structural changes. They, in turn, produce people changes such as the need for new skills, knowledge bases, attitudes, and motivations. No matter what the opportunity or problem, behavioral change—or "people change"—is the most challenging.

Given the transitional state of the health care system, nurse managers need to define problems and opportunities with insight to avoid status quo management. Developing creative insight requires exercise. (See some suggested exercises for change agents later in this chapter.) Creative insight involves looking at old problems in a fresh way, from many different perspectives. Never use past history as a guide for solutions. The manager concentrates on moving beyond the habitual, comfortable ways of experiencing a phenomenon to arrive at new insights, new possibilities (Hickman & Silva, 1984). Problems can become opportunities for change that will not only solve the immediate problem, but reshape and stimulate the system.

Situation one: Staffing.   One example of creative insight in defining a problem occurred in a medium-sized medical center. Upper management had acknowledged a staffing problem that they solved by using temporary agency nurses, pulling staff from one floor to float to another, and requesting nurses to remain on duty for an additional eight hours (for overtime pay). However, the pediatric unit supervisor saw the problem differently. After conferencing with her staff, she perceived that staffing levels indicated upper management's unwillingness to give the staff control, accountability, and respect. The problem, in her view, was inadequate staffing due to mismanagement of human resources. Nurses who are experts in the care of children resent being pulled to a unit that does not require this expertise, or to a unit that requires an expertise the child care specialist does not have. During periods of frequent pulling, these nurses were more likely to call in sick themselves.

With this problem in focus, ideas were generated. The problem was refashioned into an opportunity to create a "Children's Center," a decentralized unit encompassing pediatric and pediatric intensive care services. The proposal was to staff and manage this unit autonomously with collaboration between the unit supervisor and the pediatric nurses under her jurisdiction. No nurses would float into or out of this unit. Rather, a contingency schedule was developed to provide staff coverage for sick calls from within. Such a schedule provided a stable plan for adequate human resources to maintain optimal client care, and, at the same time, promoted collegial relationships and accountability. It also lowered overtime costs. Nurses were less likely to call in sick needlessly when they knew their colleagues would be required to cover for them. The depersonalization of coverage is eliminated.

Situation two: Communication.   This second example is hypothetical, though based on an actual organizational problem. A community health agency servicing 22 municipalities in a large semirural county had one main office and two branch offices, about 30 miles apart. The nursing staff was divided among the three offices, but the main office housed all administrative staff and support therapy staff (physical therapy, social workers, etc.). This main office was the site for most meetings, referral intake, and billing decisions.

A new director of professional services was hired after the former director of 20 years retired. The first problem the new director identified was poor communication among these three offices and between each office and other community agencies that provided client services. She associated this problem with *structure* (three offices) and proposed reorganization into one central office (a completely new location). After three years, she was still unable to persuade the executive director or the board of directors to adopt such a change. There was little agreement on the problem, and therefore no movement toward a solution.

An alternate definition of the problem is needed. Poor communication may indeed be the central issue, but it may not be tied to a structural problem. It may be a *process* problem that could be solved by changes in the pattern of communications or the technology used to communicate. Perhaps administrative staff and therapists need to make frequent visits to the branch offices, for example. A more innovative change would be to introduce teleconferencing equipment that would permit interactive electronic meetings between two or more groups of people at multiple locations. Each office would need similarly equipped conference rooms (speaker phones, interactive writing equipment, or a facsimile machine) connected by commercially available communication network services. Other organizations with similar technology (such as medical centers) could also access any of the three agency offices for meetings, inservice education, or client care conferences.

2. Collect data.

Once the problem or opportunity has been clearly defined, the change agent collects data external and internal to the system. This step is crucial to the eventual success of the planned change. All "driving" and "restraining" forces are identified so that the driving forces can be emphasized and the restraining forces reduced. It is imperative to assess the political pulse. Who will gain from this change? Who will lose? Which of these have more power and why? Can those power bases be altered? How?

The nurse manager can best assess the political climate by examining the reasons for the present situation. Who is in control that may be benefitting now? The ego involvement, commitment of the involved people, and personality likes and dislikes are as important to assess as the formal organizational structures and processes. The innovator has to gauge the potential resistance.

The costs and benefits of the proposed change are obvious focal points. The nurse manager also needs to assess resources—especially those she or he can control. One who has the respect and support of an excellent nursing staff has access to a powerful resource in today's climate. Current research findings are also helpful data in the change process.

Situation one: Staffing. To introduce her proposal for a decentralized unit with autonomous staffing prerogatives, the pediatric unit supervisor introduced earlier had to collect data to support her arguments. Examples of external data included: state, regional, and local supply and demand statistics for general and pediatric nurses; consumer demand for expert pediatric nursing services; staffing policies from competing hospitals; and research data regarding motivation of professional employees.

Internal data were derived from different system levels (organizational, group, and personal). At the organizational level, the supervisor examined the hospital's philosophy, goals, and marketing plans. She sought evidence that the hospital would benefit from marketing a Children's Center with a stable staff of specialist nurses. There was no competing focus— which would have been the case if the board of directors had had long-range plans to market a different unit. At the group and personal levels, the supervisor consulted her own staff and discussed the idea with nurses from other specialized units. If the staff had been organized into a bargaining unit, she would have had to investigate the bargaining unit's negotiated staffing policies and potential support for the idea. The goal was to collect data to support the idea that this change fits into the goals, norms, and values of the organization and its members. As a nurse leader, this supervisor was also interested in demonstrating how her idea reflected the goals and values of the nursing department and the profession.

Quantitative data help document needed change. Historical staffing and turnover data for this unit were compiled. Records were kept demonstrating higher absenteeism during periods of frequent pulling. Incident reports of unit and nonunit members documented the higher quality of care provided by seasoned specialists as opposed to temporary nurses. Finally, she estimated the cost savings expected from not hiring temporary nurses.

Situation two: Communication.   In the three-office community health agency, a cost-benefit analysis of regular teleconferences would focus on time, communication, equipment, and quality of care. Estimates of the cost of equipped conference rooms and training are straightforward. They should be outweighed by estimates of projected benefits such as:

1. Savings in *time* (translates into savings in costs) for travel to meetings

2. Savings in *time* in shorter, better managed, or teleconferenced meetings

3. Savings in transportation expenses

4. Maximized third-party reimbursement because of timely decision making (key persons can be gathered quickly and conveniently) and expeditious referrals among providers (nurses, therapists, social workers, etc.)

5. Improved productivity from key persons because their interactions are facilitated—there is more participation when distance is removed as a constraint to interaction and participants maintain access to important sources of information at their usual locations of work

6. Improved *quality* of care from productive interdisciplinary communication within the agency and between the agency and selected organizations (medical centers that have teleconferencing capacity, for example)

Quantitative data include: deployment of staff (time spent in traveling); percentage of meetings that have full versus partial participation of key persons; numbers of third-party payer rejections related to delayed or inappropriate decision making; numbers of meetings (and time associated) that had to be repeated in each branch in order to communicate essential information. Qualitative data include examples of miscommunication related to the inability to gather participants at one time for important messages and examples of delays in decision making that influenced quality of care. These examples are not exhaustive, but illustrate the need for thorough (and sometimes creative) data collection.

3. Analyze data.

The kinds, amounts, and sources of data collected are important, but they are useless unless they are analyzed. The change agent should focus more energy on analyzing and summarizing the data than on running around collecting it. The point is to flush out resistance, identify potential solutions and strategies, begin to identify areas of consensus, and build a case for whichever option is selected. When possible, a statistical analysis should be made; it is worth the effort, especially when the change agent will need to persuade persons in power who are comfortable with financial analyses, statistics, and probabilities. Themes from the data can be pulled out and threaded together to make a cogent case. These should be presented succinctly using bar graphs and charts.

Planning

4. Plan the change strategy.

Planning the *who, how,* and *when* of the change is a key step. What will be the target system for the change? Members from this system should be active participants in this planning stage. The more involved they are at this point, the less resistance there will be later. Lewin's "unfreezing" imagery is relevant here. Present attitudes, habits, and ways of thinking have to soften so members of the target system will be ready for new ways of thinking and behaving. Boundaries must melt before the system can shift and restructure.

This is the time to "rock the boat" by making people uncomfortable with the status quo. The seeds of discontent are planted by introducing information that may make them feel dissatisfied with the present and interested in something new. This information comes from the data collected—research findings, quantitative data, surveys of clients and/or staff, etc. The proposed change should be couched in comfortable terms as far as possible. Anxiety about the new change should be minimized.

Managers need to plan the resources required to make the change and establish feedback mechanisms to evaluate its progress and success. Establish control points with people who will provide the feedback. Work with these people to set specific goals with time frames. Develop operational indicators that signal success or failure in terms of performance and satisfaction.

Situation one: Staffing. Potential control points and indicators for the Children's Center proposal might be stated as:

1. Within 6 months, the head nurse will develop a contingency schedule, in collaboration with staff members, on a monthly basis.

2. Within 8 months, there will be a 20% decline in sick-outs.

3. Within 10 months, the staff will meet with upper management to report the effect of the new staffing policy on their professional identity and sense of control.

4. Within 12 months, the unit supervisor will submit a recommendation to continue or discontinue the new staffing policy based on such evidence as staff turnover, sick-outs, and use of agency personnel.

Situation two: Communication. Similar statements relevant to the community health agency situation might be:

1. Within 1 month, the executive director will obtain estimates from three competing telecommunications organizations and recommend one to the board of directors for trial.

2. Within 2 months, the director of professional services will appoint a staff member to be trained in teleconferencing.

3. Within 3 months, the trained staff member will begin training supervisors.

4. Within 4 months, two interdisciplinary meetings will take place.

5. Within 10 months, the director of professional services will report to the executive director tracking data regarding usage patterns, changes in staff deployment/time expenditures, etc.

6. Within 12 months, the board of directors will decide to extend the rental, discontinue it, or purchase the equipment.

Implementation

5. *Implement the change.*

The plans are put into motion (Lewin's "moving stage"). Interventions are designed to gain the necessary compliance. The change agent creates a supportive climate, acts as energizer, obtains and provides feedback, and overcomes resistance. Managers are the key change process actors. They use implementation tactics "to install planned changes, whether they be novel or routine" (Nutt, 1986:233). The specific activities undertaken to induce organizational change comprise the method of change (Katz & Kahn, 1978)—what is actually done. Depending on the change strategy selected (see the next section), the method might include giving a lecture or forming task forces. Some methods are directed toward changing individuals in an organization while others are directed toward changing the group.

Methods to change individuals. The most common method used to change individuals' perceptions, attitudes, and values is *information giving* (Nutt, 1986; Katz & Kahn, 1978). External expert consultants or internal organizational staff persons prepare and disseminate the information—usually in a top-down communication flow. Providing information is prerequisite to change implementation, but it is inadequate alone unless the lack of information is the only obstacle to effecting change. Information provision does not address the motivation to change.

Training combines information giving with practice in skills. As a socialization strategy, it is more of a system maintenance mechanism than an adaptation mechanism. Training typically shows people how they are to perform in a system, not how to change it. *Counseling* or *psychotherapy* is most effective for the troubled organizational member or the person who holds a powerful organizational position. *Selection, placement,* or *termination* of key people may be useful tactics for altering the forces for or against change.

Methods to change groups. Some implementation tactics use groups rather than individuals to attain compliance to change. The power of an organizational group to influence its members depends on its authority to act on an issue and the significance of the issue itself. The greatest influence is achieved when group members discuss issues that are perceived important and make relevant, binding decisions based on those discussions. Research on the use of *sensitivity groups* has not demonstrated effectiveness in implementing organizational change, most likely because these groups are not necessarily composed of members who occupy closely related positions in the organization. A more successful strategy has been the use of the *survey feedback*, in which organizational groups who do share closely related positions discuss issues as an "organizational family."

Individual and group implementation tactics can be combined. Whatever methods are used, participants should feel their input is valued. They should be rewarded for their efforts. Some people are not always persuaded a change is beneficial before it is implemented. Some undergo "cognitive dissonance," which means behavior changes first and attitudes are modified later to fit the behavior. In this case, the change agent should be aware of participants' conflict and reward the desired behaviors. It may take some time for attitudes to catch up.

Situation one: Staffing.   The pediatric supervisor recognized that she was initiating a unit-level change that would have systemwide implications. Both individual and group methods of change were needed. Providing "fact sheets" to her own unit members heightened their interest and offered a common ground for later discussion. To reduce resistance from other unit supervisors, she met informally with them one by one. Her tactic was to change attitudes by appealing to their professional values. Group meetings followed in which she suggested a trial program and requested participation in developing guidelines for contingency scheduling. She began to screen staff nurse applicants as to their desire for autonomy. Additionally, she persuaded the director of nurses and the nurse recruiter to visit another hospital that had already instituted a similar policy in its critical care unit.

Situation two: Communication.   Individual and group methods could also be used to implement a teleconferencing system. The director of nursing could hire a new manager experienced in this technology. Information and training would be necessary for all managers. A task force approach might stimulate participation from within the ranks. A seminar given by expert consultants and present users would also be beneficial. Time and costs would be limiting factors.

Evaluation

6. Evaluate effectiveness.

At each control point, the established operational indicators (step 4) are monitored as planned. The change agent determines if presumed benefits were achieved from a financial as well as a qualitative perspective. The extent of success or failure is determined and explained. There may have been unintended consequences and undesirable outcomes.

For example, in *Situation one*, the manager might obtain evidence that the new Children's Center attracts clients and retains expert staff. She would also need to measure staff satisfaction. It is possible the staff resents covering for one another and that conflict is brewing. In *Situation two* the director would evaluate if the teleconferencing process reduces wasted time and increases quality of care by improving interdisciplinary communication. She might also discover that the staff is intimidated by the technology and is wasting valuable time using it.

7. Stabilize the change.

The change is extended past the pilot stage and the target system is "refrozen." The change agent terminates the helping relationship by delegating responsibilities to target system members. The "energizer role" is still needed to reinforce the new behaviors through positive feedback. A degree of permanency is cultivated by writing formal policies and making sure staff repeat the new behavior frequently.

CHANGE AGENT STRATEGIES

Regardless of the setting or proposed change, the seven-step change process should be followed. However, specific strategies can be used, depending on the amount of resistance anticipated and the degree of power the change agent possesses. The three classic models of strategies were first described by Bennis, Benne, and Chinn (1969). They remain useful categories to consider in deciding which strategies the change agent should select depending on the circumstances.

Power-Coercive

Power-coercive strategies are based on the application of *power* by legitimate authority, economic sanctions, or political clout. For example, changes are made through law, policy, or financial appropriations. Those in control enforce changes by restricting budgets or creating policies. Those who are not in power may not even be aware of what is happening. Even if they are aware, they have little power to stop it. The change process continues through the seven steps just detailed, but there is little, if any, participation of the target system members. Resistance is handled by authority measures: accept it or leave.

The federal government's enactment of the prospective payment system for Medicare clients' hospitalizations was a power-coercive strategy for changing the economic incentives. The hospital is not paid for a client's care based on the number of days hospitalized. Rather, the hospital receives a *predetermined* fee based on the client's DRG (diagnosis-related group) regardless of the length of stay.

Power-coercive strategies are useful when a consensus is unlikely despite efforts to stimulate participation throughout the change process. When much resistance is anticipated, time is short, and the change is critical for organizational survival, this group of strategies may be necessary. A vice-president of nursing, for example, might have to exert legitimate authority to *appoint* a specific person to be a unit supervisor because the unit is leaderless during a critical time (a local epidemic of measles). Though the professional autonomy of the unit's members would be better served if they were given the opportunity to interview and vote on a candidate, organizational and unit survival needs might supersede this goal for the short run.

Of course, the potential negative consequences of this unilateral approach cannot be ignored. If the unit members have been practicing in a decentralized framework and value the accustomed autonomy, they are not likely to react positively. Resistance to the appointed leader and decreased morale can be anticipated. These strategies should not be used lightly or often if the nurse manager wishes to foster a climate of openness to change.

Empirical-Rational

In the empirical-rational model of change strategies, the power ingredient is *knowledge*. The assumption is that people are rational and will follow their rational self-interest if that self-interest is made clear to them. It is also assumed that the change agent who has *knowledge* has expert power to persuade people to accept a rationally justified change that will be beneficial to them. The flow of influence moves from those who know to those who do not know. New ideas are *invented* and communicated or *diffused* to all participants (like Rogers's "diffusion of innovation"). It is a matter of educating and disseminating information. Once enlightened, rational people will either accept or reject the idea based on its merits and consequences.

Because people do not always respond rationally, this strategy should not be used alone (Haffer, 1986). However, empirical-rational strategies are often effective when there is little resistance to the proposed change and it is perceived as reasonable. Introduction of new technology that is easy to use, cuts nursing time, and improves quality of care would be accepted readily after inservice education and perhaps a trial use. The change agent can direct the change. There is little need for staff participation in the early steps of the change process, though input is useful for the evaluation and stabilization stages. The benefits of change for the staff and perhaps research findings regarding client outcomes are the major driving forces. Well-researched, cost-effective technology can be implemented through this group of strategies.

Normative-Reeducative

In contrast to the rational-empirical model, normative-reeducative strategies of change rest on the assumption that people act in accordance with social norms and values. Information and rational arguments are insufficient strategies to change people's patterns of actions. The change agent must focus on noncognitive determinants of behavior as well. People's roles and relationships, perceptual orientations, attitudes, and feelings will influence their acceptance of change.

In this mode, the power ingredient is not authority or knowledge, but *skill in interpersonal relationships*. The change agent does not use coercion or nonreciprocal influence, but collaboration. Members of the target system are involved throughout the change process: people must participate in their own reeducation if they are to be reeducated at all. Change, or reeducation, is a *normative* change as well as a cognitive and perceptual change, and *participation in groups* is an essential change strategy (Bennis, Benne & Chinn, 1969).

Normative-reeducative strategies are well suited to the creative problem solving needed in nursing and health care today. The change agent consciously uses the change process based on theories of change that emphasize a human relations approach. Members of the target system are involved throughout all the steps of the change process. Value conflicts from all parts of the system are brought into the open and "worked through" so change can progress.

With their firm grasp of the behavioral sciences and communication skills, nurses are comfortable with this model. In most cases, the normative-reeducative approach to change will be effective in reducing resistance and stimulating personal and organizational creativity. The obvious drawback is the time required for group participation and conflict resolution throughout the change process. When there is adequate time or when group consensus is fundamental to successful adoption of the change, the manager would be well advised to adopt this framework. Examples include changing from a team to a primary nursing system (or the reverse) or initiating a new service.

CHANGE AGENT SKILLS

Making changes is not easy, but skill in doing so is mandatory for managers. Successful change agents demonstrate certain characteristics that can be cultivated and mastered with practice. Among these are:

1. The ability to combine ideas from unconnected sources (Kanter, 1983)

2. The ability to energize others by keeping the interest level up and demonstrating a high personal energy level

3. Skill in human relations—well-developed interpersonal communication, group management, and problem-solving skills

4. Integrative thinking—the ability to retain a "big picture" focus while dealing with each part of the system

5. Sufficient flexibility to modify ideas when modifications will improve the change, but persistent enough to resist nonproductive tampering with the planned change

6. Confidence and the tendency not to be easily discouraged

7. Realistic thinking

8. Trustworthiness—a track record of integrity and success with other changes

9. Ability to articulate a "vision" through insights and versatile thinking

10. Ability to handle resistance

HANDLING RESISTANCE

Why do people resist change? A generalized resistance stems from fear of losing the comfort of the familiar, no matter how inadequate it is. There is comfort in clinging to the present and uncertainty about the consequences of change. Change can threaten those with vested interest in the status quo. People view new ideas with selected perceptions—"How will this change affect me?"

For example, the change may represent a social loss when the organization is restructured and social relationships altered. Decentralization may abolish positions and decrease promotion opportunities—an actual or potential economic loss to some people. Unions may resist change that threatens job security for some of its members, even if other members of the organization as a whole will benefit. Even the *inconvenience* of learning new behaviors can be at the root of resistance.

The change agent should anticipate, ameliorate, and use resistance to change. Look for resistance. It will be lurking somewhere, perhaps where least expected. It can be recognized in such statements as:

1. "We tried that before."

2. "It won't work."

3. "No one else does it like that."

4. "We've always done it this way."

5. "We can't afford it."

6. "We don't have the time."

7. "It will cause too much commotion."

8. "You'll never get it past the board."

9. "Let's wait awhile."

10. "Every new boss wants something new to do."

11. "Let's start a task force to look at it . . . put it on the agenda."

Expect resistance and listen carefully to who says what, when, and in what circumstances. Verbal resistors are easier to deal with than "closet" resistors. Look for nonverbal signs of resistance such as poor work habits and lack of interest in the change.

Resistance has positive and negative aspects. On the one hand, resistance forces the change agent to be clear about *why* the change is needed. The agent must know the change inside and out because she or he must defend it against challengers. The positive part of resistance is the sharper focus and problem solving it encourages. It prevents the unexpected. It forces the change agent to clarify information, keep the interest level high, and answer the question "Why is this change necessary?" Resistance is a stimulant as much as it is a force to be overcome. It may motivate the target system to do *better* what it is doing presently, so it does not have to change. In this case, resistance can *produce* a change in behavior.

On the other hand, resistance is not always beneficial, especially if it persists beyond the planning stage and well into the implementation phase. It can "wear down" supporters and redirect system energy from implementation of the change to dealing with resistors. Morale can suffer (see Chapter 22 on conflict).

When handling resistance, the change agent must first be sure that she or he *wants* to reduce it. It can be used to sharpen decisions, for example, and eventually gain consensus. If it is necessary to minimize it, do not personalize the resistance. Remain rational, stick to the problem-solving change process and proceed with the following guidelines:

1. Communicate with those who oppose the change. Get to the root of their reasons for opposition.

2. Clarify information and provide accurate feedback.

3. Be open to revisions, but clear about what must remain.

4. Present the negative consequences of their resistance (threats to organizational survival, compromised client care, etc.).

5. Emphasize the positive consequences of the change and how the individual and/or group will benefit. However, do not spend too much energy on rational analysis of why the change is good and why the arguments against it do not hold up. People's resistance frequently flows from feelings that are not rational.

6. Keep resistors involved in face-to-face contact with supporters. Encourage proponents to empathize with opponents, recognize valid objections, and relieve unnecessary fears.

7. Maintain a climate of trust, support, and confidence.

8. Divert attention by creating a different "disturbance." Energy can shift to a "more important" problem inside the system, thereby redirecting resistance. Alternatively, attention can be brought to an external threat to create a "bully phenomenon." When members perceive a greater environmental threat (such as competition or restrictive governmental policies), they tend to unify internally.

9. Follow the "politics of change."

POLITICS OF CHANGE

Energy is needed to change a system. Power is the main source of that energy. Though few nurses will use coercive power sources, they will rely on information, expertise, and possibly positional power to persuade others. They should be "politically astute" by using these classic "political" strategies:

1. Analyze the organizational chart. Know the formal lines of authority. Identify informal lines as well (see Chapter 8 on communication).

2. Identify the key persons who will be affected by the change. Pay attention to those immediately above and below the point of change.

3. Find out as much as possible about these key people. What are their "tickle points"? What interests them, gets them excited, turns them off? What is on their personal and organizational agendas? Who typically aligns themselves with whom on important decisions?

4. Begin to build a coalition of support *before* you start the change process. Identify those key people who will most likely support your idea, and those who are most likely to be persuaded easily. Talk *informally* with them to "flush out" possible objections to your idea and potential opponents. What will the costs and benefits be to them—especially in political terms? Can your idea be modified in ways that retain your objectives but appeal to more key people?

This information will help the change agent develop the most "sellable" idea, or at least pinpoint probable resistance. It is a broad beginning to the data collection step of the change process and has to be fine-tuned once the idea is better identified.

The politics of change continue through all the steps of the change process. The astute change agent keeps one ear to the ground at all times to monitor power struggles. All change agents must follow the cardinal rule: Don't try to change too much too fast. But the savvy change agent develops a sense of "exquisite timing" by pacing the change process according to the political pulse. For example, she or he "unfreezes" the system during a period of coalition building and high interest—while resistance is low or at least unorganized. She or he may stall moving the project beyond a pilot stage if resistance solidifies or gains a powerful ally. In this case, the change agent will exercise mechanisms to reduce resistance. If resistance continues, she or he may consider several options: (a) the change is not workable and should be modified to meet the strongest objections (compromise); (b) the change is fine-tuned sufficiently but can be "placed on the back burner" until resistance subsides; (c) the change must proceed now and resistance must be overcome. If the last option is selected, energy is focused on overcoming resistance. Supporters are mobilized, and constant, consistent pressure is exerted to move ahead.

How the change agent uses the politics of change depends on whether she or he is an "insider" or "outsider." Someone who is part of the system being changed knows that system, has a stake in the outcome, and is familiar with the people, language, and politics. However, being an insider can restrict one's ability to move freely throughout the system. The agent may be "locked" into certain roles, authority structures, and expectations. Perspective may be limited. An outsider offers a fresh perspective and is independent of internal politics, but is unfamiliar with the system, people's values, and personal agendas. Either can accomplish change but must assess and use the politics of change differently.

Exercises to Stimulate Creative Thinking

Having "vision" is not mysterious. It is hard work. The "discipline of innovation" (Drucker, 1985) involves a deliberate, conscious search for innovative opportunities. Nurses can become innovators. To do so, they cannot cling to the status quo but must nurture the risk takers in their midst. This is not the time to rely solely on logic and pragmatic, careful, small steps to solutions to the complex problems we face. Nurses cannot continue to do more with less, and do it well. They have to do it *differently*.

Hickman and Silva (1984) offer exercises for removing blinders to insight. Nurses would do well to follow them:

1. Write down one new idea a day for a month. It can pertain to work, research, professional activities, family, or leisure, but it must be new. Consider some action on each idea (discuss it with colleagues, experiment with it, or implement it).

2. Break out of the mold. Do something unexpected, even "against the rules." Learn to tolerate ambiguity.

3. Routinely look at things differently. Read a book on creativity or attend a creativity seminar. See Steele and Maraviglia, *Creativity in Nursing* (1981), for example, and many others. *Do not stick to nursing references.* Try *A Whack on the Side of the Head* by Roger von Oech (1983).

4. Engage in wild thinking. Build in time for "unfettered thinking" in your meetings (supervisors' meetings, for example)—at least one hour several times a month.

5. Make things complex and ambiguous. Every day for a month, choose one problem or situation and look for multiple meanings, rich possibilities. Break it apart and put it back together in a different way. Check out all the angles.

The *practice* of divergent thinking prepares one to use the process almost automatically in day-to-day situations, such as in solving a difficult problem. Refer to Chapter 12 for a more detailed discussion of creativity in decision making.

SUMMARY

- Whether managing in a hospital, health maintenance organization, industry, or community health setting, the nurse manager links together subsystems of an organization to meet organizational objectives. In this role, the nurse must deal with change because it is inherent in an open system.

- There are inevitable conflicts and stresses as the organization strives to adapt and grow in a changing environment.

- Whether the nurse is managing or initiating change, she or he must have knowledge and skill in the change process within a systems framework. She or he has to analyze the many interrelating factors that influence the system's response to change. If she or he is to "manage" change conceived by top management, the nurse may not become involved until the late planning and implementation stages. Nonetheless, the change agent has to understand how to "move" a change plan, how to use and reduce resistance, and how to evaluate outcomes before "stabilizing" the change.

- A seven-step process for implementing change is summarized from several researchers.

- Nurses will continue to implement change. They can choose to survive it or manage it. The challenge is to expand their influence by initiating change at all levels of the health care system.

- Nurses must think creatively and act accordingly. They need to be *connected with their colleagues.*

- The professional association is a forum for the exchange of new ideas and experiences in change. Ideas from disconnected sources can combine, percolate, and produce innovation.

- There are many strategies for implementing change.

BIBLIOGRAPHY

American Nurses Association (ANA). (1980). *Nursing: A social policy statement.* Kansas City, MO: ANA.

Bennis, W., Benne, K., and Chinn, R. (1969). *The planning of change.* 2nd ed. New York: Holt, Rinehart & Winston.

Chinn, R. (1969). The utility of systems models and developmental models for practitioners. In: *The planning of change.* 2nd ed. Bennis, W., Benne, K., and Chinn, R. (editors). New York: Holt, Rinehart & Winston. Pp. 297–312.

Drucker, P. (1985). The discipline of innovation. *Harvard Business Review,* (May–June) 63(3): 67–72.

Drucker, P. (1985). *Innovations and entrepreneurship.* New York: Harper & Row.

Drucker, P. (1974). *Management: Tasks, responsibilities, practice.* New York: Harper & Row.

Haffer, A. (1986). Facilitating change: Choosing the appropriate strategy. *J Nurs Adm,* (April) 16(4): 18–22.

Havelock, R. (1973). *The change agent's guide to innovation in education.* New Jersey: Educational Technology Publications.

Hickman, C., and Silva, M. (1984). *Creating excellence: Managing corporate culture, strategy and change in the new age.* New York: New American Library.

Kanter, R. M. (1983). *The change masters: Innovation for productivity in the American corporation.* New York: Simon & Schuster.

Kast, F. E., and Rosenzweig, J. E. (1970). *Organization and management: A systems approach.* New York: McGraw-Hill.

Katz, D., and Kahn, R. (1978). *The social psychology of organizations.* 2nd ed. New York: Wiley. Chap. 19.

Lancaster, J., and Lancaster, W. (1982). *The nurse as change agent.* St. Louis: C. V. Mosby.

Lewin, K. (1951). *Field theory in social science.* New York: Harper & Row.

Lippit, R., Watson, J., and Westley, B. (1958). *The dynamics of planned change.* New York: Harcourt, Brace.

Nutt, P. (1986). Tactics of implementation. *Academy of Management Journal,* 29(2): 230–261.

Rogers, E. (1983). *Diffusion of innovations.* 3rd ed. New York: Free Press.

Schermerhorn, J. R., Jr. (1984). *Management for productivity.* New York: Wiley.

Steele, S., and Maraviglia, F. (1981). *Creativity in nursing.* New Jersey: Charles B. Slack.

von Oech, R. (1983). *A whack on the side of the head.* New York: Warner Brothers.

PREVALENCE OF ETHICAL ISSUES

The practice of nursing is a moral enterprise based on a commitment to provide care. Throughout history, nurses have confronted ethical dilemmas. Traditionally, issues such as confidentiality and informed consent have required the nurse's attention to safeguard patient rights. These issues are with us still today and require even more focus, as the complexity of care and treatment makes interpretation more important.

Innovations in health care technology give today's professionals the tools to keep bodies alive almost indefinitely. As we question even the definition of life and the definition of death, we face many decisions fraught with ethical dilemmas. Treatment provides cure or comfort and at the same time often costs a great deal physically, financially, and emotionally. Our clients require assistance to make difficult decisions and to balance the costs and benefits in terms of their own beliefs and values. Nurses address intrapersonal and interpersonal conflicts in their daily practice. Nurse managers face these same dilemmas and in addition must address the ethical implications of their management decisions. The ability to address ethical issues is at the heart of the practice of nursing today.

ETHICS IS INTEGRAL TO NURSING MANAGEMENT

How we operate in a management role is influenced by our beliefs and values and the experiences that form us as individuals and as leaders. Our personal values as well as the values of the profession in which we have been socialized define responsibilities to our clients and to society. The American Nurses' Association *Code for Nurses* (Figure 6–1) and its interpretive statements and the ANA social policy statement (available from ANA) provide a framework for making ethical decisions from the point of view of the profession. The Patient's Bill of Rights (Appendix B) clarifies rights for patients in institutional settings and implies an obligation on the part of the nurse to assist the patients in securing them.

As one reviews these documents, it is clear that the nurse manager has an obligation to:

1. Provide safe and respectful care

2. Not discriminate

3. Assure privacy and confidentiality

4. Ensure that the patient has enough information for informed consent

5. Support continuity of care

6. Safeguard the public from unethical or illegal practice

7. Support the welfare of the nursing profession

8. Follow physician's orders

9. Support the policies of the hospital

10. Maintain conditions of employment conducive to high quality care

11. Collaborate with other health professionals

12. Act in accord with one's own values

13. Promote efforts to meet the health needs of the public

What is obvious as one scans the list is that in the process of meeting one obligation the nurse may become unable to meet another. Consider the case of an AIDS patient who requests that the nurse not inform his spouse of the diagnosis. This creates a conflict between the duty of safe-

Figure 6—1 American Nurses' Association Code for Nurses

Preamble

The *Code for Nurses* is based on belief about the nature of individuals, nursing, health, and society. Recipients and providers of nursing services are viewed as individuals and groups who possess basic rights and responsibilities, and whose values and circumstances command respect at all times. Nursing encompasses the promotion and restoration of health, the prevention of illness, and the alleviation of suffering. The statements of the *Code* and their interpretation provide guidance for conduct and relationships in carrying out nursing responsibilities consistent with the ethical obligations of the profession and quality in nursing care.

Code for Nurses

1. The nurse provides services with respect for human dignity and the uniqueness of the client unrestricted by considerations of social or economic status, personal attributes, or the nature of health problems.

2. The nurse safeguards the client's right to privacy by judiciously protecting information of a confidential nature.

3. The nurse acts to safeguard the client and the public when health care and safety are affected by the incompetent, unethical, or illegal practice of any person.

4. The nurse assumes responsibility and accountability for individual nursing judgments and actions.

5. The nurse maintains competence in nursing.

6. The nurse exercises informed judgment and uses individual competence and qualifications as criteria in seeking consultation, accepting responsibilities, and delegating nursing activities to others.

7. The nurse participates in activities that contribute to the ongoing development of the profession's body of knowledge.

8. The nurse participates in the profession's efforts to implement and improve standards of nursing.

9. The nurse participates in the profession's efforts to establish and maintain conditions of employment conducive to high quality nursing care.

10. The nurse participates in the profession's effort to protect the public from misinformation and misrepresentation and to maintain the integrity of nursing.

11. The nurse collaborates with members of the health professions and other citizens in promoting community and national efforts to meet the health needs of the public.

American Nurses' Association, Inc. (For a complete statement of standards write the Publications Fulfillment Center, 2420 Pershing Road, Kansas City, Missouri 64108.)

guarding the client's right to privacy and the duty to protect the public health.

Another dilemma occurs as nurses are faced with an agonizing decision regarding whether to go on strike. The ANA *Code for Nurses*, statement 9 states: The nurse participates in the profession's efforts to establish and maintain conditions of employment conducive to high quality nursing care, while the obligation to provide safe care requires that we not abandon the patient.

Conflicting obligations are a major source of stress for nurses, and without help in addressing them, are also a source of nurse burnout (Cameron, 1986). Ethical dilemmas, by definition, seldom have right or wrong answers. The nurse manager can deal with them by preparing herself and her staff to participate in decision making. A knowledge of the theories and principles of biomedical ethics and a model for decision making will assist in analyzing issues and in the ability to articulate ethical positions.

ETHICAL APPROACHES

The field of biomedical ethics is a fairly new one that has become more important as health care decisions have emerged into the public arena. The abortion debate, questions related to stopping ventilatory support for Karen Ann Quinlan, and brain death legislation are examples of issues from the health care arena that have spurred public interest in ethical decision making. Philosophers, theologians, and social scientists are now contributing to the analysis of ethical issues.

Theories and principles used to address biomedical problems are drawn from the discipline of moral philosophy. Biomedical ethics applies these philosophical concepts to problems encountered in the delivery of health care. Deontology and teleology are two theoretical approaches frequently used to address issues in biomedical ethics.

Deontology (derived from the Greek word *deon*, meaning duty) focuses on duties or obligations and holds that the features of actions themselves determine whether they are right or wrong. It assumes that there are universal principles or rules that are inherently good or right, independent of their consequences. Examples of such duties are "tell the truth," "do not kill," and "keep promises."

Teleology (derived from the Greek term *telos*, meaning end), also called utilitarianism, gauges the rightness or wrongness of actions by their ends or consequences. The basic principle is that of utility. It asserts that the goal of morality is to produce the maximum benefits and minimum harm for the greatest numbers. Right conduct and duty are defined in terms of what is good or that which produces goods (Beauchamp & Childress, 1983). Whether we consider the good or harm in terms of the individual, family, or society will influence the decisions we make.

Codes of ethics and philosophical frameworks for professions have been developed by applying these theoretical bases to the practice of the professions. Thus, the philosophical premise chosen defines the obligations or duties of the professions. Leah Curtin has proposed the concept of human advocacy as a philosophical foundation for nursing practice. Since the purpose of nursing is the welfare of other human beings, she posits that the end or goal of the profession is a moral, not a scientific one. The "good" that it seeks involves our relationships with other human beings. "The wise and human application of our knowledge and skill is the moral art of nursing" (Curtin, 1979:130). This ideal of advocacy is based on our common humanity, our common needs, and our common rights. To operate as an advocate, we need to understand both the clinical and moral dimensions of the issues our patients and we, as professionals, are facing. Diseases have a physiological impact and they damage our humanity as well. Our abilities to be independent, to act freely, and to exercise our right to make choices are influenced by both medical problems and by the bureaucratic institutions with which the client must interact when he or she is ill.

The nurse in this advocacy role has a responsibility to provide appropriate information, to assist patients to make decisions within their value system, and to help them find meaning and purpose in the issues they must confront.

These philosophical positions provide divergent frameworks for addressing ethical dilemmas, i.e., defining which right or obligations apply or identifying the harm or good produced by the action. The principles addressed in the next section help conceptualize issues to make them understandable.

PRINCIPLES OF BIOMEDICAL ETHICS

Principles of biomedical ethics provide concepts and language that can be used to identify issues, to reflect on them, and to articulate the ethical positions we take. A concept is "an abstraction or generalization that helps attach meaning to a phenomenon which is observed in the clinical setting" (Rossman, 1985:52). It helps us to recognize what is occurring. If we say a patient is in shock, a fairly representative picture will appear in our minds. In the same way, if we identify an issue as one of patient autonomy, an entire range of questions will arise. Respect for persons as a basis for practice underlies the principles of autonomy, nonmaleficence, beneficence, and justice.

The Principle of Autonomy

Autonomy is derived from the Greek term *autos* (self) and *nomos* (rule), and is defined as self-rule or self-governance. Personal autonomy is "being one's own person, without constraints either by another's action or by psychological physical limitations" (Beauchamp & Childress, 1983:59). This principle requires that we respect individuals in our care as autonomous agents who have a right to control their own lives. To make one's own decision requires accurate information. Thus, informed consent is based on the principle of autonomy. Nurses often encounter situations where a person has not received information or has not heard or remembered it. We are frequently in the position of providing information to patients, seeking information for them, or letting them know that they have a right both to receive information and/or to refuse treatment. Differences of opinion between patients and families or among caregivers arise as we ask questions such as: "Should we tell him he has cancer?" "Does she know that the treatment will be painful and expensive and may be futile?"

In the spirit of respect for autonomy, we must help people to be involved to the extent they are able in decisions that affect them. To be self-governing, one must be competent to act. Competency assessment is a critical feature in determining who makes decisions. In cases of incompetency or emergency, health care professionals act in the "best interest" of the person.

When possible, we reflect the patient's values in these decisions. The competent patient has the right to decide, even if the outcome of refusing treatment may be death. For example, Jehovah's Witnesses refuse blood transfusions because in their belief system risking their eternal souls is a greater threat than death.

It is difficult to allow someone to make a decision that is "noncompliant" or likely to be harmful from our point of view. However, because of the risk of paternalism, in order to override their decision, we need to have *strong* evidence that the person is indeed incapable. *Paternalism* is a term that refers to doing what is in the "best interest" of those for whom we are providing care. Health care professionals have acted in accordance with this concept out of good will. The human rights movement in this country brought with it a major focus on individual rights. Since that time the value of patient autonomy has become increasingly important.

The right to privacy and confidentiality also arise from the principle of autonomy. The issue of AIDS has created some new questions regarding confidentiality: "How can I protect the health of other hospital staff without disclosing the person's diagnosis?" "Who has the right to information in the medical record?" In these instances, the right to autonomy and confidentiality needs to be weighed against the health and well-being of others. Autonomy is a basic right, but it is not overriding in all cases.

The Principle of Nonmaleficence

Nonmaleficence is the principle that requires that we "do no harm." This is often considered a most stringent duty for the health professional. Our contract with society requires that we provide safe care. To act in accordance with this principle, we must act thoughtfully and competently. "Due care" requires that we have adequate knowledge and skill to perform the tasks we undertake. The American Nurses' Association *Code for Nurses* states that "the nurse maintains competency in nursing."

The concept of harm can extend to infliction of emotional and financial costs as well as of pain, death, or disability. Dilemmas occur when differing perceptions of harm arise. Death may be perceived by the staff as the worst option but the patient may disagree, or vice-versa. In the case of chemotherapy administration or transplantation, it is obvious that pain and illness are harms that one may choose to sustain in order to prevent the even greater injury of profound illness or death.

The Principle of Beneficence

Beneficence—the doing of good—is on the same continuum as the principle of nonmaleficence. It is more active, however, and requires action that contributes to the welfare of others. It also includes prevention and removal of harm. Mercy, kindness, and charity are concepts related to the principle of beneficence.

The first tenet of the ANA *Code for Nurses* states "The nurse provides services with respect for human dignity and the uniqueness of the client. . . ." This means that to not provide available services would be a breach of this professional obligation and the principle of beneficence.

There have been years of discussion regarding whether a nurse has an obligation to provide care to patients having abortions when the nurse believes it is wrong. The outcome of these discussions most often is that a nurse may transfer to another unit where abortion is not routinely encountered. However, in the short term, if one is assigned to the patient, the nurse may not abandon the patient. This discussion exemplifies the higher obligation to do no harm, or nonmaleficence. Beneficence and nonmaleficence are extreme ends of the same scale. The distinction between the two comes in the degree of activity required to act. The nursing profession has a special contract to provide care for the sick. Our active involvement in providing or arranging for appropriate care is an act of beneficence.

NONMALEFICENCE $\longleftrightarrow$ BENEFICENCE
To do no harm   To do good

The Principle of Justice

Justice, in concept, is often equated with fairness, or more precisely "dessert"—giving each his or her right or due. To receive a license to practice nursing is fair because you earned it by study and effort.

Distributive justice—the just distribution of burdens and benefits in society—is a recurring theme in health care today, as advanced technol-

ogy and increased cost control create challenges for many policy decisions. Resource allocation discussions have increased in recent years with
the recognition that available resources are not limitless. On an individual
level, establishing the criteria for receiving an organ for transplant is an
example of a discussion of justice. On a macroeconomic level, issues are
addressed with questions such as: Is there a right to health care? What
does that right mean? The uninsured and underinsured have been added
to the ranks of the disenfranchised who cannot obtain health care. Policymakers discuss a "safety net" and/or providing catastrophic insurance to
assist those whose resources are expended.

Nurse managers participate in decision making as to institutional programs that will be developed or discontinued. They participate in budget
development and strategic planning. Because they wear the "two hats" of
institutional administrator and nursing manager, in their decisions they
must consider the obligation to provide quality care as well as the necessity to operate in a cost-effective manner so the institution can continue
its mission.

Nurse managers address justice questions as they consider staff mix
and the percentage of staff assigned to each shift, and as daily assignments
are made. Judgments reflect the needs of the clients, the skills of the
nursing staff, and the determination as to how the best care can be provided. The ANA *Code for Nurses* says that these decisions will be made
"unrestricted by considerations of social or economic status, personal attributes, or the nature of health problems." For most nurses, *their* best
interest would come into play if, with two equally ill people—one of them
a "bag lady" and the other, the hospital's director—they had to decide
who was assigned the best qualified staff. Beliefs and values and self-
interest do play a role in many decisions.

Therefore, nurse managers, in order to prevent discrimination and
unfairness to the greatest extent possible, need to have an awareness of
their own values and biases. We are human as well as professional, and we
make value decisions all the time. We can make our decisions more consciously, but probably not perfectly. Since there are seldom clear "right"
answers, but rather options to be weighed, a model for decision making
can help us analyze the ethical issues we confront.

A MODEL FOR ADDRESSING ETHICAL ISSUES

Most models for ethical decision making utilize the nursing process and
incorporate the principles of biomedical ethics discussed in the last section. Crisham (1985) developed and refined a model for decision making
based on her work with hundreds of staff nurses in acute care settings.
The model is a tool that can be used to clarify the issues when nurses face
conflicting obligations. It outlines a process for identifying and articulating a position so they can participate in the process of decision making.

The model involves five steps represented by the mnemonic MORAL:

M = massage the dilemma

O = outline options

R = review criteria and resolve

A = affirm position and act

L = look back

To illustrate the steps of the model, we will review the case of Mrs. Y.

Case Study

The nurse manager of an intensive care unit identified an ethical dilemma when the staff nurses caring for Mrs. Y said that she was communicating verbally and nonverbally (by resisting treatments) a wish that she be allowed to die. As her condition worsened, they anticipated that a cardiac arrest might occur and they believed it would be abusive to the patient to perform resuscitation efforts. There was no "do not resuscitate order" in the medical record. Until an order could be obtained, they were obligated by policy to initiate resuscitation efforts.

When Mrs. Y's sons were approached with this information, they indicated that a discussion of death would take away Mrs. Y's hope and thus might actually hasten her death. They wanted all possible efforts to sustain her life continued. As discussions were occurring between the nursing and the medical staff, Mrs. Y's condition worsened. She slipped into a coma and was unable to communicate.

How does the nurse manager address this dilemma?

Massage the Dilemma

The first step, as in any process, is to be aware that an ethical dilemma exists. Nurses feel discomfort less often when they are able to identify the specific conflict. *Massaging the dilemma* (or collecting data) helps one to identify the dilemma and who is, or who should be, involved in the process of decision making. Collecting all the relevant data possible is the most crucial component in ethical decision making.

It is important to remember that conflicting wishes and values may occur among several parties—patient, family, nurse, doctor—or a conflict may exist *within* the nurse's own values. A dilemma means that one believes there are reasons to do two opposing actions. Phrased another way, reasons exist to do and to not do the same thing, e.g., to respect the patient's wishes and to not violate institutional policy. In this case, the nurse manager's conflicting obligations are to:

1. Do no harm (not abuse)

2. Provide treatment (good)

3. Support the patient's autonomy and act according to his or her wishes

4. Support the family in a crisis time

5. Follow orders and hospital policy (e.g., to resuscitate since there was no order to the contrary)

6. Assist staff to act professionally and to make an ethical decision.

In collecting data for decision making, some issues for consideration are:

1. What is the prognosis at this point?

2. Who has the information regarding the prognosis?

3. Who can make the decision?

4. Was Mrs. Y competent when she indicated her wish to die?

5. What are the relationships among family members?

6. Can the sons represent Mrs. Y's best interest?

7. How capable are the sons of making the decision? Are they "in denial" regarding their mother's prognosis?

8. Can hospital policy be of assistance in this instance?

9. What is my primary obligation as a nurse manager?

As the nurse manager attempts to unravel the confusion, it is helpful to consider the nursing options and the manager's tools. Ultimately, nurses cannot write a "do not resuscitate" order, but they participate with others (e.g., family, physicians, chaplains) in the decision making. Nurses have concerns about the family system and the survivors as well as the dying patient and her autonomy. In this dilemma, the nurse manager's goal becomes to assist the decision makers and the family to share their information and their values in the hope of arriving at a consensus.

Outline Options

The process of outlining the options can be done with staff involvement in order to help them (the staff) clarify the options available and the consequences of their potential actions. Options one may identify include:

1. Do nothing

2. Discuss the medical diagnosis, prognosis, and medical plan with the primary physician

3. Discuss with the family their perceptions of diagnosis and prognosis, their values and beliefs, and what their mother would have wanted; this may include questions such as what is quality of life for her—is it awareness, productivity, spending time with grandchildren, etc.?

4. Discuss the nurses' values and clarify their rationale for not wanting to resuscitate; clarify whose "best interest" they are representing

5. Schedule a care conference with the family, nurses, physicians, and whoever else may be helpful, e.g., minister, chaplain, social worker.

Review Criteria and Resolve

To determine appropriate actions, one needs to weigh the options generated against the principles or primary values of those involved. Crisham (1985) provides a decision matrix (Figure 6–2) that includes the principles as well as practical considerations. The alternatives (options) listed in the preceding section can be put on this graph and weighed against the criteria the nurse manager believes are important. Value considerations for the nurse manager may include: respects staff, acts fairly, etc. Practical considerations such as legal impact, effectiveness, and likelihood of success can also be included in the grid.

A plus (+) or minus (−) grid or applying numerical weighting can give the nurse a visual indication of the positive and negative outcomes of various choices. Many ethical decisions are approached by weighing options because there is seldom one right or wrong answer when dealing with an ethical dilemma. Listening and attempting to understand the values of those parties involved is essential to collaborative decision making.

Figure 6–2   Decision Matrix

| Options | VALUES | | | | | | | | PRACTICAL CONSIDERATIONS | | | |
	Patient Autonomy	Beneficence	Nonmaleficence	Staff Autonomy	Interdisciplinary Relationships	Family Comfort	Compliance with Policy		Reduce Legal Risk	Time	Clarity of Issues	
Do Nothing	−	−	−	−	NA	+	+		+	+	−	
Discuss with M.D.	+	+	+	−	−	?	+		+	−	±	
Discuss with Family	+	+	+	±	NA	+	NA		+	−	±	
Discuss with Nurse	+	+	+	+	−	±	NA		+	−	±	
Schedule a Care Conference	+	+	+	+	+	±?	+		+	+	+	

Crisham, P. MORAL: How can I do what's right? *Nursing Management* (March) 1985, 16, 3.

Different individuals assess positives and negatives differently and weigh choices differently. Thus, the tool, when used with staff, can help in understanding the frame of reference of those involved.

Affirm Position and Act

Once one has decided the next appropriate action, a strategy needs to be developed. Literature in biomedical ethics indicates that knowing the correct action does not have a great deal of influence on whether health care workers act in accordance with what they believe to be correct. To enhance appropriate action, one may look at the organizational forces that assist or impede an action plan.

Questions to be considered in planning for action in Mrs. Y's dilemma include:

1. Are the nurses able to risk stating their opinion and rationale?

2. What are the consequences of following and not following institutional policy?

3. Will the physician be willing to attend a conference?

4. Can we "live with" all potential outcomes of the conference?

5. Do we need additional resources to assist with the process?

Planning the specifics of the conference is part of the nurse manager's facilitating role in ethical decision making. He or she can help the staff determine the appropriate time, place, and participants that will allow them to participate in decision making and to feel supported. Participating in the conference also will help the staff develop new skills they can use in dealing with future dilemmas as they occur.

Look Back

In Mrs. Y's case, the staff had a care conference. During the conference, it became clear that the family was acting on information obtained weeks earlier and were assuming that if treatment were successful, Mrs. Y would have two years or more of "normal" life. The nurses and doctors had seen her failing and becoming infected and septic. They now believed that the best they could do would be to prolong a painful and brutal process of dying. When family members were able to hear the new prognostic information, they agreed that extraordinary efforts would cause more harm than any possible good and agreed that if Mrs. Y arrested, she should not be resuscitated. Mrs. Y died a few days later.

In this instance, the resolution was successful in that it prevented harm to Mrs. Y and promoted the good of respect and participation for all involved. If disagreements persist, however, one may need to recycle through the process to define the problem, to generate options, and to identify consequences with all the decision makers. The nurse manager also may involve resource people to assist with the problem-solving process.

Application of the Model to Management Decision Making

As a nurse manager addresses dilemmas in his or her management practice, the same grid format that lists options, values, and practical considerations can be used as a basis for reflection. Additional values such as fairness, honesty, supporting staff autonomy and growth, or improving interdisciplinary relationships can be included. These can be listed along with the ethical principles that we applied to cases or they can replace them on the decision matrix, depending on what values are applicable to the situation.

The field of business ethics addresses issues such as corporate responsibility, conflict of interest, and honesty in dealing with consumers. The nurse manager addresses relationships with staff and colleagues, responsibility to the patients and to the organization, cost effectiveness, and sometimes community relations, in their management decisions and their supervisory relationships. Articulating the issues clearly, defining the issue one wishes to achieve, and analyzing its impact is a way of increasing the consciousness with which we make decisions. It also enhances our ability to articulate the rationale for directions we intend to pursue.

SPECIAL ISSUES FOR THE NURSE MANAGER

Provision of Safe Care

The primary ethical obligation of the nurse manager is to provide safe care. With the increasing complexity of care and the increasing complexity of technology, the nursing staff requires sophisticated assessment skills and up-to-date knowledge about new treatments and procedures. The skills discussed in Chapter 14 on training and education are important for nurse managers to use in addressing patient care from the perspective of "at least, do no harm" (nonmaleficence). The development of patient education skills allows the nurse to support patients in caring for themselves, and also provides information essential for autonomous decision making.

Confronting Unsafe Practice

The "due care" standard requires the nurse manager to deal with the unsafe or impaired practitioner. The nurse manager needs to know the institution's procedures for addressing issues of safety and professional conduct—whether the impaired practitioner is a nurse or other health care professional. It is also crucial to remember that "respect for persons" underlies all the principles of biomedical ethics. To deal humanely and gently while providing accurate data requires the nurse manager to employ his or her best communication and leadership skills while confronting this most painful issue.

Supporting Patient and Staff Autonomy

To address ethical issues, we must know our own values and goals. This knowledge assists us in articulating our own positions when we take an ethical stand. It also increases objectivity and the possibility of helping the client or staff member make decisions related to *their own* value system, not ours. We need to avoid paternalism. Language that identifies the "noncompliant" patient sometimes provides a clue that we are facing a value system that differs from our own. A patient's definition of "quality of life" and ours may be greatly disparate. To act as an advocate, the nurse must understand patient values and support patient decisions. "So often by trying to do what we think is right by our value system, we trespass upon the authenticity of the person" (Curtin, 1979:132). The nurse manager must hear and understand the values and goals of the staff in order to avoid "trespassing" on the individuality of staff and colleagues, as well.

Ethics Education and Resource Management

Since ethical issues are commonly discussed in our institutions, many facilities have created resources to deal with them. These resources can provide education, consultation, and support.

Individuals who can be of assistance are line supervisors and staff resources such as clinical specialists or ethics consultants. Also, many institutions now have ethics committees whose purposes are to develop policies that protect patient rights and to provide education and consultation for difficult cases. Most committees are interdisciplinary and thus can supply objectivity as well as an overview of the process in order to ensure "due care" in decision making.

Ongoing staff education and discussion of ethical issues when a crisis is not looming are effective tools in preparing the staff to address ethical dilemmas when they do arise. Formal classes as part of inservice education will provide a framework for discussion. Open discussion of ethical dilemmas at staff meetings will help identify issues and patterns of issues that occur frequently.

An effective method for approaching ethical issues is to use "ethics rounds." These are interdisciplinary rounds that include nursing staff and members of other disciplines who interact with patients and personnel in a unit. Principles can be presented and discussed or cases can be retrospectively reviewed and discussed. Through this process, participants develop a common language as well as an awareness of one another's values, which are then known and understood when a difficult issue arises. As staff members gain skills and awareness, ethical issues are often identified at an earlier stage and crises are more often averted. The goal of ethics education is to develop in the staff skills they can use to handle issues that arise in professional practice.

By initiating educational opportunities, the nurse manager indicates that such issues are open to discussion and are an important part of nursing practice. By listening and participating in problem solving and/or soliciting additional resources, the manager makes it possible for the staff to risk raising an issue.

The nurse manager who knows his or her own values, who respects staff members, and expects high quality care is the nurse manager who creates an environment in which ethical issues can be addressed and resolved. The time and skill required to resolve conflict and encourage creative problem solving are scarce resources in the nursing department. The capable nurse manager, therefore, is the institution's best asset in developing professional, ethical nursing practice.

SUMMARY

- Beliefs, values, and experiences influence one's ethical decision making.

- The nursing profession has delineated its code of ethics in the American Nurses' Association *Code for Nurses*. Along with the interpretive statements (available from ANA), the *Code* guides nurses' ethical decision making.

- Ethical principles include autonomy, nonmaleficence, beneficence, and justice.

- Use of a model for addressing ethical issues assists the nurse in the process of decision making.

- The nurse manager has additional ethical dilemmas including obligations to provide safe care, confront unsafe practice, support patient and staff autonomy, manage resources, and provide ethics education to staff.

- The staff's ability to deal with ethical issues is directly related to the nurse manager's skills in conflict management, willingness to allow risk taking, and support of staff acting in a professional manner.

- Nurse managers communicate interest in ethical issues by assisting staff in generating alternatives and developing strategies for action.

BIBLIOGRAPHY

American Nurses' Association (ANA). (1976). *Code for nurses with interpretive statements.* Kansas City, MO: ANA.

Aroskar, M. (1980). Anatomy of an ethical dilemma: The theory and practice. *American Journal of Nursing,* (April) *80*:658–634.

Aroskar, M. (1980). Establishing limits to professional autonomy: Whose responsibility? *Nursing Law and Ethics,* (May) *1*:5.

Aroskar, M., and Davis, A. J. (1983). *Ethical dilemmas and nursing practice.* Norwalk, CT: Appleton-Century-Crofts.

Beauchamp, T., and Childress, J. F. (1983). *Principles of biomedical ethics.* New York, Oxford: Oxford University Press.

Beauchamp, T., and Walters, L. (1982). *Contemporary issues in bioethics.* 2nd ed. Belmont, CA: Wadsworth.

Cameron, M. (1986). The moral and ethical component in nurse-burnout. *Nurs Mngmt,* (April) *17*:4.

Cranford, R. E., and Daudera, A. E. (1984). *Institutional ethics committees and health care decision-making.* Ann Arbor, MI: Health Administration Press.

Crisham, P. (1985). MORAL: How can I do what's right? *Nurs Mngmt,* (March) *16*:3.

Curtin, L. L. (1982). Ethics in nursing administration. In: *Contemporary nursing management.* Marriner, A. (editor). St. Louis, MO: C. V. Mosby.

Curtin, L. L. (1979). The nurse as advocate: A philosophical foundation for nursing. *Advances in Nursing Science,* (April) *1*.

Deciding to forego life-sustaining treatment: A report on the ethical, medical and legal issues in treatment decisions. (1983). President's Commission for the Study of Ethical Problems in Medicine and Biomedical and Behavioral Research.

Fry, S. T. (1986). Moral values and ethical decisions in a constrained economic environment. *Nurs Econ,* (July–August).

Gortner, S. R. (1985). Ethical inquiry. In: *Annual review of nursing research.* Vol. 3. Werley, H., and Fitzpatrick, J. (editors). New York: Springer.

Hunt, R., and Arras, J. (1977). *Ethical issues in modern medicine.* Palo Alto, CA: Mayfield.

Ketefian, S. (1985). Professional and bureaucratic role conceptions and moral behavior among nurses. *Nursing Research, 34*(4): 248–253.

Mappes, T. A., and Zembaty, J. S. (1986). *Biomedical ethics.* 2nd ed. New York: McGraw-Hill.

Mayberry, M. A. (1986). Ethical decision making: A response of hospital nurses. *Nursing Administration Quarterly, 10*(3): 75–81.

Nelson, J. B. (1976). *Human medicine.* Minneapolis, MN: Augsburg Publishing.

Rossman-Jillings, C. (1985). Concepts relevant for critical care nursing: The knowledge-practice connection. *Critical Care Nurse, 5*:2.

Yarling, R. R., and McElmurry, B. J. (1986). The moral foundation of nursing. *Advances in Nursing Science, 8*(2): 63–73.

Managing the
Chemically Dependent Nurse

CHEMICAL DEPENDENCY IN nursing has recently begun to come to the attention of the profession (ANA, 1984). The number of nurses with a problem of chemical dependency is not known, but what is known is: (a) 67% of all cases handled by state boards of nursing are related to alcohol or drug abuse (National Council of State Boards of Nursing, 1980; Chesney & Sullivan, 1987); (b) nurses whose licenses are sanctioned represent only a small portion of those who are addicted to alcohol and/or drugs (Bissell & Haberman, 1984; Sullivan, 1987); (c) nurses' professional futures as well as their lives are put in jeopardy when they become addicted; and (d) little help, until recently, has been available to assist nurses with recovery. Further, identifying and assisting chemically dependent nurses to return to work has been found to be cost-effective (Sullivan, 1986).

The nurse manager is responsible for the care given to patients by nurses on the unit. When a nurse is addicted to alcohol or other drugs, professional functioning is impaired and, thus, patients are put at risk. The manager is the front-line representative of the hospital, communicating to patients, their families, and the public the institution's competency. Further, the manager is responsible for providing a safe working environment and for being responsive to staff problems. Few managers are prepared to handle the very difficult and sensitive situation of a staff member who has become addicted. When an impaired nurse has been working on a unit and has been absent or not working to capacity, other staff have usually been carrying a heavier work load and/or been working overtime to cover the absenteeism. Consequently, staff morale may have suffered. So, not only does the manager need to handle the nurse suffering from chemical dependency but also must help the staff deal with their feelings about the situation.

POLICIES AND PROCEDURES

The institution assists the nurse manager in many duties by designating policies and procedures to be followed in various circumstances. Institutions also have policies regarding the chemically dependent employee. Chemical dependency has been recognized as a disease by the American Medical Association for many years, but few hospitals, unfortunately, acknowledge that addiction is a disease in their employees and that sufferers of that disease should be treated as those with other illnesses. That is, the person is not blamed for contracting the illness but is expected to obtain treatment for it, is given a medical leave of absence to do so, and can return to work when treatment is completed. If the employee refuses treatment, the institution may discharge the employee if the person's performance is not satisfactory (which is usually the case), or if safe patient care is in jeopardy.

Most people use either a legal drug (e.g., alcohol) or a readily available illegal one (e.g., marijuana or cocaine). However, because nurses are familiar with prescription drugs, know how the drugs act, and have used them themselves, they often turn to these chemicals. It has been found that health care professionals usually begin use therapeutically, taking an analgesic for headache or back pain or sedatives for sleep. Infrequent use becomes regular use and, finally, addiction may set in. At this point, the addicted person takes drugs to maintain normalcy.

Some hospital policies deal with chemical dependency issues only from the standpoint of drugs used or stolen. Thus, they ignore the reality of chemical dependency as an illness and confuse the actions of a person who steals drugs to survive (death in withdrawal is not uncommon) with the person who steals hospital property for other reasons.

There are other reasons chemical dependency among nurses is troubling to institutions, the profession, practicing nurses, and the public. One is that nursing is a female-dominated service profession; that is, nurses are expected to put the needs of others before their own. They are the caretakers of others and often deny that they need caretaking.

Another is the tendency toward "pharmacological coping"—that is, the tendency to think that whatever is wrong can be fixed with some kind of medication. Nurses see patients improve, sleep, and get pain relief when they take medications. Over time, the not too subtle message is that drugs work wonders. Also, nursing is a high-tech profession today. That instrumental skill is valued more highly than affective ability is apparent from the high esteem that intensive care nurses command compared to nurses whose specialty is, for example, psychiatry. With such values placed on technical expertise, it is not surprising that medications (the products of technological development) are used to cope, and that dealing with emotional problems and stress in any other way is not considered.

Access to highly potent drugs makes their use even more likely than for others living in today's "chemical culture." While members of the general public can easily obtain alcohol and are only sanctioned for using it if they become intoxicated or drive, nurses who become addicted to controlled substances are violating the law.

Probably the most important reason why chemical dependency in nurses is so problematic is that nurses place great expectations on themselves and others. The "super-nurse" demands that one does anything and everything well. The terms *pedestal syndrome* and *angel of mercy* connote invincibility. Nurses expect their colleagues to know about drugs and, therefore, to not become addicted. That assumption is similar to expecting a person to learn about diabetes in order to avoid contracting the disease. Will power is assumed to control addiction. Nursing deals harshly with those who do become addicted. Very often they are discharged and, if reported to the state board of nursing, they often lose— maybe forever—their license to practice. Seldom have nurses known how to or been willing to help their employees and their colleagues get help.

Now, fortunately, that has been changing. In 1982, the ANA House of Delegates passed a resolution recognizing that chemical dependency is a disease and that nurses with the disease deserve treatment prior to losing either their jobs or their licenses. (A similar resolution failed two years previously.) Since that time, the ANA has appointed a task force to delineate the problem and to formulate some strategies for assistance. The result of their work is reported in a monograph (ANA, 1984).

The ANA board of directors has since appointed a permanent committee to continue monitoring implementation of assistance programs around the country. Today, nearly every state nurses' association either has an assistance program for nurses or is planning one. These programs operate, primarily, with volunteers, supplemented by state association staff. The use of volunteers, of course, limits the amount of work that can be done, but the effort is beginning.

In addition, some hospitals have initiated recovery programs of their own for nurses either through an employee assistance program (EAP) or a program designed especially for nurses. These programs have been found to be cost-effective in saving the institution the direct costs related to absenteeism, tardiness, overtime, and turnover, and the indirect costs related to quality of care, staff morale, incidents, and the chance of litigation (Sullivan, 1986). Thus, identifying and intervening with chemically dependent nurses becomes even more crucial in today's cost-conscious environment.

IDENTIFYING THE CHEMICALLY DEPENDENT NURSE

It is not easy to identify anyone as chemically dependent. The primary symptom of chemical dependency is denial, which is present in the sufferer as well as in those around him or her. In denial, the person *really* does not believe what seems obvious. Further, alcohol or drug problems in women in general, as well as in nurses, in particular, are a stigma in contemporary society. This stigma, added to the profession's own negativeness regarding the disease, encourages nurses—even those who break through their own denial—to continue to conceal their problem. The result is that chemically dependent nurses go on practicing, endangering both patients and their own lives. However, the nurse manager can be alert to signs and symptoms that may signal a possible problem for further investigation.

Signs and Symptoms

Prior to the development of obvious serious consequences, some general signs and symptoms may become evident as a nurse's chemical dependency progresses. Some of these signs and symptoms are:

1. Family history of alcoholism or drug abuse

2. History of frequent change of work site, in same or other institution

3. Prior medical history that required pain control

4. Conscientious worker, usually responsible and hard working, with recent slippage in performance quality

5. Increasing carelessness about personal appearance

6. Frequent complaints of marital and family problems

7. Reports of illness, minor accidents, and emergencies

8. Complaints from others about the person's alcohol/drug use or poor work performance and unexplained brief absences

9. Blackouts (memory losses while conscious)

10. Mood swings—depression or threats and/or attempts of suicide (sometimes thought to be accidental overdoses)

11. Strong interest in patients' pain control, the narcotics cabinet, and use of pain control medications

12. Frequent trips to the bathroom, often taking purse

13. Irritability or withdrawn from patients and colleagues

14. Increasing isolation from others—requesting night shifts, eating alone, avoiding socializing with staff

15. Elaborate excuses for behavior such as being late for work

16. Difficulty in meeting schedules and deadlines

17. Charting illogically or sloppily

18. Increasingly missing work with inadequate explanations (such as taking long lunch hours or sick leave after days off)

Physical signs may be present, such as:

1. Shakiness, tremors of hands, jittery

2. Slurred speech

3. Watery eyes, dilated or constricted pupils

4. Diaphoresis

5. Unsteady gait

6. Runny nose

7. Nausea, vomiting, diarrhea

8. Weight loss or gain

The *drug abusing* nurse may show other signs and symptoms. For example:

1. Rapid mood change from irritation to depression to euphoria

2. Wears long-sleeved clothing continuously, even in warm weather

3. Comes to work early or stays late, or comes in on days off; may request assignment that facilitates access to drugs

4. Waits until alone to open the narcotics cabinet and then disappears into the restroom immediately afterward

In addition to individual signs and symptoms, the nurse manager should be alert to the following signs and symptoms on the unit:

1. Narcotics counts are frequently incorrect.

2. Narcotics' vials appear altered.

3. Increasing number of patients report that pain medications are not effective.

4. Patient reports on pain medication differ from those on the records

(e.g., patient reports he takes pain medication only during the day, but the record shows nighttime administration as well).

5. Physician's orders, progress notes, and narcotic records indicate discrepancies.

6. Large amount of narcotics is wasted, or many corrections are noted on the records.

7. Patterns of narcotics discrepancies are erratic (these may be timed with the substance abusing nurse's work schedule).

8. There is a marked variation in quantity of drugs required on a unit by who is on duty for that particular shift.

If the manager discovers individual signs or symptoms or is aware of the unit changes suggested, he or she should investigate further. Often, with unit discrepancies, that simply means checking the schedule to see who was working when most of the errors occurred. Usually, one or two people emerge as those most likely to have been available during the time of the discrepancies. Further checking and observation may reveal individual behaviors suggesting a person has a chemical abuse problem.

Even if the manager is unsure of his or her perceptions, or if the actions are so vague that the manager has many doubts about the identity of the person, he or she can be certain that the situation will be clarified, nonetheless, in time. Untreated, addiction will continue and, as tolerance increases, the person is likely to increase use and become increasingly careless about covering up actions. Thus, the manager will become increasingly more certain about a person's abuse problem. However, the longer the time before identification, the longer time the nurse may be practicing with impaired professional functioning, jeopardizing both patients and himself or herself. Thus, it behooves the manager to carefully assess the information about possible dependency problems but to not wait too long. When this decision is made is a matter of judgment, and the manager and his or her supervisors are responsible for making it.

The manager's supervisor should be informed about the situation and should help the manager verify perceptions and clarify procedures. One note of caution: the supervisor may not be well informed about the disease of chemical dependency and may need education regarding symptoms and intervention. In that case, higher administration may be able to help. Regardless, the first-line manager should not attempt to handle such a case without at least informing a superior.

INTERVENING

Once the manager has identified a nurse with a chemical abuse problem, intervention with that nurse must be planned. With the assistance of a superior, the manager should examine the institution's policies and proce- dures and prepare for the intervention. Preparation should include col- lecting all documentation or information about the nurse's behavior that would lead one to believe that an abuse problem exists. This includes col- lecting records of absenteeism and tardiness (especially recent changes), records of patient complaints about ineffective medications or poor care, staff complaints about job performance, records of controlled substances, and physical signs and symptoms noticed at different times. Dates, times, and behaviors should be carefully noted. Any one behavior means very little; it is the composite pattern that identifies the problem.

Next, the manager should obtain appropriate resources to help the nurse. Internal resources include an employee assistance program (EAP) counselor (if the institution has one) or other nurses identified as recover- ing from chemical dependency who have offered to help. External re- sources include the names and phone numbers of treatment center staff and the names and phone numbers of other recovering nurses and/or indi- vidual contacts with Alcoholics Anonymous. It is absolutely essential that several sources be provided so the nurse is able to contact someone who knows how he or she feels and also knows that help is available and how to get it. **This support is so important that it cannot be emphasized enough.** Not having this assistance is like telling the diabetic he has diabetes and not telling him where he can get insulin.

In addition to assistance for the nurse, the manager should check on health insurance provisions for chemical dependency treatment. Many in- surance carriers have recognized that successful treatment reduces the use of other health care facilities and, thus, reduces the cost of health care. Accordingly, they offer coverage for chemical dependency treatment to encourage participants to enter recovery programs. Others, unfortu- nately, do not. Since many of an institution's employees may be covered under the same health care plan, the manager should check these provi- sions. If the policy does not cover inpatient care, the nurse may be able to afford outpatient care, which is considerably less expensive. So, the manager should not assume treatment is unavailable even when there is little or no coverage. Alcoholics Anonymous and Narcotics Anonymous are free, and many people recover with only these programs. However, for the nurse addicted to narcotics, some period of time, even a few days, is needed in a hospital to monitor withdrawal, and most policies do cover this.

Before initiating the intervention, the manager must examine his or her own attitudes about the abuse problem. Probably the chemical abuse has gone on for some time, and both the manager and the staff may have lost patience with the person, whose performance and attendance has forced others to do more than their fair share of the work on the unit. It has likely appeared as though the nurse were shirking duties, and if chemical abuse was suspected, others may have felt that he or she should just "pull himself or herself together," stop "doing it," and, as last resort, he or she should "know better." Once the disease process is understood, however, it is apparent that none of these behaviors are possible since will power and education have not prevented others from becoming addicted as well. The manager will need to deal with staff feelings later, but at this time it is enough to be certain that one's own attitudes will not imperil the intervention. It is important that the message be clearly one of help and hope.

The goal of the intervention is to get the nurse to an appropriate place for an evaluation of the possible problem. Treatment centers or therapists who specialize in chemical dependency are sources recommended for conducting the evaluation. They have the necessary experience for diagnosing and, if indicated, treating the disease.

The manager must also decide, beforehand, what action on the part of the nurse will be acceptable. If the nurse refuses to go for an evaluation, what will be the consequence? Termination? Discipline? Report to the state board of nursing? The institution's policies and the state board of nursing requirements must be met, but, beyond that, the manager must be clear about the consequences and willing to carry them out. Most experts in treating addictions in nurses recommend that the nurse be offered the option of chemical dependency evaluation and, if needed, treatment, and if he or she does not agree to that, then termination and a report to the state board of nursing should follow. Remember, the disease of chemical dependency kills its victims, and nurses care for very sick patients whose health and safety is in their hands. It is imperative that managers protect both.

Once preparations have been made, the intervention should be scheduled as soon as possible. Others may be asked to join the manager, but the group should be small and restricted to only those involved in past problems or to the manager's supervisor. In some institutions, the top nursing administrator conducts all interventions with chemically dependent nurses and, in that case, the nurse manager must fully inform the administrator of all circumstances leading to the intervention and provide all the documentation needed. Also, the manager should participate in the intervention so that all relevant information is presented and denial is kept to a minimum.

The intervention should be scheduled at a time and place when interruptions can be avoided. It is best to surprise the nurse with a request to come to the office. Denial can build, rationalizations can be developed, and defensiveness can increase when the nurse has time to consider the problem.

The manager should present the nurse with the collected evidence showing that a pattern of behaviors has emerged that suggests an abuse problem *might* be occurring and that an evaluation must be undertaken in order to know for sure. It is important to focus on the problem behaviors, not on the inadequacy of the person. He or she has already experienced shame and guilt about his or her use, and the manager has an opportunity to help the nurse regain some perspective by pointing out that chemical dependency is a disease. He or she is responsible for doing something about it once it is diagnosed; however, the nurse will be better able to accept that a problem exists.

Often, the nurse's response to an intervention is one of relief at finally being stopped. One nurse said, "Thank God it's over," and this sentiment is expressed often. In the best case scenario, the nurse admits the problem, is grateful to be getting help, and goes willingly to treatment. It is best to go directly to treatment from the worksite if this can be arranged beforehand. A family member or friend can bring a suitcase from home later. The important thing is to move quickly before denial resurfaces.

Other nurses, of course, will continue to deny the obvious, in which case the manager must continue to confront the nurse with the reality of the circumstances. If the nurse refuses to go for an evaluation, the manager must follow the disciplinary process for discharging him or her. If the nurse is using alcohol or drugs at the time, he or she must be removed from the patient care setting immediately. The manager should arrange to have someone (either a family member or another staff member) drive the nurse home whether the nurse is going to treatment or not. Not only do alcohol or drugs make the nurse an unsafe driver, but the stress of the intervention may distract the nurse even more.

If the nurse goes for an evaluation and/or treatment, specific plans must be made for this to occur. It should be clear to all parties (chemically dependent nurse, manager, supervisor) when the nurse will contact the treatment center (the sooner the better even if he or she is not using mood-altering chemicals at this time) and when he or she will report back to the manager the recommended course of action. It is possible to arrange with a treatment facility that reports be made directly to the manager, but federal regulations regarding confidentiality prohibit the staff from reporting a patient's status to anyone without that person's written consent. Since the goal of treatment is recovery, which includes returning to work, most facilities request that the nurse give this consent.

REENTRY

The nurse manager should be involved in planning for reentry to the workplace. It is especially important for the manager and higher administration to recognize the threat to recovery that access to one's drug of addiction poses. Not all treatment staff are familiar enough with nursing to be aware of the danger of putting the nurse in constant, daily contact with these drugs. However, it is vitally important to the nurse's recovery that he or she return to work, preferably in the same setting. This dilemma has often been dealt with in two ways. One method is to reassign the nurse for a period of time (possibly as long as two years) to a job or a unit where few mood-altering drugs are given. Some choices have been the nursery, department of education, rehabilitation, or patient care audits. Although reassignment presents a problem for the institution and is disappointing to the nurse, it is far better to make this accommodation than to jeopardize the nurse's recovery.

Another method is to retain the nurse on the unit but not allow him or her to administer mood-altering medications. This method requires that other staff not only know about the nurse's problem but that they be willing to give pain and sleep medications to that nurse's patients. Since this would require giving the staff an explanation and, thus, possibly disclosing the nurse's addiction, management and staff must decide if this is reasonable to accomplish.

These methods are usually necessary only for the nurse who was addicted to narcotics, but each case should be individually decided based on the amount of stress in the job, the need for rotating shifts, and other factors that may inhibit recovery.

Contingency Contracting

Hospitals with successful programs of assistance to chemically dependent nurses utilize some type of agreement with those nurses when they return to work. These agreements, often called contingency contracts, spell out the nurse's responsibilities regarding his or her recovery and what the institution will do if those responsibilities are not carried out. Such "return to work" contracts cover a period of time, usually one to two years, and include activities such as: attendance at self-help recovery groups (Alcoholics Anonymous, Narcotics Anonymous, recovery group for nurses); appointments with treatment staff for aftercare counseling; meetings with one's immediate supervisor regarding job performance criteria; meetings with an inhouse EAP counselor (if available); random urine screens for drugs and alcohol; and regular reports from the treatment facility to the nursing administrator. Figure 7–1 illustrates a typical "return to work" contract.

Monitoring

The returning nurse must be monitored during the period of recovery. Monitoring includes reporting on the behaviors spelled out in the contract, and often involves collecting random urine samples for drug screening. Although there is considerable controversy surrounding the issue of drug screening, most of the disagreements concern using the tests on the public without cause. For nurses recovering from chemical dependency, random urine screening is used for cause and because it is an objective measure of abstinence, it provides some assurance of continuing recovery.

Figure 7—1 Typical "Return to Work" Contract

_____ HOSPITAL

Employee Assistance Program

AGREEMENT BETWEEN EMPLOYEE AND _____ HOSPITAL*

I, _____, agree to the following conditions upon my continuing employment at _____ Hospital. These conditions will apply for a period of two years, beginning on _____ and ending on _____.

1. If it should be determined that I am using any mood-altering chemicals, (except under the direction of a physician who will keep the Employee Assistance Program informed as to reason and specific period of time), I will be immediately terminated and reported to the State Board of Nursing.

2. I agree to cooperate in any random urine check requested by _____ Hospital. The results will be sent to the Employee Assistance program. If at any time mood-altering substances are found, my employment will be terminated immediately and I will be reported to the State Board of Nursing.

3. I agree to follow the prescribed program of aftercare, including attendance in AA. I will be responsible for giving documentation of attendance to the Employee Assistance Program and if I do not comply, either in attendance and/or documentation, my employment will be terminated immediately and I will be reported to the State Board of Nursing.

4. If I should voluntarily terminate from _____ Hospital, I agree to keep the Employee Assistance Program informed as to my compliance with prescribed program of aftercare, my address and place of employment. I further agree to inform my new employer of my condition and request my new employer to keep the Employee Assistance Program at _____ Hospital informed of my progress. Unless other arrangements are made which are mutually agreeable to the new employer and the Employee Assistance Program at _____ Hospital, if the above conditions are not met I will be reported to the State Board of Nursing.

These four conditions have been read and agreed upon by:

_____   _____
(Employee Signature)   (Date)

In the presence of:

_____   _____
(Director of Nursing _____ Hospital)   (Date)

_____   _____
(EAP Coordinator _____ Hospital)   (Date)

*Courtesy of The Jewish Hospital of St. Louis

The nurse manager may be the person to collect the specimen. The nurse should be approached privately and asked to produce a specimen immediately. The manager should observe the nurse voiding into the container, if possible. Procedures for handling the specimen should be meticulously followed to avoid contaminating the specimen. Some hospitals have the report sent to the administrator, the manager, or to an EAP counselor. In any case, the manager should be informed if a positive report is received and plans made for deciding future action with the nurse. Sometimes an error is made (less than 5% of the time), but more often the nurse may have used alcohol or drugs on one occasion. The manager should handle this situation carefully, consulting with the nurse's counselor and deciding if this is probably a single incident or signals a return to chemical abuse.

The manager must also deal with the staff's concerns when the nurse returns, especially to the same unit where the abuse took place. As mentioned previously, staff members may be reluctant to accept the nurse because of past behavior, and the manager can help explain the disease and recovery processes. The returning nurse should be treated as anyone else with a chronic but treatable illness. He or she may have some limitations (not administer drugs) but otherwise be well and able to work.

If the staff was not aware of the nurse's problem, then the chemically dependent nurse, in consultation with the treatment counselor, should decide whether to share this information or not, especially if the nurse's drug of choice was alcohol. The nurse can simply say he or she was away on personal business and then share the experience with close friends, if with anyone. Unless others' jobs are affected, this decision is the nurse's.

Reporting to the State Board of Nursing

A report to the state board is not an accusation. It is simply a letter stating what has occurred and asking for an investigation. Any nurse who knows of another nurse who is practicing while impaired by alcohol or drugs is charged with reporting that person to the state board of nursing. However, a nurse is not required to report those nurses who are recovering and are not endangering patients, *except in a few states*. In the states with mandatory reporting laws, it is a violation of one's own license not to report a chemically dependent nurse, even when he or she is recovering. Hospitals with successful recovery programs, utilizing contingency contracts, and doing random urine screens to be reasonably certain the nurse is remaining abstinent usually do not report a nurse to the state board *unless the nurse violates the conditions of the contract*.

Managers, again, must follow state statutes and hospital policy regarding reporting but, either way, the nurse can continue to work until the state board rules on the case. In fact, a sustained work record is the best assurance of a favorable ruling from the board. The board is charged with protecting the public, and if they are assured that the nurse is continuing with recovery, they are more apt to agree to mild, if any, sanctions. This does vary, however, from state to state and, again, the manager must know the practice in his or her own state and must know how the law is interpreted by the board. This varies considerably between states.

Health care today requires that every employee function at peak efficiency and effectiveness. Health care cannot afford to protect an employee whose professional functioning is impaired by chemical abuse. Discharging the employee and allowing him or her to go to another institution to continue practicing and endangering patients as well as himself or herself cannot be allowed to continue. The nurse manager is the front-line contact with staff. He or she can be alerted to the signs and symptoms of chemical abuse problems, can learn intervention techniques and skills, and can help recovering nurses return to the workplace. The reader is referred to *Chemical Dependency in Nursing* (Sullivan, Bissell, & Williams, in press) for more information. Concern for patients' safety mandates intervention, and humane concern for nurse colleagues mandates that such assistance be made available.

SUMMARY

- Identifying, intervening, and returning chemically dependent nurses to practice helps the institution, the manager, and the affected nurse.

- Physical, behavioral, and environmental signs can alert the nurse manager to the presence of a chemically dependent nurse.

- The goal of intervention is to get assistance for the chemically dependent nurse and to return the nurse to practice.

- The nurse manager should consult experts in chemical dependency for assistance in conducting interventions.

- Contingency contracting is a method of monitoring the returning nurse's progress with recovery.

BIBLIOGRAPHY

American Nurses' Association (ANA). (1984). *Addictions and psychological dysfunction in nursing: The profession's response to the problem.* Kansas City, MO: American Nurses' Association.

Bissell, L., and Haberman, P. W. (1984). *Alcoholism in the professions.* New York: Oxford University Press.

Chesney, A., and Sullivan, E. J. (1987). *1985 survey of state boards of nursing: Violations and actions involving alcohol and drugs.* Manuscript submitted for publication.

National Council of State Boards of Nursing. (1980–1981). Preliminary sample of board actions. Unpublished data.

Sullivan, E. J. (1986). Cost savings of retaining chemically dependent nurses. *Nurs Econ*, 4(4): 179–182, 200.

Sullivan, E. J. (1987). A descriptive study of 139 chemically dependent nurses. *Archives of Psychiatric Nursing*, 1(3): 194–200.

Sullivan, E. J., Bissell, L., and Williams, E. (In press). *Chemical dependency in nursing: The deadly diversion*. Menlo Park, CA: Addison-Wesley.

3

KEY SKILLS IN NURSING MANAGEMENT

THE ABILITY TO communicate well is an essential skill for the nurse manager who must communicate with many individuals: patients, their families, individual employees, groups of staff, administrative personnel, medical staff, other health care workers, and the public. The nurse manager must also be able to express ideas and plans both orally and in writing and be able to listen attentively and accurately to others. Often, the institution's public relations depends on the quality of the manager's ability to communicate a positive image of the organization. This is no small task; the success of most management tasks depends upon this major set of skills.

By definition, managers work through others, and their ability to do so makes effective management possible. Nurse managers carry out the classic management functions of planning, controlling, organizing, and decision making, and also perform the modern functions of management, which include motivation, leadership, and the human resource management functions of selection, training, performance appraisal, coaching, discipline, and labor relations. Communication is the essential tool by which the nurse manager performs the other tasks that will be described in this book.

Learning communicative skills may be compared to learning a technical skill, such as aseptic technique. Once a nurse understands the principles of asepsis and can maintain a sterile field, she can learn any procedure that requires asepsis. But, lacking this understanding of the basic principles, he or she might perform any procedure requiring sterility in a way that could possibly be harmful to the patient. And so it is with communication skills. Once nurse managers understand the principles of communication and develop the ability to communicate well, they can learn how to plan, organize, and manage people.

In addition, the health care setting contains some unique characteristics that sometimes limit the nurse manager's effectiveness in communicating with others. For one thing, the organizational structure of a hospital differs from other institutions in that there are multiple power centers: physicians, administration, and nursing. For example, physicians hold a great deal of power and influence, although they are not employees of the institution. Residents, interns, and students from many disciplines participate in patient care decisions but are not permanent employees.

Second, nursing has a great deal of potential power but it is primarily a woman's profession; this can lead to very real difficulties. The traditional female role in society, particularly the nurse's role, has been one of subservience and of service to others. The nurse's orientation to service and the institution's expectation that the nurse is there to serve others do not establish an environment conducive to the sharing of authority. Also, women's roles in society have taught them patterns of communication that have enabled them to exert some control over their environment, but often in a manipulative and indirect way.

Management is a matter of controlling one's environment and the persons within it to achieve results in the unit. Nurses need to feel good about exerting this control; however, nurses have seldom learned these management skills; they concentrate on patient and peer communication with little thought to using communication as a tool for control.

Communication consists of both talking and listening. By developing effective communication skills, nurse managers are able to articulate their ideas in a manner that their listeners can understand. And, through careful listening, nurse managers learn to hear others' ideas accurately and can intervene appropriately in interactions with others.

THE NATURE OF COMMUNICATION

A message that is sent does not appear out of thin air. Many steps go into generating that message, as shown in Figure 8–1. Communication is a

Figure 8–1   Communication Model

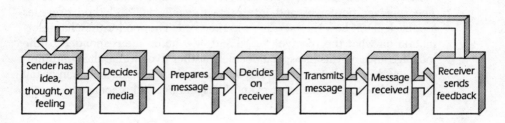

transaction between a sender and a receiver. However, the complexity involved in developing an idea, presenting it in oral or written form, sending it, and the receiving of that message produces many opportunities for distortion and interference. Many factors influence both the sender and receiver—among them, verbal and nonverbal expressions, past experiences, perceptions of each other, and meanings attributed to the other's message.

Coding the message is a primary source of possible distortion. The sender encodes the message, translating the meaning into words, expressions, and gestures, while the receiver decodes the message so that it has meaning for her or him. The processes of encoding and decoding are affected by multiple meanings of words and by expressions or nonverbal behaviors that may have very different meanings for sender and receiver. Often the meaning of a communication that is misinterpreted by the receiver can be as fraught with error as an incorrect translation of a foreign language.

Words have different meanings based on the roles of the sender and receiver. For instance, the words "let's go into the examining room" have an entirely different meaning to the participants when received by one nurse from another nurse who is escorting a patient, than when spoken by a nurse to a patient. In the first instance, the nurse sender could be requesting assistance with a procedure for the patient; in the latter instance, the patient receiver might expect that the nurse will perform a procedure that is best done in the examining room. The two emotional responses would be totally different, yet both receivers heard identical words.

COMMUNICATION AS PROCESS

Communication is far more complex than a message sent in a straight line between a sender and receiver. It is a *process* that involves give and take between the participants. Verbal and nonverbal messages are transmitted back and forth between sender and receiver. For example, an employee can be silent while a supervisor is explaining a new hospital policy; however, the employee may be communicating a response to the supervisor's message by body stance, facial expression, and eye contact (or lack of it). The receiver perceives and interprets the message and then provides feedback about how the message was received. The sender then has information on what the receiver heard and how he or she responded to the message and, on this basis, can decide whether to continue the communication and, if so, how to proceed. The following dialogue between a staff nurse and her nurse manager exemplifies a nonverbal response:

STAFF
NURSE: "Mary, can I see you?"

NURSE
MANAGER: (Nods affirmatively and frowns.)

STAFF
NURSE: "You look busy. I only need a few minutes. It can wait till after lunch."

NURSE
MANAGER: "OK."

Although the nurse manager nodded affirmatively and said nothing when she heard the staff nurse's request, she gave a nonverbal message that indicated she was unavailable to attend to the staff nurse's request. The staff nurse "heard" the nurse manager's nonverbal message accurately and responded to it appropriately, thereby gaining agreement with the nurse manager for a future appointment.

Many factors contribute to one's success, or lack of it, in communicating. The circumstances leading up to the communication, the setting, the relationship of the participants, their relative positions of power, timing, and external forces all play a part in the context in which communication occurs. Is the setting a restaurant, an office, or a patient's room? Are the participants colleagues, strangers, patients, or employees? Is one the boss, the physician, or the administrator? The key point is that where, when, and how communication occurs influences the outcome as much as words themselves.

CHANNELS OF COMMUNICATION

Messages are transmitted, received, and responses formed by both formal and informal channels. The formal channels are represented by the organizational chart shown in Figure 2–3, which depicts the relationships between various departments and supervisory personnel. The connecting lines represent the formal communication channel between them. For example, the director of nursing service communicates with the nursing supervisor for the fourth floor, and the supervisor communicates with the nurse manager who relates information to the staff. Or the director may communicate directly with the nurse manager.

Even when information passes through as few as four people, the opportunity for distortion and misunderstanding is great. Formal channels operate upward, downward, and horizontally, and a great deal of filtering of information occurs in that process. Kossen suggests that "filtering" of communication occurs as messages are transmitted from person to person. Filtering is the "straining out of ingredients in a message that are essential to a more complete understanding of its meaning" (Kossen, 1981). Due to the number of formal channels through which communication is transmitted and the large number of messages received, employees at all levels often selectively receive what they expect to hear and tune out much of the rest.

One way to understand how difficult it is for accurate communication to be disseminated through several people is to try this simple exercise.

1. Put 10 to 20 people in a circle.

2. Have one person tell a story to a second person (or read it) in a whisper.

3. Have the second person whisper the story to the next person and so on around the circle.

4. Have the last person say the story out loud; it is likely to be entirely different from the original!

Horizontal and lateral communication refers to communication between people on the same level and with comparable authority. Coordination of activities and planning are facilitated by effective communication among staff within a unit or between various units within an institution. Horizontal communication can be effective in cutting across the vertical lines of authority and in developing plans for a specific project or task without the often lengthy delay of acquiring approvals within each authority channel. However, this very process can also strain the relationships between those in authority and subordinates, depending on the norms of the institution and the expectations of the participants.

Marriner describes an additional channel within organizations—diagonal communication—which is similar to horizontal communication but refers to communication between units that are on different levels of the hierarchy, such as nursing service and housekeeping (Marriner, 1984). Additionally, diagonal communication is more often informal in nature while horizontal communication is formal. In addition to established organizational channels, information is also communicated to larger groups via conferences, memoranda, policy announcements, and procedure manuals. The nurse manager may participate in conferences and in preparing written materials for dissemination.

Informal communication, sometimes referred to as "the way things really get done," also moves vertically, horizontally, and diagonally. Informal communication is commonly known as the grapevine, deriving its name from the intelligence system used during the Civil War, which consisted of telegraph lines strung between trees like grapevines. Messages in a grapevine are often distorted. Reese and Brandt, in discussing communication channels in organizations, state that the grapevine satisfies several essential needs for people. First, it satisfies a basic need for social interaction; second, it fulfills an individual need for recognition; and, third, it can serve as a method of communicating or acquiring information that might not be available through any other channel (Reese & Brandt, 1981).

For example, the grapevine is one way for an employee to find out about events before they are announced officially. Thus, the staff nurse who has been waiting for an opening in the labor and delivery unit hears, via the grapevine, that a nurse on that unit is leaving, so she decides to approach the maternity floor supervisor to ask about a potential opening. She may enhance her possibility of getting the job by showing her interest in it. The manager must always be aware that the grapevine is operating when he or she talks with anyone. This is a way to use the grapevine to communicate informally with the organization.

COMMUNICATION MODES

Written Communication

Most people think of communication in terms of spoken interaction. However, written communication is also used to interact with others, and a combination of written and spoken communication is often used by the nurse manager in day-to-day management tasks. The nurse manager's skills must include the ability to receive oral or written information, decode that information, select information to give to appropriate people, and present that information in an effective way, written or oral, to the required person(s). Also, the nurse manager often must report back to a source the results of the activity. Generally, the nurse manager is responsible for the written work of staff members and must be able to assist them in expressing information clearly and accurately. For example, when a staff member fills out an incident report, the nurse manager must determine the accuracy and completeness of the report and communicate effectively with the staff member to ensure that the incident is reported with sufficient detail and clarity to be understood by others.

Although nurse managers may use informal modes of written communication, most written communication in management is formal. Formal written communication tasks include: (a) preparation of employee records and materials, job descriptions, performance appraisals, or anecdotal notes; (b) documentation of activity reports or justification reports; (c) a record of committee activities, including agenda and minutes; and (d) development of written policies and procedures for the unit or institution.

Memos are one way that the nurse manager communicates with others. Although the manager sometimes does this carelessly, he or she must remember that a memo is a written representation of the author to others, and the organization, clarity, style, tone, and content will be judged accordingly. Following are key behaviors to remember in writing memos:

1. Analyze the situation by determining the subject, the purpose, the form, the audience, and the voice.

2. Closely analyze the needs of the audience and the impact of possible types of voice.

3. Use this analysis to decide on the particular writing skills to be used, such as what words to use, what thoughts or sentences to write, what kinds of material to include or exclude, and how it should be organized.

4. Select words that are appropriate to the audience and are objective. Don't use "nursing jargon" when writing to nonnurses.

5. Use sentence tone to convey meaning: e.g., for a command, say directly what you expect without being overbearing or, conversely, don't ask if people want to do what you are asking such as, "No one will go to lunch before 11 am" (too harsh) or "Does anyone object to going to lunch after 11 am?" (too lenient) or "Lunch hours should be scheduled after 11 am" (just right).

6. Refer to yourself by title ("Sue Brown, RN") and include your position if writing outside your unit; refer to the audience by their titles, "nursing staff."

7. Arrange material logically by presenting the topic, purpose, what needs to be done, rationale, and time frame.

8. Include enough detail to inform but not too much to confuse or overwhelm.

Writing job descriptions and employee performance appraisals are difficult and disliked management tasks, yet are essential to maintaining high productivity on a nursing unit. Accurate and current job descriptions enable an institution to implement its purposes and ensure efficient use of human resources. Job descriptions delineate appropriate tasks to be performed that are congruent with the institution's needs. Accurate job descriptions make the job of performance appraisal easier by reducing the influence of personality factors and focusing the appraisal on the tasks performed and the quality of the performance. The face-to-face appraisal interview, a follow-up to the written appraisal, is usually more effective in specifying areas of strength and detailing needed improvement. But both written and oral communication skills are essential to carry out this task effectively.

The nurse manager utilizes anecdotal notes—"critical incidents," as they are frequently referred to—in assessing staff performance. The critical incident technique is an effective way to document events as they occur without a formal structure. They reduce both the incidence of "selective remembrance" and the influence of personal bias in appraisal. Skill in using accurate, clear language to report specific behavior is essential (see Chapter 15).

The nursing clinician who becomes a manager is familiar with the need for documentation, since a large part of her or his job in patient care is to document observations, patients' subjective reports, nursing actions, and patient responses to procedures, treatments, or medications. Nurses in practice for any length of time have most likely documented at least one incident involving a patient accident or medication error. Charting and nurses' notes are daily documentation activities. With the need to demonstrate nursing effectiveness in today's cost-conscious environment, accurate documentation can help to improve productivity and reduce risk (Deane, McElroy & Alden, 1986).

The nurse manager also has a frequent need to explain current unit conditions and future unit needs. This calls for written justification reports requesting specific resources and reporting data to justify the request. For instance, a nurse manager, in discussion with staff, may identify the need for some additional resource such as equipment, supplies, staff, or space and then develop a justification report requesting these resources. Included in the report is the background of the situation, rationale to explain the need, and specific details of how the resources will be utilized. Last, but not least, the benefit the needed resource will have for the institution is explained.

Oral reporting to a group or to specific administrators accompanies most written proposals. The value of the latter is that it provides a report that higher administration has for future reference; it also helps the nurse manager focus on specific points regarding the proposal. (More details on preparing a proposal to justify new equipment expense may be found in Chapter 19.)

Additionally, the nurse manager may be involved in developing a proposal to gain authorization for a major change or course of action. Such proposals are similar to justification reports except that the changes proposed are generally of a larger magnitude. They may involve several or all areas of the institution, and may have far-reaching and more complex consequences, both internally and externally. Essential to the development of a proposal is whether it is solicited or unsolicited, who the developers are, and their influence in effecting change within the institution. Most first-line managers participate with others in the preparation of proposals.

First-line managers are often responsible for writing or presenting activity or productivity reports. For example, the nurse manager may be required to prepare a monthly report of the activities carried out on her unit, accounting for the productive use of both human and material resources. An example of a monthly report of staff hours, expense, and the budgeted amounts is shown in Chapter 19.

The nurse manager must collect and report accurate information on the use of staff time, salaries, equipment, and supplies. Quantity, however, is not always an indication of quality. For instance, if the nurses' notes say, "A.M. care given," one can be fairly certain that the care was given but observations and patient responses are unknown.

Oral Communication

Another mode of communication is oral, which includes both verbal and nonverbal messages.

Verbal communication refers to the words that are used in interaction between two or more people. In nursing management, verbal communication is used to give and receive information, to report results, to give directions, to provide feedback, and to maintain continuity in the day-to-day tasks of managing a unit.

All nonspeech communication that transmits information about the message and the relationship of the communicants is nonverbal communication. It consists of four areas of nonspeech: (a) kinetics, or the body movements and gestures that accompany speech; (b) spatial relationships between communicants; (c) paralanguage, or nonlanguage verbalizations that affect speech, including pitch, tone, timing, pace, and voice; and (d) cultural attributes and appearance, including clothing, grooming, and hair style.

The nonverbal message comes through more powerfully and effectively when there is incongruence between what is actually said and the nonverbal message. Generally, the listener will believe the nonverbal message. For example, if you ask your supervisor, "Am I doing a good job?" and the reply is, "Yes," you will be more likely to listen to the manner of response than the *word* used. If the supervisor establishes eye contact with you and emphasizes the word "Yes," you are more likely to believe that your manager does indeed think you are doing a good job than if he or she appears distracted and walks away. In the latter instance, the nonverbal message is ambiguous and tends to leave the words open to interpretation by you. *This incongruence is the most significant difficulty in communicating effectively.*

Distorted communication occurs when the message the sender thinks he or she sent is misunderstood by the receiver. In this case, the receiver tends to respond according to his or her interpretation, and the original sender may receive distorted feedback. Consequently, the ability to prepare and present ideas, feelings, and thoughts accurately, and to respond to others' messages accurately reduces distortion in interpersonal transactions and fosters conditions conducive to problem solving and negotiation.

The nurse manager often must clarify the written words of others to staff—for instance, to explain a new hospital policy—by comprehending messages and decoding them in a manner, style, and choice of words that the audience understands. In other words, the nurse manager often acts as a conduit and a filter for communication between others and staff. The ability to assist both parties to understand and work with each other is probably the greatest asset the manager can possess. For this, the manager needs skill in both written and oral communication.

The cultural experiences of the participants control, to a great extent, the expression and understanding of messages. Since such elements as body movement, gestures, tone, and the human's response to spatial orientation are culturally defined, the participant can be expected to comprehend words within her or his own cultural context. A great deal of miscommunication is a result of the participants' lack of understanding of each other's cultural expectations.

The nurse manager must also consider the nonverbal aspects of communication in presentation of self and in others. Posture, dress (including such items as a nursing cap and a stethoscope in one's pocket), mannerisms, and gestures all contribute to the way others "hear" the manager's words in the context of nonverbal cues. Although people generally think they pay close attention to someone's words, the context and the nonverbal elements set the stage, and words have impact only as they relate to the setting. When there is incongruence between the verbal and nonverbal message, the listener will attend to the nonverbal. Therefore, the nurse manager must attend to the nonverbal behaviors of subordinates, peers, and superiors, and consider the total picture of words and their meaning within that context.

LISTENING

A central part of the ability to communicate is the ability to listen effectively. Although much has been written in recent years about active listening skills as they pertain to therapeutic skills with patients, little attention has been focused on the need for effective listening skills for nurse managers. The difficulty in receiving messages as the sender intended them lies in the fact that one must decode the message within one's own frame of reference. This includes both verbal and nonverbal elements as well as the listener's past experiences, attitudes, biases, and preconceptions regarding the sender.

In addition to the problems that most people have in listening effectively, the nurse manager has additional barriers to overcome. One of these is the complexity of her responsibility and the diversity of the nurse manager's relationships with staff and colleagues in daily interactions. Another barrier is the nursing setting with all the accompanying stimuli that often overload the nurse manager whose attention is being demanded by a number of people and in several places and situations simultaneously. This may create a lack of confidence on the part of others that the manager is really listening and responding to them.

Actually, to learn active listening skills requires paying more attention to another's message than to forming a response. The listener must pay attention to the words, expressions, gestures, and context of the message and check out with the speaker impressions of the message. Take the following example:

Ms. Jones, nurse manager, has received complaints about a staff nurse, Mary Smith. She approaches Mary and the following interaction takes place.

Ms. JONES: "Mary, could I see you?"

MARY: "Sure."

Both go to Ms. Jones's office and Ms. Jones gestures to Mary to be seated in a chair next to the desk. Ms. Jones takes a chair next to Mary.

MARY: "Is there something wrong?"

Ms. JONES: "Yes, Mary, I have received several complaints about your behavior toward the nursing assistants. They say you have been excessively critical of their patient care."

Mary scowls and looks away. She doesn't say anything. Ms. Jones allows a few minutes of silence.

Ms. JONES: "You look upset." (Reflecting Mary's expression and lack of response.)

MARY: (Nods affirmatively.)

Ms. JONES: "Do you want to talk about it?"

MARY: "There's nothing anyone can do. It's settled."

Ms. JONES: "Settled?" (Encouraging Mary to explain further.)

MARY: "Yes, you see, my husband's being transferred to California." (She starts to sob.)

Ms. JONES: "How do you feel about that?" (Eliciting the cause of Mary's distress and trying to confirm it.)

MARY: "I love my job here. Now I'll have to start all over with a new hospital, new people, new friends!"

Ms. JONES: "Oh, Mary, I'll hate to lose you but I know some hospital is going to get a very good nurse." (She pauses to let Mary realize she is appreciated.) "Mary."

MARY: "Yes?"

Ms. JONES: "Maybe you thought it would be easier to leave if you put some distance between you and the staff by being so critical?"

MARY: "Maybe. I didn't mean to be so cross with everyone."

MS. JONES: "Let me help you with your résumé and begin your letter of reference." (Showing Mary her actions will follow her words.)

In the preceding example, the nurse manager followed active listening principles. They are:

1. Find a place to talk with a minimum of distractions or interruptions.

2. Sit or stand so that you can look directly at the other person.

3. Listen to words but pay closest attention to nonverbal cues.

4. Ask questions to develop points further.

5. Be empathic—try to put yourself in the other's place.

6. Obtain feedback for your impressions of the other's thoughts or feelings.

7. Acknowledge positive contributions of the other.

8. Respond to the other's message and meaning.

9. Be patient.

Muller (1980) reported positive results when nursing service administrators used active listening techniques in meetings with hospital employees. They stated that increased feelings of being understood were reported by the staff when nursing administrators practiced active listening.

ASSERTIVENESS

Assertiveness is a term used to describe behaviors that a person can use to stand up for himself and his rights without violating the rights of others. Assertiveness training has become popular as women have become aware of their rights and have recognized that they can be assertive without being aggressive. It is especially appropriate for nurses and nurse managers to learn to assert themselves within a system that has encouraged nurses' subservience. In some cases, feminine role conditioning has been so powerful that female nurses who have achieved positions of power have gone to extreme lengths to conceal that power in order to conform to sex role appropriate behavior. In the health care field, women must not only learn to be assertive in general, but especially so in relation to hospital administrators and physicians, who are often very powerful men.

Melodie Chenevert (1985, p. 236) identified Ten Basic Rights for Women in the Health Professions. They are:

1. You have the right to be treated with respect.

2. You have the right to a reasonable work load.

3. You have the right to an equitable wage.

4. You have the right to determine your own priorities.

5. You have the right to ask for what you want.

6. You have the right to refuse without making excuses or feeling guilty.

7. You have the right to make mistakes and be responsible for them.

8. You have the right to give and receive information as a professional.

9. You have the right to act in the best interest of the patient.

10. You have the right to be human.

She states that nurses have these basic inalienable rights but that each individual is responsible for acquiring these rights for herself or himself; no one else is responsible for "giving" them to anyone else (Chenevert, 1985).

Assertive behavior is situation specific and can be differentiated from nonassertive and aggressive behavior in which participants respond in a certain manner regardless of the situation.

The results of using assertive techniques in communication can benefit the individual nurse manager, her or his staff, patients, and the institution. As the manager develops skill in clear, accurate, and honest expression of ideas and feelings, others are encouraged to respond in kind. Take the following example.

Ms. Jones, nurse manager, enters Mr. Wilson's room to find him scowling. He promptly states, "That stupid nurse forgot my medicine *again!*" Ms. Jones could respond in one of the following ways:

1. "There now, don't worry, I'm sure it will be all right."

2. "Oh, really! Well, I'll take care of her!"

3. "Tell me what you missed and I'll check on it."

If she uses the first response, she negates the patient's rights with a verbal pat on the head. She is responding nonassertively and accepting responsibility for her staff nurse's actions even without finding out the facts. With the second response, she assumes the staff nurse is to blame and plans to chastise the nurse. The third response indicates she has heard the patient and is going to take action in his behalf, but she has done this without taking the blame herself and without blaming others. She has accepted his emotional response without reacting to it.

Often people who learn assertive communication report a decrease in somatic symptoms such as headaches and abdominal distress. Since stress is known to contribute to a number of psychosomatic illnesses, it seems reasonable to assume that an honest expression of feelings would reduce a great deal of internal stress.

Another benefit that persons derive from the use of assertive techniques is that they become more likely to respond at the appropriate time. With nonassertive behavior, the person often attempts to avoid problems by remaining silent, although still angry; the aggressive person responds to the emotional aspect of the situation, thereby alienating others. But the assertive person responds in an appropriate manner to the specific situation and at the appropriate time. Participants may not agree with each other's responses, but they clarify what the other's position is and accept the other's right to differ.

Open, direct, and timely interactions between employees encourage problem identification and facilitate problem solving and decision making. Assertive communication techniques are valuable tools for the nurse manager to use in carrying out these tasks.

Assertiveness in any situation employs several rules that guide behavior (Smith, 1975). They are:

1. Avoid overapologizing.

2. Avoid defensive, adverse reactions such as aggression, temper tantrums, backbiting, revenge, slander, sarcasm, and threats.

3. Use body language that is appropriate to and matches the verbal message (e.g., eye contact, body posture, gestures, facial expression).

4. Accept manipulative criticism while maintaining responsibility for your decision.

5. Calmly repeat a (negative) reply without justifying it.

6. Be honest about feelings, needs, ideas. Use "I" statements.

7. Accept and/or acknowledge your faults calmly without apology.

DISTORTED COMMUNICATION

There is ample opportunity for distortion in the complicated process of sending, receiving, and responding to messages, as demonstrated by the following correspondence between a plumber and an official of the National Bureau of Standards (Donaldson & Scannell, 1979).

Bureau of Standards
Washington, D.C.
Gentlemen:

I have been in the plumbing business for over 11 years and have found that hydrochloric acid works real fine for cleaning drains. Could you tell me if it's harmless?

Sincerely,
Tom Brown, Plumber

Mr. Tom Brown, Plumber
Yourtown, U.S.A.
Dear Mr. Brown:

    The efficacy of hydrochloric acid is indisputable, but the chlorine residue is incompatible with metallic permanence!

                    Sincerely,
                    Bureau of Standards

Bureau of Standards
Washington, D.C.
Gentlemen:

    I have your letter of last week and am mightily glad you agree with me on the use of hydrochloric acid.

                    Sincerely,
                    Tom Brown, Plumber

Mr. Tom Brown, Plumber
Yourtown, U.S.A.
Dear Mr. Brown:

    We wish to inform you we have your letter of last week and advise that we cannot assume responsibility for the production of toxic and noxious residues with hydrochloric acid and further suggest you use an alternate procedure.

                    Sincerely,
                    Bureau of Standards

Bureau of Standards
Washington, D.C.
Gentlemen:

    I have your most recent letter and am happy to find you still agree with me.

                    Sincerely,
                    Tom Brown, Plumber

Mr. Tom Brown, Plumber
Yourtown, U.S.A.
Dear Mr. Brown:

    Don't use hydrochloric acid, it eats the hell out of pipes!

                    Sincerely,
                    Bureau of Standards

    For communication among more than two people, the chance of distortion increases proportionally.

    The source of the communication may be the origin of the distorted message. The sender may write or speak without adequate reasoning or use inadequate or very strong, judgmental words. She or he may be too fast or too slow, or the receiver may be busy or distracted. The sender may use words unfamiliar to the receiver or spend so much time on detail that the receiver misses the main point. Consider the following example of a sender's use of inadequate words at an inappropriate time.

    Supervisor (speaking to nurse manager): "Ms. Green, your unit's absenteeism is too high."

Ms. Green can interpret this message several ways: her staff is missing work more often than those on other units; the supervisor thinks the absentees are not really ill; or Ms. Green is doing something she should not, or not doing something she should, thereby causing her staff to call in sick.

Ms. Green responds by becoming defensive and thinking to herself, "I'd like to see her manage these people and take care of all our sick patients," or, "It isn't my fault people get sick."

If the supervisor offers her comment as she is passing through the unit on a busy day and if she does not sit down with Ms. Green to discuss possible underlying problems and how they can work together to solve them, the problems will remain and Ms. Green will now see her supervisor as an adversary. This will set the tone for their next interaction.

The sender may even distort the message based on his or her relationship with the receiver. In communicating with a supervisor, for instance, the sender is much more likely to report in a way that will minimize weaknesses and emphasize strengths and accomplishments. Given the previous interaction, Ms. Green may be reluctant to report future staff problems, especially if they might reflect negatively on her.

As discussed previously, the context of the interaction significantly determines its meaning and result. *Where, why,* and *how* an interaction occurs is as influential in the outcome as *what* was said. Since the sender is the initiator of the interaction, he or she is often responsible for selecting the time and place—two usually controllable aspects of the context.

The sender can reduce the amount of distortion in the message by choosing words that clearly express the intended meaning, by speaking in a manner that can be easily understood, and by selecting an appropriate time and place for the interaction. The sender cannot control many aspects of the situation but can try to minimize distortion.

The receiver has less control over the situation because he or she receives an already developed message and responds to it; consequently, the receiver has more opportunity for distorting the message. In fact, the receiver's attitude toward the sender and perception of the meaning of the message bias the message even before it is sent. The receiver is also influenced by past experiences with the sender and others. One hears it said, for instance, that a particular employee who cannot get along with a supervisor seems to "have a problem with authority figures," the connotation being that the person has displaced residual feelings toward someone in authority in the past, to the supervisor in the present situation. The receiver then selectively listens, with his or her biases and preconceptions acting as filters to allow in only the words that fit with predetermined expectations.

Douglass suggests that commonality of experiences influences the effectiveness of communication, and that the greater the number of common experiences, the more likelihood that the sender and receiver will effectively communicate with each other (Douglass, 1984). For instance, if the nurse manager has a life style similar to those of staff, they will be more likely to understand her or his words and actions accurately. In turn, the nurse manager will be more likely to present her ideas in a way that staff will understand.

Organizational determinants also influence the effectiveness of communication. For instance, status and role expectations are contextual aspects of transactions. Most nurses can remember the awe they felt as beginning students for the registered nurse in her all-white uniform, cap, a stethoscope around her neck and, of course, the very prestigious keys to the narcotics cabinet that she carried. (Since most nurses are female, most role models are female.) Soon the student learned how to imitate the nurse's behavior: carrying the stethoscope, the "right" type of pen, and the model's manner of walking and talking. Near graduation, the difference in uniform was often the only thing to distinguish between student and practicing nurse, so accomplished had the student become at "being a nurse." By that time the student had also moved from a subordinate to a collegial role. The interactions between the two had also changed, as they shared as colleagues and problem solvers together. Earlier, the student assumed the nurse "knew everything" and that she, the student, had little to offer. Consider how the communication between them had changed over that period of time.

In addition to status and role differences, the responsibilities of the participants impinge on their interaction. The nurse manager of a busy surgical unit on most weekday mornings has a hectic schedule, with several patients scheduled for surgery, preoperative medications to be administered, families and patients to be reassured, and postoperative cases from the previous day to be monitored. It is not the time for the supervisor to initiate a talk about staff nurses' absenteeism; the supervisor must consider the nurse manager's responsibilities and status. The nurse manager may think any request from his or her superior is an order and neglect patient care to attend to the supervisor's questions.

People translate or convert messages into their own language on the basis of their previous experiences and acquired knowledge. The limiting nature of experiential learning, however, creates the possibility of incomplete interpretation or erroneous translation of the message's meaning. It therefore behooves both sender and receiver to attend carefully to each other's responses, meanings, and interpretation, and to request and provide clarification and feedback frequently in transactions with others.

PRINCIPLES OF EFFECTIVE COMMUNICATION

In order to develop and increase her or his communicative skills, the nurse manager must understand the principles of effective communication. Many interfering influences have been discussed in this chapter, but these can be kept to the minimum if the manager is aware of and adheres to the following guidelines for specific interactions in management.

Principle one: Information giving is not communication. Communication requires that the participants share a mutual interaction, with the receiver providing feedback to the sender. Although much of management is giving directions and sharing information, the manager must remember that the receiver's response is necessary for communication to have taken place.

Principle two: Responsibility for clarity resides with the sender. Frustration with others' actions is built into the manager's job, and nursing management is no exception. However, this frustration can be reduced if the nurse manager makes messages to staff clear. Remember, the responsibility for communicating her or his ideas clearly is the manager's, not the staff person's. In advertising, if a new ad fails to increase sales, the fault is assumed to lie with the advertising agency, not with the customer. This assumption of responsibility of outcome belongs with the sender.

Principle three: Simple and exact language should be used. In both written and spoken communication, words used precisely and in the simplest terms possible will be more likely to be understood by the listener. This means selecting explicit words in terms of the listener's (not the sender's) experience, and it is the sender's responsibility to determine those words that will be most understandable to the listener.

Principle four: Feedback should be encouraged. The best way to be sure one's message has been accurately interpreted is to obtain feedback; lack of it is a common source of misunderstanding. Feedback has been defined as "the process of adjusting future actions based upon information about past performance" (Wang & Hawkins, 1980). Some information may be disturbing to the receiver. In this case, the feedback received may not be complimentary to the sender, or the ideas of the receiver may be in conflict with those of the sender. Nurse managers also must learn how to evaluate feedback, putting it into the total picture so that any disturbing aspect can be dealt with constructively. To respond effectively, they must learn to be skillful in encouraging feedback and in observing and evaluating verbal and nonverbal responses to their communications.

Principle five: The sender must have credibility. The personal and professional credibility of the information giver has been shown to be more important in effecting the desired outcome than the content (Costley, 1973). Being trustworthy, reliable, and competent are characteristics of a credible professional. Remember the rule, "Say what you mean and mean what you say."

Principle six: Acknowledgment of others is essential. The nurse manager may sometimes be reluctant to acknowledge the contributions of others because of fears of their responses; this is especially likely to be true if work is viewed as competitive. However, if the employment atmosphere is one of cooperation and individual contributions are viewed as complementary in nature, acknowledgment is encouraged.

Although it is easier to acknowledge staff members' contributions when their opinions match those of the manager, it is just as important, if not more so, to acknowledge those with opposing opinions. Fulton suggests that the sharing of opposing opinions can provide satisfaction for the participants if each explicitly acknowledges each other and if the entire truth is told by each (Fulton, 1981). Acknowledgment of opposing opinions is discussed in more detail in Chapter 22, *Dealing with Conflict.*

Principle seven: Direct channels of communication are best. Whenever possible, communicate directly with the individual for whom the message is intended. The more people through whom the message must be filtered, the more opportunity for distortion. Additionally, face-to-face communication is preferable to written and phone communication. Immediate feedback, both verbal and nonverbal, is obtained, thereby reducing the chances for misunderstanding, and enabling both participants to engage in facilitative dialogue to conclude the discussion and save time for the busy manager and staff member. You can also read the body language and facial expressions of the other person in a face-to-face discussion.

Adherence to all of the above principles can be expected to save time for the manager. In contrast, distorted communication and misunderstandings usually result in unproductive use of time, poor patient care, and frustration for both staff and managers. Settling problems after they have occurred takes more time than preventing them through clear and appropriate communication.

APPLICATIONS FOR THE NURSE MANAGER

Communication with Subordinates

Depending on the institution's policies, the nurse manager's responsibilities may include selecting, interviewing, counseling, and disciplining employees, handling their complaints, and settling conflicts. The principles of effective communication are especially pertinent in this relationship because good communication is the adhesive that builds and maintains an effective work group.

The communication channels utilized by the nurse manager may be downward, upward, or diagonal as demonstrated in Figure 8–2. Downward communication (between a manager and a subordinate) is often directive and includes specific instructions for the subordinate. This is an effective method to coordinate activities among personnel and to use resources of time and abilities effectively.

Figure 8–2 Communication Channels

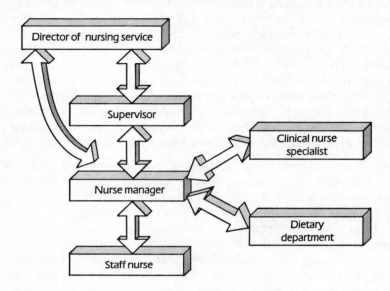

In order to give directions and achieve the desired results, however, the nurse manager needs to develop a "message strategy." The strategies suggested below should help to increase the chance of effective responses from others.

Know the context of the instruction. Be certain you know exactly what you want done, by whom, within what time frame, and what steps should be followed to do it. Be clear in your own mind what information a person needs to carry out your instruction, what the outcome will be if the instruction is carried out, and how that outcome can or will be evaluated. When you have thought through these questions, you are ready to give the proper instruction.

Get positive attention. Avoid the factors that can interfere with effective listening. Informing the receiver(s) that the instructions will be given is one simple way to try to get positive attention. Highlighting the background, justification, or the importance of the instructions may also be appropriate.

Give clear, concise instructions. Use a nonoffensive/nondefensive style and tone of voice. Be precise, but give all the information needed to carry out your expectations. Follow a step-by-step procedure if several actions need to be completed.

Secure verification through feedback. Make sure the receiver has understood your specific request for action. Ask for a repeat of the instruction.

Give follow-up communication. Understanding does not guarantee performance. Follow up to determine the outcome of your instruction, and give feedback to the receiver.

As stated earlier, direction giving is *not* communication. However, if the manager receives an appropriate response from the subordinate, communication has occurred.

The nurse manager has responsibility both for the quality of work life of individual employees and for quality of patient care of the entire unit. It is essential that a balance between these two sets of needs be pursued and that staff assignments be distributed equitably. If a few employees can influence the nurse manager to give them assignments of choice, patient care may suffer or some employees receive an unequal share of undesirable assignments.

To carry out this part of the job, the nurse manager can utilize the communication principles that have been discussed by acknowledging the needs of individual employees, especially if the needs conflict with needs of the unit; speaking directly with those involved; and by stating clearly and accurately the rationale for the decisions made. The staff may not agree with the manager's decision but will at least have heard the reasons for the decision and be more likely to comply with the decision.

Communication with Superiors

The manager's interaction with higher administration is comparable to the interaction of the manager and subordinate except that the manager is now the subordinate. Upward communication also is shown in Figure 8–2. The nurse manager must recognize that higher administration has responsibility for the consequences of decisions made for a larger area, such as all of nursing service or for the entire institution. However, the principles used in communicating with subordinates are equally appropriate in this situation. Managers must state their needs clearly, explain the rationale for requests, suggest benefits to the larger unit, and utilize the appropriate channels. They must also be prepared to listen objectively to the response of their supervisors and be willing to consider reasons for possible conflict with needs of other areas. This is, of course, a description of an ideal communication between nurse manager and supervisor, with both participants practicing good communication skills. The manager can serve as role model to both subordinates and supervisors by consistent and daily use of appropriate communication skills.

Communication with Medical Staff

Communication with the medical staff is often difficult for the nurse manager because of the nature of the physician/nurse relationship: (a) the medical staff, although not employees, have enormous power in the health care setting; (b) the historical relationship of physicians and nurses is that of superior and subordinate; and (c) there is a gender disparity within both professions with a great preponderance of male physicians and female nurses.

In addition, the medical staff is in itself diverse. The medical staff may consist of physician employees, interns, residents, physicians in private practice, and consulting physicians. Some physicians, such as pathologists, radiologists, and anesthesiologists, work on a contractual basis. Obviously, the principles of effective communication are very important in interactions with the medical staff. For more on the nurse manager's role in working with physicians, see Chapter 24.

Communication with Other Health Care Personnel

The nurse manager has the overwhelming task of coordinating the activities of a number of personnel with varied levels and types of preparation and different kinds of tasks. In addition, the manager is responsible for the care given to each patient on her unit. However, patients also receive care from personnel assigned to other units of the hospital. For instance, one patient may receive nursing care from a registered nurse who also directs care given by a nursing assistant. This patient may also receive regular care from a respiratory therapist, a physical therapist, and a dietitian.

The nurse manager must utilize considerable interactional skill in communicating with personnel and managers in other departments; in this situation the communication moves in a horizontal or diagonal direction (see Figure 8–2), depending upon whether the nurse manager is communicating with managers of other departments (at the same level on the hierarchy as the nurse manager) or directly with staff in other departments. As previously discussed, horizontal communication usually follows formal channels while diagonal communication is more often informal.

In interacting with persons from other departments, the nurse manager must recognize and respond to the differences between the goals of their departments and her or his nursing unit. This recognition can help the nurse manager to search for commonality of purpose.

Communication in Groups

The development of groups is an inevitable part of human activity. People join groups for a variety of reasons: as a way to fulfill affiliative needs (e.g., security, belonging, companionship), as a source of information, as a source of rewards, and as a means for accomplishing a goal. Individuals in groups behave in ways that are systematically different from behavior of individuals not in a group setting. The nurse manager can do a great deal to facilitate the individual benefits of group membership. For example, through planning work and making assignments, she can increase the interdependence of group members upon one another. She can foster the sharing of common interests and exert considerable control over rewards and punishments for the attainment or nonattainment of work goals. These functions of group membership for individuals operate regardless of whether or not there is a formal leader, but the nurse manager can do a great deal to foster effective individual and group performance by exercising constructive influence on these functions through her leadership behavior. Indeed, this is one of her primary roles in a nursing organization.

The nurse manager also acts as an observer of the direction in which the group is moving. She brings the attention of the staff members to the goal, clarifies issues in terms of how they relate to the unit's goals, and evaluates the group's progress toward its goals periodically. This evaluation and the subsequent planning and execution of group goals frequently includes the assistance of staff members.

All of this occurs within a context that is usually referred to as "group dynamics." Behavioral scientists have known for a long time that group interaction and group output are different from what is produced by individuals working alone. For one thing, group members are aroused by the presence of others. Frequently, this increased arousal is trans formed into increased motivation, especially when the individual's contribution to the task is fairly clear or easily measured. In addition, groups tend to make more risky decisions than individuals, i.e., work groups are more likely to go on record as supporting unusual or unpopular positions than are individuals. They tend to be less conservative than individual decision makers and frequently display more courage and support for unusual or creative solutions to problems.

Despite frequent intentions that all group members are equal, in fact some people have more influence on group processes and group decisions than do others. Inevitably, groups affect the nature and process of communication and engender a degree of competition and political activity much greater than might be expected by examining individual behavior alone. In short, groups are greater than the sum of their parts; they can bring out the best and the worst in individuals.

Clearly, however, groups are different from individuals. Influencing group processes toward the attainment of organizational objectives is the direct responsibility of the nurse manager. A viable group atmosphere is one in which staff members feel free to talk about what concerns them, feel free to critique and offer suggestions, and feel free to experiment with new behaviors without threat. For more on group communication, see Chapter 10 on leadership skills.

Communication in Public Relations

The nurse manager is a visible sign of the institution's image. His or her appearance, manner of speaking with groups as well as with individuals, and his or her nonverbal communication (body movements, tone, timing, pace, voice, and pitch) convey powerful messages about the ability of the institution to provide competent and professional care. In today's competitive health care environment, it is critical that every message about the institution be professional. Obviously, it also must depict an accurate image of the institution.

SUMMARY

- Effective communication skills are essential tools for the nurse manager to use in the task of managing her unit. These skills, like many others, can be learned.

- Communication is an interactive process that occurs between a sender and a receiver. It includes oral, verbal and nonverbal communication, and written communication.

- Communication channels operate as both direct (formal) and indirect (informal) lines in an organization.

- Nurses have only recently become aware of their need to express their ideas, opinions, and desires without violating others' rights. Assertive communication training provides the necessary skills.

- Distorted communication occurs because the communication process is complicated and is affected by extraneous variables. Understanding the source of some of these variables can help reduce distortion in the message sent and received.

- Principles of effective communication include accepting responsibility for sending a clear message, using exact language, and encouraging feedback.

- Communication between the nurse manager and subordinates, superiors, and physicians revolves around their mutual tasks.

- The nurse manager conveys the institution's image of competency and professionalism to the public.

BIBLIOGRAPHY

Blondis, M. N., and Jackson, B. E. (1982). *Nonverbal communication with patients.* New York: Wiley.

Bloom, L. Z., Coburn, K., and Pearlman, J. (1975). *The new assertive woman.* New York: Dell.

Butler, P. (1976). *Self assertion for women.* New York: Harper & Row.

Camuñas, C. (1986). Using public relations to market nursing service. *J Nurs Adm, 16*(10): 26–30.

Chenevert, M. (1985). *Pro-nurse handbook.* St. Louis: C. V. Mosby.

Chenevert, M. (1983). *Special techniques in assertiveness training for women in the health professions*. 2nd ed. St. Louis: C. V. Mosby.

Costley, D. L. (1973). Basis for effective communication. *Superv Nurs*, (January).

Deane, D., McElroy, M. J., and Alden, S. (1986). Documentation: Meeting requirements while maximizing productivity. *Nurs Econ*, 4(4): 174–178.

Donaldson, L., and Scannell, E. E. (1979). *Human response development: The new trainer's guide*. Reading, MA: Addison-Wesley, pp. 47–48.

Douglass, L. M. (1984). *The effective nurse*. 2nd ed. St. Louis: C. V. Mosby.

Edwards, B. J., and Brilhart, J. K. (1981). *Communication in nursing practice*. St. Louis: C. V. Mosby.

Fulton, K. (1981). Acknowledgment supports effective communication. *Superv Nurs*, (March).

Jacobs, B. C., and Rosenthal, T. T. (1984). Managing effective meetings. *Nurs Econ*, 2(2): 137–141.

Kossen, S. (1981). *Supervision: A practical guide to first line management*. New York: Harper & Row, p. 25.

Kreps, G. L., and Thompson, B. C. (1984). *Health communications: theory and practice*. New York: Longman Publications.

Marriner, A. (1984). *Guide to nursing management*. 2nd ed. St. Louis: C. V. Mosby.

Muller, P. A. (1980). Using an active listening model. *Superv Nurs*, (April).

Reese, B. L., and Brandt, R. (1981). *Effective human relations in business*. Boston: Houghton Mifflin.

Smith, M. J. (1975). *When I say no, I feel guilty*. New York: Bantam Books.

Wang, R. Y., and Hawkins, J. W. (1980). Interpersonal feedback for nursing supervisors. *Superv Nurs*, (January).

Motivating
Staff

THE TERM *motivation* comes from the Latin word *movere*, which means
"to move." All human behavior is motivated by something; very few behaviors in normal human beings are completely random. Some behaviors
are instinctive (genetically caused), but most human behavior is goal directed. People do things for some reason, to get a certain result. The reasons may not always be logical or rational, but they do tend to be systematic or predictable. It is this latter characteristic of human behavior that
makes the study of motivation possible and even utilitarian, particularly
from an organizational point of view. While the concepts discussed in this
chapter are relevant to human behavior in general, the chapter will focus
on motivational problems frequently encountered by nurse managers in
motivating staff members.

WHY MOTIVATE PEOPLE?

Motivation is unquestionably important in a hospital setting. Hospitals, like any other organization, require people to function effectively if they are to provide adequate patient care. This implies, first, that a hospital must motivate qualified personnel to seek employment in the institution and, then, motivate them to remain on the job. Continual turnover means wasted training costs, inconvenience, and disruption of staff functions, as well as continual recruiting. (Recruitment, selection, and retention of staff are dealt with in Chapters 13 and 16.) Once the employees are on the job, it is the nurse manager's responsibility to motivate them to produce both quantity and quality of work.

Beyond this, an understanding of motivational processes is essential for a fuller understanding of the effects of such other factors as leadership, job design, and incentives (e.g., salary) systems as they relate to employee performance and satisfaction. Indeed, most other techniques and programs are designed primarily to influence motivation—that is, individual and group performance. The question for the nurse manager is how to utilize these tools most effectively to motivate effective nursing performance.

WHAT MOTIVATES PEOPLE?

All motivational theories have the same three characteristics: they are concerned with what mobilizes or energizes human behavior; they are concerned with what directs behavior toward the accomplishment of some objective; and they suggest how such behavior is sustained over time. In various ways, all of the motivational theories to be considered here attempt to address these issues. The relative success or failure of any of these perspectives on motivation depends upon its ability to explain motivation adequately, to predict with some degree of accuracy what people will actually do, and, finally, to suggest practical ways of influencing people to accomplish organizational objectives.

There are some distinct differences among motivational theories, however, which allow them to be classified into at least two different groups—content theories and process theories—in terms of practical application. In general, *content* theories emphasize individual needs or the rewards that may satisfy those needs, whereas *process* theories emphasize *how* the motivation process works to direct an individual's effort into performance.

CONTENT THEORIES OF MOTIVATION

Instinct Theories

Content theories have generally taken two different forms: instinct theories and need theories. Instinct theories are much older, dating from the 1890s. While some theorists saw instincts as purposive and goal directed, other instinct theorists defined the concept more in terms of blind, mechanical action. However, all of them characterized instincts as inherited or innate tendencies that predispose individuals to behave in certain ways. One version of the instinct theories dates from Sigmund Freud, who noted that individuals are not always consciously aware of their desires and needs. Thus, Freud tended to focus on the notion of unconscious motivation (Freud, 1949).

In the early 1920s, however, instinct theories came under increasing attack on several grounds. First, the list of instincts by this time had grown to well over 6,000, making it very difficult to pinpoint the specific motivation for a given behavior in terms of one or some combination of instincts. Second, while every individual was assumed to have a complete set of instincts, researchers became increasingly aware that these instincts varied in strength across individuals. In addition, the relative strength of various instincts did not seem to be strongly related to subsequent behavior. Finally, some psychologists began to question whether Freud's unconscious motives were really instinctive or were, in fact, learned behaviors.

This latter criticism led, in part, to the development of a second class of content theories focusing on the concept of learned needs. While there are many need theories, the most popular are those of Abraham Maslow, Clayton Alderfer, and Frederick Herzberg.

Need Hierarchy Theory

Maslow attempted to bring a greater degree of order to the concept of needs by restricting the list to five needs and organizing them into a hierarchy of prepotency. That is, the needs identified by Maslow were assumed to operate in a particular order, the lower level needs being prepotent for controlling behaviors until those needs were satisfied and then the next higher need becoming responsible for energizing and directing behavior. The hierarchy, from lowest to highest level, is as follows: (a) physiological needs (e.g., hunger, thirst), (b) safety needs (e.g., bodily safety), (c) belongingness or social needs (e.g., friendship, affection, love), (d) esteem needs (e.g., recognition, appreciation, self-respect), and (e) self-actualization (e.g., developing one's whole potential) (Maslow, 1943; Maslow, 1954).

Maslow's need theory is frequently used in nursing to provide an understanding of human behavior. That is, a patient's needs are viewed in this hierarchical order, with nursing care directed toward meeting the lower level needs before higher ones. Although Maslow's theory provides an explanation of human needs, it is less useful in management, where predicting behavior and directing appropriate change is the focus.

Existence–Relatedness–Growth Theory

Alderfer has suggested three, rather than five, need levels: (a) existence needs (including both physiological and safety needs), (b) relatedness needs (Maslow's belongingness and social needs), and (c) growth needs (including the needs for self-esteem and self-actualization). Alderfer's ERG (Existence–Relatedness–Growth) theory is similar to Maslow's in assuming that the satisfaction of needs on one level activates the next higher level need. Alderfer suggests, however, that frustrated higher level needs cause a regression to and reemphasis upon the next lower level need in the hierarchy (Alderfer, 1969, 1972).

Alderfer's model, however, suggests that more than one need may be operative at any point in time. Thus, it is somewhat less rigid than Maslow's hierarchy. In essence, Alderfer presents nothing really new or substantially different from Maslow, and the criticisms of Maslow's theory in management are essentially applicable to Alderfer's modified need hierarchy theory as well.

Two-Factor Theory

Herzberg's two-factor theory explains motivation as identical to job satisfaction (Herzberg, 1966; Herzberg, Mausner & Snyderman, 1959). Herzberg states that job satisfaction and job dissatisfaction are not opposite ends of the same continuum; rather, they are two different continua. The factors that lead to no job satisfaction are quite different from those that lead to no job *dis*satisfaction, and the resulting behaviors from these two states are also quite different.

Herzberg regards job dissatisfiers as, essentially, the lack of such extrinsic factors as satisfactory pay, adequate technical supervision, enlightened company policies and administration, good working conditions, and job security. Herzberg suggests that employees need the presence of most, if not all, of these extrinsic factors in order not to experience job dissatisfaction. Dissatisfied employees are more likely to be absent, file grievances, or quit the job.

The presence of these factors, however, will not necessarily create job satisfaction or motivation. Rather, satisfaction and motivation result from such intrinsic on-the-job factors as a sense of achievement for performing a task successfully, recognition and praise, responsibility for one's own or another's work, and advancement or changing status through promotion. To the extent that these intrinsic factors are present, an employee is assumed to experience job satisfaction and hence will be highly motivated to perform the job effectively.

Herzberg's results, however, appear to be quite specific to the research methodology that he used. That is, other researchers have found little or no relationship between satisfaction and motivation. Thus, while Herzberg's hygiene factors (generally lower order needs) and satisfiers (generally higher order needs) have enjoyed a popularity among managers second only to Maslow's need hierarchy, the weight of research evidence indicates that it, too, is inadequate for conceptualizing motivation in the work setting.

PROCESS THEORIES OF MOTIVATION

For all their popularity, the content theories only explain why a person behaves in a particular way. In contrast to the content theories, process theories do much more than just *explain* behavior; they assist in *understanding* behavior. Understanding results in a manager's ability to predict what an employee will do on the job. Prediction, of course, implies being able to control or influence employee behavior.

Reinforcement Theory

One process approach to motivation is reinforcement theory, which views motivation as a learning process (Skinner, 1953). According to this theory, behavior is learned through a process called *operant conditioning*, in which a behavior becomes associated with a particular consequence. In operant conditioning, the response–consequence connection is strengthened over time—that is, learned. The behavior is called an "operant behavior" because the individual is seen as operating on his or her environment in order to obtain a desired consequence.

Thus, to produce a desired behavior with operant conditioning, one must be able to control or manipulate the consequences of behavior. Consider, for example, a nursing student who correctly administers an intramuscular injection. The patient remarks that "it didn't hurt at all," and the instructor says, "Well done!" In this instance, the praise of both patient and instructor are desired consequences that occur only when the behavior (giving the injection) is properly performed. Each time this behavior–consequence sequence occurs, the behavior is strengthened or better learned.

The focus on desirable consequences (e.g., praise, money, favored task assignments), refers to *positive reinforcement*. A positive reinforcer is a stimulus that when added to a situation, strengthens the likelihood of an operant response. Thus, behavior that leads to positive consequences tends to be repeated, while behavior that leads to negative consequences

Figure 9–1   Types of Reinforcement

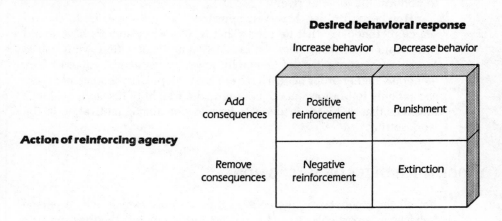

tends not to be repeated. Obviously, both processes are important in an organization. There are times when we wish to have employees do things that they are not currently doing and there are also times when we wish employees would not do things that inhibit effective performance.

Reinforcement increases the frequency or magnitude of a behavior. This is shown in the left column of Figure 9–1, which indicates that the frequency or magnitude of a behavior may be increased by either positive or negative reinforcement. In the former, some positive consequence or reinforcer (e.g., praise) is applied for the express purpose of increasing a desired behavior. However, behavior may also be increased by removing something from the environment, as shown in the lower left quadrant of Figure 9–1. This is known as *negative reinforcement* and is sometimes called escape or avoidance learning. If the individual's performance can terminate the noxious stimulus, it is called escape learning. When behavior can prevent the onset of a noxious stimulus, the procedure is called avoidance learning. Both are types of negative reinforcement.

A simple example should make the difference between positive and negative reinforcement quite clear. For example, a staff nurse does a complete job of charting, which is reinforced by the nurse manager with praise. This is positive reinforcement. In contrast, negative reinforcement might occur when a staff member stops engaging in an undesirable behavior in order to avoid a reprimand. For example, a nurse who has been tardy repeatedly arrives for work on time and, therefore, is not reprimanded for tardiness. In this case, the staff member has engaged in avoidance learning by increasing effective or desirable performance.

As shown in the right column in Figure 9–1, there are different ways to decrease the frequency or magnitude of a behavior as well. In the second example, the nurse manager wishes to stop a behavior—i.e., lateness—that is incompatible with effective job performance. When a nurse manager applies pressure to reduce the occurrence of a behavior, the procedure is known as *punishment*. However, when a reinforcer is simply removed from a situation in order to reduce the occurrence of a given behavior, the procedure is known as *extinction*. Punishment is an active response, while ignoring the behavior is a passive response.

Nurse managers should emphasize positive reinforcement, since repeated studies have demonstrated that this is the best way to change behavior. This is not to say that other reinforcement procedures are inappropriate. To be sure, punishment, especially if severe enough, will produce an immediate and drastic change in behavior, which is why it is used so much. However, research has shown that the cessation of undesirable behavior in the face of punishment is generally not permanent. The undesirable behavior will be suppressed only as long as the reinforcing agent is monitoring the situation and the threat of punishment is present. Punishment is negative in character and may lead an employee not only to avoid exhibiting a given behavior but to avoid the reinforcing agent and the job as well. In short, reliance upon punishment as a primary means of changing behavior is likely to result in lower job satisfaction, greater absenteeism, and, eventually, greater turnover without necessarily producing better performance.

Extinction means that there is no consequence at all for a behavior. With extinction, the behavior will eventually cease. This is a relatively inefficient way to go about changing employee behavior because it may take a long time. The best combination of reinforcing actions is to ignore (i.e., extinguish) the undesired behavior *and* simultaneously to positively reinforce the appropriate behavior when it occurs. For example, ignore lateness and praise punctuality. This is much easier for the employee to understand and much more effective from a managerial point of view. After all, only rarely do we want individuals to do nothing; rather, we want them to do something different. That something must be appropriate and constructive in terms of job performance.

The problem with operant conditioning in the minds of many managers is that there is no sure way to elicit the desired behavior so that it can be reinforced. That is, the manager must wait for the employee to perform in the desired manner before a positive reinforcer (consequence) can be administered. However, one can simply *tell* employees what they should be doing and what they should not be doing. In most cases, this should be sufficient to elicit the desired behavior, which then should be positively reinforced.

Sometimes, however, this procedure is simply not sufficient. For example, consider the case of Mrs. Armstrong, a nursing assistant, who never came to work less than 20 minutes late. Her uniform was always wrinkled and sometimes soiled, her personal hygiene left something to be desired, and her general attitude was quite unpleasant. The nurse manager decided that a procedure called *shaping* would be the most appropriate remedy. Shaping involves selectively reinforcing behaviors that are successively closer approximations to the desired behavior. For Mrs. Armstrong, it was not a matter of not knowing what to do; she had been reprimanded and counseled innumerable times on appropriate job behavior. Her problem did not appear to be lack of knowledge, but a simple lack of motivation.

The nurse manager, Ms. Ernest, tried for a week to find a single, positive behavior to reinforce. The following week, she found occasion to praise Mrs. Armstrong several times. One day, for example, Mrs. Armstrong came to work only ten minutes late, and her relative punctuality was promptly reinforced by the nurse manager. Similarly, she seemed to have made at least an attempt to comb her hair, so she was positively reinforced for its improved appearance. On every occasion, however, the nurse manager was met with a grunt and an occasional icy glare from Mrs. Armstrong, who continued about her own business. After a few weeks, however, she seemed to respond more favorably to the praise and increased interest (rewards) of the nurse manager. Her comb appeared to have wandered through her hair at least twice on most days and, while wrinkled, her uniform was relatively clean.

Within a period of approximately two months, Mrs. Armstrong's performance, although not perfect, was substantially improved and she had ceased to be an embarrassment to her colleagues and the hospital. Moreover, her disposition had improved and she had actually begun to develop some friendships with other members of the staff. Her appearance and hygiene were, for the most part, quite acceptable, although her punctuality had improved only slightly. While she was clearly no superstar, she had come to be regarded as a valuable and necessary member of the staff.

The main point of this actual story is that behavior modification via the principles of positive reinforcement may take some time, especially when shaping procedures must be implemented. That is, each successively closer approximation to the desired behavior was reinforced and well established before progressively reinforcing only closer approximations to the desired behavior. When people become clearly aware that rewards are contingent upon a specific behavior, their behavior will change eventually.

Behavior modification works quite well provided: (a) rewards can be found that, in fact, are seen as positive reinforcers by employees; and (b) such rewards can be controlled or made contingent upon performance by supervisory personnel.

This does not mean that all rewards work equally well or that the same rewards will continue to function effectively over a long time. Were a nursing manager to praise someone four or five times a day every day, the praise would soon begin to wear thin; that is, it would cease to be a positive reinforcer. Care must be taken not to overdo a good thing. For this

Figure 9–2   Effects of Different Reinforcement Schedules

Arrangement of reinforcement contingencies	Schedules of reinforcement contingencies	Effect on behavior when applied	Effect on behavior when removed
	Continuous reinforcement	Fastest method to establish a new behavior	Fastest method to extinguish a new behavior
	Partial reinforcement	Slowest method to establish a new behavior	Slowest method to extinguish a new behavior
	Variable partial reinforcement	More consistent response frequencies	Slower extinction rate
	Fixed partial reinforcement	Less consistent response frequencies	Faster extinction rate
Positive reinforcement Avoidance reinforcement		Increased frequency over preconditioning level	Return to preconditioning level
Punishment Extinction		Decreased frequency over preconditioning level	Return to preconditioning level

Adapted from Behling, O., Schreisheim, C., & Tolliver, J. Present theories and new directions in theories of work effort. *Journal Supplement Abstract Service* of the American Psychological Corporation. In Steers, R. M. & Porter, L. W. (1979) *Motivation and Work Behavior.* New York: McGraw-Hill.

reason, a *continuous schedule* of reinforcement—that is, reinforcement every time a desired behavior occurs—may result in the reinforcer losing its effectiveness over time (see Figure 9–2).

Partial schedules of reinforcement, however—reinforcing the behavior upon every second or third occurrence—may be quite helpful. This is known as a *fixed ratio schedule* of reinforcement. However, this requires very close monitoring by the nurse manager to reinforce *every nth* response and is obviously not very practical. However, reinforcing on a fairly regular basis, labelled a *variable ratio schedule*, might be quite feasible. In this instance, every second or every third response *on the average* over a period of time would be positively reinforced. It is also common in organizations to use a *fixed interval schedule* of reinforcement, as in the distribution of weekly or monthly paychecks.

Some rather interesting research findings have emerged over the years on continuous and partial schedules of reinforcement. For example, we know that the continuous schedule of reinforcement (i.e., every response is reinforced) is the fastest method of establishing a new behavior, while any kind of partial schedule of reinforcement is much slower. On the other hand, behaviors established under a continuous schedule also extinguish very quickly once the reinforcement stops, whereas a behavior that has been established on a partial schedule of reinforcement continues for a much longer time. In addition, continuous schedules of reinforcement are probably better when money is used as the reinforcer rather than other reinforcers such as praise.

Although reinforcement definitely changes behavior, there is nothing to indicate what is reinforcing to a given individual, or why. That is, a reinforcer is effective only if it is a reward for *that* individual. Most people are motivated by different kinds and amounts of rewards, but reinforcement theory does not explain such individual differences in response to reinforcers and punishers.

Expectancy Theory

Victor Vroom introduced expectancy theory in 1964 to explain work motivation (Vroom, 1964). In contrast to behavior modification, which focuses strictly on observable behaviors, expectancy theory suggests that people's thoughts about and evaluation of the environment and events—in other words, their expectations—are important in determining behavior. Thus, the major difference between expectancy theory and behavior modification is that expectancy theory regards people as reacting consciously and actively to their environment, while behavior modification suggests that people passively react to forces (reinforcement contingencies) in their environment. Expectancy theory is concerned with conscious choice behavior, while behavior modification focuses on the learned stimulus-response bonds that are formed as a result of positive reinforcement. Both theories, however, place a strong emphasis on the role of rewards and their relationship to the performance of desired behaviors.

Expectancy theory asserts that a person is motivated on the basis of expectancies or beliefs about future outcomes (consequences of behavior), and by the value the individual places on those outcomes (Vroom, 1964; Mitchell, 1974). In order to know when and where a person will put forth maximum effort, three components are important: expectancy, instrumentality, valence. *Expectancy* is the perceived probability that an action or a behavior will lead to a specific performance. *Instrumentality* is the belief that performance will lead to some outcome (reward or punisher). *Valence* is the value or desirability of an outcome. These three combine to indicate an individual's level of effort expended toward task performance.

The manager must determine individuals' beliefs regarding their expectancy that work will yield achievement (*E*xpectancy), that achievement will yield rewards (*I*nstrumentality), and how the rewards are valued (*Va*lence) (see Figure 9–3). These three components are multiplied together— Effort = [$E \times (I \times V)$]—to determine the amount of effort an individual will exert. Thus, when *any one* is drastically reduced, so is motivation

Figure 9–3   Expectancy Theory

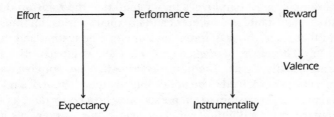

(effort). For example, if persons do not believe that they are capable of performing a task (expectancy), *or* they believe that there will be little chance of reward for work (instrumentality), *or* the value of the outcome (valence) is low, motivation is reduced. In fact, the multiplication of these components indicates that a zero value for *any one* of them results in zero motivation.

Expectancy theory also considers multiple outcomes. For example, consider the possibility of a promotion to nurse manager. Even though a staff nurse believes that such a promotion is positive and a reward for competence and performance in patient care, he or she also may realize that there are some possibly negative outcomes: for instance, working longer hours, losing the close camaraderie enjoyed with other staff members, and being the person to whom everyone (staff, administrators, patients, and physicians) comes with complaints. Therefore, when considering rewards, the nurse manager must always ask: What does this staff member believe about her or his ability to do the work (expectancy), the probability that the work will lead to outcomes (instrumentality), and the desirability of those outcomes (valence)?

Equity Theory

Equity theory suggests that effort and job satisfaction depend upon the degree of equity that an individual perceives in the work situation (Adams, 1963, 1965). Equity simply means that a person perceives that her or his contribution to the job is rewarded in the same proportion that another person's contribution is rewarded. Since contributions may differ, rewards may differ. Contributions include ability, education, experience, and effort, while rewards include pay, prestige, and fringe benefits. Thus, equity theory is concerned with the conditions under which employees perceive their contributions to the job and the rewards obtained therefrom as fair and equitable. Equity does not in any way imply equality; rather, it suggests that those employees who bring more to the job deserve more in the way of rewards.

As long as one's perceived *ratio* of outcomes to input is approximately equal to that of a relevant comparison person, a state of equity is said to exist. For example, most employees understand that the registered nurse and the nursing assistant have different and unequal salaries, but most also understand that each brings different and unequal education and experience to the job. Therefore, perceived equity in their assigned duties and in their salaries usually exists. Inequity occurs when an employee's outcome/input ratio is perceived to be noticeably unequal to that of a relevant comparison person. The comparison person may be a co-worker, a person doing a similar job for a different employer, an "ideal worker," or it may actually be the person himself or herself at some other time or in some other job situation.

Equity does not motivate a change in behavior; rather, inequity motivates a *change* in behavior that may either increase or decrease actual effort and job performance. Equity simply motivates the status quo. The nurse who sees the nursing assistants' salaries raised while nurses' salaries are not may be motivated to attempt some change, while no or equal percentage salary changes will motivate everyone to continue as they are now. Performance levels, be they high or low, are likely to remain constant. Again, one must be aware of the difference between behavior and performance. Reducing inequity may or may not change performance.

It is very difficult to predict exactly what a given individual will do in response to perceived inequity. However, there are some basic principles which may help in predicting reactions.

First, it is assumed that people will try to maximize rewards and minimize increasing contributions. Second, they will be more resistant to changing their ideas about their own rewards and contributions than to distorting their perceptions of the contributions and rewards of the comparison person. Moreover, perceived contributions and rewards central to an individual's self-esteem and self-concept will also be more resistant to change than those that are less central to these concepts. In the previous example, if nurses perceive that the increased salaries of the nursing assistants imply a loss of their own status, they will be more apt to attempt some type of change. Changing a person's reactions to the comparison person also will be more difficult once this comparison has stabilized over time. In other words, a nurse must act when the salary increase is announced, or a change will be unlikely to occur.

Finally, the least likely thing an individual will do is to leave the situation. Usually this occurs only after all other attempts to restore perceived equity have failed and the individual perceives a great deal of inequity.

Individuals can try to restore what they perceived as equity in a variety of ways. First, they can increase or decrease actual contributions, especially effort. Nurses can attempt to increase their status by assuming more patient care assignments, spending more time on charting, or exhibiting other behaviors reflective of added effort. Second, they may attempt to persuade the comparison persons to increase or decrease their inputs—persuading the nursing assistants to work less, for instance. Third, they may attempt to persuade the organization to change either their own rewards or those of the comparison persons (salary changes). Fourth, they may psychologically distort the perceived importance and value of their own contributions and rewards ("How could they run this unit without me?"). Fifth, they may distort the perceived importance and value of the comparison person's contributions or rewards—for instance, "What can you expect of assistants?"

The latter two are probably among the easiest ways in which to restore equity without actually changing performance levels. In addition, the employee may select a different comparison person, someone who is seen as more relevant for the comparison being made—say, the nurse manager. Finally, the individual may actually leave the organization.

The most extensively researched aspect of equity theory is the use of pay as a reward. Pay is an important reward to most people. Assuming that altering job effort is more feasible than other reactions to inequity, certain predictions regarding pay inequity can be made. Predictions of employee effort vary according to perceived underpayment inequity or overpayment inequity. In general, most of the research has been focused on overpayment inequity, probably because it is more controversial. It is easy to understand why individuals might change their behavior if they feel they are being cheated or underpaid, but it seems less likely that they should change their behavior (i.e., increase performance) when they feel they are being inequitably overpaid. Nevertheless, equity theory suggests that any kind of inequity, either underpayment or overpayment, will motivate changes in behavior.

Thus, the concept of equity may be seen as one of several potential social norms that operate in groups, particularly with respect to the distribution of rewards. Figure 9–4 contrasts some distribution rules regarding allocation of rewards in small groups (Leventhal, 1976). The appropriate distribution rule (equity versus equality) is dependent upon the goal of reward allocation. For example, when the goal is to maximize individual productivity in a group, rewards should be distributed equitably: that is, based on individual expertise and contributions. If the goal is to maximize harmony and minimize conflict in a group, however, then rewards should be equally distributed to all participants regardless of their contribution.

The degree of cooperation required for task performance is another important factor in the distribution of rewards. If tasks are essentially individual in nature—that is, staff members carry out tasks on their own without a high degree of cooperation required—then equity should be the rule for allocating organizational rewards. On the other hand, if a high

Figure 9—4 Distribution Rules for Allocating Rewards

Distribution rule	Situations where distribution rule is likely to be used	Factors affecting use of distribution rule
Equity/contributions (outcomes should match contributions)	1. Goal is to maximize group productivity 2. A low degree of cooperation is required for task performance	1. What receiver is expected to do 2. What others receive 3. Outcomes and contributions of person allocating rewards 4. Task difficulty and perceived ability 5. Personal characteristics of person allocating rewards and person performing
Equality (equal outcomes given to all participants)	1. Goal is to maximize harmony, minimize conflict in group 2. Task of judging performer's needs or contribution is difficult 3. Person allocating rewards has a low cognitive capacity 4. A high degree of cooperation is required for task performance 5. Allocator anticipates future interactions with low-input member	1. Sex of person allocating rewards (e.g., females more likely to allocate rewards equally than males) 2. Nature of task

Adapted from Leventhal, G. S. Fairness in social relationships. In J. Thibaut, J. Spence, & R. Carson (Eds.), *Contemporary Topics in Social Psychology.* Morristown, N.J.: General Learning Press, 1976. Used with permission.

degree of cooperation and coordination is required for effective task performance (i.e., group or team tasks), then rewards should be distributed equally among group members.

In other words, it is important to differentiate between rewarding individual performance versus group performance. If the nurse manager wants individual staff members to perform individual tasks (e.g., patient care, record keeping) competently and productively, then rewards should be individualized. If the task is essentially a group task (e.g., surgical nursing team), however, then performance will be maximized when staff members are rewarded for group rather than individual performance.

The important point is that perceived fairness of rewards does affect the manner in which individuals view their jobs and the organization and can affect the amount of effort they expend toward task accomplishment. Moreover, the research evidence seems to indicate that inequitable rewards, especially underpayment inequity, lead to increased psychological tension and lower job satisfaction and may have an adverse impact on job performance. In times of economic retrenchment, when no one receives a salary increase, people may perceive the situation as equitable if they believed it to be equitable prior to the retrenchment. In this case, job satisfaction may not be adversely affected. Similar to Herzberg's notion of extrinsic factors, pay equity is important to keep a good motivational situation from going sour, but distributing rewards equitably will not necessarily improve an otherwise poor motivational environment.

Goal Setting Theory

There are three basic propositions in goal setting (Locke, 1968). The first is that specific goals lead to higher performance than do general goals such as "Do your best." The second proposition states that specific, difficult goals lead to higher performance than specific, easy goals provided the goals are accepted. Finally, incentives such as money, knowledge of results, praise and reproof, participation, competition, and time limits affect behavior only if they cause individuals to change their goals or to accept goals that have been assigned to them. Thus, unlike expectancy theory and equity theory, goal setting suggests that it is not the rewards or outcomes of task performance per se that lead to the expenditure of effort, but rather the task goal itself. The only two functions of rewards are to help ensure the acceptance of an assigned task goal or to induce an individual to set a more specific and more difficult goal for himself or herself. It is the specificity and difficulty of the goal which mobilizes energy and directs behavior toward goal accomplishment.

Studies indicate that setting specific goals produces higher levels of performance than does the use of general goals or no goals (Locke, Shaw, Saari & Latham, 1981). Moreover, the higher the goal, the higher the performance. The relationship between goal difficulty and performance typically predicts 50–75% of the differences in individual performance levels. Of course, all of this is useful only to the extent that individuals accept performance goals. In practice, employees working at their normal job duties rarely completely reject their performance goals. The legitimacy of the nurse manager/staff nurse relationship is one that is readily accepted by most nurses. As long as tasks and duties are seen as reasonable or not totally impossible, specific, difficult goals will very likely produce higher performance as long as such performance is rewarded and the individual is held accountable for task accomplishment.

There is some evidence that the continuing presence of supervision helps to ensure goal acceptance. Supervisors who are frequently absent or not available for large periods of the working day are likely to have employees with substantially lower productivity than those of supervisors who are on the job with their employees.

Specific, difficult goals will likely lead to higher levels of job performance regardless of whether the nursing staff participates in every decision regarding the setting of performance standards. In some hospitals and with some nurse managers, participation is a natural and encouraged form of management; in other hospitals and with other nurse managers less emphasis may be placed on participative management. Either method is likely to be appropriate and productive, provided the manager is supportive of the employee. In other words, supportiveness and encouragement, particularly in the face of difficult or undesirable tasks, go a long way toward engendering acceptance of high performance goals and subsequent high levels of performance.

SUMMARY OF MOTIVATIONAL THEORIES

It is obvious that no single approach to motivating staff members is likely to maximize staff performance and satisfaction. Some methods may work better than others with different people or in different settings. However, all the various perspectives on what motivates individuals in work settings contribute something to our understanding of and, ultimately, our ability to influence employee motivation. All of the motivational theories can be integrated to some extent by recognizing the *need basis* in every theory, including the process theories. For example, reinforcement theory does not specify what a reinforcer is or why it works. However, it seems reasonable that reinforcers change behaviors simply because they lead to the fulfillment of some underlying need. Similarly, in expectancy theory there is nothing to say why an outcome has a strong positive or negative valence. We simply measure valences and assume that some outcomes are indeed motivational.

It may well be that self-competency, or self-efficacy, a need to cope successfully with the environment, can be used to integrate the various motivational perspectives (Locke & Schweiger, 1979; deCharms, 1968; Bandura, 1977, 1982). Viewed in this way all of the theories, both content and process, can be viewed as linked by this common human need. While it may be most useful to specify particular needs or processes (e.g., reinforcement, equity, expectancy) to describe human motivational behavior more precisely, recognizing a common basis such as self-competency does point out that there is utility to be gained from a variety of theoretical approaches.

It is this utility in practice that is particularly important for managers in organizations. The content theories recognize that people do have particular needs and that to some degree these needs must be fulfilled. People have needs for money, or at least the things that money can buy, and to some extent they may have higher order needs that can be fulfilled through proper job design and assignment of tasks (e.g., professionalism, altruism). Content theories indicate that people have needs but do not say much about *how* to satisfy them. In contrast, the process theories focus specifically on techniques and methods to improve performance and satisfaction, even though these are not phrased in the terminology of need fulfillment. Nevertheless, to the degree that all motivational theories are based upon an underlying need such as self-competency, the techniques and methods of the process theories represent useful means for providing need fulfillment.

INCREASING STAFF MOTIVATION

The question still remains: "How does one motivate staff?" Figure 9–5 shows a simple model of the manner in which the various motivational theories are related. First, there is a task to be accomplished. If this task is expressed in terms of a specific, difficult goal that is accepted by the staff member, then one may realistically expect a reasonably high degree of performance in most situations. How does this happen? Goals, perceived ability, and perceived situational constraints all combine to form the perceived likelihood that effort will lead to a given level of performance (goal accomplishment). This expectancy, when combined with the promise of valued rewards following goal attainment, leads to effort or motivation. Thus, goal setting and expectancy theory suggest not only that staff members should know exactly what they *should* be doing but also that they perceive rewards as contingent upon performing their assigned tasks.

Actual ability and situational constraints combine with effort to produce performance levels. Actual ability levels may be used by the nurse manager in assigning tasks that are commensurate with the nurse's ability, education, and experience. Performance may also be enhanced by removing situational constraints such as rotating shifts or providing assistance in overcoming them, for example by assignment to the same shift for more consecutive days. Careful management of these factors by the nurse manager will help ensure that staff members' efforts or motivation will actually be translated into effective job performance.

Expectancy theory focuses on anticipated rewards. If these rewards are not received, then subsequent expectancies and instrumentalities will be lowered. Performance should, in fact, lead to valued rewards that are perceived as being fair and equitable by staff members. Extrinsic rewards or reinforcers help to satisfy lower order needs, while intrinsic rewards or

Figure 9–5 Integrated Model of the Motivational Process

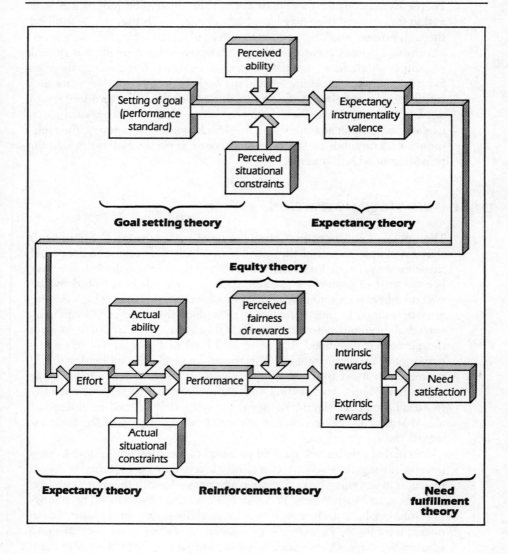

reinforcers are likely to satisfy higher order needs. For example, pay helps to satisfy the need for food, clothing, and shelter, while praise helps satisfy esteem needs.

In terms of future performance, rewards that are made contingent on performance and are perceived as being equitable will do a great deal to increase motivation. Thus, the effective management of staff motivation relies upon a combination of approaches, taking into consideration individual needs. Such an approach is far more likely than any single method or technique to produce effective job performance. The key to effective motivation is really the nurse manager's attitude that it *can* be done, given a little thought and effort. Motivation of staff members is not always easy, but it is certainly one of the most important parts of the nurse manager's job. With practice and a little ingenuity, most managers find that far more can be done than they had initially realized to motivate their staff to high levels of performance.

Motivation in Organizational Change

Why do some people resist change while others seem to welcome it? A very simple answer, but one that applies to most situations in which job changes are being contemplated, is simply that people like to know what is going on. A job is a very important part of a person's life. Not only is considerable time spent on the job, but one's social standing and prestige, in addition to personal identification, are very frequently related to the nature of one's work, job title, and, to some extent, the organization in which one is employed. This is especially true of professionals such as physicians, registered nurses, physical therapists, and the like.

Changes that are not understood or are seen as unnecessary will, at best, "rock the boat" and, at worst, actually threaten one's sense of stability and ability to cope with the environment. Thus, it is not surprising that change is frequently regarded as a threatening experience, especially when one is unsure why a change is being made and what will be expected once the change is implemented. This is tantamount to giving someone a general goal, such as "do your best," and then expecting specific types and levels of performance.

In terms of expectancy theory, the perceived likelihood that effort will lead to high performance is irrelevant unless "high performance" is specifically defined. Moreover, if an individual does turn in a "high performance," he or she may not be sure whether valued rewards or negative social pressure from peers will result. In short, people do not understand what choices to make because they do not understand what choices they actually have. Small wonder, then, that change can have such a devastating impact on both performance and employee satisfaction.

However, change does not have to be a negative force. Properly managed, change can be one of the nurse manager's best tools for influencing employee performance and job satisfaction, if the manager adheres to the following key rules in introducing change.

First, implement change only for a good reason. Change for change's sake is likely to be perceived as arbitrary, unnecessary, and an unreasonable use of the nurse manager's power and influence. For example, a nurse manager may complain that staff members actively resisted her leadership from her very first day on the job. She felt that the staff resented both her and anything that she attempted to accomplish that was different from "the way things used to be." Consequently, she had begun to arbitrarily change procedures just to "get them out of their rut." Of course, the result was quite predictable; things went from bad to worse.

Why did the staff members so actively resist this nurse manager's leadership efforts? There are many potential reasons, but the most likely is that staff members knew the rules of the "old" game. They knew the things they must do to please the previous nurse manager as well as the things they could reasonably get away with. The standards of the new nurse manager were different; the rules of the game had changed and the staff members still wanted to play the old game. Making arbitrary changes just for the sake of change is an excellent way to invite the active resistance and resentment of staff members.

So what is a "good" reason for change? There are three "good" reasons that are applicable to a wide variety of situations. The first is change in order to solve some problem. Eliminating problems, either real or perceived, is an open invitation for change and one readily accepted by most individuals. A second "good" reason involves making work procedures more efficient so that time will not be wasted on relatively unimportant tasks. A third readily accepted reason is to reduce unnecessary work load. No one wants to do more work than he or she has to or needs to do in order to accomplish a job. Focusing the need for change on one of these "good" reasons will go a long way toward decreasing resistance and increasing acceptance of change efforts.

A second cardinal rule in introducing change is to do so gradually. Do not try to change everything all at once. If there is anything worse than a feeling of ambiguity and powerlessness over what to do in one situation, it is the total confusion of what to do in ten different situations. The nurse manager should introduce change in only one or two areas at first and then build upon the success of that effort as a means of developing the trust and cooperation of the staff. This doesn't mean dragging one's feet in order to get anything done. It does mean, however, that change should be an orderly and planned process undertaken in manageable increments.

The third cardinal rule in introducing change is to plan it. Changes that are devised and implemented on the spur of the moment are likely to result in unexpected problems for the nurse manager as well as for staff. By planning the change and the strategy for introducing it carefully, the likelihood that the change will be accepted and will be successful is greatly increased.

Strategies involve introducing change and gaining the support and commitment of staff members in implementing it. The first step of a successful strategy is the introduction of a felt need for change. Again, solving a problem, making procedures more efficient, or reducing unnecessary work are excellent ways to do this. In terms of gaining the acceptance and support of individual nurses, explicit procedures and methods for on-the-job training, coaching, and performance appraisal (discussed in Chapters 14 and 15) are proven managerial tools that will greatly increase success in introducing change and modifying employee behavior. (See also Chapter 5 for a more complete discussion of organizational change.) When introducing change to an entire group of employees, the same principles apply. First of all, a felt need for the change must be established by involving the staff in the recognition of a problem or in discussing ways to increase efficiency and reduce unnecessary work. Through group participation, staff members are more likely to become actively involved in solutions and in creating change than resisting it. The same key behaviors used for individual coaching and performance appraisals, as discussed in Chapter 15, can be easily adapted for use in group problem-solving discussions.

An effort should be made to focus the group's discussion and effort on a single problem or change and upon the specific actions to be taken by each member of the group before attempting to deal with other problems or changes. It is important to keep the group discussion from wandering before closure on specific actions has been reached.

Undesirable Jobs

In any organization there are undesirable jobs which someone must perform from time to time. There is a strong tendency to assign these "bad" jobs to the best employee simply because this increases the likelihood that the job will be done properly. This practice, however, may give the high performing staff member the impression that the rewards of high performance are disagreeable tasks. While the staff member may accept them in the short run as a necessary evil, this practice will serve only to lower that person's motivation and increase dissatisfaction with the job in the long run. Assigning desirable tasks or, better yet, allowing the staff member a choice of tasks as a reward for high performance will be much more motivating.

Serious consideration should be given to making the assignment of undesirable tasks contingent upon poor performance insofar as possible. However, there should not be anyone on the staff who is doing an exceptionally poor job. Punishing consistent but not outstanding performance with the assignment of an undesirable job can be damaging to the motivation of some individuals.

If staff members are performing at approximately the same level of performance above some minimal standard, equity and positive reinforcement become critical issues. If the same people always get the undesirable jobs simply because they do them so well, feelings of inequity will mount rapidly, but if everyone understands that the undesirable job is regularly rotated so that no one is unduly penalized by having to repeatedly perform it, inequity is less likely to occur. Even better is to provide

some incentive for completion of undesirable tasks in a timely and professional fashion. This may be accomplished by allowing the staff member
a choice of favored tasks contingent upon completion of the undesirable job.

Individual preferences are important and cannot always be anticipated by the nurse manager. What is desirable or undesirable to one person may be viewed quite differently by another. The nurse manager who
knows individual preferences among potential incentives has a powerful
tool for motivating employees and fostering their job satisfaction. Task assignment is only one of many potential incentives or reinforcers, but
it can be a very powerful incentive when properly used (see Lancaster, 1985).

Job Design

The early history of job design was one of increasing specialization and
fragmentation. In the very early history of industry, well before the Industrial Revolution, general craftsmanship was plagued by problems of
inefficiency. This led to the specialization of jobs to increase efficiency and
production. However, labor costs rose and completion of products was
delayed as a result of the specialization, in part because of the increased
necessity for coordination among specialists in completing tasks. With the
advent of the Industrial Revolution and mass production, increased efficiency was brought about by further fragmenting the work into highly
specialized movements that were repeated over and over during the
course of the working day. Increased worker monotony produced increased absenteeism. The managerial reaction to this problem was an increased emphasis on discipline.

Thus, the scope of jobs has decreased steadily through specialization
and fragmentation of the total work effort. In the early days of nursing, for
instance, nurses assumed all the duties involved in caring for patients, including cleaning the room. Today, however, they increasingly specialize in
highly specific areas or somewhat fragmented job duties, so that we now
have the "IV nurse" or the "ICU nurse," for instance.

One problem with the specialization of professionals is that highly
specialized training does not allow one to change emphasis or specialties
easily within a professional career field. After several years, many highly
talented nurses become bored with extreme specialization and the monotony of doing the same things over and over or dealing with the same types
of patients day after day. The problem in industry was simply that the
work remained unchanged, so the solution to this was job redesign. In
health care there is a corresponding trend back toward more general versus highly specialized health care professionals. The concept of "holistic
health" and a concern for the psychological as well as the physical patient
have become increasingly important within the past decade. Consider

also the trend from team to primary nursing. Thus, the movement is away from job simplification and toward job enlargement.

Job enlargement and job enrichment describe two attempts to reduce the negative effects of specialization. *Job enlargement* may be defined as the addition of tasks in order to increase the variety of skills and talents that staff members must use in the performance of their jobs. This not only increases variety on the job but also provides a sense of completion by allowing an individual to do a larger, and thus more identifiable, piece of the entire task. The problem with job enlargement, however, is that it is frequently just "more work," rather than "better work" or work that entails greater responsibility and a higher level or different kind of professional skills. Intrinsic, higher order needs are particularly strong among professionals, and simply giving them more work as opposed to better work does little to satisfy their higher order needs or to stimulate outstanding job performance.

In contrast to job enlargement, *job enrichment* focuses on closing the gap between the doing and controlling aspects of the job. In job enrichment, employees are given greater latitude in selecting work methods, evaluating their work, or participating in decisions affecting either their job or the organization as a whole. Thus, job enrichment is characterized by greater responsibility and control over the job, as opposed to simply adding more mundane tasks to be accomplished.

The purpose of job redesign is to create jobs that provide a high degree of internal work motivation, high quality of work performance, high satisfaction with the work, and low absenteeism and turnover (Deci, 1975). These results are more apt to occur in individuals who experience the following psychological states: (a) greater meaningfulness in their work; (b) a sense of responsibility for the results of their work; and (c) feedback regarding the effectiveness of their work (see Figure 9–6).

One might assume that professional employees, such as nurses, would experience these rewards as a result of their work. However, if motivation, absenteeism, and turnover were not problems among professional staff, there would be no need for this chapter. Clearly, motivational systems must be developed and implemented to retain highly talented and productive nurses in jobs where their services are particularly needed. Job redesign tries to increase the degree to which an individual experiences meaningfulness, responsibility, and effective feedback, which lead to high performance and high job satisfaction, by dealing with a specific set of core job dimensions that research has shown to be related to the presence of these psychological states.

Core job dimensions. According to job redesign theory, five core job dimensions (Figure 9–6) activate the critical psychological states (Hackman & Oldham, 1980; see also Guthrie et al., 1985). The first core job dimension is *skill variety*, the degree to which a job provides activities

Figure 9-6 Job Characteristics Model of Work Design

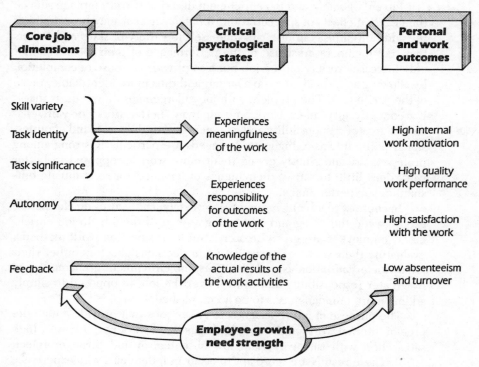

Hackman, Oldham. "Motivation through design of work: test of a theory." *Organizational Behavior and Human Performance, 16,* 250–279, 1976. Reprinted by permission of Academic Press.

which involve the use of different skills and abilities. The second core job dimension is *task identity*, the degree to which a job requires completion of a whole and identifiable piece of work. This entails doing a complete task from beginning to end. These two dimensions are generally representative of job enlargement. However, job enrichment adds three additional core job dimensions that are important for creating the desired psychological states. In particular, *task significance* is the degree to which a job has importance for the lives and work of other people both inside and outside the organization. The dimension of *autonomy* is important in that such a job provides considerable freedom, independence, and discretion to the staff member in scheduling the work to be accomplished and choosing the procedures to be used in carrying it out. Finally, *feedback* is the degree to which individuals are able to obtain clear information regarding the effectiveness of their performance. This may be apparent from the task itself or may be available from other individuals—particularly patients, other nurses, and the nurse manager.

There are several principles to guide the redesign of jobs to enhance these five core job dimensions. The first principle is that of forming natural work units, combining tasks which logically fit together. This helps employees to see the significance of their tasks and to feel a greater sense of responsibility for the outcome of what they do. A second and related principle is that of combining tasks, which helps to increase perceptions of skill variety and task identity. By carefully combining tasks, natural work units may be formed, and both principles become available for motivating and satisfying staff members.

A third principle is that of establishing client relationships. This already exists in nursing, where the nurse/client relationship is a prerequisite to providing care. Clients provide direct feedback to the nurse on their perception of the nurse's work. In addition, client relationships increase skill variety because the nurse must practice the interpersonal skills necessary for effective communication with different patients. Finally, client relationships affect autonomy in that the nurse must decide how to manage the relationships with patients and co-workers in the unit.

The fourth principle concerns added control over one's work. Again, allowing staff nurses to participate in decision making, selecting work methods, and evaluating their own work increases the amount of autonomy experienced from the job.

The fifth principle is that of opening feedback channels. This involves essentially two things, the first being feedback from the nurse manager regarding job performance, a topic discussed in Chapter 15. However, feedback coming from the job itself (including patients), is even more important in that it is both immediate and specific. For example, staff nurses may be made responsible for evaluating their own performance, such as patient response to their ministrations. Such nurses are continually reminded of performance quality without the potential interpersonal problems inherent when negative feedback is provided by the supervisor. Proponents of primary nursing have argued that staff who work in such units have greater satisfaction as a result of these principles.

Barriers to job redesign. There are some common problems in the redesign of jobs of which the nurse manager should be aware. The first may actually be the most important in that the nurse manager's role may change from leader and director of unit staff to that of coordinator of staff activities. Somehow, the notion of "coordinator" seems inconsistent with our cultural stereotypes of "leadership." We tend to think of a leader as the person in charge, or "the boss." That stereotype of leadership tends to include the unilateral and unquestioned use of power, with objectives, strategies, and evaluation defined strictly from the leader's perspective. Some authors treat this issue as a matter of "leadership style" and tend to regard it as a personality characteristic. This particular barrier, however, is one over which the nurse manager can exercise direct and explicit control.

There are a number of factors involved in effective leadership other than the power afforded by virtue of job title and reporting relationships. Effective leadership is accepted leadership, and there are many ways in which to foster acceptance of the nurse manager's legitimate organizational power (see Chapter 10). The strategies and techniques described in this chapter, however, are tools meant to help in achieving individual and unit effectiveness. If effectiveness means being a coordinator as opposed to "the boss," then those strategies and techniques are what the nurse manager should use.

Another barrier to job redesign is that the values implicit in job redesign may be at odds with those of hospital administration. The notion of providing autonomy, feedback, and greater responsibility and self-direction in the performance of jobs may not be in tune with the philosophy and the history of the hospital hierarchy—matters that are not under the nurse manager's immediate discretion or control. However, different management areas afford different degrees of responsibility, and there may be a good deal of flexibility within the limits of the rules. Job redesign is just another tool to use within the limits of the situation at hand.

In some cases, staff members are reluctant to engage in job redesign or other motivation efforts because they fear that increased productivity may have implications for their job security. That is, if productivity increases sufficiently, some people may lose their jobs because they are no longer needed to accomplish the work within the unit. In nursing, however, this is seldom a problem since most nursing units are chronically understaffed. Increased productivity not only eases the work load but, if properly managed (e.g., rewarded), is likely to result in greater satisfaction and organizational commitment and less absenteeism and turnover. Second, there is a tendency to focus on quantity and to ignore the quality of work as a separate but equally important dimension. Fears regarding job security tend to focus solely on the quantity issue and ignore quality. Effective motivation of staff members involves both of these dimensions, but job enrichment most consistently increases job satisfaction and work quality rather than the quantity of work produced.

The fourth major barrier to job redesign is that not everyone desires change or "growth" on his or her job. Some people prefer to have their work very clearly prescribed, unvarying in its content or procedure, and highly predictable from day to day. Job redesign is only appropriate when their jobs are not structured enough to suit their needs.

Still another major barrier to job redesign is the frequent lack of predetermined goals: that is, exact specification of what is to be accomplished by redesigning an individual's job. Expectancy theory suggests that people know exactly what it is they *should* do to make a given level of performance as high as possible. Thus, in implementing any job redesign measures, clear goals and objectives, planning with respect to how these goals can and should be attained, and periodic monitoring of progress to identify needed changes in strategies or objectives are essential. Job redesign may seem somewhat complex, but it is simply another technique that encompasses a variety of motivational strategies with an eye toward overall nursing effectiveness.

Climate and Morale

Climates are clusters of employee perceptions of an organization's events, practices, and procedures; when taken together, these perceptions are useful in characterizing the organization or subunit. There are many climates in an organization: for example, a productivity climate, a climate for safety, a climate for patient care, and so on. One must specify the climate to which one is referring. Thus, a nursing unit is characterized as having a climate for high productivity to the extent that the work is usually completed at the end of each shift and that patient satisfaction is generally good. When such a climate exists, nurse managers may be reasonably sure that their managerial efforts have been relatively effective in motivating staff to high standards of performance.

Just as climate refers to group versus individual perceptions, morale refers to the combined attitudes of all work group members versus individual job satisfaction. Morale is essentially a matter of "group spirit" or cohesiveness. It is important because cohesiveness reflects the attractiveness of group members to the group and indicates the degree to which group values and expectations (norms) are adopted as one's own. Group norms are common expectations held by the members of a work unit with regard to decision making, productivity, and the like, and become increasingly important as group cohesiveness increases.

Group norms may be productive, provided they are congruent with or support organizational goals. High morale can aid in pursuing productivity or effectiveness goals. In contrast, low or negative morale may lead to or be associated with active resistance on the part of group members to leadership and motivational efforts. For example, there may be a norm to restrict productivity, a low standard for a "fair day's work" that is enforced by subtle group pressures. This is not uncommon in some nursing units.

The phenomenon of "groupthink" is an example of nonproductive group norms, such as the failure to prepare for an attack on Pearl Harbor and the decision to institute the Bay of Pigs invasion. Groupthink occurs frequently in organizations when there are shared norms or expectations that: (a) the group is invulnerable to outside pressure; (b) the group believes itself to be morally right, which inclines members to ignore the ethical and moral consequences of their decisions; (c) the group rationalizes warnings and other forms of negative feedback; (d) there is direct pressure upon any individual who expresses doubts about the group's shared illusions or who questions the validity of arguments supporting an alternative favored by the majority; (e) there is self-censorship—that is, pressure for individuals to conform to the group consensus; and (f) there is a shared illusion of unanimity within the group.

Under these conditions the group limits its discussion to a few alternative courses of action, fails to reexamine the course of action initially preferred even after learning of risks and drawbacks not previously considered, and makes little or no attempt to obtain information from experts. Group members are interested in facts and opinions that support their preferred policy but ignore facts and opinions that do not; they fail to develop contingency plans to cope with foreseeable setbacks that could influence or endanger the overall success of their chosen course. Thus, groupthink can be not only counterproductive but potentially dangerous as well.

High morale can, however, be used as a positive force for productivity under more favorable conditions. Again, the feeling of "togetherness" or group cooperation is the strongest determinant. A second factor is agreement on goals. Third, there must be progress toward those goals and, finally, each member should have specific and meaningful tasks necessary for goal achievement. While not all of these are absolutely essential in bringing about group cohesiveness and commitment toward organizational objectives, they can all be fostered by careful planning, inclusion of staff members in diagnosing problems, developing action plans for their solution, and carefully managing performance based on the principles and techniques outlined in this chapter. In short, morale can be a significant factor in either helping or hindering the nurse manager's efforts to motivate staff members.

SUMMARY

- Content theories of motivation define motivation primarily in terms of need satisfaction.

- Process motivation theories describe how motivational processes operate and prescribe specific actions for implementation by the nurse manager. Thus, content and process theories provide different perspectives on what mobilizes, directs, and sustains effort (motivation).

- Reinforcement theory views motivation as a process of learning which specific behaviors lead to rewards and which behaviors are either unrewarded or punished. Positive reinforcement (reward) is more effective in changing behavior (motivation) than punishment.

- Expectancy theory regards conscious choice as the determinant of motivation, either in what a nurse will do or in how much effort will be exerted on a given task. Three components are necessary: the perception that the nurse can actually perform the task (expectancy), the perception that task performance will actually result in some outcomes (instrumentality), and the perceived value of the outcomes (valence, i.e., rewards or punishers).

- Equity theory deals with the perceived fairness of an employee's ratio of outcomes/inputs relative to the same ratio perceived for a comparison person. Inequity may occur either for underpayment or overpayment (outcomes) and motivates an individual to do something to restore perceived equity.

- Goal setting theory indicates that specific, difficult goals lead to higher performance levels than either general goals or specific easy goals.

- No motivation theory provides a complete description of the motivational process; each theory/technique brings a different perspective and contribution to understanding and influencing motivation. Effective staff motivation is best accomplished by combining the theories and techniques so that their effects are complementary.

- In implementing change, the nurse manager should: (a) introduce change only for a good reason; (b) implement change gradually; and (c) plan change strategies carefully.

- Job design includes job enlargement and job enrichment, both of which may be used by the nurse manager to increase employee motivation.

- Barriers to job design include: stereotyped perceptions of the nurse manager as the "boss" rather than as "leader" of a professional staff; organizational policies and values; fear of change; job security; personal characteristics; and a lack of predetermined goals.

- Group cohesiveness or "teamwork" can lead to either effective or ineffective individual and unit performance, depending on the behavior expectations (norms) the group holds for its members.

BIBLIOGRAPHY

Adams, J. S. (1965). Injustice in social exchange. In: *Advances in experimental social psychology*. Vol. 2. Berkowitz, L. (editor). New York: Academic Press.

Adams, J. S. (1963). Toward an understanding of inequity. *J. of Abnorm and Soc Psychol*, 67:422.

Alderfer, C. P. (1972). *Existence, relatedness, and growth*. New York: Free Press.

Alderfer, C. P. (1969). A new theory of human needs. *Organizational Behavior and Human Performance*, 4:142.

American Academy of Nursing, Task Force on Nursing Practice in Hospitals. (1983). *Magnet hospitals: Attraction and retention of professional nurses*. Kansas City, MO: ANA Publication.

Bandura, A. (1977). Self-efficacy: Toward a unifying theory of behavioral change. *Psychol Rev*, 84:191.

Bandura, A. (1982). Self-efficacy mechanism in human agency. *Am Psychol*, 37:122.

Bonaquist, P. (1986). From job satisfaction emerges new leadership. *Nursing Success Today*, 3(10): 15–21.

deCharms, R. (1968). *Personal causation; the internal affective determinants of behavior*. New York: Academic Press.

Deci, E. L. (1975). *Intrinsic motivation.* New York: Plenum.

Floyd, G. J., and Smith, B. D. (1983). Job enrichment. *Nurs Mngmt, 14*(5):22.

Freud, S. (1949). The unconscious. In: *Collected papers of Sigmund Freud.* Riviere, J. (translator). London: Hogarth Press. (Original edition, 1915.)

Guthrie, M. B., Mauer, G., Zawacki, R., and Cougar, J. (1985). Productivity: How much does this job mean? *Nurs Mngmt, 16*(2):16–20.

Hackman, J. R., and Oldham, G. R. (1980). *Work redesign.* Reading, MA: Addison-Wesley.

Haw, M. A., Claus, E. G., Durbin-Lafferty, E., and Iverson, S. M. (1984). Improving morale in a climate of cost containment. Part 1. Organizational assessment. *J Nurs Adm, 14*(10):8–15.

Herzberg, F. (1966). *Work and the nature of man.* Cleveland, OH: World.

Herzberg, F., Mausner, B., Snyderman, B. (1959). *The motivation to work.* New York: Wiley.

Lancaster, J. (1985). Creating a climate for excellence. *J Nurs Adm, 15*(1):16–19.

Leventhal, G. S. (1976). Fairness in social relationships. In: *Contemporary topics in social psychology.* Thibaut, J., Spence, J., Carson, R. (editors). Morristown, NJ: General Learning Press.

Locke, E. A. (1968). Toward a theory of task motives and incentives. *Organizational Behavior and Human Performance, 3*:157.

Locke, E. A., and Schweiger, D. M. (1979). Participation in decision making: One more look. In: *Research in organizational behavior.* Vol. 1. Staw, B. (editor). Greenwich, CT: JAI Press.

Locke, E. A., Shaw, K. N., Saari, L. M., and Latham, G. P. (1981). Goal setting and task performance: 1969–1980. *Psychological Bulletin, 90*:125.

Maslow, A. H. (1954). *Motivation and personality.* New York: Harper.

Maslow, A. H. (1943). A theory of human motivation. *Psychol Rvw, 50*:370.

Miner, J. B. (1980). *Theories of organizational behavior.* Hinsdale, IL: Dryden Press.

Mitchell, T. R. (1974). Expectancy models of job satisfaction, occupational preference, and effort: A theoretical, methodological and empirical appraisal. *Psychol Bull, 81*:1096.

Mitchell, T. R. (1982). *People in organizations.* New York: McGraw-Hill.

Skinner, B. F. (1953). *Science and human behavior.* New York: Free Press.

Steers, R. M., Porter, L. W. (1979). *Motivation and work behavior,* 2nd ed. New York: McGraw-Hill.

Vroom, V. H. (1964). *Work and motivation.* New York: Wiley.

ASSUMPTION OF A nurse manager position brings with it new rights, privileges, and responsibilities. Among the latter are, for instance, managing the health care of patients, directing the work and activities of employees, implementing and controlling a budget, serving as a vital link in the organizational chain of communication and control, and managing the functions that keep the unit running. The position demands effective leadership—that is, the exercise of power and influence through interpersonal interaction processes—for the execution of these tasks.

Some people use the term *leadership* as a synonym for management, but the two terms do not have the same meaning. *Leadership* is an interpersonal relationship in which the leader employs specific behaviors and strategies to influence individuals and groups toward goal setting and attainment in specific situations. The leader is a group member who influences and directs the contributions of other members toward individual or group achievement. *Management*, in contrast, refers to the coordination and integration of resources through planning, organizing, directing, and controlling in order to accomplish specific institutional goals and objectives. Thus, the manager is primarily concerned with scheduling and coordinating resources and tasks. An implicit prerequisite for effective management is the establishment of leadership behaviors or style(s) to achieve the objectives of management activities.

Supervision, too, is often confused with leadership. *Supervision* is the coordination of the basic work activities of the organization in accordance with plans and procedures. It involves overseeing the work activities of others and is directly concerned with leader/subordinate interaction. It is possible for either a manager or supervisor to also be a leader. However, there are managers with little or no leadership ability and supervisors with no management skills. Management refers to certain task-oriented activities in a job. Supervision refers to certain people-oriented activities in a job. Leadership is the effective combination of management and supervision in a manner that invites or even inspires people to strive toward the attainment of organizational goals. In this chapter, the processes and behaviors of effective leadership are developed.

LEADERSHIP DEFINED

Leadership is the use of one's skills to influence others to perform to the best of their ability. Although everyone has a different potential for leadership, the skills can be identified and learned, thereby improving the leader's performance.

Leadership has been considered an interaction among people, a process of influencing the activities of an organized group toward goal setting and goal achievement (Stogdill, 1959). Historically, the nurse manager has been identified as the person who oversees all activities on the unit, including making patient care assignments, scheduling staff time, and planning inservice education. How nurse managers accomplish these activities depends upon their leadership styles and skills.

Leadership requires the presence of other people (followers) and is the relationship between those people and the person who is leading. Mere appointment to a leadership position does not ensure that a person will be accepted by the group or that the person is capable of giving leadership. A leader must be able to make people want to accomplish something. Thus, leadership is an interpersonal process of influencing the activities of an individual or a group toward goal attainment in a given situation (Moloney, 1979). Leadership does not mean domination; it is the leader's job to get work done through other people. For example, the nurse manager who accurately identifies a personality conflict between two employees and still is able to achieve agreement on a vacation schedule is using effective leadership skills.

Leadership can be formal or informal, regardless of the hierarchical position or status of the nursing staff involved. Leadership is *informal* when practiced by a team member who is not designated as the nurse in charge. Whenever one nurse exerts more influence than another in accomplishing the work of the unit, that nurse is described as a leader. This action can be complementary or contradictory to the goals of the unit or the hospital. Leadership is *formal* when practiced by the designated nurse in charge of the unit.

BASES OF POWER

Leadership, or the exercise of power and influence, involves one individual trying to change the behavior of other individuals. It usually means bringing some kind of force to bear on those individuals to persuade them to act in accordance with the leader's wishes and goals. A leader has power to the extent that: (a) the group members think the leader controls and will use rewards or punishments to back up requests; (b) the group members either greatly fear or value highly the outcomes that may result; and (c) the group members have few alternatives—that is, little way to change or decrease the pressure that the leader can exert.

What are some of the resources that the leader can bring to bear in a leadership situation? Studies of power have led to the development of six bases of power (French & Raven, 1960; Mitchell, 1982):

1. **Reward power** is based upon a number of incentives that the leader can provide for group members and upon the degree to which the group members value those incentives. For example, a nurse manager may have considerable influence in determining the salary or vacation time of a staff nurse. Thus, reward power is largely based on a leader's formal job responsibilities.

2. **Punishment**, or coercive power, is based upon the negative things that the leader might do to individual group members or the group as a whole. For example, the nurse manager might give a staff nurse very undesirable job assignments, a formal reprimand, recommend that her or his pay be docked, or even that she or he be fired.

3. **Information power** is based upon "who knows what" in an organization and the degree to which they can control access to that information by other individuals. The nurse manager, for instance, is frequently privy to information obtained at meetings with the nurse supervisor or through other informal channels of communication that are either not available to or are unknown to members of the nursing staff. Thus, information can be either formally or informally gathered and distributed.

4. *Legitimate power* stems from the group members' perception that the nurse manager has a legitimate right to make a request; this power is based on the authority delegated to the nurse manager by virtue of her job and position within the management hierarchy.

5. *Expert power* is based upon particular knowledge and skill not possessed by the staff. Nurse managers, by virtue of their experience and, possibly, advanced education, frequently qualify as the persons who know best what to do in a given situation. For example, newly graduated nurses might look to the nurse manager for advice regarding particular procedures or for help in using equipment on the unit.

6. *Referent power* is based upon admiration and respect for an individual as a person. For example, a young nurse asks the advice of the nurse manager regarding a personal problem at home. Thus, referent power is largely a function of the leader's personal qualities.

This is a fairly impressive list of power bases that are potentially available to the nurse manager. Moreover, it indicates that power and influence may be derived from a number of different sources; that is, rewards and punishment are basically organizationally determined, while information power and legitimacy are primarily based upon the nurse manager's position within the organization. Referent power and expertise are based primarily on personal characteristics. While all of these sources of power are used at one time or another, the most effective combination seems to depend upon the situation at hand and the people involved.

There are some general principles underlying the use of power. For example, managers seem to prefer using expert and legitimate power rather than punishments or appeals to friendship. By the same token, subordinates are more likely to comply with legitimate, expert, and referent power than they are with reward and coercive power. Fortunately, there is considerable agreement between what managers prefer to use and what subordinates prefer to have used in a leadership situation. Nevertheless, there are some important differences, both in individuals and in organizations. For example, some managers are more authoritarian and others are more participative in their leadership styles. The latter managers tend to rely more on expertise and referent power or social pressure to get things done. Similarly, more formally structured organizations tend to emphasize a greater degree of autocratic control in their management systems.

LEADERSHIP: PERSONALITY, BEHAVIOR, OR STYLE?

The search for effective leadership characteristics as personality traits or personal attributes has not been productive. For every example of a great leader with certain characteristics, ten examples of leadership failure on the part of individuals possessing those same characteristics can easily be found. By the early 1950s, it had become clear that the situation itself is a major determinant of the extent to which leadership characteristics have any influence at all in determining leadership effectiveness.

At about this same time, researchers at several major universities began to focus more on what leaders do rather than on what personal characteristics they possess. Thus, leadership behavior research in laboratories at Harvard University found "activity," "taskability," and "likability" leadership behaviors. Studies at Ohio State University were conducted in field settings and asked subordinates to describe the behaviors exhibited by their leaders. Two major dimensions were identified, one called "consideration" and the other "initiation of structure." Researchers at the University of Michigan also conducted their research in the field but asked leaders themselves to describe what they did. This effort also produced two major dimensions of leadership behavior: "job-centered behavior" and "employee-centered behavior."

The similarities across these research efforts are remarkably consistent. In each case, concern for the task was identified as a major aspect of leadership behavior (task ability, initiation of structure, job-centered behavior), and a second major dimension dealing with interpersonal relationships also emerged (likability, consideration, employee-centered behavior).

Specifically, *initiating structure* refers to behavior in which the nurse manager organizes and defines the work to be accomplished and establishes well-defined, routine work patterns, channels of communication, and methods of getting the job done. For example, the nurse manager provides a detailed manual of job descriptions, personnel policies, and procedures for requesting time off on certain holidays. *Consideration*, on the other hand, refers to behavior that conveys mutual trust, respect, friendship, warmth, and rapport between the nurse manager and the staff. In this situation, the employee learns to expect that the nurse manager will hear a complaint openly without any reprisal.

While the consistency of these research efforts was encouraging, the relationship of leader behaviors to leader effectiveness proved very puzzling. It soon became clear that more of either task behavior or interpersonal behavior does not necessarily lead to greater leadership effectiveness. Nor did either interpersonally oriented or task-oriented leadership styles or any combination thereof consistently lead to higher performance and productivity. Instead, it became clear that the situation has a profound influence in determining the relationship between leadership behavior and performance.

Nevertheless, this earlier focus on leadership behavior was a significant advance in understanding leadership effectiveness. Soon, the search for leadership styles or clusters of leadership behaviors began, in an attempt to identify particular patterns or styles of leadership that would be more effective in most situations.

Leadership Styles

Leadership styles can be identified as *sets or clusters of behaviors* (see Levenstein, 1985). Thus, for nurse managers leadership style is the manner in which they use interpersonal behaviors to influence the accomplishment of goals for the unit.

Since an individual's behavior is influenced both by his or her formative years and lifetime experience, leadership style reflects these prior experiences. Having found that it was not possible to identify specific characteristics or traits present in all successful leaders, researchers began studying ways in which successful leadership is accomplished—that is, how leaders delegate tasks and how they communicate with workers. One result has been the recognition that, unlike traits or other specific characteristics, leadership behaviors can be learned.

The fact that a leader's personality or past experience helps form a leadership style does not mean that that style is unchangeable or that a nurse manager always uses the same, single style of leadership. Styles of leadership range from very authoritarian to very permissive and change according to the situation. For example, a nurse leader may use one style when responding to an emergency situation such as a cardiac arrest. Another style may be used to encourage creative problem solving to plan the care for a multi-problem patient, while a third style may be used to generate ideas for use of a new procedure. An effective nurse manager leadership style is one that best complements the organizational environment, the tasks to be accomplished, and the personal characteristics of the people involved.

Authoritarian leadership style.   Sometimes called autocratic, the authoritarian style represents primarily directive behaviors. Autocrats make decisions alone and, although they may be essentially correct in their thinking, they may lack the group support that results from decisions made with consultation. They tend to be more concerned with task accomplishment than with concern for the people who perform those tasks; they consider themselves to be in positions of authority and expect their followers to respect them and obey their directions. Such a leader may listen to suggestions, but may not necessarily be influenced by them. This kind of leader does little to encourage individual initiative or cooperation among the staff members.

Autocratic leaders frequently exercise power with coercion. Their personality is firm, insistent, self-assured, dominating (with or without intent), and they keep the center of attention. Such leaders are thought to view workers as naturally lazy, lacking ambition, disliking responsibility, and preferring to be led. Furthermore, autocratic leaders are assumed to be self-centered, indifferent to organizational needs, resistant to change, not very bright, and lacking creative potential (McGregor, 1960). This type of leader has little trust or confidence in workers and vice-versa.

While autocratic leadership is not always the best form of leadership, it is necessary in times of crisis when there is no time for group decision. During a cardiac arrest, for example, being self-assured, firm, and dominating the actions of others are appropriate leadership behaviors. Autocratic leadership is also useful when the leader is the only one who has the essential information or skills in areas in which the staff nurses are inexperienced. In these situations staff members expect to be told what to do. During a disaster drill or in an actual disaster, a new employee would best be informed of correct procedures by direct commands, issued with the expectation of blind obedience.

Democratic leadership style. In the democratic or participative style of leadership, the leader is people-oriented, focusing on human relations, teamwork, and the building of an effective work group. Here, "togetherness" is emphasized and the leader is viewed as a helper who belongs to the group and is the organizer of teamwork. Workers are made to feel that they have important contributions to make. Communication is open and usually goes both ways, and a spirit of collaboration and joint effort exists. Consequently, the members of the team have a greater feeling of satisfaction and freedom.

For example, a patient with a very recent myocardial infarction is repeatedly found walking in his room even though he is supposed to be on bed rest. The nurse manager, using a democratic leadership style, could call a case management conference in which the staff could collectively explore methods to encourage the patient to remain in bed and to promote his participation in his recovery.

The democratic leader's primary goal is to keep the group headed in the right direction. The main assumption made by those who use this style is that if people are treated as adults, they are likely to respond as adults. Democratic leaders try to give workers a feeling of self-worth and importance.

Some decisions do not permit the leader to be totally democratic, but participation can help staff members identify with the work setting. Participation promotes the acceptance of goals and thereby elicits the staff's cooperation in carrying out decided-upon activities; it also provides the opportunity for them to change or improve their work methods, encourages their professional and personal growth, and helps them learn from their mistakes. Although research studies have found that this style of leadership does not consistently lead to high productivity, it does enhance employee job satisfaction (Locke & Schweiger, 1979).

Permissive or laissez-faire leadership style. In this style, leaders have no established goals or policies and deliberately abstain from leading their staff. The general climate is one of permissiveness with no central direction or control. The leader wants everyone to feel good, fosters freedom for everyone, and avoids responsibility by relinquishing power to the staff.

The effectiveness of this style depends upon the people within the group. In some instances, an informal leader takes over and the unit runs smoothly when that person is present. Permissive leaders often assume workers are ambitious, responsible, dynamic, flexible, intelligent, creative, and accepting of organizational goals. This style can sometimes be effective in highly motivated professional groups, but is not generally useful in a highly structured health care delivery system composed of people from a variety of professions and paraprofessions and in which organization and control form the basis of most operations.

There are still other styles of leadership in clinical settings. *Bureaucratic leaders* are similar to autocratic ones in that they may be insecure about their own ability to lead and find security in following established policies. They wield power by fixed rules and are deficient in initiative and flexibility. They allow no variations; as long as the rules are followed, there are no problems. Such a leader acts in an official capacity, relates impersonally to the staff, and seldom makes a decision if there are no standards or norms for guidance.

The *mollifying autocrat* is halfway between the bureaucratic and democratic leader. She is concerned about too much independence within the staff, but is also concerned about the staff as people. This nurse manager communicates well with the staff, listens, and asks for their ideas. Once they have had the opportunity to speak, this leader does what she had planned to do prior to discussion with the staff.

The *parental style* describes leaders who never discipline and are too good to their staff. Staff dependence and obedience are fostered and rewarded. Communication usually occurs in a downward direction, but some upward communication occurs. Controls are loose when all goes well but, when problems occur, these nurse managers are ineffective.

The *multicratic style* of leadership combines the best points of the three traditional styles: autocratic, democratic, and laissez-faire. The multicratic leader combines flexibility of approach and concern for people to achieve the goal of effective administration.

An understanding of leadership styles does not explain which style will be most effective under which circumstances, nor does any of these approaches consider the specific and systematic effects of the leadership situation. This recurrent deficiency in leadership research eventually led to the development of several contingency theories of leadership that attempt to incorporate leadership traits, leadership behaviors, and leadership situations into a unified theoretical framework. This framework helps us not only to understand more about effective leadership but also to predict what kinds of leader behaviors will be most effective under which circumstances.

THEORIES OF LEADERSHIP

The Contingency Model

In the mid 1960s, Fiedler published his contingency model of leadership effectiveness, which suggests that a leader's style must be matched with the requirements of the situation in order for the leader to be effective (Fiedler, 1967). Effectiveness is very carefully defined as the performance of the group itself, not some rating of the leader's effectiveness. Fiedler differentiates two leadership styles, which he calls relationship-oriented and task-oriented leadership.

These leadership styles are assessed with a questionnaire that he calls the Least-Preferred Co-worker scale (LPC). The leader rates his or her least preferred co-worker on a set of 17 bipolar scales anchored at either end by adjectives (e.g., efficient-inefficient, friendly-rejecting). If the leader's least preferred co-worker is described in relatively positive terms, then the leader is said to have an underlying relationship-oriented motivational style. If the least preferred co-worker is described in relatively unfavorable terms, then the individual is said to be a basically task-oriented leader.

Since Fiedler (1967) defines leadership as a process of influence, the leadership situation is described on a dimension that represents the ease with which the leader can influence group members. This dimension, called Situation Favorability, is made up of three components: (a) *leader-member relations*, or the degree to which the leader enjoys the loyalty and support of her subordinates; (b) *task structure*, or the degree to which the task or finished product is clearly described or that there are standard operating procedures that guarantee successful completion of the task and make it easy for the leader to determine how well the work has been performed; and (c) *position power*, or the degree to which the leader is able to administer rewards and punishments (essentially a matter of legitimate power).

When leader-member relations are relatively good, when the task is relatively structured, and when the leader has high position power, it is relatively easy for the leader to influence the group toward the accomplishment of organizational objectives. Similar to the leadership behavior research, Fiedler states that the leader-member relations component is the most important, the task structure the next most important, and the leader's formal position power the least important determinant of situation favorability.

Figure 10–1   Predictions From Fiedler's Contingency Theory of Leadership

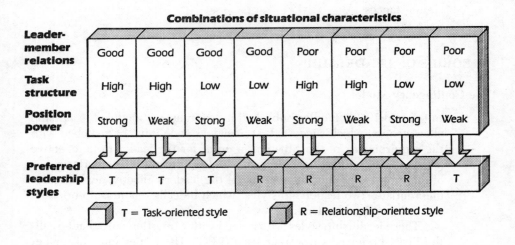

Figure 10–1 illustrates the preferred leadership styles given certain combinations of situational characteristics. According to Fiedler, a leader is most effective when leadership style and situation match, and he suggests that leaders should attempt to seek situations in which their predominant style is most appropriate. Should a mismatch occur, Fiedler suggests that the leader should either attempt to change characteristics of the situation or to change his or her own leadership style to better fit the situation.

Path-Goal Theory

Path-goal theory, developed by House, is an effort to apply a theory of human motivation and task performance to the realm of leadership effectiveness (House & Mitchell, 1974). That is, one of the primary functions of leadership is to motivate group members toward the attainment of organizational objectives. Path-goal theory suggests that this motivational function can best be carried out by the leader's engaging in behaviors that remove obstacles to goal attainment and by making personal rewards for employees contingent upon attainment of those goals. Thus, a leader's function is to coach, guide, and provide performance incentives to ensure high work performance. Furthermore, the theory suggests that leader behavior directly affects group members' job satisfaction to the extent that the leader makes rewards available and that the leader's behavior itself is a source of satisfaction to subordinates.

The motivational functions of leadership are built directly on the expectancy theory of work motivation (see Chapter 9). Briefly, employees should work for rewards that they find attractive and that are very likely to be awarded for successful performance. However, expectancy theory also suggests that the perceived probability that effort will lead to high performance must be strong before the individual will actually be highly motivated. In this case, the leader's role is one of clarifying the nature of the task (the performance objective), facilitating the employee's attainment of that objective by providing the necessary materials and training, and ensuring the coordination and cooperation of the other individuals required for task accomplishment.

Forms of leadership behavior. To accomplish these ends, according to path-goal theory, leader behavior takes one of four basic forms: (a) supportive leadership—behavior that includes considering the needs of subordinates, displaying concern for their well-being, and creating a friendly climate in the work unit; (b) directive leadership—letting subordinates know what they are expected to do, giving specific guidance, asking them to follow rules and procedures, scheduling and coordinating the work; (c) achievement-oriented leadership—setting challenging goals, seeking performance improvements, emphasizing excellence in performance, and showing confidence that subordinates will attain high standards; and (d) participative leadership—consulting with subordinates and taking their opinions and suggestions into account when making decisions.

Additionally, leader behavior will be interpreted and responded to in different ways depending upon such situational factors as characteristics of subordinates and of the task and environment. Specifically, subordinates' needs for achievement, affiliation, and autonomy, their ability to do the task (job skills, knowledge, experience), and their personality traits, such as self-esteem, form a background or context within which leader behavior produces its effects. Task and environmental characteristics also form a part of the background and include task structure (defined the same as in Fiedler's contingency model), the extent to which the job is mechanized, and the degree of formalization imposed by the organization (e.g., written job descriptions, rules, standard operating procedures, and performance standards). In other words, the effect of leadership behavior on subordinate satisfaction and effort depends upon the situation in which the leadership behavior occurs.

For example, *supportive leadership* behavior should be especially effective when subordinates perceive the job as boring, frustrating, stressful, or otherwise unpleasant. By trying to make the job more tolerable, the leader can directly affect employee satisfaction and perhaps even increase the desirability of the intrinsic aspects of the work. Of course, when the work is perceived as interesting and enjoyable, supportive behavior will not necessarily increase the amount of job satisfaction or motivation. When an employee has relatively high self-esteem or little fear of failure, supportive leadership may have little or no effect on that person's motivation.

Directive leadership should reduce role ambiguity, provided staff nurses do not already know what to do in a particular situation and are therefore dissatisfied. Directive leadership can dissolve the ambiguity and increase the nurses' satisfaction. When the nurse manager explains the relationship between performance and rewards, for instance, these expectancies should increase. In addition, directive leadership can affect the desirability of outcomes for task success by directly affecting the size or magnitude of rewards and punishments. However, these effects will be successful only to the extent that the nurse manager actually has control over specific rewards and punishments. As noted in Chapter 9, money is not the only incentive that can be used to successfully motivate staff members. In addition, the situation determines whether or not the nurse manager who exhibits directive leadership behaviors is likely to increase staff motivation and satisfaction.

Achievement-oriented leadership behaviors should increase the confidence of subordinates in their ability to achieve challenging goals. As noted in the discussion of goal setting theory in Chapter 9, the higher the goal, the higher the performance, even when the goal is not always attained. Thus, the simple act of setting a goal, in addition to the expression of confidence in subordinate ability, should increase employee motivation. Of course, this should be more evident when the task is fairly ambiguous and nonrepetitive—that is, when the task is relatively unstructured.

Similarly, *participative leadership* behavior should have its greatest effect with unstructured tasks. Participation gives subordinates an opportunity to learn more about a task with which they are unfamiliar, and participating in decision making regarding goals, plans, and strategies to attain those goals directly affects employees' understanding of what has to be done and how they must go about accomplishing it. Staff members who have high achievement or autonomy needs should respond more favorably to participative leadership behavior than staff members who have less need for achievement and autonomy and prefer structured tasks with little responsibility for decision making. In fact, such persons may find participation to be threatening and rather unpleasant, leading to less satisfaction with the nurse manager.

In short, the effect of specific leadership behaviors on employee satisfaction and motivation depends directly upon the situation (particularly the degree of task structure) and employee characteristics.

Focusing on nurse manager behaviors in order to improve staff performance is supported by research conducted by Jenkins and Henderson (Jenkins & Henderson, 1984). This study concentrated on how staff nurses, who perform the bulk of patient care, perceived the behaviors of charge nurses. Nurse manager behaviors that recognized the staff nurse's need for belonging, love, social activity, self-respect, status within the organization, recognition, dignity, and appreciation were viewed as essential for motivation and quality patient care.

How well does the path-goal theory of leadership actually work? It is difficult to answer with certainty, because the majority of studies testing this theory have had conceptual or methodological flaws and the theory itself is quite complex. Moreover, the definitions of the four categories of leadership behavior are relatively imprecise and very broad and, while the notion of task structure is logically important, the degree of structure in any given task depends not only on the task itself but the manner in which it is introduced to the employee and the degree of preparation needed for task accomplishment.

To be sure, many nursing tasks are highly structured; however, many aspects of nursing (e.g., patient relationships, orienting new staff members, some special projects) are relatively unstructured. Thus, it is difficult to prescribe a given leadership behavior that would be most successful for a particular task and employee combination. In short, there is no substitute for good common sense and the judicious application of motivation and leadership principles on the part of the nurse manager. There simply is no formula that will work in every situation with every staff member or which can be applied across the board by anyone.

The task of leadership is complex and requires continuous problem solving. To use the path-goal theory of leadership effectively, the nurse manager will need to engage constantly in diagnosing and predicting employee responses to given leadership acts. What path-goal theory does provide, however, is a framework that casts some light on the effects of specific leadership behaviors and the types of situations in which such behaviors are or are not appropriate. It can therefore be an effective leadership tool for nurse managers who regard their leadership responsibilities realistically.

The Normative Model of Decision Participation

Vroom and Yetton have provided a normative, or prescriptive, model for determining the amount of participation in decision making to be used in different situations (Vroom & Yetton, 1973). In essence, this model helps one "to decide how to make a decision." In operation, the model attempts to consider two characteristics that determine the effectiveness of the decision: (a) the quality or rationality of the decision and (b) the acceptance or commitment on the part of subordinates to execute the decision effectively. What follows is a brief synopsis of the model.

Vroom and Yetton suggest that (a) managers' decisions can be made with varying degrees of subordinate participation and (b) the amount of participation depends upon whether subordinates' acceptance of the decision is required to implement it effectively and on whether or not the manager has all of the information needed to make the decision. As Figure 10–2 shows, these latter dimensions combine to form a two-by-two table which can be used to help nurse managers decide when to allow

Figure 10–2 Variables Affecting Use of Participation in Leadership

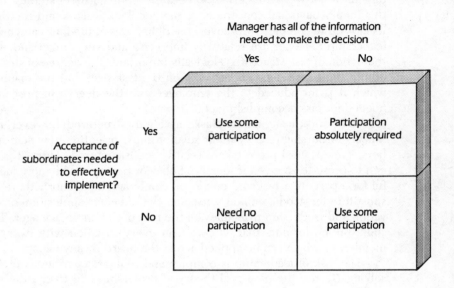

their staff to participate in decision making and to what degree their participation is appropriate, i.e., group problem solving versus delegation.

Participation is not simply present or absent; it varies and can be represented by many different leadership styles. For instance: a nurse manager may (a) delegate all decision authority to a group meeting of staff and agree to live with their decision (delegate); (b) delegate to a staff meeting but participate in the meeting as an "equal" member (join); (c) consult with the staff individually or in a group, make the decision, and then inform the staff (consult); (d) make the decision and then "sell" it to the staff by providing information or other arguments (sell); or (e) simply decide (tell).

It makes sense that the effectiveness of each of these styles differs by the type of decision. Figure 10–3 is a decision tree designed to help nurse managers decide when to use each style of making leadership decisions.

The nurse manager needs to ask herself only three questions: (a) Do I have all the information needed to make the decision? (b) Is acceptance of subordinates required for effective implementation? and (c) If I delegate, will subordinates make a decision that I can live with? Figure 10–3 also indicates the time consideration in each style. Less participative styles usually take less of the manager's time per decision.

Let's look at an example: Ms. Jones, nurse manager of the cardiac intensive care unit, is interested in changing her unit from team nursing to primary care. She has the support of administration and now must consider her staff's reactions. Following Figure 10–3, she asks the following questions:

1. Do I have all the information needed to make the decision? Ms. Jones decides "no"; she needs to know, for example, what staffing patterns would be required and how that would affect personnel costs.

2. Is acceptance by subordinates required for effective implementation? In this case, the answer is obviously yes.

3. If I delegate, will subordinates make a decision I can live with? Ms. Jones decides, no, she is ultimately responsible for the outcome of such a major change and, therefore, must make the final decision.

According to Figure 10–3, the leadership style to use in this case is either sell or consult. Ms. Jones could convince her staff that primary nursing would have many benefits and gain their acceptance (sell). Or she could discuss with the staff the pros and cons of implementing primary

Figure 10–3 Use of Participative Leadership Styles

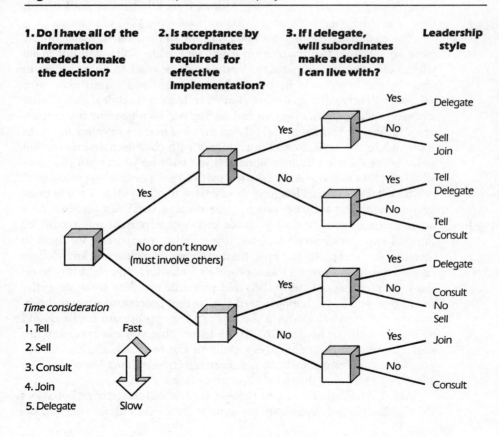

nursing, gather information on staffing, costs, and other possible consequences to the unit and the hospital, ask for their recommendations, and
then make a decision (consult).

A SOCIAL LEARNING APPROACH TO LEADERSHIP

Social learning theory recognizes that although education is one way in
which human beings learn what to do in various situations, most of what
people learn throughout life does not come from formal classroom training or even on-the-job coaching. Indeed, the average child of two or three
has learned an incredible array of behavior, most of it without the aid of
formal parental training. Rather, the child's behaviors are learned vicariously by observing models (e.g., parents, siblings, television) and then
rehearsing these behaviors either covertly or overtly until they are well
practiced. Indeed, the expression "Out of the mouths of babes . . ."
largely reflects instances in which children practice new behaviors without having yet learned fully why they are done or when to do them. The
point is that social learning processes begin at a very early age and continue throughout our entire lives. Although such behaviors are learned,
they cannot be effectively performed without some kind of practice.

For example, reading this book on how to be a nurse manager, or,
more specifically, this chapter on using leadership skills, will not make
you an effective nurse manager. You may know what to do and even to
some extent how to do it, but without practice and experience, your
learning will be minimal. You can, however, learn a great deal about being
a nurse manager (both effective and ineffective) by observing nurse managers for whom you have worked and nurse managers in other units. In
short, while this book should provide you with considerable information
about being a nurse manager, none of it will truly be yours until you actually put it into practice and make it a part of your personal experience.

So what does social learning theory have to offer you as a nurse manager in managing and supervising your nursing staff? Simply this: As a
nurse manager you are a very visible and very important role model for
the staff members whom you lead. If you feel it is important for them to
accomplish some particular task, then use your expertise as a knowledgeable model. Demonstrate the appropriate behaviors, the right way to do
the task, pointing out the pitfalls and potential problem areas along the
way. Once you have demonstrated the correct procedure several times,
ask the staff nurse to perform the task, giving appropriate feedback and
guidance as she or he does so. To the extent that you can involve other
staff nurses in such training (especially in the feedback and social support for task accomplishment), the more effective training becomes. (See
Chapter 14 for more detail on these processes.)

What about nontraining situations? What about the nursing behaviors
that, although not technical, are critical to successful nursing perfor-

mance? What about being at work on time or even a few minutes early to allow time for report without inconveniencing the departing shift? What about displaying cooperation, sensitivity, and tact with other nurses, doctors, and patients? Remember that your behavior as a role model always serves as a guide for the behavior of others. By becoming more consciously aware of what you yourself do, how you do it, and when you do it, you can more easily begin to diagnose the successes and failures of your staff.

When your nurses do not accomplish the job according to your expectations, first ask yourself whether you have provided the appropriate behaviors as a role model. If you have, simply draw their attention to the appropriate behaviors (without necessarily holding yourself up as a supreme example), but gently remind them of what they should be doing and reinforce them with praise when they do the right things. If, on the other hand, your analysis shows that your behavior as role model is deficient, acknowledge your own deficiency to your subordinates and explain the importance of behaving in the appropriate manner and your intention to do so in the future. This requires courage. If you can do it and, in fact, change your own behavior, your new behavior will be noticed and, in most instances, emulated.

Pygmalion Effect

The Pygmalion effect is so named after George Bernard Shaw's play by that name that was popularized on Broadway as "My Fair Lady" (Patton & Giffin, 1981). The Pygmalion effect refers to self-fulfilling prophecy, in which an individual or a situation becomes what one expects it will be. In "My Fair Lady," the professor envisioned the poor, illiterate flower girl as an erudite princess, which she in fact eventually became. A fairy tale, perhaps, but its effect has been demonstrated to be both subtle and profound.

For example, elementary school children were tested at the beginning of the school year and matched in terms of their measured intelligence quotients (IQs). Within each "same IQ" pair, one child was randomly assigned to the "high expectation" group, while the other was randomly assigned to the "low expectation" group. Only the researchers knew that the children in each pair had identical IQs; their classroom teachers were given the expectation of high or low performance for each student in the coming school year. The teachers tried to treat each child as an individual, giving each one the particular attention and training required for his or her own development on the basis of their expectations about each child's potential for improvement.

At the end of the school year, each child's intelligence was again tested. The children who had been placed in the "high expectation" group increased their IQs significantly above those children who were placed in the "low expectation" group. How and in what subtle ways the teachers' expectations were reflected in intelligence scores at the end of the school year is unknown. The fact is that the teachers' expectations produced differences in the children's test-taking behavior.

It is fairly easy to understand how a self-fulfilling prophecy can affect human beings who have a high capacity for perceiving and interpreting the responses of others around them. The power of this effect, however, becomes even more apparent in a study in which graduate students who were conducting research with laboratory rats were given expectations about how smart or how stupid the particular rats were. The rats had presumably been bred for effective learning (smart rats) or slower learning (stupid rats). In fact, the rats were litter mates, born of the same mother and reared in exactly the same environment. The only difference lay in the expectations given the graduate students.

The students trained the rats to learn a sequence of left and right turns in a standard laboratory maze. The rats in the "stupid group" were given the same number of trials to learn the maze as those in the "smart group." At the end of the study the "smart" rats were found to have learned the correct sequence of turns significantly faster than the rats in the "stupid group."

How the graduate students conveyed their expectations to the rats in each group is unknown. Obviously, the behavior of the researchers was very subtle and could not have involved formal language as cues or hints regarding their expectations. Nevertheless, the behavior of the rats was distinctly different, illustrating the very potent effect that our expectations of other individuals actually have.

The Pygmalion effect is closely related to social learning, the focus of which is that behaviors are observed and learned vicariously. The Pygmalion effect demonstrates that not only modeled behaviors but also attitudes, particularly attitudes toward the performer, are learned as well. If these attitudes are so easily learned by rats, then how easily can subtle behaviors of which the nurse manager is unaware be perceived and responded to by staff nurses?

How do the nurse manager's expectations show up in the motivation and performance of the staff nurse? Consider the motivation theories that were discussed in Chapter 9. Why should a staff nurse expect to perform well if she or he perceives that the nurse manager really does not think that she or he can accomplish the task? It is very difficult for most people to hide their true feelings and expectations. If the nurse manager really does not think the staff nurse can accomplish the task, then perhaps the task is much too difficult. The key is to have *realistic expectations* about an individual's ability, to expect a performance that is demanding but attainable for that individual. Leader behaviors must be expressed with a "can do" attitude, the kind of behavior which conveys to the staff nurse, "I expect you to be what you *can* be."

Chapter 9 discussed the shaping of behavior—that is, positively reinforcing approximations to the behavior that is desired. A key factor in shaping, as in the Pygmalion effect, is to have realistic expectations regarding the degree of approximate behavior to be achieved while maintaining conscious efforts to develop the actual kind of behavior that is desired. In short, do not accept "close" as "good enough"; only "acceptable or better" is "good enough." Of course, "good enough" today may not be "good enough" two weeks from now; the realistic expectation can realistically change. But realistic expectations are never impossible to achieve. Realistic expectations or goals should be challenging and should be supported by the nurse manager's coaching and expressions of confidence and pleasure with subordinate successes.

How does this occur? For example, achievement-oriented leadership behavior stresses the attainment of challenging goals. Directive and/or participative leadership behaviors should help to clarify not only what the staff nurse should do but also to understand how to do it. Again, modeling is an excellent way to facilitate this kind of learning. Finally, supportive leadership behavior can be employed to express confidence in the staff nurse's ability to do the job and to express pleasure with the subordinate's success.

After all, the subordinate's success is ultimately the leader's success. If the nurse manager takes pride in the staff nurse's success and does everything in his or her power to bring about that kind of success, then the nurse manager will, indeed, be an effective leader. The important point is that our attitudes are expressed very subtly in our behaviors. Realistic expectations and genuine help in trying to develop employee performance will go a long way toward achieving that end.

LEADERSHIP IN GROUPS

Hospital nursing is a continuous problem-solving, interacting group task. Because staff nurses work in close proximity and frequently depend upon each other to accomplish their jobs, the character or climate of group interaction is extremely important. A viable group atmosphere is one in which staff members feel free to talk about what concerns them, to critique and offer suggestions, and to experiment with new behaviors without threat. Such an atmosphere can only be maintained in a work group that is warm and supportive and is relatively unhindered by interpersonal conflicts and political infighting. Maintaining such an atmosphere or climate is a difficult task for nurse managers.

In order to gain a clearer understanding of this leadership task, we must first consider in detail what we mean by a group, how and why groups are formed, and what factors influence group effectiveness.

What Is a Group?

One can conceive of a group in terms of (a) *perception*—if individuals see themselves as a group, then a group exists; (b) *structure*—if two or more individuals interact so that they perform some function, have a set of rote relationships, and have a set of norms to regulate their behavior, then a group exists; (c) *motivation*—if a collection of people exist whose existence as a collection is rewarding to each individual, then a group exists; or (d) *interpersonal interaction*—if several individuals communicate and interact with one another regularly over time, then a group exists (see Steers, 1981).

An integration of these definitions provides us with the following definition: A group is two or more individuals who, over time, share a common set of norms, have different roles, and interact with each other or together to pursue common goals.

Group Formation

There are two primary types of groups. *Informal* groups evolve naturally as a result of individuals' self-interest. They are not part of any organizational design or appointed leadership. An example is a group of people who regularly eat lunch together. *Formal* groups are work units developed by the organization either temporarily or permanently. Examples are sections of departments and committees. Often informal groups form and work against formal groups. Most individuals are simultaneously members of many formal and informal groups both in and out of the organization that employs them.

People join groups for many reasons:

1. *Security*—People want protection from threats; groups provide support.

2. *Proximity*—People often come together because they are located together.

3. *Group goals*—People form groups to pursue goals that cannot be pursued alone.

4. *Economics*—People often form groups (e.g., collective bargaining organizations) to pursue economic self-interest.

5. *Social needs*—People often join groups because they want to belong, be needed, or because they want to lead.

6. *Self-esteem needs*—People often join prestigious groups to increase their self-esteem.

Finally, groups typically in developing follow a set pattern of activities: they *form*, come together; *storm*, develop leaders and roles; *norm*, accept goals and rules for acceptable behavior; and *perform*, agree on basic purposes and activities and start working.

Group Effectiveness

Many factors determine a group's effectiveness once it emerges or is formed by the institution. These characteristics are reviewed in the following sections.

Group task. The task of a group can influence effectiveness by influencing an individual's motivation and imposing requirements or group process. If a task is boring, inefficiently designed, frustrating, or does not fulfill members' needs (such as autonomy, feedback, or task significance), each group member's effort will decrease.

The more people who work on an additive task (group performance is the sum of individual performance), the more resources can be used. On a disjunctive task (the group succeeds if only one member succeeds), more people provide a greater likelihood that someone in the group will be able to solve the problem. With a divisible task (tasks with a division of labor), more people provide a greater opportunity for specialization. However, with a conjunctive task (the group succeeds only if all members succeed), more people increase the likelihood that one person can slow up the group. Consequently, group productivity often depends on the group task.

On many divisible tasks, the level of interdependence is important. There are three kinds of interdependence: (a) *pooled*, where each individual contributes, but none are dependent on any other member (e.g., a committee discussion); (b) *sequential*, where each member must coordinate his or her activities with the members on each side or above and below them (e.g., an assembly line); and (c) *reciprocal*, where each member must coordinate his or her activities with every other individual in the group (e.g., a hockey team).

Finally, task uncertainty plays a role in group effectiveness. Tasks that are highly uncertain require individuals to process more information, identify multiple goal paths, increase effort, and coordinate activities more precisely. Consequently, task uncertainty places more demands on group members.

Group size. Though adding group members typically increases productivity, sometimes a phenomenon called *social loafing* occurs, in that as the size of a group increases each member contributes less of his or her potential. Also, large group size has been found to be associated with low satisfaction, higher absenteeism, and turnover.

Group composition. Groups tend to perform better the higher the abilities of each member. But coordination of effort, proper utilization of abilities, and task strategies must be considered. Furthermore, homogeneous groups tend to function more harmoniously while heterogeneous groups may experience conflict. Homogeneity has its risks, however, in that members may fall into what is called *groupthink*—a failure to explore alternative approaches or ways of thinking. Also, homogeneous groups may contain redundant strengths and weaknesses.

Spatial arrangement.   Who interacts with whom is an essential consideration in groups. It is considered in detail in Chapter 8. Closed groups—those whose members rarely interact with outsiders—are not as creative as open groups. Interactive patterns within the group must also be related to group task as just seen. Open communication will also facilitate performance on complex or uncertain tasks. It has also been found that a person's feeling of participation is related to her position in a communications network; that group leadership is more likely to emerge from the more central positions in communications networks; that overcentralized communications are effective in implementing tasks but not in developing new strategies; and that information is lost or distorted if it must travel through too many people.

Reward structure.   American organizations are prone to reward individuals rather than groups, but competitive or individualistic reward systems can be destructive in groups requiring members to cooperate to achieve success.

Group cohesiveness.   Group cohesiveness is the extent to which members of a group are motivated to remain in the group. Members of highly cohesive groups put more effort into group activities, are more satisfied, are absent less, and are more influenced by group goals. Group cohesiveness can be increased by several means: (a) making it more difficult to join the group; (b) rewarding the group as a unit; (c) increasing group status; (d) allowing participation in goal identification; (e) increasing frequency of interactions; and (f) developing member trust in each other. Nursing organizations have used many of these means to increase organizational cohesiveness.

Group norms.   Norms are expectations shared by group members that define proper conduct and attitude for group members. Norms are critical for group functioning in that they allow members to predict each other's behavior to some extent. Also, norms serve as standards against which the behaviors of group members can be judged. Those who deviate from the group norms are likely to find overt and covert pressure brought to bear for conformity. The key to considering group norms for the nurse manager is that which relates to level of work effort of members. If these norms conform to organizational goals the group will be seen to be effective.

Consequently, groups will be effective when:

1. The members are attracted to it

2. Members trust each other

3. Norms and goals of the group are congruent with organizational goals

4. Group size and structure and heterogeneity match the task to be accomplished

5. Group members are motivated to communicate openly and cooperate

6. The group is rewarded for goal attainment

7. Social loafing is reduced

Groups can often solve problems that individuals cannot because they bring more expertise to bear and are more likely to take risks and be creative. However, groups may engage in groupthink or defuse responsibility—groups tend to be less responsible than individuals. Groups are not a universal solution to all problems but can be used effectively in many situations. However, to be used, the leader must understand the dynamics of the group formed.

Intergroup Conflict

Most groups must interact with other groups; intergroup relations are an important element in organizations. Organizations require coordination between groups to be productive, yet groups often develop rivalries and antagonisms. Groups often compete for rewards, status, resources, and privileges. Schein (1980) has suggested that the following may be observed of groups in competition:

1. Within the competing group:
   a. Group cohesion increases
   b. Members become more task-oriented
   c. Authority becomes more centralized
   d. Activities become more organized

2. Between the competing groups:
   a. The other is viewed as an enemy
   b. One's own group's strengths are overestimated and vice-versa
   c. Communication between groups decreases
   d. When forced into interaction with the other group, only that which reinforces the original predisposition toward the other group is heard

According to Schein, there are two approaches to managing intergroup conflict: (a) deal with the competition after it occurs, and (b) prevent its occurrence in the first place.

Strategies for minimizing ongoing competition are:

1. Identify a common enemy.

2. Appeal to a common goal.

3. Bring representatives of the competing groups into direct contact with one another.

4. Train members of the competing groups to minimize conflict.

Actions to be taken to prevent intergroup conflict include:

1. Reward groups for contributions to the organization.

2. Reward groups for cooperating with other groups.

3. Stimulate frequent interaction between members of various groups.

4. Reduce isolation and withdrawal of groups from other groups.

5. Rotate members between groups.

6. Avoid situations of lose-lose or win-lose competition between groups (see Chapter 22)

7. Emphasize sharing of resources.

Conferences and Committees

The nurse manager participates in both formal and informal groups. Formal groups include conferences and committees while informal groups occur whenever people gather for some period of interaction. Conferences are usually one-time affairs, held for a limited time and purpose such as to deal with a specific patient's problem, while committees may have an ongoing assigned task.

Both can be classified in relation to their purpose, membership, and leadership. Figure 10–4 shows various types and purposes of conferences; the purpose usually determines the members and the leader. For example, a nurse manager might call a report conference to request an up-

Figure 10–4 Types of Nursing Conferences and Their Purposes

Type	Purpose
Direction-giving conference	give job assignments specify areas of responsibility give client care information
Client-centered conference	analyze one client's problem discuss alternative solutions plan for implementing solutions
Content conference	learn new information related to nursing care
Report conference	inform leader about member activities
General problems conference	discuss communication problems among group members

Adapted from content in Douglass, L. M. & Bevis, E. O. *Nursing Management and Leadership in Action.* St. Louis: C. V. Mosby, 1983. Used with permission.

Figure 10–5 Advantages of Assigning of Tasks to Groups or Individuals

Assignment to Groups	Assignment to Individuals
Utilizes diversity of member resources and opinions	Reduces pressure toward conformity
Recognizes and corrects errors sooner	Encourages individual initiative
Increases members' motivation	Centralizes responsibility and authority
Makes group decisions more acceptable to those who helped make them	Facilitates faster problem solving and decision making

date from staff members regarding the effectiveness of a new staffing procedure.

Committees are relatively permanent groups with institutional or organizational sanction. They are usually directed toward a specific purpose, have some mechanism for selecting members, and have authority to make recommendations or decisions. Committees are usually formed when the input of various people is necessary for information gathering and decision making and when persons representing several units will be instrumental in implementing the decisions made. However, assignment of a given task to one or two individuals, rather than a committee, may be preferable if the nature of the task is complex and requires a high degree of coordination. According to Vroom and Yetton, the decision to utilize groups is based on the quality of the decision, the acceptance of the decision by subordinates, and the time required to make the decision (Vroom & Yetton, 1973). The advantages of assigning tasks to groups or individuals are shown in Figure 10-5. The structure of the organization, the nature of the task, and the preference of the manager and other administrators influence the choice between committees versus individuals.

The disadvantages of committees must be weighed against their advantages. Committees are expensive considering the hourly pay per member, preparation time, secretarial help for minutes, and calls or memos reminding members of the time and place. These disadvantages must be compared to advantages such as group input, participative decision making, and other factors such as those listed in Figure 10–5.

A number of group characteristics influence the nature and effectiveness of small group communication. For one thing, the status and authority of each member in relation to the other, their past experiences together and current relationships both individually and as a group, and the expectations and preconceptions they have of each other will influence the communication patterns they use. Second, the structure of the group imposes certain patterns of interaction. If one's supervisor is chairperson of a committee, for instance, the member will tend to interact with that chairman in the same pattern as the two normally interact in their superior/subordinate pattern. Time and place characteristics are additional determinants of communication. When and where meetings are scheduled may facilitate or hinder specific member participation. And a final consideration is the expertise of each member in relation to the assigned task.

The behavior of each member may be positive, negative, or neutral in relationship to the group's goals. Members may contribute very little or they may use the group to fill personal needs. Some members may assume most of the responsibility for the group action, thereby "helping" the less participative members to be noncontributing members. Appropriate behaviors, listed below, can facilitate the group's action.

1. Come prepared with necessary information.

2. Listen to others with an open mind.

3. Contribute information, ideas, and opinions.

4. Ask other members for ideas and opinions.

5. Request clarification of information.

6. Recognize opposing points of view.

7. Keep remarks on the topic.

8. Be willing to state disagreement and give rationale.

9. Volunteer to help with the implementation of decisions, when appropriate.

Leadership behaviors facilitate group communication and movement toward acceptable decisions. Facilitative leader behaviors are as follows:

1. Establish an atmosphere conducive to participation and cohesiveness.

2. Encourage participation by all members.

3. Keep the group focused on the task assigned.

4. Do not allow one person to dominate the group.

5. Focus the discussions on one topic at a time.

6. Allow persons with dissenting opinions to explain their point of view.

7. Summarize discussion and ask the group to arrive at a decision.

8. Determine the plan of action for implementing the decision.

9. Request arrangements for follow-up and individual members.

Just as in one-to-one interactions, the nurse manager can use her or his participation in a group, as either leader or member, to effectively perform all of the other tasks of management including motivation, training, and conflict resolution. The nurse manager's skills are most challenged in group interactions. The manager must attend to individual interactions as well as group process. However, the nurse is only one part of an interaction, and the context, the roles of participants, past experiences, and institutional determinants are other influences on a communication system made up of two or more people.

GROUP MEETINGS

Thompson and Wood (1980) have described a meeting as a play calling for a script, preparation of the actors, and a competent director to insure a successful performance. They summarize the contributions of the various components as follows:

1. *The director*, known as the chairperson, who is responsible for planning the meeting, preparing the agenda, directing the meeting, and for follow-up of plans made.

2. *The script*, known as the agenda, which is important in determining the effectiveness of the group's activities. Thompson and Wood suggest the following guidelines for agenda preparation: "(a) if you can put it in a memo, don't put it on the agenda; (b) have a clear purpose behind every meeting you hold and behind every agenda item on the agenda; and (c) every item should require some kind of action by the group" (Thompson & Wood, 1980).

   Chairpersons should have in mind what kinds of outcomes they expect in terms of group discussion, a plan of action, smaller subgroups formed for specific purposes, or policy decisions to be reached. In addition, they should plan the agenda so that the meeting will move along and keep the participants involved. Careful planning, such as determining items in order of priority and their potential impact on the group, is essential. Thompson and Wood also suggest sending out the agenda and all necessary material a week prior to the meeting so that all people can be prepared.

3. *The actors*, otherwise known as the group members, are not in the audience to be entertained; they are the participants. Their responsibility is to come prepared, to respond to others' ideas and comments, and to make contributions in a clear, concise, and logical manner.

4. *The stage*, or meeting room. Where the meeting is held and where people sit affect what happens in the meeting and the outcomes. If conflict between participants is expected or if one participant is a great deal more powerful than the other(s), then the site chosen for the meeting should be in neutral territory.

   The head of the table is the most powerful position and should usually be occupied by the chairperson. Those who sit on the sidelines may see themselves as of lesser importance to the group's activities or may be antagonists. The seat at the foot of the table may also be selected by an antagonist.

Management is a very complicated, multifaceted function that demands extensive knowledge and skill—but one thing must be very clear: managing others in today's health care institutions is a *communication process*. The inability to communicate automatically leads to the inability to manage, no matter how much one *knows* about leadership, organizational theory, or nurse management. Communication is a skill and can be learned. Nurse managers must learn to communicate succinctly and effectively and with widely diverse groups of people. Furthermore, the financial and consumer relations responsibilities newly added to the job of nurse manager require new types of communication skill. Who knows what tomorrow will bring—but if one continues to learn and *can* communicate what is learned, that person will be successful.

SUMMARY

- One of the responsibilities of a nurse manager is leadership—the employment of specific behaviors and strategies to influence individuals and groups toward goal attainment in specific situations.

- Leadership differs from management, which is a more global term encompassing processes of planning, organizing, directing (supervising), and controlling. Leader behavior can be learned.

- Leadership is the exercise of power. Power can come from several sources: control over rewards, control over sanctions, control of information, authority given by the hospital, expertise, and referent power.

- The search for leadership characteristics has focused on personality traits, leader behaviors, and leadership styles. None of these approaches has adequately defined successful leadership.

- Leadership styles include authoritarian, democratic, permissive, bureaucratic, mollifying, autocratic, parental, and multicratic.

- Fiedler took leadership beyond identifying styles/behaviors with his contingency theory. He said that successful leadership was an interaction of leadership style and situation.

- House developed path-goal theory, which says that a leader is effective to the extent that she helps subordinates identify goals and paths to those goals.

- Vroom and Yetton provide a model of participative leadership that is prescriptive—it tells the nurse manager which style of leadership to use in different situations.

- Nurse managers must pay attention to the examples they provide staff and their expectations of staff members. These will both influence staff behavior.

- Hospital nursing is a team effort. The nurse manager must develop an understanding for group communication and interpersonal attraction and use that understanding to develop a supportive climate to foster group cohesiveness.

- Nurses interact in many groups, conferences, and committees. A knowledge of group theory and dynamics is critical.

BIBLIOGRAPHY

Fiedler, F. E. (1967). *A theory of leadership effectiveness*. New York: McGraw-Hill.

French, J. R. P., and Raven, B. (1960). The bases of social power. In: *Group dynamics*. 2nd ed. Cartwright, D., Zander, A. (editors). Evanston, IL: Row, Peterson.

Hoffman, G., and Graivier, P. (1983). *Speak the language of success*. New York: G. P. Putnam.

House, R. J., and Mitchell, T. R. (1974). Path-goal theory of leadership. *J of Contemp Bus*, 3:81.

Jenkins, R. L., and Henderson, R. L. (1984). Motivating the staff: What nurses expect from their supervisors. *Nurs Mngmt*, 15(2):13.

La Monica, E. (1983). *Nursing leadership and management: An experimental approach*. Monterey, CA: Wadsworth Health Sciences Division.

Levenstein, A. (1985). So you want to be a leader? *Nurs Mngmt*, 16(3):74–75.

Locke, F. A., and Schweiger, D. M. (1979). Participation in decision making: One more look. In: *Research in organizational behavior*. Vol. 1. Staw, B. (editor). Greenwich, CT: JAI Press.

McGee, R. F. (1984). Leadership styles: A survey. *Nursing Success Today*, 1:26.

McGregor, D. (1960). *The human side of enterprise*. New York: McGraw-Hill.

Mitchell, T. R. (1982). *People in organizations*. 2nd ed. New York: McGraw-Hill.

Moloney, M. M. (1979). *Leadership in nursing: Theory, strategies, action*. St. Louis: C. V. Mosby.

Patton, B. R., and Giffin, K. (1981). *Interpersonal communication in action*. 3rd ed. New York: Harper & Row.

Schein, E. H. (1980). *Organization psychology*. Englewood Cliffs, NJ: Prentice-Hall.

Steers, R. M. (1981). *Introduction to organizational behavior*. Santa Monica, CA: Goodyear.

Stogdill, R. M. (1959). *Individual behavior and group achievement*. New York: Oxford University Press.

Thompson, A. M., and Wood, M.D. (1980). *Management strategies for women*. New York: Simon & Schuster.

Vroom, V. H. (1976). Leadership. In: *Handbook of industrial and organizational psychology*. Dunnette, M. D. (editor). Chicago: Rand McNally.

Vroom, V. H., and Yetton, P. W. (1973). *Leadership and decision making*. Pittsburgh, PA: University of Pittsburgh Press.

Personal Organization

Setting Priorities

The Role of Objectives

Nurse Manager's Time Wasters

Interruptions

Telephone Calls

Paging and Beeping

Drop-In Visitors

Respecting Time

Scheduling

Paper Work

Delegation

Authority

Assignments

Underdelegation

What Not to Delegate

Summary

TIME MANAGEMENT IS a misnomer. No one manages time. What is managed is how time is used. The nurse manager, like all other managers, must use time wisely. The work time of the nurse manager may be broken into many increments, the most common of which is a work shift: typically, an eight-hour period beginning and ending with reports and filled with numerous activities and events. A given shift could involve time spent on many activities: staff scheduling, conducting daily rounds, counseling a patient's family, reading and responding to mail, training a new staff member, or writing an incident report, to mention only a few. Some days, unexpected emergencies and crises must be absorbed into the schedule, and the eight-hour shift may become a nine- or ten-hour workday.

It is a mistake to think of a work shift, or even a workweek, only in terms of activities and events. The nurse manager may become involved in a myriad of activities and events, out of which must come some sense of organization. That means effectively planning and scheduling work time to ensure that the most important work is completed and sufficient time is left for the unexpected emergencies and crises that are sure to happen. Good time management can ensure clearly measurable outcomes, and the well-organized nurse manager is one who realistically plans and schedules. The focus is not on activities and events, but rather on the outcomes that can be achieved in the allotted time. Activities are scheduled within the hours and minutes available.

Time is the most scarce resource of the nurse manager. If an hour or a minute of the work shift is wasted, or allowed to be wasted by others, it is lost forever. The nurse manager may lengthen a workday to complete some important tasks, but time has not been affected. Time cannot be lengthened or shortened, only more or less of it used.

It is possible for the nurse manager to become overloaded with responsibilities, with more to do than should be expected in the time available. This is typical. There is never sufficient time to get involved in all the activities, situations, and events in which the nurse manager might like to become involved. No one has the time to do everything he or she wants to do but, although there is not time for everything, there is always time to do the most important things. Thus, effective planning and scheduling of the nurse manager's work shift begin with establishing priorities.

PERSONAL ORGANIZATION

Personal organization occurs when the nurse manager has clearly defined priorities that are based upon well-defined, measurable, and achievable objectives. The nurse manager does not work alone. Priorities and objectives are often related to those of many other professionals, as well as to objectives of patients and their families. How time will be used is often a matter of resolving conflicts among competing needs.

Setting Priorities

Nurse managers may want to do more than is actually possible, and others may expect or demand more from nurse managers than is actually possible. They must therefore determine the highest priorities and make sure the most important things get done on a timely basis. Setting priorities becomes easier when the term, priority, is understood. Most dictionaries consistently list two connotations of the word priority: (a) that which is most important or most valuable; and (b) that which comes first. Priorities cannot be set effectively without considering both meanings. When there are several competing functions, activities, or events to which time must be given, two questions must be asked. First, "What is the relative importance of each?" For example, what is the relative importance of the annual division report, a subordinate's performance report, a patient's complaint, and a routine staff meeting? Second, "What is the relative urgency of each?" Considering both of these helps one decide which will be first to receive attention.

Figure 11–1   Importance-Urgency Chart

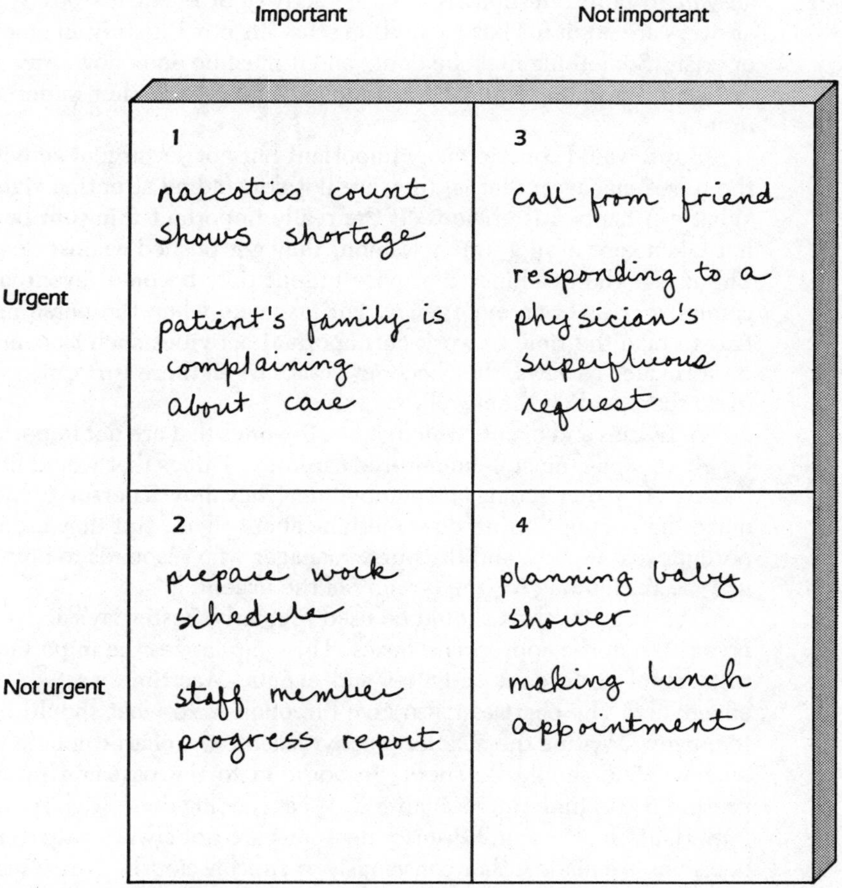

	Important	Not important
Urgent	**1** narcotics count shows shortage patient's family is complaining about care	**3** call from friend responding to a physician's superfluous request
Not urgent	**2** prepare work schedule staff member progress report	**4** planning baby shower making lunch appointment

How time will be used is based on the priorities established. Postponing or cancelling a routine staff meeting with nothing really urgent on its agenda might be a wise decision if that time could be spent on preparing the annual division report due next week. Setting priorities also involves deciding what not to do as well as what to do. In addition, some activities and demands are so unimportant that a nurse manager should not give them any time at all.

Figure 11–1 is a chart that can be used to analyze how priority decisions are now being made, as well as to determine the relative priorities of activities to be planned and scheduled. For any activity or event, ask, "Is it important?" If the answer is yes, it fits the left-hand vertical column of the chart; if the answer is no, it fits the right-hand column. To decide if it fits in the first or second horizontal column, ask, "Is it urgent?" If the answer to both questions is yes, the activity or event fits box 1; if both answers are no, it fits box 4. Anything that fits box 1 is truly an emergency or crisis. Something must be done, and it must be done now. Any activity or event fitting box 4 may be a waste of time. It is neither important nor urgent.

Box 2 would contain many important but not yet urgent activities for the nurse manager; that is, they are not demanding attention right now. What can happen is obvious. If the really important things in box 2 are not taken care of in a timely fashion, they get pushed against deadlines. The closer the deadline, the more urgent they become, eventually becoming a crisis or an emergency. For instance, when the nurse manager fails to take the time to work on important activities such as completing performance reviews, they become a crisis when there isn't time available to do them and do them well.

Activities and events which fit box 3—ones that are not important but highly urgent—must be monitored carefully. Things that would fit in this box are often demanding and compelling. They draw a person to them and make the person want to do something about them. But they are not important, just urgent, and the nurse manager who responds to box 3 items may be responding to "the tyranny of the urgent."

This priority chart should be used regularly. Yesterday's activities can be written in the appropriate boxes. This emphasizes the importance and urgency of yesterday's activities and events. Was time wasted, or used effectively? The chart can also give direction as to what should be done tomorrow. Writing the next day's activities into the chart can help to focus on how time should be spent. In addition to the past and future, the present use of time can be analyzed. What is being done "right now"? Is it important? Is it urgent? Priority decisions are not always easy, but these decisions are made either consciously or subconsciously. Nurse managers must make these decisions conscientiously.

The Role of Objectives

Personal organization is the key to using time effectively. Well-organized nurse managers place primary emphasis on planning and scheduling those activities that fulfill their role responsibilities and result in the achievement of the unit's objectives. These are covered in Chapter 3. The nurse manager's personal objectives are derived from these role responsibilities and unit objectives. Defining personal objectives and achieving them are keys to success.

Objectives of the nurse manager may be subdivided. Subobjectives may be shared with an assistant nurse manager, unit clerks, or staff nurses.

When these subordinates achieve their own objectives, the nurse manager's objectives are achieved. A manager works through others.

Without measurable, realistic, and achievable objectives it is difficult to determine achievement and evaluate performance. The nurse manager is evaluated in terms of accomplishing specific objectives and fulfilling role responsibilities. The nurse manager's subordinates are evaluated on their accomplishment of the subobjectives assigned to them and fulfillment of their role responsibilities.

Five major questions must always be answered if the nurse manager is to be organized:

1. What are the specific objectives to be achieved?

2. What are the specific activities necessary to achieve these objectives?

3. How much time is required for each activity?

4. Which activities can be planned and scheduled for concurrent action and which must be planned and scheduled sequentially?

5. Which activities can be delegated to staff?

All objectives are not equally important. Also, some are more urgent, as are the activities required to achieve them. Activities must be planned and scheduled in terms of priority, and it must be estimated how long each activity is going to take. Once this is decided, the activities can be planned with sufficient time scheduled for each one. Completing these activities as scheduled is critical to managing time effectively. Without personal planning it is easy to become involved in "activity traps"—i.e., any activity that cannot be related to an important objective. Usually, activity traps are neither planned nor scheduled. They waste the nurse manager's time (see Figure 11–1, box 4).

In all cases, the relative importance and urgency of objectives and role responsibilities of the nurse manager must be considered. Personal organization for the nurse manager is synonymous with clearly defining priorities and working on the highest priorities first.

Plans and schedules should be written with an important point in mind. They usually will not work out as written, since it is almost impossible to have a perfect plan and a perfect schedule; unexpected events and problems are bound to occur. Some activities take longer than expected; emergencies occur. A major purpose of a plan and schedule of activities is to give its user "a track to run on." If for one reason or another the nurse manager is side-tracked, there is a plan and schedule to which to return. Priorities for the day can be reviewed. If activities have to be rescheduled, the remainder of the work shift can be devoted to those items with the greatest importance and urgency.

Figure 11-2 Interruption Log

Employee Karen Tarbell, RN HN   Date 9-12   Department Medical-Surgical

WHO	T/V	I/T	TIME	HOW LONG	TOPICS DISCUSSED	IMP	TIME SAVING ACTIONS
Unit Clerk	V	T	8:40	6m	plastic bag shortage	B	Let unit clerk know she has authority to order bags
Social Worker	T	T	9:00	4m	wants info for a transfer patient	C	Refer to patient's RN
Dr. Nelson	V	T	9:09	14m	request extended treatment time ball game and his new car	A	Stand up during conversation especially to reduce socializing.
Alice, RN	V	T	9:33	15m	pickup light meter - not available talked about boyfriend problem	A U	Should not have asked leading questions about boyfriend.
Dr. Nelson	V	T	10:10	2m	lost otoscope	U	
Carol, HN	T	T	10:15	2m	call for lunch appointment at 12:15	U	
Marsha, LPN	V	T	10:25	3m	request time off return light meter	C B	Find someone else to check out equipment — maybe unit clerk
Alice, RN	T	I	10:30	2m	light meter available	B	
Unit Clerk	V	I	10:42	4m	go to see if Dr. Nelson found his otoscope	U	Could've called him & saved time. Did I need to check at all?
Barb, RN	T	I	10:55	10m	call for lunch appointment talked about movie Barb saw	U U	Save movie conversation for lunch
Alice, RN	V	T	11:15	1m	pickup light meter	B	Check out procedure above
Sharon, LPN	V	T	11:30	7m	dropped in about "?" as usual	U	Discuss this habit with Sharon.
Marsha & Sue	V	T	11:34	30s	report they are going to lunch	B	Do I encourage too much socializing?
Dr. Nelson	T	T	11:37	17m	concerned about a patient's treatment	A	
Patient's Family	V	T	12:06	15m	good PR talk with patient's husband	A	

WHO = Who discussion was with

T = Telephone   I = I initiated T or V
V = Visit   T = They initiated T or V
TIME = Time of interruption

HOW LONG = Length of interruption
TOPICS DISCUSSED = List items discussed vertically
IMP = A-high, B-moderate, C-low, and U-unimportant
TIME SAVING ACTIONS = What can be done to save time

Note: It may require more than one line to record a single interruption.

NURSE MANAGER'S TIME WASTERS

Time is wasted by the nurse manager when it is devoted to something that really need not be done. Time is also wasted when more time than is actually necessary is spent in doing something. Interruptions and distractions are major time wasters. Many should not receive the attention of the nurse manager, and often those given attention could be dealt with in less time.

Interruptions

Not all interruptions are negative. An interruption occurs any time the nurse manager is stopped in the middle of one activity to give attention to something else. An emergency or crisis, for instance, may cause the nurse manager to interrupt daily rounds. These emergencies and crises may be more important and urgent than completing rounds at that time.

The nurse manager's work shift is subject to many interruptions, many of which have a negative impact on the nurse manager's performance. A staff member who drops in or telephones when the nurse manager is in the middle of writing a report is likely to be a time-wasting interrupter. One must first determine the interruptions that are actually experienced so that positive action can be taken to eliminate as many as possible and more effectively control those which cannot be eliminated. However, an interruption that is more important and urgent than the activity in which the nurse manager is presently involved is a positive interruption; it deserves immediate attention.

The nurse manager should keep an interruption log (see Figure 11–2) for several days. In the log should be recorded who interrupted, the nature of the interruption, when it occurred, how long it lasted, what topics were discussed, the importance of the topics, and time-saving actions to be taken. Analysis of these data may identify patterns that can be used to plan ways to reduce the frequency and duration of interruptions. These patterns may indicate that certain staff members are the most frequent interrupters and greatest sources of distraction. They call on the telephone or drop in frequently to discuss a number of topics.

The nature of the topics discussed may follow some definite pattern, too. For example, a major part of all conversations might be spent discussing current events, family activities, or personal matters rather than topics related to work. On the other hand, some interruptions and topics discussed might relate to important hospital policies or nursing concerns that need resolution or clarification. The interruption patterns may indicate that most of them occur during a certain part of the work shift or during a certain part of the week. They may also demonstrate that some staff members and co-workers are more likely to waste the nurse manager's time than others. Figure 11–2 presents the interruptions experienced by one nurse manager between 8:00 A.M. and lunch. The nurse manager must consider what time-saving actions, if any, should be taken.

Any patterns identified should help in taking corrective action. One must recognize that the nurse manager is an essential part of whatever patterns are found; it is possible to be a part of the problem and not even realize it. He or she is either causing these patterns to develop or is allowing others to create them. It is the nurse manager's responsibility to control how time is used.

Behavioral patterns are habits. People often act and react without even being aware. Interruption patterns may result from vicarious learning or direct positive reinforcement. Nurse managers may reinforce unnecessary interruptions, which increases the probability of their recurrence. Or nurse managers may model behavior that may be imitated by others. If nurse managers do not demonstrate respect for time, then neither will those with whom they interact.

Effective communications between the nurse manager and others are essential. Undercommunication can have a devastating effect upon the success of a unit, as can overcommunication. The latter often occurs today because of a misunderstood and abused organizational concept called the "open door" policy. In many organizations an "open door" policy has come to mean that any person may walk in or telephone any other person at any time and take as long as they choose. This is "open communications," not an "open door." An "open door" policy means that when there is something important to discuss, time will be made available to discuss it. It does not necessarily mean right now.

Telephone Calls

Telephone calls are a major source of interruption, and the interruption log will provide considerable insight for the nurse manager regarding the nature of telephone calls received. Today it is not possible to function effectively without a telephone. Unfortunately, some people do not function effectively with a telephone. A ringing telephone is highly compelling; it draws a person to it and makes it necessary to do something about it immediately. Few people allow a telephone to ring unanswered. The nurse manager has many telephone calls, some of them time wasting. Almost all telephone calls can be controlled by the nurse manager; but if she or he does not control a telephone conversation, then the other party will. Here are some tips on how to handle telephone calls effectively:

Minimize small talk and socializing. Many telephone conversations start with, "Hello . . . how are you?" The caller may take more time than available to answer this question. Try, "Hello . . . what can I do for you?" This approach gets to business first. It is always best to be warm, friendly, and courteous, but not allow others to waste time with inappropriate or extensive small talk.

Plan calls. The nurse manager who plans telephone calls does not waste anyone's time, including that of the person called. A small pad or note paper kept by the telephone is essential. Topics to be discussed are written down before the call is made. Less time is spent calling back to inform the other party of an important point or ask a forgotten question.

Set a time. The nurse manager may have a number of calls to return as well as calls to initiate. It is best to set aside a time—perhaps each day or half day—to handle routine phone calls. An attempt should be made not to interrupt what is being done at the moment. If an answer is necessary before a project can be continued, then phone; if not, phone for the information at a later time. Often, getting needed information later will not impede the progress of a project.

Use a timer. The time a call is received or placed should be written on the note pad. Telephone conversations usually last much longer than expected. Recording the length of telephone conversations is important for an interruption log, and it is important to be aware of the length of all telephone conversations. Timing calls makes the nurse manager more time conscious.

State and ask for preferred call times. If a party called is not available, ask for two time frames in which the call might be placed again. Ask, for example, "Would it be best if I called back between 11:00 and 12:00 this morning or between 3:30 and 4:00 this afternoon?" If neither choice is good, a better time can be negotiated. When the other party is to return a call, preferred times should also be stated. Say, for example, "Could you have her return my call between 1:00 and 2:00 this afternoon or between 9:00 and 11:00 tomorrow morning?" This approach gives the caller more control. It prevents what is commonly called "telephone merry-go-round."

Paging and Beeping

For years, paging and, more recently, beeping have been important communication tools in hospitals. In an emergency or crisis, immediate messages are essential. Unfortunately, paging and beeping frequently interrupt activities that should not be interrupted. Often, more discretion should be used in determining when a person should be paged or beeped. High priority activities should not be interrupted by low priority messages. There are times when persons should inform the paging and beeping service that they are not to be interrupted unless there is an emergency or crisis. As soon as they are free, they can check the service for messages. Those who carry beepers should inform the service when they are turning the beeper off, where they can be reached during the time it is off, and when it is turned back on. Paging and beeping will continue to be important to the nurse manager, but they should not be misused or abused.

Drop-In Visitors

The nurse manager may have many visitors. All who visit are important, but what they wish to visit about may not be. Even the topics that are important may not be urgent. It may be necessary to spend time with a visitor, but it may not be so urgent that the time be "right now." Below are several important ideas for handling visitors and visiting others.

Meet visitors outside of office. When possible, visitors should be met in a reception area or hall. The nurse manager can then decide when a visitor should be invited to the office for longer conversations.

Keep visits short. Standing up when a drop-in visitor appears will help. Standing conversations are likely to be shorter than sitting ones. If the visitor has an important and urgent topic, he or she can be invited to sit down. Standing up is also more courteous than remaining seated and increases control. When the conversation should end, a short step and gesture toward the door, or standing up if seated, communicates that point to the visitor.

Give a few minutes, but stay in control. If interrupted and a few minutes are available, ask the visitor if the message is brief and tell him or her how much time can be given. When that time is up, decide if the discussion should continue or be terminated, and assert control. If the conversation should continue, tell the visitor the time you allowed is up but the situation is too important to stop now. If the situation is less important and urgent than other pressing matters, end the conversation and set up a later appointment, if necessary.

Encourage appointments. Routine matters should be dealt with during routine appointments. Emergencies and crises are not routine and should not be treated as such. The nurse manager will have many conversations a day with co-workers, staff, and superiors. If regularly scheduled meetings are established with those who need to see the nurse manager, they will hold routine matters for those appointments. Drop-ins are most likely to occur when others are not certain when they will be able to see the nurse manager. Their philosophy becomes "Catch them when you can." A well-organized nurse manager lets others know in advance "when they can."

Keep staff informed. Visits can be minimized if the staff is kept informed. Use memos; try memos with response copy or space for responding. Use routing slips when materials are to be sent to only a few staff members.

Reduce interruptions by arranging furniture. The nurse manager whose desk is arranged so that immediate eye contact is made with passersby or drop-in visitors is asking for interruptions. A desk turned 90 or even 180 degrees from the door minimizes the potential eye contact. An office without a visitor's chair can also help keep conversations short. An offer to get a chair for a visitor with an important or urgent topic can be a courteous approach. Placing visitor chairs behind the nurse manager's desk almost requires an invitation before visitors will be comfortable in seating themselves.

Go see them. Who are "them"? "Them" are the long-winded people with whom every nurse manager might have to deal. Some people don't know when to quit talking or when to leave. A nurse manager facing this situation should consider going to that person's office. When business is completed, it is easier to say, "I've got to go now," rather than, "You've got to go now."

RESPECTING TIME

The key to effectively managing interruptions and distractions is respect for one's own time as well as that of others. Nurse managers who respect their own time are likely to find others respecting it also. It takes the same values and attitudes to respect one's own time as that of others. Using the above suggestions regarding telephone calls and drop-in visitors will communicate to those who interact with the nurse manager that respect for time is demanded. The nurse manager, however, must reciprocate, by respecting the time of others. If the nurse manager needs to talk to someone, it is appropriate to arrange an appointment, particularly for routine matters. This approach can become contagious. Remember, emergencies and crises are always handled immediately.

SCHEDULING

Once objectives and priorities have been established, the nurse manager can concentrate on scheduling activities. Some system to keep track of regularly scheduled meetings (staff meetings), infrequently occurring events (annual report due dates), and appointments is necessary. This system could include both a calendar and a file. On the calendar is information on the purpose of the meeting, who will be attending, the time and place. A file might contain correspondence or reports related to the meeting. The file can be arranged by date so that it is readily available at the time needed. Further, if the manager needs to prepare for the meeting (reading correspondence or preparing a response), the file can be placed at an earlier date (e.g., one week ahead) to allow for preparation time.

Using a calendar makes it easy to always know what is coming up in the future, and helps one in thinking about ideas for future events. For example, if the nurse manager knows that he or she will be meeting with a superior next week to discuss plans for the unit for the coming year, he or she could jot down ideas as they occur. Some managers have two calendars: a larger one at work with room for details and a smaller one to carry to meetings and home. By always having a calendar handy (e.g., while waiting in the dentist's office), there is more opportunity to jog one's memory.

PAPER WORK

Hospitals cannot function effectively without good information systems. In addition to telephone calls and face-to-face conversations, nurse managers spend considerable time writing and reading communications. Increasing government regulations, avoidance of legal action, new treatments and medications, data processing, word processing, and electronics continuously place greater pressure on the nurse manager to cope with increasing paper work. Overcommunication and the related waste of time, money, and effort may become as much of a concern as undercommunication.

Computer terminals are routinely found at the nurses' station and in the offices of the nurse manager and other administrators. In computer terminology, the nurse manager of today and the future must know how to interface with these new technologies. Chapter 20 explains computer systems for the nurse manager.

Word processing, electronic mail, and other information processors are replacing many of the traditional hand methods for processing information. Regardless of the state of the technology, the nurse manager must be able to process information. Whether that information be handwritten, type printed on a high speed printer, or flashed on a computer terminal, there are some basic principles to be followed.

Plan and schedule paper work. Writing and reading reports, forms, letters, and memoranda are essential elements of the nurse manager's job. They cannot be ignored. They will, however, become a major source of frustration if their processing is not planned and scheduled as an integral part of the nurse manager's daily activities. Nurse managers should learn the hospital's information system and requirements immediately, analyze the paper work requirements of their position, and make significant progress on that part of the job daily.

Sort paper work for effective processing.   A system of file folders or large envelopes in which to sort mail can be very helpful. For instance, all paper work requiring action is placed in the file labeled "A"; it can then be handled according to its relative importance and urgency. All paper work that is informational in nature and related to present work is placed in a file labeled "I." Other reading material such as professional journals, technical reports, and other items to read that do not relate directly to the immediate work should be placed in a file labeled "R." The "I" file contains those things that must be read immediately. The "R" file materials are not as urgent and can be postponed to a later time.

Don't be afraid to throw things away, or erase them from the memory of your electronic information system. When they no longer have value, don't let them become clutter. Every nurse manager needs a waste basket. Have a big one; fill it often.

Share paper work responsibilities.   Don't be afraid to delegate some paper work to others; both routine and nonroutine paper work functions can be delegated. Teaching staff members to handle paper work effectively strengthens a unit's capacity to handle this important element of its responsibilities.

Write effectively.   Handwrite less and dictate more, providing that dictating equipment is available. The person with average dictation skills can dictate on a machine at least five times as quickly as he or she can handwrite. Dictate all letters, memos, and reports. The keys to successful dictation are outlining, good grammar, and clear enunciation. Improved typing skills are essential for operating computer terminals.

Analyze paper work frequently.   Review filing policies and rules regularly, and purge files at least once each year. All standard forms, reports, and memos should be reviewed annually. Each should justify its continued existence and its present format. Don't be afraid to recommend changes and, when possible, initiate the changes.

Don't be a paper shuffler.   There is a saying, "Handle a piece of paper only once." This is often impossible if taken literally. What it really means is each time a piece of paper is handled, some action is taken which furthers the processing of that paper. Paper shufflers are those who continuously move things around on their desks. They unreasonably delay action; the paper problem mounts. A desk top is a working surface; it is not for files and piles.

DELEGATION

Delegation is a major tool in time management. Delegation is not the same as direction. Delegation is defined as sharing responsibility and authority with subordinates and holding them accountable for performance.

Figure 11–3 Delegation and the Hierarchy of Hospital Positions

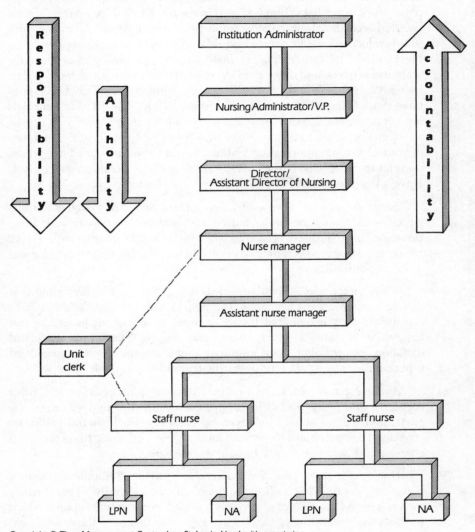

Delegation is a high-level skill relying on trust that subordinates have all the skills and knowledge to know *how* to do something. Direction is telling someone what to do; delegation is giving them the task and asking them to do it. Delegation is a two-way process (see Figure 11–3). Those at higher levels of administration share their responsibilities and authority with subordinates who in turn share with their subordinates. Accountability always flows upward. The small sign that President Harry S. Truman kept on his desk—"The buck stops here"—exemplifies the true meaning of accountability.

At every level each supervisor is accountable for the successes and failures of subordinates. Nurse managers have the right to share in the successes and achievements, and also the problems and failures, of every employee in the unit. Obviously, those who delegate effectively will have more opportunities to share in successes and achievements than in problems and failures.

Within the hierarchy of health care organizations, the nurse manager is both a subordinate and a superior. Work is delegated to the nurse manager by a superior; the nurse manager in turn must decide which of many job responsibilities will be shared with subordinates. "What to do?" and "What to delegate?" are questions to be answered by every nurse manager.

The role description for the nurse manager presented in Chapter 1 can aid in making these decisions. Additionally, formal job descriptions for the nurse manager, assistant nurse manager, registered nurses, licensed practical nurses, nurse assistants, and unit clerks help in making delegation decisions. The nurse manager must understand the full range of job responsibilities for the unit and delegate appropriately to assure that all responsibilities are met.

The nurse manager's job itself must be thoroughly understood. Along with planning and organizing for personal performance, nurse managers have a major responsibility for planning, organizing, and controlling the work within the unit. Thinking time is essential for these activities. Nurse managers are responsible for managing, not carrying out, the details of the unit's work; they must work with and through staff members and motivate them to *want* to do their job effectively.

This does not mean the nurse manager never gets involved in the work of subordinates. In smaller hospitals with limited staff, during emergencies, or when there is a staff shortage due to vacations and illness, nurse managers often find themselves involved in the detailed and routine work of the unit. However, the more time spent in these activities, the less time there is to carry out those functions and activities specific to the job of the nurse manager.

Through effective delegation, nurse managers can also develop staff members' potential, but they must know their staffs. The more they know about staff members' backgrounds, experiences, knowledge, and skills, the better prepared they will be to delegate specific responsibilities. Developing a skills profile for each staff member can help identify strengths as well as those areas in which delegation can be used to train and develop. Nurse managers who do not develop their staffs' abilities are the nurse managers who will be more and more involved in the daily routine and detail work of the division.

Just as effective delegation leads to the development of a confident staff, so it reduces the risk of errors and mistakes. Working with others always involves additional risks, risks resulting from poor communication, skill deficiencies, or differences in values and attitudes. These risks can be reduced if the nurse manager knows both the competencies of subordinates and how to delegate effectively.

Becoming an effective delegator involves a thorough understanding and use of three basic concepts: responsibility, authority, and accountability. Each is different; yet, it is not unusual for them to be confused with each other (see Figure 11–3 and the simplified version of the Vroom and Yetton model presented in Chapter 10). The Vroom and Yetton model tells you how to choose a delegation style in solving a management problem.

Authority

Authority is most frequently thought of as legitimate power. It is the power that goes with the position of nurse manager. Authority resides in the position, not the person.

Authority, like responsibility, can be shared with subordinates. When subordinates are assigned responsibility, they must also be assigned sufficient authority to carry out that responsibility. For example, asking the assistant nurse manager to participate in a decision-making meeting regarding new procedures without giving the authority to represent the unit would lead to frustration. Staff members should never be given responsibilities for which the necessary authority cannot also be delegated.

When authority is delegated, there are two decisions to be made. First, what areas of authority, or what resources, must the person control to achieve the expected results? Second, what will be the limits, boundaries, or parameters for each area of authority or resource to be used? A unit manager having the responsibility for maintaining adequate supplies will need budget authority. The authority to spend money on supplies, however, may be limited to a specific amount for specific supplies or may be allocated for supplies in general. Authority may also be delegated for assigning staff. Limits may be made regarding how many personnel may be assigned and regarding how long or for which assignments they might be used. Authority to work on a specific assignment should be limited by a deadline for completion.

The power associated with formal authority is an essential tool for the nurse manager in effective functioning. However, it does have one major pitfall; it is consumable. The nurse manager can "use up" formal power. It can be depended upon too greatly. The tendency to do so can often be associated with a lack of confidence in subordinates, and even a lack of self-confidence on the part of the nurse manager. The nurse manager who constantly emphasizes authority in relationships with staff members may create animosity, frustration, possibly hostility, or even sabotage. Subordinates do not like to feel that they are being pushed, ruled, or forced. A "heavy hand" may create negative reactions.

Not using authority when it should be used can also be detrimental. The nurse manager must be willing to take corrective action on procedural problems, discipline a subordinate for excessive absenteeism, make decisions in a timely manner, and take control during emergencies or crises.

Authority must be used in the right way at the right time but should never be abused. Proper use of authority increases the nurse manager's credibility with both superiors and subordinates. It ensures their confidence and trust and protects the staff; i.e., the nurse manager should immediately discipline an employee who is excessively absent, then others don't have to do extra work or, if they do have to assume additional work, they may feel better about doing it. The nurse manager's credibility is based on confidence, fairness, and consistency.

Controlling an assignment means holding the subordinate accountable for the use of resources over which he or she has been delegated authority. It must be continuously decided if the assigned resources are sufficient or if additional resources are needed. Are the limits placed on the use of those resources adequate, and what could be done to assure sufficient authority for the subordinates to carry out the assigned responsibilities?

To establish effective controls, the nurse manager must also make decisions about the feedback and information needed to control work delegated to others. She or he must decide what feedback is needed and how it is to be presented. It is important to control—that is, to determine— the results expected and the authority to be shared without impeding the development of a subordinate. Control should be thought through when objectives are established, not as an afterthought. For example, a nurse is responsible for administering medications and given authority for access to drugs, drawing up medications, and administering them to the patients. The nurse is held accountable through several controls, which might include the narcotics key control, end of shift drug counts, and review of patients' records, medication charts, and shift reports.

Assignments

The primary means through which nurse managers can free time to do their own work is their ability to delegate effectively. The most common manifestation of delegation in the day-to-day activities of nurse managers is patient care assignments. To the degree that they can make these assignments effectively, they will be equally effective in reserving valuable time for those activities that they alone can do.

The major responsibility for clarifying an assignment lies with the person delegating the work. If the nurse manager does not know the specific results desired from the subordinate's activities, it is virtually impossible for the subordinate to know them. A subordinate should not be expected to commit to an assignment that is not understood. Thinking about an assignment, analyzing it thoroughly, and being able to state it in specific measurable terms are essential.

A subordinate's restating the assignment just received does not necessarily mean that the assignment was understood; it could simply mean the assignment was remembered long enough to restate it. For other than the simplest assignment, probing questions and discussion on the part of the nurse manager and the subordinate will minimize misunderstandings and make both parties to the assignment feel more confident.

When the nurse manager gives an assignment to a subordinate, a team relationship develops. Together they will have a winning or losing experience. The nurse manager's success is determined by subordinates. All members of any team must work together. In delegation the nurse manager is both the coach and captain.

Planning assignments, making them effective, and following up to ensure successful performances can be fulfilling experiences for all parties concerned. These tasks draw on the nurse manager's leadership, motivation, communication, and analytical skills. Helping subordinates grow and expand professionally can be a gratifying experience.

There are several steps which can assure more effective delegation.

Plan before delegating.   Thinking time saves time. The nurse manager should take time to analyze and write out assignments before they are delegated. Figure 11–4 can be used for this. The more complex the assignment, the greater the need to plan it. Even the simplest assignments require thought and analysis, and reducing the possibility of errors and omissions for simple assignments can be just as crucial as for complex assignments. All assignments should be subjected to the thought processes required by the steps to follow.

Define the responsibility to be assigned in terms of specific results to be achieved.   Write down specific results to be achieved. Ask, "Do they make sense? Are they measurable, realistic, and achievable? Will the subordinate understand what is to be accomplished? What questions could be asked of the subordinate or could the subordinate ask to ensure common understanding?"

The more complex and critical the task and the less skilled and experienced the subordinate, the greater the need to structure the assignment. Stating only "what is to be achieved" is not adequate for many assignments. The nurse manager may provide more structure and reduce the risk involved by discussing how it is to be done, when things are expected, where it is to be done, and specifically who may do what. Too much structuring, however, can involve the nurse manager in too many details of an assignment. The nurse manager must decide the trade-offs between personal involvement and the risk involved with critical assignments.

Figure 11—4 Delegation Analysis and Planning Form

Describe responsibility in terms of results to be achieved:	
Assignment date _____ Due date(s) _____ _____ _____	Level of importance A B C D E F
Authority-parameters: 1. 2. 3. 4. 5. 6. 7. 8. 9. 10.	Accountability—what, when, and how: 1. 2. 3. 4. 5. 6. 7. 8. 9. 10.

Determine the authority to be delegated and the appropriate limits. This means considering what resources must be available to the subordinate to achieve the expected results, and the necessary limits, boundaries, or parameters that should be placed on the use of each resource. Too little authority may make it impossible for the subordinate to accomplish what is expected; undefined authority may be taken as unlimited authority and the subordinate may take action or make commitments which are unacceptable. Limits help identify exceptions with which the nurse manager can assist the subordinate. Handled properly, limits do not appear to subordinates as excessive restrictions; they can actually create a "comfort zone" within which the subordinate functions independently.

Don't complete the assignment for the subordinate. Often nurse managers' concern about staff members' lack of progress on an assignment leads them to "take over" for subordinates, rather than guide them to complete the task themselves.

Hold the subordinate accountable and stay in control. Decide what information or feedback is required to stay in control of the assignment without impeding a subordinate's progress and without getting too involved in the assignment. The nurse manager should be able to state with confidence, "I never delegate a task to a subordinate or delegate it in such a way that it can be messed up so badly that I can't fix it." Gaining the confidence required to make this statement results from planning effective controls for an assignment, and letting the subordinate know what information or feedback is needed and when it is expected.

Decide if written reports are necessary or if brief oral reports are sufficient. If written reports are required, state if tables, charts, or other graphics are necessary. Be specific about reporting times. Identify critical events or milestones that might be reached and brought to the nurse manager's attention. The nurse manager has to decide how closely the assignment will be supervised. However, controls should never be so tight that they limit subordinates' opportunity to grow and expand.

Subordinates have to learn what not to do as well as what to do. They must be given the opportunity to make mistakes within defined limits— limits that never allow them to go so far that the nurse manager cannot fix it.

Troublesome statements to be avoided when giving assignments are ones like "as soon as possible"; "do what's necessary to get the job done"; and "let me know if you have any problems." Never say, "as soon as possible." Give a specific deadline. If a subordinate is told, "Do whatever is necessary," she or he just might! It is not possible to anticipate or discuss with a subordinate *every* problem that might arise; it is usually not worth the time or effort and no one has perfect knowledge, anyway. It is important, however, for the nurse manager to think about problems that may occur and discuss how they might be resolved by this subordinate.

Select the subordinate for the assignment carefully and know why that subordinate was selected. The results to be achieved, the authority to be delegated, and how closely the nurse manager wishes to supervise an assignment are important factors in determining whom to select. Also to be considered are the education, experience, abilities, and work habits of the subordinates. Review the subordinates' skill profile.

The nurse manager may choose to give some assignments to the most experienced, best qualified person on the staff. New staff members might be given certain assignments designed specifically to test their knowledge and skills. Information in job applications, résumés, and reference letters do not always tell the whole story. Specific assignments yield proof that what is said about employees on paper is a true representation of their ability to perform.

All staff members should be given the opportunity to grow professionally. The nurse manager should select subordinates for assignments that will expand their experiences and skills. Most staff training and development will occur through actual experience. Personal growth and achievement can occur within definable and controllable limits without excessive restrictions.

Make the assignment effectively. The nurse manager makes many simple yet important assignments every day. Giving even brief consideration to the six points discussed above will reduce ambiguities and confusion. Assignments will be made and carried out more effectively. Highly complex and important assignments require considerable preparation before they are delegated to subordinates.

When the nurse manager's homework has been done in advance of meeting with a subordinate, making the assignment can be an enjoyable and gratifying experience for both. Set aside sufficient time to make the assignment, make an appointment with the subordinate, and minimize interruptions or distractions during this time. Give the subordinate an overview of the assignment and explain why he or she was chosen. Thoroughly explain and discuss the results expected. Describe the authority the subordinate will have and the limits within which the subordinate will work. Emphasize the control arrangements necessary for a successful assignment. Listen carefully to the subordinate's questions. The right answers can eliminate ambiguities and confusion. They can also strengthen the subordinate's confidence in dealing with highly complex or critical assignments.

Don't demean the subordinate or be critical of the questions asked. Be supportive. The subordinate's questions are likely to center on major concerns and may bring anxieties to the surface. It is best that these be resolved at the time the assignment is made, rather than allowed to become serious issues later.

Underdelegation

Many attitudes—some valid, some not—can lead to underdelegation. Risk factors, time constraints, feelings about subordinates' capabilities, and a strong need to prove oneself are some of the attitudes commonly expressed by nurse managers to explain why they do not delegate more. Poteet (1984) identified some obstacles to delegation (Figure 11–5).

If a nurse manager has doubts about being an effective delegator, the following questions should be asked: Do you work long overtime hours? Are you unable to get to important projects? Are you doing the staff

Figure 11—5 Obstacles to Delegation.

1. Ignorance about the delegation process

2. Incomplete transition from staff nurse to nurse manager

3. Anxiety over prospect of losing technical competence

4. Fear of losing control

5. Crisis management orientation

6. Failure to set goals and timetables

7. Job confusion

8. Desire to control upward communication

9. Competition for managerial positions

10. Personal job insecurity

11. Poor time management

12. Lack of commitment to employee development process

13. Lack of confidence in subordinate's abilities

14. Fear of managerial incompetence

Poteet, G. W. (1984). Delegation strategies: A must for the nurse executive. *Journal of Nursing Administration, 14*(9):18–21. Used with permission.

nurses' job? When you come back from days off, do you find your desk stacked with work? Have no innovative plans been developed recently? If the answer is yes to most of these questions, then the individual must explore ways to delegate more effectively.

Delegation is a major skill for nurse managers and failure to delegate can lead to many negative results. If nurse managers constantly solve problems that subordinates could well take care of, they have little time left to do those things that require more knowledge, skill, and authority—in short, to manage. In addition, nurse managers who deprive staff of opportunities to grow as professionals and as persons contribute only a fraction of what managers have to offer.

What Not to Delegate

Just as a nurse manager cannot do everything that must be done, so there are many functions and activities that cannot be delegated. In some hospitals nurse managers may conduct daily rounds—a responsibility that perhaps cannot be delegated to the assistant nurse manager or a staff nurse. Or the nurse manager may be required to conduct all performance reviews of staff. In some situations the nurse manager may be personally required to issue or even administer certain drugs. The nurse manager may be required to write the annual objectives for the division, collect the information for and submit drug usage reports, or write all incident reports. With effective delegation of those functions and activities that can be shared, the nurse manager will have enough time to carry out the responsibilities specifically required of her or him.

Three important areas of responsibility, however, should never be delegated. The first is responsibility for disciplining an immediate subordinate. Few things can destroy the staff's confidence more quickly than the inability of the nurse manager to discipline effectively. This responsibility should never be delegated upward to a supervisor or to the personnel department, even though either or both might have some involvement in the disciplinary procedure. Staff members must view the nurse manager as the key person responsible for maintaining control of the unit.

Second, the nurse manager should not delegate responsibility for handling morale problems within the unit. Obviously, advice may be sought from superiors and other professionals, but it is primarily up to the nurse manager to create a satisfactory work environment and working relationships among all employees in the unit. Being an effective delegator is an essential element in maintaining a highly disciplined staff with high morale. Chapters 9 and 10 provide additional information and approaches to these topics.

Third, the nurse manager should not delegate anything for which he or she has legal accountability. Terminating an employee or handling a potentially litigious patient complaint are examples of the manager's tasks that should not be delegated.

SUMMARY

- Nurse managers must use time wisely to accomplish everything that is expected of them. This takes planning. Without time management, only more time will help.

- Time management begins with the establishment of priorities. Role duties and objectives can be used to guide priority listing.

- Setting priorities includes deciding what not to do as well as what to do. Writing out the next day's activities in a prioritized list is important. Written plans rarely work out as planned. Schedule in open time to allow for emergencies.

- The nurse manager's work shift is subject to many interruptions. An interruption log will help identify patterns that can be used to plan ways to reduce unnecessary interruptions.

- Telephone calls are a major source of interruption. They can be controlled by minimizing small talk, planning calls, using a timer, and stating preferred call times.

- Drop-in visitors are also a source of interruption. One should meet visitors outside the office, keep visits short, encourage appointments, keep staff informed, and arrange furniture to discourage unscheduled visitors.

- Nurse managers who respect their own time are likely to find others respecting it also.

- Written communication can also cause interruptions. These can be minimized by planning and scheduling paper work, sorting, delegating, writing effectively, and using an effective filing system.

- Delegation is a major tool in time management. The nurse manager must understand her role and her staff's abilities in order to effectively delegate. When authority is delegated, the nurse manager must set the limits of responsibility. Assignments must be given clearly and precisely.

- Several steps can be taken to ensure effective delegation: plan before delegating, define responsibility in terms of results, define authority limits, don't complete subordinates' assignments, hold subordinates accountable, and select subordinates who are capable.

- Three things should never be delegated: disciplining immediate subordinates, handling morale problems within the unit, and responsibilities for which the manager has legal accountability.

BIBLIOGRAPHY

Eliopoulos, C. (1984). Time management: A reminder. *J Nurs Adm,* 14(3):30.

Kossen, S. (1981). *Supervision.* New York: Harper & Row.

Lakein, A. (1973). *How to get control of your time and your life.* New York: Signet.

Miller, M. L. (1984). Implementing self-scheduling. *J Nurs Adm,* 14(3):33.

Poteet, G. W. (1984). Delegation strategies: A must for the nurse executive. *J Nurs Adm,* 14(9):18–21.

Problem Solving and Decision Making

THE NECESSITY FOR nurse managers to use advanced problem-solving and decision-making strategies has become increasingly apparent to hospital administrators. Latz found that nurse managers generally utilized short-term planning, made decisions alone, under stress, and seldom solved potential or nonroutine problems (Latz, 1977). The result was problem solving on a crisis basis; potential and long-term problems were not identified; and decision making was a solitary process.

Nurse managers must think, as well as act, to solve problems. They must make decisions based on objective evidence to reduce failure and to decrease personal prejudices or lack of experience and knowledge. This chapter focuses on problem solving and decision making as a diversified process nurse managers can use daily.

The label "problem solving" is used inconsistently and often interchangeably with decision making in the literature. While the two processes appear similar and may depend in some instances on one another, they are not synonymous. Solving a problem may involve a set of decisions; conversely, a major decision may have involved the solving of several related problems. However, some decisions are not of a problem-solving nature, such as decisions about budgets, equipment, or other matters that have no immediate bearing on selecting future courses of action. In contrast, some problems do not involve decision making as a deliberate process. Habitual action or a pure behavioral response may be modes of problem solving, but they do not require much in the way of higher mental processes—holding onto the wall when walking down a wet hospital corridor, for instance, or stopping a patient from pulling out his IV. Most of the time, however, decision making is a subset of problem solving, which in turn comes out of a dynamic situation in which there is a recognition that something is wrong and a reaction or solution to it is needed. Decision making is the behavior exhibited in selecting and implementing a course of action from among alternatives that may or may not involve a problem.

PROBLEM SOLVING

Defining the Problem

The most important part of problem solving is defining the problem. The problems nurse managers perceive will determine the solutions or changes they implement. For our purposes, a problem can be identified as a departure from a desirable state of affairs as perceived by the nurse manager, who is responsible for dealing foresightedly with the situation.

Suppose the nurse manager had mandated that all patient care plans be updated each week, but the majority of staff nurses were unable to complete this task. The problem might be identified as the fact that the care plans were not completed. The causes may have been noncompliance or, perhaps more correctly, fatigue; the staff may have been working long hours due to the admission of a large number of critically ill patients. A problem should be a descriptive statement of a state of affairs, not a judgment or conclusion. If one begins the statement of a problem with a judgment, the solution will be equally judgmental and could overlook critical descriptive elements of the deviation. For instance, if the nurse manager defined the problem as noncompliance and proceeded to write anecdotal notes before further fact finding, a minor problem could develop into a full-blown crisis.

Therefore, the most important step in problem solving is the first one: identification of a situation that appears to be a problem and the classification of the problem as potential, actual, or critical (Stevens, 1980). A *potential* problem is one that can emerge at any time but may not need to be dealt with immediately. *Actual* problems need prompt action, and *critical* problems, crisis intervention. The solution will depend upon the exactness with which the problem has been identified. The problem should be stated in descriptive, nonjudgmental terms. If the problem is prematurely or incorrectly diagnosed, the solutions will be inadequate or the unidentified problem may lead to a crisis situation. The three principles for diagnosing a problem are: know all the facts; separate facts from interpretations; and determine the scope of the problem.

For example, an RN on the night shift has complained that an LPN consistently omits taking vital signs for her group of patients but charts that she has done so. Since the problem concerns two levels of staff, the nurse manager must gather facts from reliable sources at both levels. She or he must question the RN as well as the LPN and can also subtly ask patients about the situation. If the nurse manager cannot separate facts from interpretations of facts, she or he should seek the assistance of an appropriate confidante. Otherwise, she or he makes the mistake of acting on the first interpretation as if it were a factual reality—i.e., the accused is lazy or dishonest.

Premature interpretation can alter one's ability to deal with facts objectively. Are there other explanations for the apparent behavior, without negative assumptions regarding the character of the LPN? Accurate assessment of the scope of the problem will also determine if a lasting solution need be sought or just a stopgap measure. Is this just a situational problem requiring only intervention with a simple explanation, or is it more complex, involving the integrity of the LPN or the reporting by the RN? Problems must be diagnosed and classified in order for action to be taken and decision making to begin.

Problem-Solving Methods

There are various methods used to solve problems. Managers with little management experience, for instance, tend to use a *trial and error* technique, applying one solution after another until the problem is solved or appears to be improving. These inexperienced managers are unable to judge from past experience and have little time for research. A "shoot from the hip" solution is put into effect, which may or may not work; if not, a new solution is substituted until the problem is resolved.

As an example, a rehabilitation unit shows an increasing incidence of decubitus ulcers. The nurse manager, using a trial and error problem-solving method, utilizes various treatments to decrease the size of the ulcers—e.g., heat lamps and Maalox, betadine and a cold hair dryer, hydrogen peroxide and Elase ointment. After a few months, when none of the treatments works, it occurs to the nurse manager that perhaps standard preventive methods would be better. A turning schedule is enforced, the problem is decreased, and the prior low level of ulceration incidence is restored. A trial and error process can be more time consuming than is desirable and may even be detrimental. Although learning does occur, the nurse manager risks being perceived as a poor problem solver who has wasted a great deal of time and money in implementing ineffective solutions.

Experimentation, another type of problem solving, is much more rigorous than trial and error; pilot projects or limited trials are examples. Experimentation may be creative and effective or uninspired and ineffective, depending on how it is used. If experimentation is used as a major method of problem solving, it may evolve into a trial and error technique. However, if the situation is one wherein all previous methods of problem solving have failed, it may be beneficial to experiment with various solutions.

For example, a nurse manager and staff nurse disagree about many management decisions; the staff nurse continually undermines the authority of the nurse manager in these matters. Constant trouble is brewing among staff due to this nurse's inappropriate comments and criticism. Counseling, confrontation, and threats have failed to bring about a desired effect—namely, mutual alliance, improved morale, and productivity. In this situation the nurse manager may wish to experiment. Rather than terminating the employee, the latter may be assigned to a special project requiring initiative and the assumption of some particular responsibility for a defined time. What will be the result? This choice might be the one that proves innovative, solves the problem, and salvages an employee. As an alternative, all concerned could accept that some disagreement is inevitable and can be useful to task accomplishment.

Still another problem-solving technique is problem *critique,* in which the nurse manager assumes the role of listener and facilitator, providing feedback and constructive criticism to assist the staff in proper identification of problems. Many times the communication process has broken down to the point that it is difficult to identify the actual problem. The nurse manager would continue with dialogue in this manner until the problem has been correctly identified, according to the participants.

For example, one nurse has been complaining bitterly about the new admission assessment form developed by the nursing service department. The nurse manager discovers, through listening, that this nurse had developed and submitted a set of forms to the policy and procedure committee that had been rejected. Resolution of this rejection had never taken place and the problem became displaced. After the nurse manager established constructive dialogue and developed a fair critique of the nurse's perception of things, the real problem was identified and brought out into the open.

Some problems are self-limiting. If permitted to run a natural course, they will be solved by those personally involved. This is not to say, though, that a uniform laissez-faire style solves all problems. The nurse manager may not ignore his or her managerial responsibilities, but will often see ideal situations when allowing the participants to discover their own solutions to a problem. This often happens, for instance, when a newly graduated RN joins a unit where most of the staff are LPNs with many years of experience. The new RN may be defensive and overly assertive in her role, and the LPNs may resent her level of education as well as her lack of experience. If the nurse manager intervenes, a problem that might have been worked out by the persons involved becomes an ongoing source of conflict. Many staffing problems, role conflicts, and interpersonal relationships can be solved by the persons involved if the nurse manager is willing to take a subsidiary position, allowing the others to solve the problem. The great skill required here is knowing *when* to do nothing! Chapters 8 and 22 discuss this issue.

Metaphor-based techniques for developing creative problem solutions are concerned with breaking conventional thinking patterns and suspending judgment so as to evoke a volume of highly original ideas within a short time through the process of forced association (Gillies, 1982). This means that certain concepts or ideas are identified and persons must form new ideas from old ones. This is an analytical approach through which analogies (including fantasy or symbolism) are used to develop creative thinking to increase output of individuals or groups. New ideas that do not necessarily fit the traditional model are discussed in an attempt to discover new alternatives, and a conscious effort is made to look at old problems from a completely different viewpoint.

For example, a terminally ill man with bone metastases has been difficult to care for due to repeated staff failures to position him comfortably. Employing metaphors, the staff imagine themselves in a magic bed, trying to find, with their own bodies, the ultimate comfortable position. They could fantasize about strings holding up their extremities or a magic carpet that would apply no pressure to their battered body carrying them off. A more direct analogy might be a tub or heated swimming pool. The usual problem is looked at differently and metaphorical solutions are discussed.

This method may at first seem simple-minded and easy. True, it is often easy (and unproductive) to just think up metaphors, but applying them requires great energy and results may be difficult to achieve. For instance, if the staff wanted to pursue the magic carpet analogy, something akin to the kinetic bed would have to be employed.

Another approach very similar to metaphor-based techniques and designed to help trigger creative ideas is called *brainstorming* (Osborn, 1953). This is the use of one's brain to "storm" a creative problem and to do so in commando fashion, with each "stormer" audaciously attacking the same objective. To obtain maximum creativity from a group with the brainstorming technique, four basic rules must be fully understood and adhered to:

1. Judicial judgment is ruled out. Criticism of ideas must be withheld until later.

2. Free-wheeling is welcomed. The wilder the idea, the better; it is easier to tame down ideas than to think them up.

3. Quantity is the goal; the greater the number of ideas, the more the likelihood of winners.

4. Imagination and improvement are sought. In addition to contributing their own ideas, participants should suggest how ideas of others can be turned into better ideas, or how two or more ideas can be joined into still another idea (Osborn, 1953).

While the ideas may be wild, they may also lead to some creative solutions. Some of the criticisms of this approach have been the high cost factor, the time consumed, and the superficiality of many solutions.

While all of the above methods utilize a qualitative process to problem solving, the decision tree attempts to quantify (express in terms of how much) the problem-solving process. A *decision tree* (Figure 12–1) is a graphic model that allows presentation of the risks, outcomes, options, preferences, and other pertinent information for specific problem solving over a period of time; it allows the nurse manager to visualize alternatives to a decision and the possible consequences.

The process begins with a primary problem with at least two alternative decision possibilities. The predicted consequence for each alternative is considered, along with the probability that that consequence will occur. The model resembles a tree as the decision points are diagrammed.

Thus, in Figure 12–1, the nurse manager decides to attempt to give the staff every other weekend off. The alternative decisions to implement this procedure are to use the float pool, go back to one weekend off a month, employ staff from temporary agencies, or work short-staffed. Each alternative has certain consequences and these are numbered according to the probability of their occurring. An arbitrary numbering system can be assigned from 1 through 5, 1 being the lowest probability and 5 the highest.

Thus, if the float pool is utilized, there is high probability that such personnel will be familiar with the hospital, moderate probability that the staff will have some weekends off and be content, and low probability that float personnel will be unable to meet staffing needs. If the nurses go back to having only one weekend off per month, there is high probability of poor morale, decreased productivity, and increased overtime and moderate probability of increased turnover.

The results diagrammed on the tree represent the nurse manager's experiences and judgment but may also be supported by computerized data. The decision tree is not a pure quantitative method that indicates the obviously correct decision, but a technique that produces a varied data base on which to make a decision based on consideration of various alternatives and their probable consequences. The user comes to realize that subsequent decisions may depend upon future events. Decision trees are useful for short- and medium-term planning as well as for decision making. The tree takes into account the probability of each of the

Figure 12–1 A Sample Decision Tree

		III. Consequences	IV. Probability
I. Problem **Staff want every other weekend off**	**II. Decision alternatives** Utilize float pool to enable staff to have every other weekend off	Familiarity with hospital	5
		Staff gets some weekends off	3
		Unable to meet staffing needs	2
		Staff content	3
	Continue to have one weekend off a month	Poor morale	5
		Decreased productivity	5
		Increased turnover	4
		Increased overtime	5
		Coverage adequate	5
		Expensive	5
	Use temporary agencies to enable every other weekend off	Unfamiliar with hospital	5
		Staff content	2
		Unable to meet staffing needs	3
	Work short staffed to enable every other weekend off	Decrease patient care	4
		Staff gets weekends off	5
		Decreased costs	2
		Increased overtime	3

consequences occurring from each alternative and the value of each alternative. The decision is made by identifying the choice that minimizes loss and maximizes gain (Marriner, 1982). Most nurse managers, however, hesitate to use the decision tree matrix due to its complicated form.

La Monica and Finch (1977) have applied the Vroom and Yetton decision-making model to nursing management situations and suggest that managers using this model have significantly more effective outcomes than managers not using the model. This model allows managers to diagnose the situation and determine the most effective means to solve the problem.

The leader asks seven questions to be answered in a yes/no format, with each question asking still more specific questions concerning the matter asked. The decision model answers the following: (a) if the decision must be accepted by all, then group involvement is essential; (b) if quality and expertise are a requirement, then persons with expertise should solve the problem; and (c) when quality and acceptance are required, then experts and group should solve the problem. The purpose of the tree is to integrate these variables and suggest a decision-making style, taking the shortest amount of time considering the difficulty of the task.

The Problem-Solving Process

The process itself consists of eight steps and is a method of arriving at the best possible alternatives. The nurse manager may not always be able to leave the floor for the library to search out topics relating to a problem. Many nursing problems require immediate action. Therefore, developing a list of principles, learning an organized method for problem solving, and enlarging the problem-solving skills that come from critical thinking are needed to select the best solutions. The eight steps are:

1. Define the problem.

2. Gather information.

3. Analyze the information.

4. Develop solutions.

5. Consider the consequences.

6. Make a decision.

7. Implement the decision.

8. Evaluate the solution.

1. Define the problem or problems clearly. The first indication of a problem may be nurse managers' concern over a number of conditions like poor staff performance, outmoded care plans, or low morale. Their first view of the problem may be a need for more nurses or more overtime. When the nurse managers examine this idea critically, however, they may discover that they are drawing conclusions too soon and have not considered other factors that may be contributing to decreased productivity such as increased patient acuity levels or a fluctuating census.

In defining a problem, the nurse manager should determine the area it covers and ask: "Do I have the authority to do anything about this myself? Do I have the knowledge? The time? Could I get someone else to do it? What benefits could be expected from solving the problem?" A list of the potential benefits provides the criteria by which to evaluate and compare alternatives. The list also serves as a means to judge costs and assign priority numbers for the solutions listed.

2. Gather information. Information must be gathered to define the problem, to work out and evaluate solutions, and to check up on the effects of the solution. The information gathered will probably be a combination of facts and feelings. Relevant, valid, accurate, detailed descriptions should be obtained from appropriate persons or sources, and the information should be put in writing; this encourages people to report facts accurately. The nurse manager may choose to have everyone involved provide information. While this may not always provide accurate information, it may reduce misinformation and it allows everyone an opportunity to tell what he or she thinks is wrong with a situation.

Experience is another source of information—the nurse manager's own experience, as well as the experience of other nurse managers and of the staff. The latter usually have ideas on what should be done about the problem, and many of these ideas represent good information and valuable suggestions. The information gathered will never be complete, however. Some data will be useless, some inaccurate, but some will be used to develop innovative ideas worth pursuing.

3. Analyze the information. Objectivity is very difficult to maintain, particularly if persons have already formulated their own opinions regarding the problem. The information should be analyzed only when all of it has been gathered and sorted into some orderly arrangement, such as one of the following:

a. Categorize the information in order of its reliability.

b. List the information in terms of most important, important, least important.

c. Set the information in a time sequence. What happened first? Next? What came before what? What were the surrounding circumstances?

d. Set information up in terms of cause and effect. Is A causing B or vice-versa?

e. Classify the information into such categories as human factors, personality, education, age, relationships among people, problems outside of the hospital; technical factors such as nursing skills, equipment, or the type of unit; and time factors such as maturity, length of service, overtime, type of shift, and double shifts. Also ask, "How long has this been going on?" Consider policy factors, such as hospital procedures or rules applying to the problem.

Since no amount of information is ever complete, assumptions will need to be made and all assumptions must be supported by critical thinking. In any problem that involves people, there will be a value system that will influence each individual's analysis. This must be considered.

4. Develop solutions. As the nurse manager analyzes information, numerous ideas about possible solutions will suggest themselves. These should be put in writing, and the nurse manager should start developing ideas about them. She or he should not limit herself or himself to a simple solution, because doing so may limit thinking and cause too much concentration on detail. Developing alternative solutions makes it possible to combine the best parts of several solutions into one superior one. Also, alternatives are valuable in case the first one is impossible to achieve.

When exploring alternative solutions, one should be uncritical of the way the problem has been previously handled. Some problems are already long-standing before they reach the nurse manager, and attempts have been made to resolve them over long periods of time.

Past experience may not always supply an answer but can aid the thinking process and help prepare for future problem solving. For assistance with decision making, nurse managers can review the literature, attend relevant seminars, and brainstorm with others. Sometimes others will have solved similar problems and their methods can be applied to a comparable problem.

5. Consider the consequences. In determining the best solution to a problem, the nurse manager should consider the short- and long-term consequences of each possible solution. The solutions may be compared in terms of the following questions:

a. How far has the situation deteriorated? Must drastic steps be taken, or can time aid as a cure? Is the problem just arising or has it existed for a long time?

b. What will be the effect of each possible solution on the quality of patient care?

c. Which solution is readily applicable and will produce the quickest results?

d. Have these solutions been used before? What have the results been?

e. What are the likely causes of severe worker dissatisfaction under this method?

f. What are the likely causes of strong worker satisfaction under this method?

g. What will be the cost of each solution?

h. How does the cost of each solution compare with the results that it will give?

6. Make a decision. Some solutions have to be put into effect quickly; matters of discipline or poor patient care need immediate treatment. Nurse managers should know in advance their authority to act in an emergency and the penalties for various infractions.

If the problem is a technical one, however, and the solution to it brings a change in the method of doing work (or new equipment), there may be resistance. All persons become disturbed by changes that reorder their habit patterns and threaten their security or status. Many plans have failed because the leader failed to recognize the change process that must be set in motion before solutions can be implemented.

Before change is introduced, those who will be affected by it should be fully informed of the goals. If more than half of the personnel are against the change, it is not likely to succeed unless an effort is made to sell them on the idea. Important staff members must be committed to the new idea. The nurse manager should spend time with the key persons involved, explain the reasons for the change, and elicit their responses. All of the outcomes, positive and negative, *must* be identified. Alternate solutions should be developed and weighted in their order of importance. Change might be tried first in a limited area where difficult elements can be ironed out. Problems can then be dealt with before the application is widened. Pilot studies and dry runs allow for positive and negative feedback, so corrections and refinements can be made before a final general application. (See Chapter 5 for a complete discussion of the change process.)

It is worthwhile to mention here what Chester Barnard refers to as the "zone of acceptance" in executive decision making (Barnard, 1937). Most employees will cooperate only with directions or orders that fit into their "zone of acceptance." Some orders will clearly be unacceptable, some will be neutral, others barely acceptable, and some fully acceptable. This last group lies within the "zone of acceptance." Thus, if an order is given that the nurse manager knows will not be obeyed, steps must be taken to educate or motivate the staff nurses to comply with it. Example: the nurse manager decides that a solution to the short-staffing problem is to utilize staff from temporary agencies. The unit's own staff, however, has preconceived ideas about agency nurses and does not wish to cooperate with them in making the transition smooth. If the nurse manager cannot educate or motivate the staff to interact positively with the agency nurses, the solution, no matter how good, will fail. It is not within the staff's "zone of acceptance."

7. Implement the decision. Implementation should follow the decided-upon action. If new problems emerge that the nurse manager had not considered, these impediments must be evaluated as carefully as the potential consequences discussed earlier. The nurse manager must be very careful, however, not to abandon a workable solution just because someone objects to the solution (which at least one person will). If the previous steps in the problem-solving process have been followed, this solution has already been carefully thought out and potential problems addressed. No perfect solution is possible and all change is disrupting. The nurse manager must keep in mind that doing nothing *is* taking action.

8. Evaluate the solution. After the solution has been implemented, the nurse manager should review the plan instituted and compare the actual results and benefits with the objectives that were established and the outcomes that were expected when the decision was made. People tend to fall back into old habit patterns or give lip service to change when actually the same old behavior is taking place. So the nurse manager must ask: "Are the objectives being fulfilled? If so, are the results better or worse than expected? If they are better, what reasons may have contributed to the success?" Such a periodic check-up gives the nurse manager valuable insight and experience to use in other situations and keeps the change on course.

The outcome should be studied somewhat as a football coach studies replays of a football game. Where were mistakes made? How can they be avoided in the future? What decisions were successes? Why? If the nurse manager evaluates and builds upon experience, problem solving will become an expert skill that can be utilized throughout a management career.

Group Problem Solving

Decision making by the individual is the traditional, status quo approach. The nurse manager is confronted with a problem and decides how to solve it. Today, both the complexity of problems and desires of staff for involvement create the need for staff participation in decision making and for group approaches to problem solving.

Participative problem solving means that others in addition to the nurse manager are involved in the decision process. The participants may include all ancillary personnel or only nurses. The problem-solving process can be formal or informal and may entail intellectual, emotional, and physical involvement.

A principal argument for group involvement is that information in quantity—and often of higher quality—can be brought to bear on the selection of alternatives. Involving numerous personnel may yield information that is more complete, accurate, and less biased than information obtained from only one person, since it has been clarified through group exposure. Discussion and participation in the process, before the decision is made, will also enhance cooperation in effective implementation. Since nurses at all levels are under time constraints, the data-gathering phase will be limited by the job setting.

In practice, the degree of participation will be determined by several factors: (a) who initiates ideas; (b) the extent that subordinate support is required for implementation of a solution; (c) how completely an employee carries out each phase of decision making: diagnosing, finding alternatives, estimating consequences, and making choices; (d) how much weight the nurse manager attaches to the ideas received; and (e) the amount of knowledge she or he has about the matter. Likert (1961) has found that when individuals are allowed to participate, they function more productively, and implementing solutions becomes easier because of the shared problem solving.

Participatory management can be time consuming. Nevertheless, because of the diverse opinions that will emerge, it may take less time for a group to make a decision than for an individual to gather information and analyze it. Another disadvantage of participatory problem solving is the emergence of benign tyranny within the group. Those members who are less informed or confident may allow stronger members to present all solutions and decisions. This sets the stage for a power struggle between the nurse manager and a few assertive members of the group. From a behavioral standpoint, however, the advantages usually outweigh the disadvantages, and each member learns to contribute to the attainment of the organizational objectives.

Another form of the participative process, called Quality Circles, is adapted from Ouchi's Theory Z (Ouchi, 1981). This has been successful in this country as well as Japan. This style, which can easily be adapted to nursing, is based on trust and worker involvement in decisions that affect them. The system emphasizes consensus-based decision making, lifetime job security, and a strong commitment to the goals of the organization. The desired results are increased job commitment, higher productivity, and lower turnover.

The group participation process in Z management is often called Quality Circles. These have been used in health care situations, but their use requires total organizational decision and commitment. Nurse managers would not ordinarily use this technique unless their institution was using it. However, it may be useful to understand the process.

As an example, nurses on each floor are divided into circles of eight or ten individuals, with a facilitator appointed for each circle. The facilitators form another circle, which interfaces with circles at higher and lower levels, so there is reciprocal representation at all levels. Circles are thoroughly disciplined operations committed to training, group skills, and rigorous step-by-step improvement procedures. There is continuous discussion within the circles whenever a policy or procedural change is made, until a true consensus has been achieved.

Many management decisions are made in circles, and no decision is final until every member has had a part in the decision and agrees with the outcome. This can be a time-consuming process, but once consensus is reached, implementation is instantaneous and the net effect is increased productivity. In other forms of participatory decision making, a majority wins, leaving a dissatisfied, obstinate minority who may sabotage implementation. In consensus-based decision making, everyone feels a part of the process, has a voice in the decision, and is therefore a winner.

While research on this theory is limited, one study has shown improved morale, decreased alienation, and greater incentives for unified productivity when Quality Circles were introduced (Moore, 1982). Likert's System 4 Theory also closely approximates management by consensus. The research he and his colleagues have done support the conclusion that the more that employees are allowed to participate, the greater the likelihood of superior performance (Likert, 1961). However, the most important limitation to its use is the extent to which it is germane to the Japanese culture, which is quite different from Western culture (Smith, Reinow & Reid, 1984). The work ethic in Japan puts high value on teamwork while in America, independent accomplishment is more highly valued. Thus, group decision making is very workable in Japanese settings and less so in American ones. Another important element here is that Quality Circles may be more useful when the membership represents various interacting units or disciplines, especially in health care. This model, because of the greater participation it provides and the long-term rewards built into the system, certainly needs to be evaluated in terms of nursing management. It shows potential for use in an area where innovative management is badly needed.

Another form of group participation is the use of committees, or a group of people chosen to deal with a problem. Formal committees are part of the organization and have authority as well as a specific role, while informal committees are primarily for discussion and have no delegated authority. An *ad hoc* committee is a formal committee appointed for a specific purpose and limited time. Committee members are often given the task of collecting data, analyzing it, and making recommendations. Committees are also useful in planning and formulating policy.

The advantages of a committee are that it represents group participation and persons with specialized knowledge as well as direct interest can provide information that will help in the search for a pertinent and timely decision. The hope is that there will be resolution of differences after these have been thrashed out in committee meetings. It is important to determine size, scope, and authority of the committee as well as appointing a chairperson who will facilitate the effectiveness of the committee (Marriner, 1984).

The significant problem with a committee is that it may reach a compromise that may not really satisfy any of the participants. Other major constraints are that the committee may be bound by organizational rules, may look for solutions and make decisions with too narrow a focus, and may take too long to make decisions.

Another example of group participation is the *Nominal Group Technique* (NGT; Delbecq, VandeVen & Gustafson, 1975). A nominal group is a group in name only because no social exchange is allowed between members. NGT consists of (a) silent generation of ideas in writing; (b) round-robin feedback from group members to record each idea in a terse phrase on a flip chart; (c) discussion of each recorded idea for clarification and evaluation; and (d) individual voting on priority ideas with the group decision being mathematically derived through rank ordering or rating.

Although research is just starting to emerge on NGT, there is some evidence that this technique may be better than the traditional committee functioning for several reasons—among them, the fact that the silent, independent generation of ideas, followed by further thought and listening during the round-robin procedure, results in a higher quality of ideas. In addition, the structured process forces equality of participation among members in generating information on the problem. NGT also minimizes the chances of more vocal and persuasive members influencing the less forceful persons. Members work and think individually, not "contaminated" by others' ideas or presence.

The nurse manager needs to assess the health team members on the unit to determine if a participatory process would enhance decision making. If staff show similar qualifications and work well together, perhaps Quality Circles could be instituted with success. If the group is extremely diversified and individualistic, however, NGT might be beneficial. If there are only a few persons with leadership potential, then a committee could be utilized with some success. It is essential, however, that the decision-making method be matched with important characteristics of the staff. (See Chapter 10 for further discussion on group activities.)

Stumbling Blocks

Among the many obstacles to problem solving, inexperience plays an important role. In some instances, the nurse manager's past experience can determine how much risk will be taken in any present circumstance. How much has been learned from these experiences, positive and negative, can affect the current viewpoint and result in either subjective and narrow judgments or in very wise ones.

Personality. The nurse manager's personality can and often does have an effect on how and why certain decisions are made. Many nurse managers are selected because of their expert clinical, not management, skills. They will often start out insecure and resort to varieties of unproductive activity. And a nurse manager who is insecure may make decisions on a primarily approval-seeking basis. When a truly difficult situation arises, rather than lose face with the staff, he or she makes a decision that will placate people rather than achieve the larger goals of the institution. On the other hand, a nurse manager who demonstrates an authoritative type of personality might make unreasonable demands upon the staff; that is, few weekend requests are granted, and no compensations for long hours are given because of the nurse manager's "workaholic" attitude. Similarly, a lazy middle manager may cause a unit to flounder because any new ideas or solutions to problems may demand action she is disinclined to take.

Rigidity. Rigidity, an inflexible management style, is another obstacle to problem solving. It may result from ineffective trial and error solutions, fear of risk taking, or may be an inherent personality trait. As discussed previously, ineffective trial and error problem solving can be avoided by the nurse manager gathering sufficient information and determining a means for early correction of wrong or inadequate decisions. Also, to minimize risk in problem solving, the goal is to have knowledge and understanding of alternative risks and expectations. Personality traits are difficult to change, but awareness tests from management seminars or evaluations from staff may indicate to an individual that her or his attitudes are not conducive to productive leadership.

The nurse manager who uses a rigid style in problem solving easily develops tunnel vision—the tendency to look at new things in old ways and from established frames of reference. It then becomes very difficult to see things from another perspective, and problem solving becomes a process whereby one person makes all of the decisions with little information or data from other sources. In the current dynamic, changing health care setting, rigidity can at times be a nurse manager's greatest barrier to effective problem solving.

Preconceived ideas. Effective nurse managers do not start out with the preconceived idea that one proposed course of action is right and all others wrong. Nor do they assume that only one opinion can be voiced and others will be silent. In short, they start out with a commitment to find out why staff members disagree, not necessarily with any preconceived idea about who has the right answers. If the staff sees a different reality or even a different problem, nurse managers need to integrate this information into a data base so as to further the problem-solving possibilities.

Most people have preconceived ideas about the nature of problems and their solutions, and those who are certain that only their perception of "what's wrong" is accurate may never accept the final decision reached and possibly the whole process of argument. Nurse managers, however, have the formal responsibility for problem solving and decision making and must put personal ideas on hold until they have gathered enough information to view the situation objectively and in the widest possible perspective.

Satisficing, Optimizing, and Maximizing

Satisficing is not a misspelled word; it is a strategy whereby the individual chooses a solution that is not ideal but either is good enough (suffices) under existing circumstances to meet minimum standards of acceptance, or is the first acceptable alternative. An *optimizing* approach first identifies all possible outcomes, examines the probability of each available solution, then takes the action that yields the highest probability of achieving the most desirable outcome. A *maximizing* strategy, on the other hand, looks at possible solutions, choosing the first one that meets minimal satisfactory standards of acceptance (Gillies, 1982).

Patient care situations present a multitude of problems that are ineffectively solved with satisficing strategy. For example, a patient, poststroke, has been placed on a busy surgical floor until a bed in the rehabilitation unit is ready. The patient needs a great deal of care and is unable to communicate with the staff or the family; early contractures are noticeable. In designing the proper care plan for this patient, the nurse manager may use a satisficing solution: reasoning that the patient will soon be on a rehabilitation unit, she or he determines that range of motion every four hours need not be done if the patient gets up in a chair every day. Or she or he may maximize the solution and implement a plan of care fulfilling all possible goals for that patient. However, the staff may satisfice, doing only what they feel is absolutely necessary. There are many examples of this nature that demonstrate how a maximizing solution can become a satisficing one in the delivery of health care.

Nurse managers who solve problems using the satisficing criterion usually lack the ability to maximize. They view their units as drastically simplified models of the real world and are content with this simplification because it allows them to make decisions with relatively simple rules of thumb or from force of habit. These techniques do not make demands upon their capacity for thought nor do they solve problems on a long-term basis.

DECISION MAKING

Risk and Uncertainty

Managers make decisions under three conditions: certainty, uncertainty, and risk. The nurse manager is no exception. Decisions that involve risk are more difficult to make than certainty decisions, since under conditions of risk only limited information and experience are available and there may be many possible outcomes for each alternative. Traditional methods break down when applied to risk decisions. It is with these decisions that the mathematical technique of probability makes its greatest contribution.

One type of probability that can be applied to risk decisions is objective statistical probability: a precise mathematical technique that permits the decision maker to calculate possible outcomes and make inferences. The probability calculation is based upon experience. Tossing a coin provides a simple example of the method and has implications for statistical probability. For instance, a person tosses an unbiased coin 100 times, with an outcome of 50 heads and 50 tails. With this experience, on the 101st toss, the decision maker will assign a probability of 0.5 (50%) that the coin will show a head (or tail).

Most nurse managers in hospitals do not have as much relevant experience as does the coin tosser. Furthermore, the coin tosser can be pretty sure that half the time the 101st toss will be heads. Yet, if he still gets several heads in a row, the probability that the next toss will be a tail is higher each time. In other words, it may take a great number of outcomes in order for the probability to work itself out.

Typically nurse managers must put all of their eggs in one basket: the next outcome. They do not have the time or resources to let the probability work itself out. Therefore, objective statistical probability has certain constraints. Despite limitations, however, statistical probability, when properly applied and interpreted, has proven effective in helping middle managers make risky decisions. For example, the director of nursing directs all nurse managers to staff for minimum requirements during the Christmas and New Year holidays. A two-year review of hospital records for this time of year could be used to estimate patient census and acuity level. The nurse manager could then, with a fair amount of precision, staff the unit based on these previous statistics.

Decision trees and utility models are also effective quantitative methods that can be used for risky decision making. There are other types of quantitative approaches which are beyond the scope of this book and may be considered when highly statistical methods are needed to make high risk decisions.

Computers and management information systems (MIS) are other important tools to help with risky and uncertain decisions, and many hospitals have computer terminals available for management. However, the nurse manager is going to have to become familiar with the decision-making software and ask three questions before the system can be of value: What data are important? What will be done with the data compiled? How will it fit into the decision-making process? (Chapter 20 discusses computer systems in detail.)

Another model used for risky decisions is minimax analysis. Under minimax, the nurse manager attempts to calculate the worst outcome possible for each alternative, then selects the alternative that will be the least offensive when everything possible goes wrong. An example is when a hospital contracts with a school of nursing to allow beginning nursing students to work on a unit that admits a large number of seriously ill patients and has a high turnover among personnel. The nurse manager lists the worst outcomes from each possible way of handling the situation and chooses the alternative offering the most acceptable results (see Figure 12–2).

It is obvious that choices 4, 5, and 7 could possibly be negotiated and implemented to bring about a positive presence in a unit already besieged

Figure 12–2   Minimax Analysis

Problem: Nursing students' participation in unit with large numbers of acutely ill patients and high staff turnover.

Nurse Manager's Alternative	Worst Possible Outcome
1. Refuse to cooperate.	1A. Dismissal from the hospital.
2. Request admission clerk to distribute patients evenly to other floors.	2A. Clerk refuses. 2B. Agrees but fails to follow through.
3. Set a maximum number of students allowed on a unit.	3A. School and hospital refuse to comply—confrontation.
4. Work closely with instructor to assign students to low-acuity cases.	4A. Instructor refuses to comply—confrontation.
5. Insist that instructor be present for all procedures and/or treatments in which student nurses participate.	5A. Instructor cannot/will not comply.
6. Assign one patient to two students.	6A. Patient irritated by increased stimulation.
7. Selectively orient students and instructor prior to clinical rotation.	7A. They refuse to participate.

with low morale and turnover. Alternative 6 could be the one choice whereby doing nothing presents the least amount of difficulty.

Uncertainty decisions are the most complex ones. No knowledge, meaningful experience, or probability of outcomes can be assigned for extreme cases of uncertainty. In such cases, the nurse manager has no rational basis for choosing one alternative over another, since rational choice is based on assessing the desirability of each identified outcome. It is important to determine, however, when decision making is really uncertain or if the nurse manager's condition of uncertainty is due to inadequate information or error. Fortunately, misinformation and lack of knowledge can be corrected, enabling the nurse manager to recognize new outcome possibilities and predict the probability of each known outcome.

NEED FOR CREATIVITY

A realistic approach, good management climate, and an environment conducive to hard thinking and evaluation are all important. But what turns a mediocre problem-solving team into an excellent one is the quality and originality of thinking that takes place. Creativity, simply defined, is the ability to develop and implement new and better solutions that are useful or satisfying. Creativity is the only way to keep an organization alive. One that functions by rule only stifles creativity, is inflexible, and is on the road to oblivion.

Steiner found general agreement among scholars and top managers regarding many of the intellectual and personality characteristics of creative persons. Some of these qualities are:

1. Generate ideas rapidly.

2. Are flexible, able to discard one frame of reference for another and/or to change approaches spontaneously.

3. Have a tendency to provide original solutions to problems.

4. Prefer complex thought processes to simple and easily understood ones.

5. Are independent in judgment, more able to believe in themselves even under pressure.

6. Exhibit distinct individualistic characteristics, seeing themselves as different from their peers.

7. View authority as conventional rather than absolute; that is, accept authority as a matter of expedience rather than personal allegiance or moral obligation.

8. Are willing to entertain and express personal whims, impulses, exhibit a more diverse "fantasy life" on clinical tests, and also inject humor into situations (Steiner, 1965).

In other words, creative people are likely to view authority as not absolute, to make fewer black and white distinctions, to have a less dogmatic view of life, to show more independence of judgment and less conformity, to be willing to give consideration to their own impulses, to have a sense of humor, and to be less rigid and freer but not less effectively controlled.

Many persons have attempted to define steps in the creative process and the results look much like the steps set forth earlier in this chapter regarding the problem-solving process. A more descriptive definition is "the creative process is that sequence of thinking leading to ideas which sooner or later will be regarded as novel and worthwhile. It is seldom completed on a step-by-step procedure, but is more often characterized by long delays, inactivity, and then large unpredictable leaps" (Steiner, 1965).

Identifying the characteristics of a creative person and the creative process are necessary before nurse managers can stimulate creativity. The following methods can help stimulate creativity:

Step 1. Nurse managers should assess their own beliefs and make sure they themselves subscribe to creative management. There is no substitute for a day-to-day example.

Step 2. A carefully designed planning program is essential. For example, creativity conferences can be planned wherein the method is basically that of questioning everything that the staff does. A method of work simplification, built on the premise that most people cannot increase productivity by working harder, but by eliminating certain steps and creating a new service or solutions, can be used at these conferences. Some organizations have instituted such conferences on a monthly or bimonthly basis, involving all employees. The focus is on problems any member of the group chooses to bring up that are creating difficulties for the unit or individual. This is not a gripe session, but problem solving in a creative way. To facilitate progress at these conferences, one should: (a) pick a specific task to improve; (b) gather relevant facts; (c) challenge every detail; (d) develop preferred solutions; and (e) implement improvements.

Step 3. The nurse manager also needs to meet with new employees routinely as part of the orientation process at which time information about solutions to problems is sought. New employees are not encumbered with the details of accepted practices and can offer prior experiences or insights before they get set in their ways or have their innovative ideas "turned off." The advantages offered by new employees should be explored, for all staff on the unit will gain from such use of human resources.

Step 4. The nurse manager must work with a philosophy (from the larger organization) that stresses creativity and takes measures to encourage it. If creativity has priority in the hospital setting, then the reward system should be geared to and commensurate with that priority. Those whose creativity is prized should not be promoted into situations whereby they lose their creativity. For example, a creative LPN who has devised innovative ways to provide nutrition to pediatric patients may be stifled when "promoted" to an outpatient clinic. Conversely, a staff nurse who has shown tremendous flexibility in working with all types of patients is held back from promotion because she is so productive on the unit. Advancement and status should be provided within the area of creativity.

Creativity demands a certain amount of outside contacts, receptivity to new and seemingly strange ideas, proper research assistance, a certain amount of freedom, and some permissive management. Continuing education of staff members should be encouraged in both formal and informal opportunities. There should be willingness to organize in a flexible fashion and to make the unit (hospital) opportunity-oriented. This means a willingness to abolish needless communications, to eliminate barriers to action, and to better identify opportunities.

Step 5. Nurse managers should try to stimulate creativity through experimentation with such devices as brainstorming or similar techniques.

Step 6. A climate must be created for the survival of potentially useful ideas. It is regrettable if good ideas are developed but never used.

A new idea is an extremely perishable thing; its creator is likely to be its sole supporter, after which it may have none, since the normal reaction is either to ignore it or seek its defects. The attitude on the unit or hospital must be favorable to giving new ideas a fair and proper hearing to reduce the tendency to destroy all creative processes within the individual or group.

The major limitation on creativity stems from the initial cost. The greater the creativity sought and the greater the departure from present practice, the greater the investment will be. In the long run, however, creative ideas can lessen costs and, in fact, may be very cost effective. The problem is to determine if and where it is important, how important it is, and to encourage the creative exchange of ideas with other units so that the new effect is to enhance vitality and productivity.

SUMMARY

- Defining the problem-solving and decision-making process is an essential component for nurse managers.

- Principles for diagnosing problems are: having all the facts; separating facts from interpretations; and determining the scope of each problem.

- Various methods of problem solving include trial and error, experimentation, problem critique, metaphor-based techniques, brainstorming, decision trees, and knowing when problems are self-solving.

- The problem-solving and decison-making processes utilize principles that enlarge problem-solving skills and develop critical thinking. To start any discussion on decision making, the proper identification of the problem must be made, being as specific as possible. Decisions cannot be made about matters unless the exact nature of the problem is understood.

- Risk and uncertainty are factors in problem solving and decision making but methods can be utilized that lead to appropriate decision making with a maximum probability of success.

- Some of the obstacles to problem solving and decision making are personality characteristics, rigidity, and preconceptions.

- Various types of group decision making are helpful for nurse managers because they require interactions with others and the perceptions and ideas of other people often provide multiple alternatives that help in approaching the problem situation.

- Creative decision making is critical but requires a supportive management climate in order to turn mediocre problem solvers into ones who develop innovative solutions.

BIBLIOGRAPHY

Barnard, C. (1937). *Functions of the executive*. Cambridge, MA: Harvard University Press.

Corcoran, S. A. (1986). Task complexity and nursing expertise as factors in decision making. *Nurs Res, 35*(2):107–112.

Delbecq, A. L., VandeVen, A. H., Gustafson, D. H. (1975). *Group techniques for program planning*. Glenview, IL: Scott Foresman.

Duxbury, M. L. et al. (1984). Head nurse leadership style with staff nurse burnout and job satisfaction in neonatal intensive care units. *Nurs Res, 33*:2.

Gillies, D. A. (1982). *Nursing management: A systems approach*. Philadelphia: Saunders.

Huber, G. P. (1980). *Managerial decision making*. Glenview, IL: Scott Foresman.

Janis, I. L., Mann, L. (1977). *Decision making*. New York: Free Press.

La Monica, E., Finch, F. E. (1977). Managerial decision making. *J Nurs Adm, 7*(5):20.

Lancaster, W., and Beare, P. (1982). Decision making in nursing practice. In: *The Nurse as change agent*. Lancaster, J., and Lancaster, W. (editors). St. Louis, MO: C. V. Mosby, pp. 146–170.

Latz, A., (1977). An investigation of the managerial techniques of nursing service directors. St. Louis University. Unpublished master's thesis.

Likert, R. (1961). *New patterns of management*. New York: McGraw-Hill.

Marriner, A. (1984). *Guide to nursing management*. 2nd ed. St. Louis, MO: C. V. Mosby.

McKenny, J., Keen, P. (1979). How managers' minds work. *Harv Bus Rvw*, (May–June): 74.

Moore, R., et al. (1982). On the scene: Quality circles at Barnes Hospital. *Nurs Adm Quart, 6*:3.

Obsorn, A. F. (1953). *Applied imagination*. New York: Charles Scribner's Sons.

Ouchi, W. (1981). *Theory Z: How American business can meet the Japanese challenge*. Reading, MA: Addison-Wesley.

Peterson, M. E. (1983). Motivating staff to participate in decision making. *Nurs Adm Quart*, (Winter) 7(2):63.

Smith, H. L., Reinow, F. D., and Reid, R. A. (1984). Japanese management: Implications for nursing administration. *J Nurs Adm, 14*(9):33–39.

Steele, S. M., Maraviglia, M. S. (1981). *Creativity in nursing*. Thorofare, NJ: Charles B. Slack.

Steiner, G. (1965). *The creative organization*. Chicago: University of Chicago Press.

Stevens, B. (1980). *The nurse as executive*. 2nd ed. MA: Nursing Resources.

Warner, D. M., Prawka, J. (1972). A mathematical programming model for scheduling nursing personnel in a hospital. *Mngmt Sci, 19*:4.

4

HUMAN RESOURCE MANAGEMENT SKILLS

Recruiting and Selecting Staff

IN SERVICE OR labor-intensive organizations such as health care organizations, the quality of personnel hired and retained will determine whether or not an organization is successful in accomplishing its objectives. The selection of personnel is therefore of vital importance because the cost of improper selection can be high. The visible cost is represented in recruiting, selecting, and training an employee who must later be terminated because of unsatisfactory performance. The hidden costs may be even more expensive and include: low quality of work performed by the unmotivated employee, disruption of the work place, and patients' ill will and dissatisfaction, which may make them reluctant to return to the particular unit or hospital.

    The selection process is one of matching people to jobs and includes the following elements: job analysis; methods of recruiting applicants; selection technique(s) that measure applicants' skill, ability, and knowledge; and assurance that the selection techniques developed and used conform to legal constraints.

    The responsibility for selection of nursing personnel in hospitals is usually shared by the personnel or human resources department and

Figure 13—1   Flowchart of the Selection Process

Activity	Responsibility
Develop/review job requirements ↓	Nursing service ↓
Develop selection systems (application, tests, interview guide) ↓	Nursing service/Personnel ↓
Initial contact with organization/ Recruiting ↓	Nursing service/Nurse manager ↓
Application blank/résumé ↓	Nursing service ↓
Preliminary interview/screening ↓	Nursing service/Personnel ↓
Selection testing or assessment center, if used ↓	Nursing service/Personnel ↓
Reference check ↓	Nursing service/Personnel ↓
Manager/Supervisor interviews ↓	Nurse manager ↓
Medical examination ↓	Personnel ↓
Integration of all information ↓	Nursing service/Nurse manager ↓
Comparison of applicants to make hire/no hire decision(s) ↓	Nurse manager ↓
Job offer ↓	Nurse manager/Nursing service ↓
Acceptance of offer ↓	Applicant ↓
Entry and processing/orientation	Nursing service/Personnel/Nurse manager

Goodale, J. G. *The Fine Art of Interviewing,* © 1982, p. 63. Reprinted by permission of Prentice-
 Hall, Inc., Englewood Cliffs, New Jersey.

nursing service. The first-line managers within nursing are the most knowledgeable about the job requirements and can best describe the job to applicants. The personnel department performs the initial screening and monitors hiring practices to be sure they adhere to legal stipulations.

Figure 13–1 shows a flowchart of the selection process and suggested responsibilities. As indicated in the chart, it is vital for the immediate supervisor or nurse manager to take part in the selection process. The personal commitment to the recruit is generally higher when the nurse manager participates in the interviews. This is because: (a) the nurse manager is generally in the best position to assess applicants' technical competency, potential, and overall suitability; and (b) it allows applicants to have their technical, work-related questions answered more realistically.

Whether involved in the selection of applicants or not, the nurse manager must keep others who are involved in selection and recruitment informed of the personnel needs of the work unit and any changes that may have taken place in the job to be filled. The nurse manager is usually the first to be aware of changes such as potential resignations, requests for transfer, and maternity leaves that require personnel replacement. She or he is also aware of changes in the work area that might necessitate a change such as the need for a night nurse instead of a day one. Communicating these needs to the appropriate recruiting person promptly and accurately helps ensure effective coordination of the selection process.

JOB ANALYSIS

Before any recruiting or selection of new staff is attempted, the people responsible for hiring should be familiar with the job description and the skills, abilities, and knowledge required to perform the job. The process of determining duties and requirements is job analysis—a research process that determines: (a) the principal duties and responsibilities involved in a particular job; (b) tasks which must be done to discharge each duty; and (c) the personal qualifications (skills, abilities, knowledge, and traits) needed for the job. The outcome of a job analysis is a job description and these, obviously, will vary from job to job and hospital to hospital. Figure 13–2 is an example.

Job knowledge is the foundation for almost all human resource functions. Before nurse managers can train an individual to do a job, they must know the tasks of the job; before they can appraise a person's performance in a position, they must know the performance that is required of that individual in the first place. Job analysis provides the means by which this can be accomplished. If no job descriptions currently exist, then the nurse manager should develop one for each job in the unit. Each person should have a copy of her own job description.

An important factor in selection is the job specification which details the personal qualifications needed. While knowledge, skill, and ability requirements can be inferred from a description of the tasks and duties to be performed, a description of knowledge, skill, and ability requirements does not necessarily permit an inference about tasks and behaviors. Consequently, a job analysis which lists tasks may be more appropriate than one which lists only personal requirements. Many commercially available instruments list only personal requirements.

A relatively large number of techniques are available for performing job analysis (Cascio, 1978). They vary substantially in complexity and in ability to deal with different kinds of jobs. Different techniques include: *supervisory conferences, critical incidents, work sampling, observation, interviewing, questionnaires,* and *checklists.*

Figure 13–2 Staff Nurse Job Description

Position: Staff Nurse

Supervised by: Head nurse

Department: Nursing Service and
Operating Room

Section: Various Nursing Areas and
4430, 3620

Job Grade: 15 **Job Code No:** 126

Purpose of Position: Provides direct patient care activities including assessment, planning implementation and evaluation.

Primary Responsibilities: Functions include admission and ongoing assessments of patients utilizing physical and psychosocial assessment skills, diagnostic data and medical evaluations. Evaluate effectiveness of care provided as related to short and long term patient goals. Develops a plan for patient care including actions in anticipation of discharge needs. Implements nursing actions and medical orders to meet complex needs of patients and important others. Documents care provided and patient responses to care in appropriate forms in the patient's record.

Assumes Charge Nurse responsibilities (once licensed) and accountability for care provided by LPNs and non-licensed nursing personnel as assigned. Leadership abilities are demonstrated in functioning as a professional role model, consumer relations and communication skills, problem solving and decision making and assistance in orienting and training personnel.

Participates in continued professional development and research activities for the improvement of patient care.

Performs other job related duties as assigned.

Training, Education, Experience or Other Requirements: Graduate of a state approved school of nursing, possesses current RN licensure with the Missouri State Board of Nursing or current RN Missouri temporary work permit or has applied for licensure examination. Required to work rotating shifts.

Physical Demands: Stands and walks most of time on duty. Lifts and pushes patients on stretchers and in wheelchairs. Usually works in a clean, air-conditioned area. May be subject to infectious patients, contaminated specimens, toxic drugs, and radiation.

Replaces Job Description: Nurse; Staff; dated June, 1985.

PERFORMANCE EXPECTATIONS
Expectation I: **Assessment/Evaluation of Patient Care**

Demonstrates the ability to assess and evaluate appropriate patient care to promote optimal levels of wellness.

Figure 13–2 (*continued*)

1. Patient Care:

   a. Assesses/evaluates patient understanding of disease process or present condition.
   b. Assesses patient utilizing a body systems approach.
   c. Identifies nursing care problems/diagnoses.
   d. Evaluates outcomes of nursing care/medical therapies related to body systems assessment.
   e. Assesses discharge and/or transfer needs based on medical, nursing, and home care problems.

2. Diagnostic Data:

   a. Correlates diagnostic data with patients' assessment and recognizes changes in patients' condition relative to that data.
   b. Interprets and utilizes diagnostic data specific to patients on the patient care area.

3. Goals:

   a. Identifies short and long term goals for patients based on acute and chronic needs.
   b. Evaluates outcomes of nursing care with specific focus on the patients' progress toward achievement of short and long term goals.

Expectation II: Planning/Implementation of Patient Care

Utilizes assessment data and problem identification to plan and provide appropriate nursing care toward patient's optimal level of wellness.

---

1. Patient Care:

   a. Plans nursing care based on medical treatment regimen, nursing assessment data, identified nursing problems and significant other/patient participation.
   b. Demonstrates competence in performance of nursing skills relative to area of practice.
   c. Collaborates with other health team members to plan and provide holistic nursing care.
   d. Provides nursing care which reflects consideration of discharge and/or transfer needs.
   e. Organizes patient care to be completed within designated shift.

2. Diagnostic Data:

   a. Reviews available diagnostic information to develop a holistic approach to patient care for assigned group of patients.
   b. Utilizes diagnostic data to report significant findings and initiate changes in therapies.

Figure 13–2 (*continued*)

3. Goals:
   a. Organizes care in order to plan for meeting both acute and chronic needs of the patient.
   b. Focuses nursing care to assist the patient/significant other in identifying and achieving short and long term goals.
   c. Establishes care plan to meet short and long term goals.

Expectation III: **Patient/Significant Other Education**

Initiates patient and significant other education of routine therapies and procedures, and begins discharge planning and teaching upon admission.

1. Performs consistent ongoing assessment/evaluation of patients' learning needs, e.g., upon admission—reason for hospitalization, basic understanding of illness/condition, understanding of relationship between illness and routine therapy.

   a. Assesses factors which enhance or interfere with teaching/learning.
   b. Evaluates success of teaching through patients' ability to verbalize implications of illness, treatment plan, and complications and return demonstration of basic health care concepts.
   c. Assesses patients'/significant others' learning needs for discharge.
   d. Evaluates patients' and significant others' understanding of patients discharge health status.

2. Develops/implements plan of care based on patients'/significant others' learning needs.

   a. Revises teaching plan as patients' needs become more complex, diverse or resolved.
   b. Explains routine therapies, procedures, and surgeries.
   c. Explains and/or reinforces teaching regarding disease process.
   d. Performs health care teaching as outlined in care plans.
   e. Provides pertinent educational resources, e.g., educational classes, audiovisual aids, booklets, and Clinical Specialists.
   f. Consults with other health team members regarding readiness for discharge.
   g. Develops/implements plan of care for discharge education.
   h. Refers to appropriate outside agencies, groups and resources for outpatient follow-up prior to discharge.

Expectation IV: **Documentation**

Documents pertinent data in a concise manner that is consistent with the approved Hospital system of documentation.

Figure 13–2 (*continued*)

1. Documents assessment of patients' physical and non-physical needs from admission to discharge utilizing nursing diagnoses.
2. Documents plan of care and patients'/significant others' response to plan.
3. Documents care given, medications, treatments and other therapeutic diagnostic measures including any omissions and patients' response to same.
4. Documents and reports patient/visitor/employee incidents.
5. Maintains current, accurate nursing care plans.
6. Documents teaching and patients'/significant others' response to teaching.
7. Charts in a manner which reflects the patients' current status and condition using pertinent nursing diagnoses.
8. Documents nursing referrals/consultations for patients' care, discharge, or support services.

Expectation V: Consumer Relations

Identifies the patient, significant others, staff, and physicians as consumers and demonstrates techniques for providing an open, professional, congenial atmosphere.

---

1. Communicates with and listens to the patient, significant others, and members of the health team in a concise, tactful, and considerate manner.
2. Demonstrates cooperative and effective relationships with all other personnel/departments.
3. Recognizes potential and actual consumer concerns in a timely manner.
4. Investigates all information pertinent to concerns to clearly define problem.
5. Assesses methods for meeting consumer needs.
6. Acts to resolve consumer problems and reports results of action taken to the appropriate manager.
7. Assists co-workers in dealing with consumer problems as needed.
8. Demonstrates effective/courteous telephone communication skills.
9. Maintains patient confidentiality in regard to the patient's Bill of Rights.
10. Encourages patient and significant others to evaluate nursing care by encouraging completion of patient questionnaire.

Expectation VI: Leadership Skills/Teamwork

Identifies potential and actual problems in patient care area. With other patient care providers, recommends solutions and intervenes appropriately. Is accountable for the care of assigned patients and the care assigned to other health care providers whom the RN covers. Communicates pertinent information to appropriate person.

Figure 13–2   (*continued*)

1. Makes rounds on assigned patients.
2. Identifies problems occurring throughout shift.

   a. Assesses/evaluates problems identified.
   b. Seeks assistance from Head Nurse/Assistant Head Nurse/designated others as needed to develop plan for intervention.
   c. Implements plan for intervention and reports to Head Nurse/Assistant Head Nurse results of action taken.

3. Assigns patients' care with patient needs and staff capability taken into account.

   a. Assesses/evaluates capabilities of nursing care providers assigned for coverage.
   b. Provides information/demonstrates skills to assigned nursing care providers as indicated.

4. Delegates tasks effectively when indicated.
5. Recognizes staff noncompliance with policies and procedures. Instructs staff regarding current policy/procedure when possible and informs appropriate manager (Head Nurse, Assistant Head Nurse, Supervisor).
6. Functions as Charge Nurse when assigned by Head Nurse/Assistant Head Nurse (after successful completion of State Board examination).

   a. Reviews/revises patient care assignments with patient needs and staff capability taken into account.
   b. Adjusts patient care assignment during shift as need arises.
   c. Revises assignments as indicated to prevent overtime.
   d. Provides adequate orientation and appropriate assignment of float pulled staff, nursing students and orientees.
   e. Assures oncoming shift of appropriate staff complement based on patient census and acuity. Takes action to arrange coverage.
   f. Communicates all pertinent information occurring during shift to Head Nurse/Assistant Head Nurse/Supervisor and/or other appropriate person.
   g. Supervises/evaluates nursing care provided during shift.

Expectation VII: Policies and Procedures

Knowledgeable and supportive of Hospital and Nursing philosophy, policies and procedures as demonstrated in personal conduct and provision of nursing care.

---

1. Demonstrates professional conduct consistent with policies and procedures.
2. Organizes time to review policies and procedures on an ongoing basis and demonstrates compliance in nursing practice.
3. Provides input to Head Nurse and/or Policy and Procedure Committee for development and revision of policies and procedures.

Figure 13-2   (*continued*)

Expectation VIII: Budgetary Awareness

Provides cost-effective, quality patient care through appropriate use of supplies and personnel.

1. Completes and signs time sheet properly.
2. Recognizes the budgetary impact of numbers and mix of personnel.
3. Makes appropriate charges.
4. Uses supplies and equipment judiciously.
5. Communicates problems in acquisition or use of supplies and services to Head Nurse/Assistant Head Nurse/Nursing Supervisor.

Expectation IX: Professional Development

Participates in continuing education programs for the improvement of patient care and demonstrates interest in professional growth.

1. Assumes responsibility and accountability for own practice.
2. Identifies strengths and limitations of professional practice.
3. Utilizes identified strengths and limitations as a basis for selecting developmental opportunities.
4. Verbalizes rationale for decisions/actions based on current principles of nursing practice.
5. Acknowledges errors or omissions in care and takes action to correct these.
6. Remains updated and current in unit activities by attending unit staff meetings/reading minutes.
7. Accompanies MD and/or Head Nurse on patient rounds when possible.
8. Attends and participates in patient care conferences and presents at least one conference or inservice per year.
9. Completes at least two continuing education programs per year relative to area of practice.
10. Incorporates new knowledge into daily nursing practice.
11. Participates in programs for career development and/or attainment of BSN.
12. Acts as preceptor for orienting personnel as requested by Head Nurse/ Assistant Head Nurse.
13. Assists Head Nurse/Assistant Head Nurse in orientation and development of students and staff unfamiliar with the patient care area.
14. Maintains and submits to Head Nurse current licensure and educational record/qualification permits as relevant to practice.

Figure 13–2 (*continued*)

Expectation X:	Problem Solving/Research
	Utilizes problem-solving methodologies for benefit of patients/significant others, the patient care area, and the nursing profession.

1. Recognizes and proposes solutions to patient and/or divisional problems.
2. Utilizes appropriate resources in investigation of problems, e.g., patient record documentation, patients/families, colleagues, journals.
3. Participates in data collection and implementation of investigational protocols as directed by Head Nurse.
4. Identifies problems on assigned patients and/or patient care area amenable to research and recommends these to Head Nurse/Clinical Nurse Specialists for investigation.
5. Implements applicable research findings relative to care of assigned patients, consistent with policy/protocols in collaboration with Head Nurse/Clinical Specialist.

Supplied by Barnes Hospital Nursing Service, St. Louis, MO. Used by permission.

Supervisory conferences are situations where the analyst brings the supervisors and/or first-line managers together in a conference to identify the critical tasks or duties required in a job. The *critical incident* technique also requires the involvement of managers, who keep records of job holders' behaviors that have contributed to particularly successful or unsuccessful job performance. Both methods are very time consuming, and the critical incidents method sometimes does not give a complete picture of the job because only the very positive or negative behaviors are listed. *Work sampling* is the process of actually doing the job. It is rarely used because it is so time consuming.

Observation is one of the most common methods used by job analysts. It is most often used for analysis of jobs that consist largely of repetitive, short-cycle, manual operations. *Interviewing* is another common method. It relies on position holders providing information to a job analyst about tasks or personal characteristics associated with the job.

Questionnaires and *checklists* also rely on job holders for most of the description of tasks and personal requirements. Checklists tend to be more structured than questionnaires and may consist of 200 or more items for the individual respondent to check off if he or she performs them. These data are then analyzed to determine the tasks performed by the majority of persons currently in the job. Questionnaires can be open-ended. Several commercial questionnaires are available. When a checklist is used as the basis for job analysis, a large number of job holders is needed to supply the data because of the statistical analysis techniques used. The nurse manager might participate in developing a job analysis, usually through a supervisory conference, interviewing, or by the use of questionnaires (Bouchard, 1976).

Assuming that they are free of error and distortion, job descriptions and specifications can be compared to a photograph: that is, they represent what the job is at the time the job analysis is performed. The tasks and duties information can be used to construct performance appraisal instruments and training programs. The job specification information can be used to develop selection procedures. Figure 13–3 is an example of a structured interview guide used for job analysis.

Figure 13–3   Interview Guide Used For Job Analysis

Job Description Questionnaire

Department: _____   **Name:** _____

Position/Title: _____

I.   Please briefly describe the main purpose or objective of your job.

II.   Respondent's Title: _____

Whom do you supervise? _____

Check this box if you do not supervise   ☐

Job Title	**Number of People**
_____	_____
_____	_____

III.   Please list, **in order of importance**, the primary responsibilities of your job. For instance: "insure medications are administered on time"....

A. _____
B. _____
C. _____
D. _____
E. _____

Figure 13–3 (*continued*)

IV. Please describe (in the same order) the steps that you go through in order to perform the above stated responsibilities. That is, what duties or tasks must you do to insure fulfillment of your responsibilities. For instance: "Check with Pharmacy to see that medications are delivered on time, check with Xray to see that patients are scheduled as ordered" etc. . . .

    A. _____

    B. _____

    C. _____

    D. _____

    E. _____

V. Please list, **in order of importance**, any specific duties which you might perform periodically.

    A. _____

    B. _____

    C. _____

VI. Who do you contact on institution-related matters (excluding supervisors and subordinates) both inside and outside of the institution? (i.e., Central Supply, Laboratory, Physical Therapy, product representatives)

    A. Inside institution? _____

    B. Outside institution? _____

VII. What equipment do you use, or need to know how to use to:

    A. Perform your job successfully? _____

    B. Train others? _____

VIII. Briefly describe the environment in which you do your work (i.e., noise level, traffic area).

IX. If a friend asked you to describe the good and bad points of your job, what would you say? Please be as specific as possible.

X. What is the **absolute minimum** education requirement for this job? (None, H.S., some college, etc. . . .) Why?

XI. What is the **absolute minimum** amount of experience a person would require, in a similar or related area, to perform this job **reasonably** well? Why?

Figure 13–3 (*continued*)

XII. What other training or courses, not easily available at school, would be absolutely required to perform your job reasonably well? Why?

_____

What training do you think would be helpful?

_____

XIII. How long should it take someone with the necessary requirements to perform your job reasonably well? Why?

XIV. What are the absolute minimum physical requirements of this job? (i.e., weight lifting, energy level, sleep cycle)

Requirements	**Reason**
_____	_____
_____	_____

XV. What skills, knowledge, or abilities **must** you have in order to be able to perform your job reasonably well and why? (i.e., communication skills, management ability, technical nursing skill)

Skill, Knowledge, Ability	**Reason**
_____	_____
_____	_____

XVI. Are there any other details about your job you think need to be stated?

_____

Adapted from a form developed by Douglass Max. Used with permission.

RECRUITMENT

Recruitment is the activity that links staff planning with selection. Its purpose is to locate and attract enough qualified applicants to provide a pool from which the required number of qualified individuals can be selected. Even though *recruiting* is primarily carried out by personnel department staff and nurse recruiters, nurse managers have an important role to play in the process.

A nurse manager's ability to create a positive work environment through her or his management and clinical expertise will help retain a higher percentage of staff. Through informal channels of communication, new workers will hear about and be attracted to a particular unit. In contrast, a weak manager is more likely to have a higher turnover rate and be less likely to attract sufficient numbers of nurses of high quality to that unit.

There are essentially four elements in any recruiting strategy: *where to look, how to look, when to look*, and *how to sell the organization to potential recruits*. For most hospitals, the best "where to look" is in their own geographic area. When hard pressed to find enough nurses, however, many hospitals make national searches, although most nurses do not look for jobs on a national level. Besides, there may be a large number of unemployed nurses in any geographic area. Inactive nurses are a potential pool of applicants, particularly in difficult economic times (Decker, Moore & Sullivan, 1982).

Obviously, organizational location plays a part in recruiting. If the hospital is in a major metropolitan area, a search may be relatively easy; if it is in a rural community hospital, however, recruitment may need to be conducted in the nearest city. In the final analysis, organizations recruit where experience and circumstances indicate they will find people with the necessary skills. Recognizing this, most hospitals adopt an incremental strategy whereby they recruit locally first and then expand to a larger and larger market until a large enough applicant pool is obtained.

There are many choices in deciding "how to look"—among them, employee referrals; advertising in newspapers, journals, and at professional conventions; educational institutions; employment agencies (both private and public); and temporary help agencies. Most applicants come from their own application and some form of advertising, although, with the current nursing shortage, some hospitals are offering bounties for employee referrals. Direct applications and employee referrals are quick and relatively inexpensive ways of recruiting people, but these methods also tend to perpetuate the current racial or social mix of the work force. There are also indirect problems related to "inbreeding" of persons who are graduates of the same educational institutions.

Advertising may be as simple as the use of classified ads in the local newspapers or of more complex advertisements in journals and at professional meetings. Advertising can be an effective recruiting tool, but it tends to be very expensive and usually requires the assistance of technical personnel.

Empirical evidence shows that a relationship exists between the recruiting source and subsequent tenure with an organization (Decker & Cornelius, 1979). Applicants referred by informal methods (e.g., recommended by friends, walk-ins, and rehires) tend to remain with an organization longer than applicants recruited by formal methods (e.g., newspaper and other advertising and employment agencies).

The recruiting source has also been shown to be related to subsequent productivity. Nurses coming from informal sources of referral are likely to have more realistic information about the job and the institution and, therefore, their expectations more closely fit reality. Those who come to the job with unrealistic expectations tend to have those expectations violated quickly, with dissatisfaction as the result. In an open labor market, these individuals will leave the organization and high turnover will result. However, in difficult economic times, more individuals will tend to stay in the organization because they need the job, but they are not likely to perform as well as other employees. Consequently, even *where* one looks for applicants may have significant consequences later on.

It has been well established that proximity to home is a key factor in choosing a job, so that nurses living near the hospital are an inviting target for recruitment (Decker, Moore & Sullivan, 1982). With some effort and probable expense, one can obtain from the state board of nursing the names of registered nurses and target those in zip code areas surrounding the hospital. Also, one could ask personnel officers in large companies or institutions near the hospital to target spouses who are nurses. Students in any local school of nursing are also an excellent potential source of employees when they graduate.

One source of new nurses that has been widely overlooked is the inactive nurse. Survey statistics show that between 27% and 40% of registered nurses in any geographic area are not working in health care and that, of those nurses, approximately 70% would consider returning to nursing, given certain conditions such as refresher training and continuing education (Decker, Moore & Sullivan, 1982). Many older nurses would volunteer their time to reenter nursing and learn the new skills. Most of these now inactive nurses would look for the following components in employment (listed by priority): proximity to home, management support, quality of orientation, salary, and opportunity to specialize.

The timing of contact in recruiting has not been a major concern in health care, since, except for brief periods of time, there has been a continuing shortage of nurses. But let's suppose that in the past it has typically taken 10 days for a hospital's recruitment advertisement to begin producing applications, 4 days for invitations to interview to be issued, 7 days to arrange for interviews, 4 days for the organization to decide whether or not to employ a given individual, 10 days for the applicants offered positions to make up their minds, and then an average of 20 days for those accepting offers to report to work. This suggests that vacancies must be advertised almost two months before they are expected to occur. Today, however, health care organizations are finding that it takes much more time to fill positions due to the shortage. So, if there is to be any personnel planning, these time lines should be considered.

The final issue to be addressed in development of a recruiting strategy is the matter of communication, since this is known to influence job seekers. Contacts with applicants require a professional approach, and appointments with personnel departments and first-line supervisors must be on time, friendly, and conducted in an organized manner. The organization must be responsive to the applicant's needs.

Overselling the organization leads to unrealistic expectations that may lead to later dissatisfaction and turnover. Realistically presenting the job requirements and rewards improves job satisfaction in that the new recruit learns what, in actuality, the job is like. To promise a nurse every other weekend off and only a 25% rotation to nights on a severely understaffed unit and then scheduling her off only every third weekend with 75% night rotations is an example of giving unrealistic job information. It would be much better to represent the situation honestly and describe the steps management is taking to improve the situation. The recruit could then make informed decisions about the job offer.

Expectancy theory suggests that applicants are motivated to apply for those jobs that they believe are attainable (expectancy) and offer a package of rewards that they find attractive (valence). This knowledge does not help pinpoint precisely the factors that influence beliefs or perceptions on the part of the applicant or the role that recruiting plays in this influencing process. However, it *is* known that job seekers are influenced by the tone of communications from the organization. So in recruiting one must look at both the medium and the message.

The medium is the agent of contact between the organization and the potential applicant. Obviously, one wants to search for a medium which gives the widest exposure. Unfortunately, the media that do that also tend to be inefficient and low in credibility. The more influential media in terms of selling an organization tend to be the more personal ones: present employees and recruiters. Acquaintances or friends of the recruit have prior credibility and the ability to communicate more subtle aspects of the organization and the job. Also, personal contact tends to be warmer.

Developing an effective recruiting message is difficult. Sometimes the tendency is to use a shotgun approach or to sugarcoat the message or make it very slick. A more balanced message, which includes honest communication with personal contact, is preferable.

Even though recruiting is primarily done by nurse recruiters, nurse managers are important in the recruiting process. Recruiting will be easier when current employees spread the recruiting message, reducing the need for expensive advertising and bounty methods. To a very large extent, proper management can serve as a recruiting tool.

Recruitment activities generate applicants from whom selections must be made. The primary purpose of any selection procedure is to assess an applicant's ability and motivation relative to the requirements and rewards of the job so that a matching process can be carried out. To the extent that these matches are made effectively, positive outcomes such as high job satisfaction and high quality performance can result.

INTERVIEWING

There are many selection methods but the most common method used for selection by nurse managers is interviewing. The interview is an information-seeking mechanism between an individual applying for a position and a member of an organization doing the hiring. During the interview, the interviewer is trying to elicit and evaluate information gathered from the application form and the interview, as well as from test results, if tests were given earlier. The applicant is trying to gather information about the job and the institution. Initial screening may be conducted by the personnel department to determine that an applicant meets the educational and experience criteria for the job. Following the initial screening, nursing supervisors and/or the nurse manager may conduct the interview, if it is for a staff nurse position. If staff from the personnel department or the nursing office conduct the interviews, mistakes may occur because these persons may be unfamiliar with specific job dimensions.

The interview is intended to:

1. Obtain enough information about the applicant to determine whether he or she is suitable for employment in the hospital and for the particular job under consideration

2. Give information about the hospital, job, and the people employed so the applicant can make a decision about joining the staff

3. Create good will toward the hospital or employing institution by the way the applicant is treated and the interview is managed

An effective interviewer must learn to solicit information efficiently and to gather relevant data. Interviews may last for one or one-and-a-half hours and, as shown in Figure 13–4, include an opening, information-gathering periods, and a closing. The opening is important because it is an attempt to establish rapport with the applicant so that the latter will provide relevant information. Gathering information, however, is the core of the interview. Giving information is also important, because that's where the interviewer can create realistic expectations in the applicant and sell the organization, if that is needed. However, this portion of the interview must come after the information has been gathered, because if it comes before, all the answers will be given away. Finally, the closing takes care of all the mechanics of possible employment.

Figure 13—4   Time Schedule of an Interview

	1½ hours	1 hour
Opening	7 minutes	3
Disclosure of interview procedure	3 minutes	2
Interests	5 minutes	5
Educational history	20 minutes	10
Job history	20 minutes	15
Future plans	10 minutes	5
Information about the organization and position	15 minutes	10
Additional questions and answers	5 minutes	2
Closing	5 minutes	3

Adapted from Decker, P. J. *Selection Interviewing Procedures for Healthcare Managers.* Copyright 1983, by Phillip J. Decker. Used with permission.

Principles for Effective Interviewing

Plan the interview.   Examine the application blank for job requirements and map out areas to be covered in the interview; plan and organize questions pertinent to optimal interviewing in an environment free from interruptions.

Personal characteristics of the interviewer, both as an individual and as a representative of the hospital, may influence the applicant's decision. First impressions of the interviewer are created by the latter's tone of voice, eye contact, personal appearance, grooming, posture, and gestures, as well as by the interviewer's impact throughout the interview.

Respond to the applicant.   Express concern for the applicant's feelings while maintaining control over the interview; respond appropriately to the applicant's comments, questions, and nonverbal behaviors; convey interest in the applicant in an atmosphere of warmth and trust; use encouragement and compliments.

Elicit information.   Use appropriate questioning to elicit relevant information; probe incomplete answers and problem areas while maintaining an atmosphere of trust; structure the interview so that comprehensive questions and follow-up comments can be explored.

Give information.   Communicate appropriate and accurate information about the hospital and available jobs for which the applicant might qualify; answer the applicant's questions truthfully.

Process information.   Gather, integrate, and analyze interview information to culminate in a final placement decision or recommendation;

identify personal characteristics by judging them in the context of the job requirements.

Staying Within the Law

Equal employment opportunity (EEO) law and succeeding court decisions have had two major impacts on selection procedures. First, organizations have been more careful to use predictors and techniques that can be shown not to discriminate against protected classes; and, second, organizations are reducing the use of tests suspected of built-in bias and relying more heavily on the interview as a selection device. However, Title VII of the Civil Rights Act of 1964 (43 Fed. Reg., 1978), to be discussed more extensively in relation to hiring, later in this chapter, applies to interviews as much as it does to tests.

Many interviewers become annoyed with what they perceive as restrictions imposed by EEO legislation, but EEO legislation does not restrict the employer from asking or measuring job-related characteristics. The legislation simply says that it is illegal to make a personnel decision based on a person's race, color, sex, religion, national origin, or other characteristics added by state law. Figure 13–5 presents questions which are appropriate and inappropriate to ask in interviews. (See also Poteet, 1984.) The basic rule of thumb in interviewing is: when in doubt about a question's legality, do not ask it. If it can be proven that only job-related questions are asked, EEO law will not be violated. The positive way of

Figure 13–5 Preemployment Questions

	Appropriate to ask	**Inappropriate to ask**
1. Name	applicant's name	questions about any name or title that indicate race, color, religion, sex, national origin or ancestry
2. Address	questions concerning place and length of current and previous addresses	any specific probes into foreign addresses that would indicate national origin
3. Age	requiring proof of age by birth certificate *after* hiring	requiring birth certificate or baptismal record *before* hiring
4. Birthplace or national origin		any question about place of birth of applicant or place of birth of parents, grandparents or spouse
		any other question (direct or indirect) about applicant's national origin
5. Race or color		any inquiry which would indicate race or color
6. Sex		any question on an application blank that would indicate sex

Figure 13–5 (continued)

7. Religion		any questions to indicate applicant's religious denomination or beliefs
		request a recommendation or reference from the applicant's religious denomination
8. Citizenship	question about whether the applicant is a U.S. citizen; if not, whether the applicant intends to become one	questions of whether the applicant, his/her parents, or spouse are native born or naturalized
	question if applicant's U.S. residence is legal and require proof of citizenship *after* being hired	require proof of citizenship *before* being hired
9. Photographs	may be required after hiring for identification purposes only	request photograph *before* hiring
10. Education	questions concerning any academic, professional, or vocational schools attended	questions asking specifically the nationality, racial or religious affiliation of any school attended
	inquiry into language skills, such as reading and writing of foreign languages	inquiries into the applicant's mother tongue or how any foreign language ability was acquired (unless it is necessary for the job)
11. Relatives	ask for the name, relationship and address of a person to be notified in case of an emergency	any unlawful inquiry about a relative as specified in this list
12. Organization	questions about organization memberships and any offices that might be held	questions about any organization an applicant belongs to which may indicate the race, color, religion, sex, national origin or ancestry of its members
13. Military service	questions about services rendered in armed forces, the rank attained, and which branch of service	questions about military service in any armed forces other than the U.S.
		request of military service records before hiring
	require military discharge certificate *after* being hired	
14. Work schedule	questions about the applicant's willingness to work required work schedule	ask applicant's willingness to work any particular religious holiday
15. References	ask for general and work references not relating to race, color, religion, sex, national origin or ancestry	request references specifically from clergymen (as specified above) or any other persons who might reflect race, color, religion, sex, national origin or ancestry of applicant
16. Other qualifications	any question that has direct reflection on the job to be applied for	any non–job-related inquiry that may present information permitting unlawful discrimination

Adapted from a document distributed by the Ohio Civil Rights Commission, 220 S. Parsons Ave., Columbus, OH 43215. Used with permission.

viewing EEO guidelines is to consider what possible relevance sex or race, for instance, have to job performance. If the object is to identify the best people to do the job, EEO legislation is not restrictive.

Preparing for the Interview

A very important facet of effective interviewing is preparation for the interview; most managers do not adequately prepare. In general, when time is limited, it is better to use part of it for planning rather than squander all of it on the interview itself. This is preferable to possibly spending more time later trying to correct the performance of a poor employee. Before the interview, the interviewer should review the job requirements, the application, and the résumé, write any specific questions for the applicants, and prepare the setting. Planning is best done immediately prior to the interview. This gives the interviewer time to relax and unwind from the pressures and distractions of the job. Also, if applicants are interviewed one right after the other, planning immediately prior to each interview allows a pause between candidates.

Lack of advance preparation may lead to insufficient interviewing time, interruptions, or failure to gather important information. Other problems include losing control of the interview because of a desire to be courteous or because a particularly dominant interviewee is encountered. This typically keeps the interviewer from gathering the needed information.

A cardinal rule is to review the application or résumé before beginning the interview. If the interviewee arrives with the résumé or application in hand, ask the person to wait for a few minutes while you review it. In doing so, consider three things. First, are there clear discrepancies between the applicant's qualifications and the job specifications? If the answer is yes, then no interview may be necessary. Second, look for specific questions to ask the applicant during the interview. Finally, look for a "rapport builder" (something you have in common with the applicant) to break the ice at the beginning of the interview.

In order to provide a relaxed, informal atmosphere, the setting is important. Both the interviewer and the applicant should be in comfortable chairs, as close as is comfortably possible. No table or desk should separate them. If an office is used, the interviewer should arrange chairs so that the applicant is at the side of the desk. There should be complete freedom from distracting phone calls and other interruptions. The applicant should not be seated so she or he can look out a window.

A selection interview should be planned just like any other business undertaking. All needed materials should be on hand, and the interview site should be quiet and pleasant. If others are to see the applicant, their schedules should be checked to make sure that they are available at the proper time. If coffee or other refreshments are to be offered, advance arrangements need to be made.

Unstructured interviews present problems; if interviewers fail to ask the same questions of every candidate, it is often difficult to compare them. With any human skill or trait, there is no standard or true score that can serve as a basis on which to compare applicants. One can only compare people against other people. Consequently, the most effective interviewing is when all applicants are seen before the decision to hire is made. But to do this, the same basic information is needed from all interviewees, and this calls for structured interviews, preferably by means of an "interview guide." The notes one makes about the interviewee can be written and retained on the same sheet. This may be needed later, to indicate the job-related reasons for the decision.

Developing Structured Interview Guides

An interview guide is a written document containing questions, interviewer directions, and other pertinent information so that the same process is followed and the same basic information is gathered from each applicant. It is usually job- or job category–specific, as shown below:

Do job analysis to determine tasks of the job
↓
Use tasks to determine personal characteristics
(skills, abilities, knowledge) required to do the tasks
↓
Write questions and develop behavioral simulations to tap whether
or not the applicant has the personal characteristics required
↓
Put these questions and ideas in the interview guide format
to guide you in the interview

Behavioral simulations differ from tests, in that they capture actual behavior, not what individuals say they would do. They are exercises designed to elicit behavior by placing the person in a controlled situation similar to the job. Examples are typing tests or administering medications. In order to be legal, simulations must: (a) have standardized administration; (b) be administered to all applicants reaching the same level of the selection process; (c) require skills which will not be provided by training; (d) be job related; and (e) provide the applicant with appropriate time for preparation.

Figure 13–6 presents an example of the process of identifying tasks, personal characteristics and, consequently, questions for the interview guide. Figure 13–7 is an interview guide format. This figure can be used to construct your own interview guide, but do not copy the questions verbatim; develop your own questions based on the categories.

Figure 13–8 is an example of "job-related questions" for an oncology unit that would be asked in area 6 of the interview guide. Figure 13–9 is

Figure 13–6 How to Determine Questions/Simulations to Use
in an Interview Guide

Task	→	Personal Characteristic required to effectively perform task	→	Question/ Simulation designed to determine if applicant has personal characteristic
type letters		type 50 wpm		typing test
compose routine letter		grammar spelling knowledge of letter format		questions about previous work experience work sample questions
open and sort mail		reading manual skills		previous experience
maintain files		know alphabet experience		questions about experience ask to recite alphabet, etc.

Adapted from Decker, P. J. *Selection Interviewing Procedures for Healthcare Managers.* Copyright 1983, by
Phillip J. Decker. Used with permission.

Figure 13–7 Interview Guide Format

1. The interviewer should record responses to each question during the interview. Immediately after the interview, indicate your reaction to each answer beneath the response. Use what is appropriate (e.g., Education questions may not be necessary for a candidate out of school 10 years with extensive work history).

Candidate: _____

Interviewer: _____

Date: _____ Position sought: _____

Review of application form:

Items of interest to you on the application:

Figure 13–7 (*continued*)

2. Open the interview and establish rapport.

___ Warm friendly greeting.
___ Names are important, yours and the applicant. (Use first or last name correctly.)
___ Break the ice—talk about his/her trip to _____, hobbies, weather etc. and/or talk briefly about yourself—position, hobbies, etc.

Outline topics to be covered in the interview.

___ Education
___ Work History
___ Miscellaneous
___ Job Preview

3. Education

I. A. High School Name _____

    B. Year Graduated _____

    C. Which courses did you like best? _____

    D. Which courses did you like least? _____

    E. Extracurricular activities you enjoyed the most: _____

II. A. Nursing School (College or Hospital) _____

    B. Year Graduated _____

    C. Additional College Work _____

    D. Additional Degrees _____

    E. Which courses did you like best? _____

    F. Which courses did you like least? _____

    G. If you had the opportunity to start your education all over again knowing what you know now, what would you do differently? _____

    H. What were some of the highlights of your years in school? _____

4. Employment History

    A. Tell me about your current job. What are your duties? What kind of decisions do you normally make? _____

Figure 13–7 *(continued)*

   B. What is there about your present position you like the most? _____

   C. The least? _____

   D. What aspects of your work is your supervisor especially pleased with? _____

   E. What areas do you feel you could improve on? _____

   F. What is there in your present job that you would change if you could? _____

   G. What things in a job do you consider to be important? _____

   H. What type of supervisor do you prefer working for? _____

   I. Why are you leaving your present job? _____

5. Self Evaluation

   A. What are the most important ways in which you've changed in the last 5–10 years? _____

   B. What do you see yourself doing in the next 10 years? _____

   C. What are some of the things you can work on to better your chance of getting where you want to go? _____

   D. What do you like to do in your spare time? _____

   E. What do you consider to be your strongest asset? _____

   F. What are other assets? _____

   G. What are 2 or 3 things that you have done in your lifetime of which you are the most proud? _____

   H. What is there in your overall background that you feel would enable you to do a good job in this position? _____

6. Job Related Situation: Tell me how you would handle this situation . . .

   (see Figure 13–8)

7. Will you work night/weekend rotations? ___ yes ___ no

Figure 13–7   (*continued*)

8. Job Preview Information

    A. Unit structure (Personnel)
    B. Orientation period
    C. Duties
    D. Available shift
        1. D/E, D/E, E, N
        2. 8 hrs, 10 hrs
    E. Tour of unit—Discussion of nursing care in general

9. Closing the Interview

    A. Is there anything you would like to add?
    B. Date available to start _____
    C. Follow-up date _____
    D. Thank you

Adapted from guides used by Barnes Hospital Nursing Service, St. Louis, MO. and from Decker, P. J. *Selection Interviewing Procedures for Healthcare Managers.* Copyright 1983, by Phillip J. Decker. Used with permission.

Figure 13–8   Oncology Unit Job Related Questions

Describe how you would intervene in the following situations:

A patient that you admitted with a diagnosis of lymphoma is going to begin chemotherapy and you are preparing to hang the first dose. When you enter the room she says, "You know I just can't believe that I have cancer. I know it is what the doctor says but it just doesn't seem possible to me."

The wife of a patient overhears some doctors caring for her husband say that the patient has received the incorrect dose of chemotherapy. You are caring for him.

A young man is diagnosed with acute leukemia and expresses anger and frustration in the presence of his wife. You witness the frequent outbursts and become increasingly aware of the sense of hopelessness on the part of both him and his wife.

A leukemia patient has been classified as a no code. On the night shift the patient develops dyspnea, becomes uncomfortable, anxious and screams out periodically. The patient is on 100% O_2 already but his wife insists that something more be done.

Figure 13–8 *(continued)*

A physician making rounds notices a discrepancy in your patient's I&O. The weights indicate that he has gained 10 pounds but the intake records do not show how this could have happened.

You are working nights and caring for an extremely seriously ill man receiving platelets and antibiotic therapy. The patient's blood pressure is continuing to drop. You have talked to the resident on call twice by telephone and he tells you to continue the present orders. The man's condition continues to decline. What would you do?

Adapted from a form used by Barnes Hospital Nursing Service, St. Louis, MO. Used with permission.

Figure 13–9 Staff Nurse Position, Burn Unit: Realistic Preview Information

Positive Information

    A. Patients are here for length of time—lots of patient and family teaching
    B. Critical as well as recovering patients
    C. Decision-making opportunities
    D. Bedside nursing
    E. Learning environment
    F. Able to assist with research
    G. Small unit, close knit, dedicated group
    H. Burns as well as other prior difficulties or concurrent problems to work with
    I. Children as well as adults

Negative Information

    A. Type of patient is sometimes difficult to deal with; i.e., young children or elderly—often alcoholics, psychological difficulties
    B. Emotionally stressful
    C. Physically difficult

Adapted from a form used by Barnes Hospital Nursing Service, St. Louis, MO. Used with permission.

an example of the type of information that would be presented in area 8, job preview information.

Interview guides reduce interviewer bias, provide relevant and effective questions, and reduce leading questions. Interview guides also provide a normative data base for applicant comparisons. Space left between the questions on the guide provides room for note-taking, and the guide also provides a written record of the interview.

The Interviewing Process

The interviewer should start on time, give a warm, friendly greeting, introduce herself or himself, and ask the applicant his or her preferred name. The interviewer should try to minimize status, not patronize or dominate, and not hide behind a desk. The objective is to establish an open atmosphere so that applicants reveal as much as possible about themselves. Rapport should be established and maintained throughout the interview. This can be done by talking about one's self, neutral and mutual interests such as hobbies or sports, and using nonverbal cues such as maintaining eye contact. Finally the interviewer should start the interview by outlining what will be discussed and setting the time limits for the interview.

The interviewer must be very careful not to form hasty first impressions and make equally hasty decisions. Interviewers tend to be influenced by their first impressions of a candidate—shaking hands with someone who has a limp, sweaty handshake, for instance—and such judgments often lead to poor decisions. First impressions also color the search for information that goes on in the interview; interviewers tend to search for information to justify their first impressions, good or bad. If the first impression is negative and the interviewer decides not to hire a potentially successful candidate, the interviewer has wasted an hour or so and possibly lost a good recruit. And if, because of a positive first impression the interviewer hires an unsuccessful candidate, problems may continue for months.

Using the structured interview guide, the interviewer should take notes, telling the candidate that this is being done to aid recall and that he or she hopes the candidate does not mind. There are various ways of asking questions, but only one question should be asked at a time and, where possible, open-ended questions should be used. These cannot be answered with a single yes, no, or one-word answer, and usually elicit more information about the applicant. Close-ended questions (what, where, why, when, how many, etc.) should only be used to elicit specific information when probing.

"Work sample questions" should be used to determine an applicant's knowledge about work tasks and ability to perform the job. It is easy to ask a secretary if she or he knows how to type. The secretary says, "yes," but this doesn't necessarily prove the ability, so the secretary could be asked to type something while the interviewer watches. Or the interviewer might ask some very specific questions about a typewriter or typing which only a typist or secretary can answer. Leading questions should be avoided because the answer is implied in the question ("We have lots of overtime. Do you mind overtime?"). The interviewer may also want to summarize what has been said, use silence to elicit more information, reflect back the applicant's feelings to clarify the issue, or indicate acceptance by urging the applicant to continue.

Next in an interview is the information-giving section, the interviewer having decided in advance what kind of information (both positive and negative) to give a candidate so that the latter will be realistically in-

Figure 13–10 The Effective Interview

---

1. Give a warm, friendly welcome.
   a. relax and smile.
   b. use appropriate name, be consistent and pronounce it correctly.

2. Talk about yourself to help applicant relax.

3. Tell applicant the purpose and structure of the interview.

4. Use your Interview Guide, follow the order and content exactly.

5. Take brief notes, and inform the applicant that you intend to.

6. Probe to get details about negative or unclear information.

7. Listen attentively.

8. Summarize what you have heard for each main section of the interview.

9. Give job preview information which is realistic.

10. Give a friendly goodbye.
    a. outline the next steps in the selection process.
    b. ask for any additional comments/questions.
    c. say goodbye and thank applicant for coming in.

Adapted from Decker, P. J. *Selection Interviewing Procedures for Healthcare Managers.* Copyright 1983, by Phillip J. Decker. Used with permission.

formed. Failure to present realistic information about the job may result in a new employee accepting employment with unrealistic expectations; this increases job turnover and may decrease productivity. Figure 13–9 is an example of realistic information for applicants.

The interviewer should also consider each applicant before reaching the information-giving part of the interview. Is the candidate promising enough to warrant the time spent in giving detailed information about the job? The interviewer must also know what information he or she should give and what is provided by others. Benefit or compensation questions are usually answered only by the personnel office. However, direct questions should not be avoided so that a realistic job preview is given.

In closing the interview, the interviewer may want to summarize the applicant's strengths and weaknesses. This is sometimes very difficult, so it may not always be done. But, the interviewer must make sure that the applicant is asked if she has anything to add to the impression that has been gained and to ask questions related to the job and the organization. Thanking the applicant and completing any notes made in the interview concludes the interview process. Figure 13–10 gives a full set of key behaviors for an effective interview to be followed whenever one is interviewing. These key behaviors can also be typed on a large index card for easy reference while interviewing.

DECIDING TO HIRE

Here are the logical steps in making a decision. First, weigh the qualities required for the job in order of importance; more emphasis should be placed on the more important elements. Second, weigh the qualities desired on the basis of the reliability of the data. The more consistent the observation of behavior from different elements in the selection system, the more weight should be given that dimension. Third, weigh job dimensions by trainability—that is, consider the amount of education, experience, and additional training the applicant can logically, not ideally, be expected to receive, and consider the odds that the behavior in that dimension can be improved with training. Dimensions least likely to be learned in training should be given the most weight.

Also, the interviewer should attempt to compare data across individuals in making a decision. It is much easier and more accurate to make decisions based on a comparison of several persons than to make a decision for each individual after each interview. This kind of data integration also prevents early impressions from affecting the decisions to hire. Time spent in selection is preferable to time spent in coaching, disciplining, and appraising a poor performer.

Interview Reliability and Validity

There have been numerous research studies on the reliability and validity of employment interviews. In general, *intra*rater reliability is fairly high, *inter*rater reliability is rather low, and the validity of the typical interview is very low. Research has also shown that: (a) structured interviews are more reliable and valid; (b) interviewers who are under pressure to hire in a short period of time or meet a recruitment quota are less accurate than other interviewers; (c) interviewers who have detailed information about the job for which they are interviewing exhibit higher interrater reliability; (d) the interviewer's experience does not seem to be related to reliability and validity; (e) there is a decided tendency for interviewers to make quick decisions and therefore be less accurate; (f) interviewers develop stereotypes of ideal applicants against which interviewees are evaluated, and portions of the stereotype are interviewer-specific, thus decreasing interrater reliability and validity; and (g) race and sex have been found to influence interviewers' evaluations.

Possibly the greatest weakness in the selection interview is the tendency for the interviewer to try to assess an applicant's "basic character" during the interview (Goodale, 1982). Judgments are made about the applicant's personality characteristics as well as knowledge and skill. Although it is difficult, if not impossible, to eliminate such subjectivity, evaluations of applicants are often more subjective than they need to be, particularly when interviewers try to assess personality characteristics. Information collected during an interview should answer two fundamental questions: (a) *Will* the applicant perform the job? and (b) *Can* the applicant perform the job?

The best predictor of the applicant's future behavior in these two respects is past performance. One should look at previous work and non-work experience, previous education and training, and current behavior, not personality characteristics, which even psychologists cannot measure very accurately. There is little reason to expect a nurse manager without any preparation to do an adequate job.

Testing for Selection

A test is any systematic standardized procedure for obtaining information from individuals. For employment purposes, a test gathers information pertaining to the applicant's abilities, skills, knowledge, or motivation believed to be required to carry out the job. There are aptitude tests, personality and interest tests, and work sample tests. *Aptitude* tests measure those individual characteristics that are likely to lead to acquiring knowledge or skill; they therefore indicate what tasks the applicant might be able to perform in the future, given the opportunity and/or training. *Personality and interest* inventories attempt to measure a person's motivation or personality characteristics, but they are not used to any great extent in employee selection. Aptitude tests are more accurate in predicting training success than job performance. In general, neither aptitude tests nor personality and interest inventories are accurate employment predictors.

Work sample tests are quite literally samples of the work performed on the job, the underlying assumption being that performance of a representative sample of the job will predict performance on the job itself. Work samples can be split into two categories: behavioral and knowledge. Behavioral work samples are those tests where a person actually does some of the behaviors involved in the job—a typing test, for instance. Job knowledge tests measure the knowledge required to do the job—for instance, a medical terminology test for an applicant for a unit clerk position.

Testing is usually the province of personnel office or nursing service staff, and the nurse manager will seldom, if ever, become involved in it because of (a) the legal requirements to validate these kinds of selection instruments, and (b) the need to ensure standardized administration policies. For the most part, paper and pencil testing will not be done in the typical hospital because of the costs and effort required in validity studies.

Education, Experience, and Physical Exams

Education and experience requirements for nurses have long been an integral part of the staffing process and bear a close relationship to work sample tests. Educational requirements represent a job knowledge sample since they tend to ensure that applicants have at least a minimal amount of the necessary knowledge. Experience requirements are very much like behavioral samples because the assumption is that, given a certain number of years of experience, the nurse would have performed a certain number of the required tasks.

References and letters of recommendation are also used to assess an applicant's past job experience, but there is little evidence that these have any validity. (Very few persons write "bad" letters of recommendation, and when applicants are almost invariably described in positive terms, one really does not know their potential for success in the job.) However, in the rare instances when candidates are described in negative terms, it does indicate future problems. Criticisms are likely to be very mild and may be indicated by omission rather than commission. Letters with any criticism, however, should be taken very seriously.

In almost every selection situation, an applicant fills out an application form that calls for previous experience, education, and references. Most application forms also ask for the applicant's medical history and other personal data. The obvious question is: Do applicants distort, either intentionally or unintentionally, their responses on an application form? Studies looking at this question indicate that there is usually little distortion, at least not on the easily verifiable information. Applicants may stretch the truth a bit, but rarely are there any complete falsehoods on application blanks. Relative to other predictors, the application form may be one of the more valid predictors in a selection process; its validity parallels that of work sample exercises.

The pre-employment physical exam serves a number of selection purposes. It screens out applicants who may have major physical or obvious mental impairments that would seriously impede successful job performance. It also identifies applicants with unfavorable attendance records or who may have excessive future claims against health insurance.

Assessment Centers

Many nonhospital organizations have turned to the use of assessment centers, especially in the selection of supervisory/managerial personnel. This is a relatively new practice for health care institutions, but some hospitals are now using such centers.

An assessment center is not a place; it is a process used for identifying individual strengths and weaknesses for a specified purpose such as selection, promotion, or development (Moses & Byham, 1977). Individuals engage in a series of exercises, both individual and group, constructed to simulate critical behaviors related to success on the job. The assessment center method is particularly appealing to organizations because judgments are based on the applicant's overt behavior in the assessment center, which parallels that required on the job. The likelihood of predicting future job performance is enhanced by using multiple assessment techniques, by standardizing methods of making inferences, and by pooling the judgments of multiple assessors.

Assessment centers are quite useful when candidates are needed for a job that is quite different from the one they now hold: selection of a staff nurse for the job of nurse manager, for instance. It is very difficult to judge how well a staff nurse who is performing mostly clinical skills will perform managerial behaviors. The hospital may very well end up with the loss of a good clinician and the inheritance of a poor manager because of an attempt to judge managerial ability by evaluating clinical skills. In this case, an assessment center is an appropriate method because it will simulate managerial behaviors.

Here are the essential elements of the assessment center process. (a) The analysis of relevant job behavior determines the attributes, characteristics, skills, abilities, or knowledge to be evaluated. (b) The techniques or exercises are designed to provide information to be used in evaluating job-related dimensions, skills, or abilities as previously determined. (c) Multiple assessment techniques are used, and at least one or more is of the behavioral simulation type. (d) Multiple dimensions that describe the relative skills, abilities, and knowledge required to do the job are used. (e) Multiple assessors (nursing service supervisors and directors) receive thorough training in order to process information in a fair and impartial manner. And (f) judgments resulting in hiring or promotion decisions are based on a pooling of the information from the different assessors and techniques and are made by consensus. Common exercises in assessment centers include interviews, organizational games, in-baskets (assessee working through the typical nurse manager's in-basket material), leaderless group discussions (staff meetings), some kind of presentation, role plays, and occasionally paper and pencil tests.

VALIDITY AND LEGALITY IN HIRING

Any selection procedure should include valid selection predictors; these are instruments (application form, tests, interviews) that are predictive of applicants' future effectiveness as employees on the job. Validity of a predictor cannot be assumed, but must be investigated scientifically. This refers to statistically measuring the connection between a predictor score and some measure of success on the job. Job analysis information will help one develop both the predictor and the measure of success. The use of valid predictors is not only desirable in choosing the best employee but also satisfies legal requirements. Staffing activities have been subject to considerable scrutiny regarding discrimination and equal employment opportunity, mainly as a result of Title VII of the Civil Rights Act of 1964, as well as the Equal Pay Act of 1963 and Age Discrimination Act of 1967.

As stated earlier, Title VII of the Civil Rights Act specifically prohibits discrimination in *any personnel decision* on the basis of race, color, sex, religion, or national origin. "Any personnel decision" includes not only selection but entrance into training programs, performance appraisal results, termination, benefits, and so on. The act applies to most employers with more than 15 employees, although there are several exemptions—among them, "business necessity" and "bona fide occupational qualification" (BFOQ). One may discriminate on the basis of national origin, religion, sex, and age, for instance, if that discrimination can be shown to be a bona fide occupational qualification or is necessary for the operation of a business. An example of a BFOQ is a male part in a play, or a male Sunday school teacher of a certain religion.

Business necessity can be claimed in the instances when not discriminating would put the organization out of business. For instance, hospitals employ a very small proportion of male nurses and hence "discriminate" against male nurses. However, since few male nurses are available on the job market, it is a business necessity. Examples of evidence generally not sufficient for a BFOQ or business necessity are claims of "customer preference" or gross gender characteristics such as "women cannot lift over 30 pounds." BFOQ claims that have been supported include the refusal to hire women as correctional counselors at a men's prison.

Title VII is also a complaint-oriented law: that is, any person who feels he or she has been discriminated against may file a complaint with the government against an employer. When a complaint is filed, the Equal Employment Opportunity Commission (EEOC) *or* the applicable state agency created to enforce the EEO law sends notice to the employer and initiates an investigation of the complaint. The EEOC has broad investigatory powers and access to all relevant employment records and documents. If it finds there is reasonable cause to believe that illegal discrimination has taken place, it will notify the employer and attempt to settle the complaint through conciliation. If this attempt fails, the EEOC or the individual may file a lawsuit against the company. Any legal action can result in reinstatement and/or back pay of up to two years for the suing party.

When an individual files a complaint of discrimination, he or she need only prove unequal treatment or that fewer members of minority than of nonminority groups are hired. The latter is known as adverse impact. The burden of proof then shifts to the organization, which must justify that its decisions were not related to the individual's race, color, sex, religion, national origin, or other categories that state laws may add such as handicap or national ancestry. There are two possible methods of justifying this claim: (a) to indicate that the hospital did not have the information on race, sex, and so forth in the first place and therefore could not have used it (this is a very difficult claim to make since most applicants are interviewed or are seen in a health care organization before hire); (b) to prove that the hire/no hire decision was based on some job-relevant criterion and not on race, sex, color, religion, or national origin.

The Equal Employment Opportunity Commission (EEOC) is charged with enforcing and interpreting the Civil Rights Act and has issued Uniform Guidelines on Employee Selection Procedures (43 Fed. Reg., 1978). The guidelines specify the kinds of methods and information required to justify the job relatedness of one's selection procedures. These guidelines will not be described in detail here; however, the methods of selection discussed in this chapter do follow their specifications. Remember that the law *does not say* one cannot hire the best person for the job or that one must hire so many whites and so many blacks. What it says is that race, color, sex, religion, or national origin must not be used as selection criteria. As long as the decision is not made on the basis of minority status, one is complying with U.S. EEO law. Canadian civil rights law parallels U.S. law, and consequently is not reviewed here.

Validation refers to the procedure used for gathering evidence that a predictor is job-related. The outcome of a validation study is information indicating the degree to which the predictor is related to job success. Two major types of validation studies are possible. *Empirical* validation is the most rigorous, costly, and time consuming. *Content* validation is considerably easier because it takes the form of a logical argument rather than an empirical argument, but it may not always make the strongest argument for job relatedness. In empirical validation studies, scores on both the predictor and the criterion measures are obtained from job applicants or employees. If employees are used, both predictor and criterion scores are obtained at the same time (concurrent validation). *Predictive* validation is a method wherein predictor scores are obtained from a sample of job applicants, and selection decisions are then made about those applicants—but not on the basis of the predictor being studied. The criterion scores for those applicants who become employees are collected later.

Concurrent and predictive validation strategies will almost always be performed by the personnel office or by consultants because they are so complicated and require precise collection of data. Not only does the nurse manager rarely become involved with statistical validity, many hospitals simply do not do it. Unless adverse impact—underutilization of a protected class—can be proven, the government will not scrutinize any part of the selection system. Therefore, if the number of minorities in a given job classification such as staff nurse or unit clerk is representative of the community at large, then there is no purely legal reason to do validation studies and many hospitals do not do them. However, content validity (being a logical argument) can always be used and should be in most situations, regardless of whether a hospital believes that there may be adverse impact or not in given job categories.

Content validity is a logical argument that says (a) the predictor is a representative sample of the tasks and duties required of a job incumbent, and (b) every measure used in the predictor is an actual part of the job. Content validity is most often used in relation to work sample or job

Figure 13—11   Validating the Selection Interview

		Marginal (25)	High (45)
Performance	High (30)	5	25
	Moderate (25)	10	15
	Low (15)	10	5

Interview Assessment

Taken from Goodale, J. G. *The Fine Art of Interviewing*. Englewood Cliffs, N.J.: Prentice-Hall, ©
  1982, Prentice-Hall, Inc. Used by permission.

knowledge predictors such as interviews, typing tests, and assessment
centers. For instance, a typing test used to select secretaries would not be
content valid because a secretary does other things besides typing. However, it is content valid for the job of clerk typist. To do content validity,
one simply has to take from a task list or job description of behaviors a
relatively small but representative number of tasks for the applicant to
perform during the selection process.

Assessing validity is not always easy, but nursing service should attempt it. The following is one way to perform a crude test of validity. To
do it, evaluations of applicants must be retained; this is advisable for legal
purposes, anyway. Also needed are some measures of performance on the
applicants that were hired. Figure 13–11 is a graphic depiction of a situation in which 70 applicants were interviewed and hired in a nursing service over a period of a year. After they had been employed for at least six
months, their performance appraisal forms were collected and grouped
into three categories of performance: high, moderate, and low.

These three *performance ratings* are listed in the left vertical side of
the table, and the *interview assessments* (whether they were rated high or
marginal for future performance) across the bottom. In this example, 45
of the applicants were assessed to be in the high category and 25 in the

marginal one. Of the 45 applicants who rated high, the performance appraisals showed 25 to be performing well, 15 moderately well, and only 5 low. This indicates a fairly good level of selection accuracy. If the same proportion was true for the 25 initially assessed as marginal, this would not indicate high validity. More sophisticated correlational analysis of validity is possible with larger numbers of applicants. See Guion (1965) for more information on statistical determination of validity.

It is important that nursing services examine the validity of their selection procedures, even if the only procedure is interviewing. Only then can one know if the selection of applicants is being done effectively.

SUMMARY

- The selection of staff is a critical function that involves matching people to jobs. Responsibility for hiring is often shared with nurse managers.

- Selection processes most often include screening application forms, résumés, medical exams, reference checks, and interviews but may include tests and assessment centers.

- Job analysis is the key to all selection because it defines the job. Selection procedures are designed to elicit information about the applicant. Then people can be placed in positions for which they are suited.

- Recruitment is the process of locating and attracting enough qualified applicants to provide a pool from which the required number of new job holders can be chosen. Poor quality applicants and/or a small pool will result in less accurate matches between job and applicants.

- Selection interviewing is a complex skill which is intended to obtain information about the applicant and give the applicant information about the hospital. The nurse manager, if involved in selection, will be involved in interviewing candidates for jobs in her area of responsibility.

- There are several principles of effective interviewing: plan and structure the interview; respond to the applicant in order to encourage rapport; elicit information through questioning techniques; give realistic job information; and process the information obtained in order to make a final placement decision.

- Developing a structured interview guide is a critical element in selection interviewing because it helps the interview "stay on track," and provides a mechanism for taking and storing notes about the applicant.

- Tests and assessment centers are complicated, standardized mechanisms for gathering application data which are sometimes used in selection. The nurse manager is not always involved in the use of these selection techniques. Assessment centers are most often used in hiring managers.

- All selection systems must be job-related. This is shown by validation studies. If selection systems are job-related, they will not discriminate on the basis of race, color, sex, religion, or national origin which is a requirement of the Civil Rights Act of 1964.

BIBLIOGRAPHY

Bouchard, T. J., Jr. (1976). Field research methods: Interviewing questionnaires, participant observation, systematic observation, unobstrusive measures. In: *Handbook of industrial and organizational psychology.* Dunnette, M.D. (editor). Chicago: Rand McNally.

Cascio, W. F. (1978). *Applied psychology in personnel management.* Reston, VA: Reston.

Decker, P. J., and Cornelius, E. T., III. (1979). A note on recruiting sources and job survival rates. *J App Psychol, 64*:463.

Decker P. J., Moore, R. C., Sullivan, E. (1982). How hospitals can solve the nursing shortage. *Hosp Health Services Adm, 27*(6):12.

Ertl, N. (1984). Choosing successful managers: Participative selection can help. *J Nurs Adm, 14*(4):27.

43 Fed Reg 38290-315 (1978).

Goodale, J. G. (1982). *The fine art of interviewing.* Englewood Cliffs, NJ: Prentice-Hall.

Guion, R. M. (1965). *Personnel testing.* New York: McGraw-Hill.

Moses, J., and Byham, W. (1977). *Applying the assessment center method.* New York: Pergamon Press.

Poteet, G. (1984). The employment interview: Avoiding discriminatory questioning. *J Nurs Adm, 14*(4):38–42.

Robertson, D. E. (1978). New directions in EEO guidelines. *Personnel J, 57*:360.

EVERY INDIVIDUAL IS unique and will, therefore, vary in education, skills, and ability. There are a few common denominators: new staff nurses will have attended nursing school and new unit clerks will have attended high school, trade school, or college. Yet many within each group will probably not have developed all of the skills and knowledge necessary to perform their jobs at the expected level. Further, new nursing practices and technology call for a continuing need for training. One of the nursing manager's major responsibilities is to assist subordinates in developing specific job skills, an activity usually referred to as training.

Most early educational theories were based on the belief that the fundamental purpose of education was the transmission of the totality of human knowledge from one generation to the next. This is a workable assumption provided that the quantity of knowledge is small enough to be collectively managed by the educational system and that the rate of change is small enough to enable the increase of knowledge to be packaged and delivered. Today, however, these conditions do not exist. Instead, we are living in a period of knowledge explosion in which cultural and technological change is rapid. This means that we simply cannot pass the totality of human knowledge from one generation to the next. We cannot even keep up year by year. The implications of this are two: first, education will no longer be primarily or exclusively directed toward children. We will see much more education of adults, and that education will be specifically formulated for adults. Second, we will see education moved to a partnership between the teacher and the learner so that it occurs everyday in an unstructured manner.

The process of education can be considered to operate constantly during conscious human activity and calls for consideration of several issues: how people learn, the content of what they need to learn, the processes of learning, and how to teach. People even need to be taught how to learn so that they can do their learning efficiently and will be prepared to learn new information as it becomes available.

Every hospital has specific goals, and their attainment requires trained personnel. Therefore, most hospitals have specialized training personnel, either assigned directly to nursing service or in special training and education departments. Such departments administer ongoing employee training and development programs and often orientation programs, yet the nurse manager, too, will often be extensively involved in the training process. A new employee, for example, must be taught specific work rules and tasks as well as new nursing or medical practices at the unit level. Nurse managers will also be extensively involved in patient education. Trained personnel are the key to success in a unit and in the hospital itself. Properly training employees will usually result in higher productivity, fewer accidents or mistakes, better morale, greater pride in work, and better nursing care.

Whether educational activities are planned for staff or patients, the basic model of the training function or the basic process of training remains the same. Figure 14–1 shows this process, which is similar to the nursing process and includes assessment, planning, implementation, and

Figure 14–1 Training Model

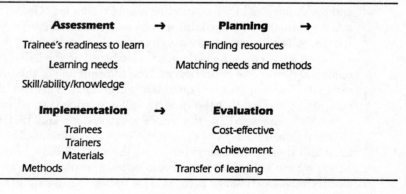

Assessment →	**Planning** →
Trainee's readiness to learn	Finding resources
Learning needs	Matching needs and methods
Skill/ability/knowledge	

Implementation →	**Evaluation**
Trainees	Cost-effective
Trainers	
Materials	Achievement
Methods	Transfer of learning

evaluation. Assessment is the process of investigation that provides knowledge about the trainee's readiness to learn and her or his specific learning needs—skill, for instance, or ability or knowledge. Planning entails obtaining training resources to present to the trainee and the matching of training needs and methods. Implementation is the gathering together of the trainers, the trainees, and all of the materials and methods needed for the training program(s). Evaluation is an investigative process in which one determines whether the training was cost-effective, whether the objective was achieved, and whether the learning was transferred from the learning site to actual use on the job.

TRAINING

Needs Assessment

The first step in training is to determine that a need for a training program exists. A hospital should commit its resources to a training activity only if, in the best judgment of its nurse managers, the training can be expected to achieve some organizational goal such as better patient care, reduced operating cost, or more efficient or satisfied personnel. Only educational institutions can legitimately view training as an end in itself.

This naturally leads to the question, On what should training resources be spent? This decision must be based on the best available data. In hospitals, these data can come from training specialists, other knowledgeable managers in the organization, and from continuous systematic and accurate analysis of the hospital personnel's training needs. In educational institutions, the decision comes from a monitoring of the needs and resources of the community and of the kinds of behaviors that are useful in the sites that employ the institution's graduates.

A health care institution will seek behavior change or increased knowledge as a means toward some organizational goal. For the educational institution, the process is fairly simple: determine what behaviors are needed by the trainees and then teach those new behaviors. To the extent that the trainees change their behavior to that which is desired, the training is successful. For the health care institution, the problem is more complex. First, those activities that can be made more effective by training efforts that change behavior must be identified. Also, a great deal of maintenance-type training is always going on in any organization. This type of training is used to instruct both new employees and current employees who are promoted. A certain amount of training resources must be assigned to such training. The remaining resources should be aimed at specific activities that will increase the effectiveness of the organization.

Too often, training programs are initiated simply because they have been well advertised and marketed or because other organizations have found them useful; however, it does not make sense for an organization to adopt an expensive training effort simply because other organizations are doing it. Such a faddish practice can be reduced by systematically determining training needs and using them as a base for developing very specific training content. In this way, organizations use training programs only for people and situations where needed.

Planning and Implementation

After the needs have been determined, the next step is to plan the training program. Nurse managers usually are involved in training their staffs and patients, but they don't necessarily have to do it themselves. They can routinely delegate it to other staff members or to a staff nurse who becomes a preceptor (a staff member who supervises the training of a trainee). It can be done through the closed circuit television system in the hospital, by training specialists assigned to either nursing service or a training and education department. Thus, the nurse manager has many resources for training at her disposal.

Wexley and Latham (1981) suggest three main questions to be considered in assessment and planning: Is the individual trainable? How should the training program be arranged to facilitate learning? And, what can be done to ensure that what is learned during training will be transferred to the job? There are no well-developed and tested theories of learning to answer these questions, so trainers must rely on some simple principles of learning and basic knowledge about training methods to develop any training interventions. Also, theories of motivation (see Chapter 9) can help ensure that the trainee has a desire to learn and to apply any skills or concepts that are taught.

Learning Principles

There are two sets of principles that guide training activities. One set of principles has been found to facilitate learning and another to determine the degree of transfer of learning from the training context to the job.

Readiness to learn. Before the learner can benefit from any formal training, he or she must be ready to learn. Readiness refers to both the maturational and experiential factors in the learner's background that are critical for further learning. Students do not take algebra, for instance, before they take basic math, and after algebra they take geometry, trigonometry, and calculus, in that order. The logic is that trainee readiness at any stage is primarily due to previous learning in particular subjects. Training programs fail if the prerequisite skills and knowledge are not considered, since it is very difficult to learn a new sequence of behaviors if the component behaviors have not been previously learned. Maturational factors also relate to readiness to learn. There are limits to the amount of information a person can acquire and retain at any one time.

Motivation to learn. Most researchers agree that motivation affects performance through an energizing function. In other words, a motivated individual will work harder to achieve a consequence. Motivation has been studied in two ways: (a) the process, which seeks to explain *how* behavior is energized, directed, sustained, and stopped; and (b) the content, which considers which specific things motivate specific people. In training, motivation exercises its influence in two areas: motivation to attend to the training content; and reinforced motivation, in the form of anticipated benefits, for accurate behavioral rehearsal and practice. If learners are informed in advance about the benefits that will result from learning the content and adopting the modeled behavior, it strengthens their motivation. Furthermore, anticipated benefits can strengthen retention of what has been learned observationally by motivating people to encode and rehearse modeled behavior that they value. Motivation, of course, is only one of the things that commands attention. It is difficult *not* to hear compelling sounds or to look at captivating visual displays.

The learner's first attempt to reproduce the target behavior may not always be successful; reinforcement from trainers and other trainees will help the behavior to endure. When individuals try to reproduce training demonstrations, they will compare their attempt with the symbolic representation they have retained. Through practice, they correct their reproduction attempts until they match the symbolic representation. This is self-reinforcement. Furthermore, maintenance of behavior can be influenced by external reinforcement (i.e., rewards or benefits) on the job.

Conditions for practice. Learning theory research has shown that when a complex task is to be learned, it should be broken down into its parts and one should learn each part separately, starting with the simplest and going on to the most difficult. However, part learning should be combined with whole learning—that is, trainees should be shown the whole performance so that they know what their goal is and where they are going. The training content should then be broken down into integrated parts, and each part should be learned in practice until it is retained intact and can be recalled accurately. Then a trainee should be allowed to put all of the parts together and practice the whole performance.

It has also been determined that spaced practice is more effective than massed practice, especially for motor skills. If the learner has to concentrate for long periods of time without some rest, learning and retention will suffer. It's a little like cramming for an examination: the test scores are usually relatively high, but rapid forgetting sets in very soon. Consequently, spaced practice seems to be more productive for long-term retention and for transfer of learning to the work setting.

Overlearning, or practicing beyond the point of first accurate recall/

reproduction, can be critical in both acquisition and transfer of knowledge and skills. Overlearning is desirable in a program when the task to be learned is not likely to be immediately practiced in the work situation and also when performance must be maintained during periods of emergency and stress. Consequently, in any training situation, practice should be encouraged to the point of overlearning.

Transfer of training. The ultimate goal of any training program, especially in organizational training, is that the learning be transferred into the context in which it will be used. Ellis has made the following suggestions for maximizing transfer. First, one must maximize the similarity between the training context and the job (ultimate transfer) context; the training should look as much like the job, or like the situation where the behavior is to be used, as possible. Adequate practice—in fact, overlearning—is recommended.

Second, transfer is not going to occur until the learning has become part of long-term memory. The training practice should include a variety of stimulus situations so that trainees will learn to generalize their knowledge. Third, transfer will occur more readily when the important features of the content to be learned can be labeled or identified to distinguish the major steps involved. Finally, the general principles underlying the specific content or behavior to be learned should be understood or coded along with the physical behavior. This can be done by asking the learner to apply the general principles in a variety of situations and by supplying her or him with a written description of the rules that underlie the behavior across contexts (Ellis, 1965).

Memory Span

The ability to retain what one has learned is obviously relevant to the effectiveness of a training program; yet generally speaking, the better the memory, the more effective the learning. There are two types of memory: short-term and long-term. Short-term memory is a system that stores information for current attention and where actual information processing is carried out. The amount of energy or capacity available to short-term memory is limited; thus, only a few storage or processing activities can be carried out simultaneously. Long-term memory, in contrast, represents the products of an individual's experience that have been processed through short-term memory and then stored for long-term use. Products in the long-term memory range from individual letter or word codes to more general things such as strategies for processing and maintaining information.

Many factors have been found to increase memory span. Rehearsal is perhaps the simplest strategy that can be used to process and store things for long-term memory. Rehearsal is generally viewed as an interactive process. It maintains information in short-term memory by ensuring a sufficiently high level of activation and it facilitates the transfer of information to long-term memory. Adults have the capacity to rehearse several different items at the same time while children under nine years old usually do not. The more rehearsal a person experiences, the better will be the performance in recall tasks.

Grouping of items or activities to be learned also tends to increase memory span. Groups of no more than three or four are best when items are presented orally; more items (four to six) can be included in a grouping when sequences are presented visually. Adults tend to group spontaneously to enhance memory. Recall is also enhanced when grouping is prompted by an experimenter.

A third facilitator of memory span is "chunking," which refers to the recording of two or more nominally independent items of information into a single familiar unit. Thus, only familiar sequences can be chunked, and the more familiar the sequence, the greater the ease with which it can be chunked. Short-term memory has only limited capacity to chunk, but the amount of information that can be stored and processed through short-term memory increases in direct proportion to the size of the chunk. Consequently, any time a given amount of information can be recoded and represented in a smaller space, memory will be enhanced.

Organization also enhances memory span. With increasing maturity, people become increasingly able to package material so that it is organizationally consistent with already stored material. The more organized the material presented, the more likely it is to be learned.

Social Learning Theory

Social learning theory attempts to integrate much of what we know about how people learn. It suggests that a person can observe her or his own behavior and that of others and use this observation to plan future action. How a person behaves over time influences what that person becomes. People think about *when* to use behavior and try to use certain behaviors so as to increase the likelihood of positive consequences. If these positive consequences occur, the response will probably be more use of the behavior.

Social learning theory is a behavioral theory and it builds on principles of reinforcement theory. Bandura (1977) explains that, except for elementary reflexes, people are not equipped with an inborn repertoire of behavior. Instead, new response patterns are acquired either by direct experience or by observation.

Positive and negative results affect the actions of people in their day-to-day functioning. Some of their behaviors are successful (rewarded or satisfying) and some are not; some actually result in punishing consequences. Through this process of differential reinforcement, the successful behaviors are retained and behavior that leads to no consequence or

Figure 14–2 Reinforcement Process

Positive Reinforcement (reward)

Stimulus → Behavior → Positive Consequences (behavior will increase)

Negative Reinforcement (punishment)

Stimulus → Behavior → Aversive Consequences (behavior will diminish)

Adapted Decker, P. J. *Health Case Management* MICROTRAINING Decker & Associates, 1983.
    Used with permission.

punishing consequence is no longer used. This is shown in Figure 14–2. In a given situation, a behavior which leads to a positive consequence (reward) will be repeated (positive reinforcement). If the consequence is negative (punishment), the behavior is not repeated. If we learned everything in this trial and error way, though, it would be impossible to explain the quickness of human learning; learning that occurs without evidence of behavior change (no-trial learning); and how the human species has survived.

In the social learning analysis of behavior, information about one's self and the nature of the environment is developed and verified through four different processes. First, people derive much of their knowledge from direct experience of the effects produced by their actions. Second, information about the environment is frequently extracted from vicarious experience—that is, observation of the effects produced by someone else's actions. Third, when vicarious experience is limited, people can develop and evaluate their conceptions about the environment in terms of the judgment voiced by others. Last, people can use the information gained from active, vicarious, and social sources of verification (all of which rely on external influences or sources) as a basis for logical determination of the nature of the environment. After people acquire rules of inference based on active, vicarious, or social sources, they can evaluate the soundness of their reasoning through logical processes, either inductive or deductive.

Social learning theory suggests that anticipation of reinforcement is one of several factors that influence what is observed and what goes unnoticed (see Figure 14–3). Knowing that a given person's (the model) behavior is effective in producing valued outcomes or avoiding punishing ones increases the observer's attentiveness to the model's actions. This suggests, furthermore, that observational learning will be more effective when observers are informed in advance about the benefits of adopting a model's behavior; this is preferable to waiting until the observers produce imitative behavior and then rewarding them.

However, attending to a model's behavior is insufficient unless several retention processes are used so that the behavior is actually learned and

Figure 14–3   Social Learning Theory

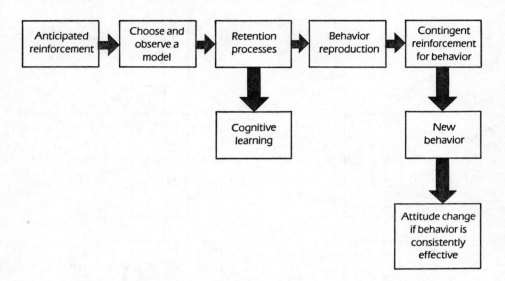

retained. According to social learning theory, behavior is learned sym-
bolically through cognitive processes before it is performed. Then, after
these cognitive processes have been completed, a person will try out the
behavior. If it leads to positive consequences, it will be used in the future.
This is the motivational process that maintains the new behavior. By observing the model, an individual forms an idea of how and in what sequence response components must be combined to produce a desired
new behavior. People guide their actions by prior notions rather than relying on the outcomes to tell them what they must do.

Modeling transmits information to observers about new responses
and how these responses can be combined into new patterns. This information can be conveyed by physical demonstration, pictorial representation, or verbal description. Much social learning occurs on the basis of
casual observation of the behavior of others. However, people also learn
desired behaviors through written descriptions of how to behave and
from different media sources such as television.

Relapse Prevention

Marx (1982) has presented a model to increase the long-term maintenance
of newly trained behaviors. This model emphasizes the learning of a set of
self-control and coping strategies (see Figure 14–4).

The first step in this model is to make trainees aware of the relapse

Figure 14—4   A Model of the Training Relapse Process

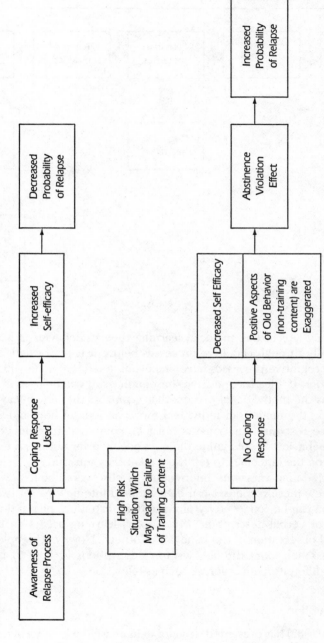

Adapted from Marx, R. D. (1982). Relapse prevention for managerial training: A model for maintenance of behavior change. *Academy of Management Review, 7*(3), 433–441. Used with permission.

process itself. Most training programs are presented as being quite successful. Awareness of what may make the program vulnerable is neglected and trainees may not consequently be able to avoid situations in which the training content will be unsuccessful. Trainees are asked to pinpoint situations that are likely to sabotage their efforts. Trainees can then be: (a) taught to anticipate high-risk situations, (b) taught coping strategies for avoiding high-risk situations, and (c) taught that slight slips or relapses are predictable outcomes of any training paradigm and need not become full-blown relapses. These techniques should increase trainees' self-efficacy (feelings of control over the situation requiring use of the training content).

The importance of this model is in showing that trainees' exposure to possible failure situations will enable them to expect and prepare for such situations in advance. This advance mental preparation for trying situations will decrease the probability of small relapses turning into absolute failure due to the "abstinence violation effect." The effect occurs when guilt over a small violation of the training content leads a trainee through cognitive dissonance to deny the possible effectiveness of the training content. Such denial almost guarantees that a small slip will end up as a total relapse or non-use of the training content. Again, the keys are: (a) awareness of the relapse process; (b) identification of high-risk situations; and (c) the development of coping responses. The trainee should not be afraid to discuss possible failure situations and ways to cope with them. Better yet, trainees should practice such situations using the training content in the neutral environment of training. In this way the trainees prepare themselves for the difficult situations. But, the trainees will not be motivated to prepare for the difficult situations unless they know about the relapse process.

Adult Education Theory

Thirty years ago, the only educational concepts and techniques available were those developed for the education of children. It was assumed that anybody who knew anything about basic education and was reasonably good at managing the development and logistics of educational programs could be a good trainer of adults. However, in the last 10 to 20 years, varying techniques for helping adults to learn have been developed, and one of the primary discoveries is that adults as learners are very different from children. Knowles suggests there are no fundamental differences in the way adults and children learn, but he does point to significant differences that come from the situations surrounding adult and child learning. He suggests there are four basic concepts (see Figure 14–5) on which differences in adult and child education can be shown (Knowles, 1970).

The first is the individual's self-concept. Children see themselves as dependent persons but, as they move towards adulthood, they become increasingly aware of themselves and their own decision making and they

Figure 14–5 Characteristics of Adult Learners and Educational Implications

Characteristics of Adult Learners	Implications for Adult Learning
Self-Concept: The adult learner sees himself as capable of self-direction and desires others to see him the same way. In fact, one definition of maturity is the capacity to be self-directing.	A climate of openness and respect is helpful in identifying what the learners want and need to learn.
	Adults enjoy planning and carrying out their own learning exercises.
	Adults need to be involved in evaluating their own progress toward self-chosen goals.
Experience: Adults bring a lifetime of experience to the learning situation. Youths tend to regard experience as something that has happened to them, while to an adult, his experience is him. The adult defines who he is in terms of his experience.	Less use is made of transmittal techniques; more of experiential techniques.
	Discovery of how to learn from experience is key to self-actualization.
	Mistakes are opportunities for learning.
	To reject adult experience is to reject the adult.
Readiness to learn: Adult developmental tasks increasingly move toward social and occupational role competence and away from the more physical developmental tasks of childhood.	Adults need opportunities to identify the competency requirements of their occupational and social roles.
	Adult readiness-to-learn and teachable moments peak at those points where a learning opportunity is coordinated with a recognition of the need-to-know.
	Adults can best identify their own readiness-to-learn and teachable moments.
A problem-centered time perspective: Youth thinks of education as the accumulation of knowledge for use in the future. Adults tend to think of learning as a way to be more effective in problem solving today.	Adult education needs to be problem-centered rather than theoretically oriented.
	Formal curriculum development is less valuable than finding out what the learners need to learn.
	Adults need the opportunity to apply and try out learning quickly.

become very capable in self-direction. This change in self-concept from one of dependency to independent autonomy characterizes maturity. Adults tend to resent being in situations where they are treated with a lack of respect, talked down to, judged, or otherwise treated like children. Thus, adult educators should be facilitators rather than dominant teachers and the adult learner should have some input into what is taught.

The second concept is *experience*. Adults have accumulated vast quantities of experience whereas children have not, and that experience can lead adults to make choices about what is taught and in what format. In adult education, this should be valued because the teacher can use theory to integrate and formalize it. The educator knows the theory, but the trainees have the experience. In contrast to child education, which is oriented toward one-way communication, assigned readings, and audiovisual presentations, adult education should therefore include experiential learning, two-way and multidirectional communication such as group discussions, role playing, teamwork exercises, and skill practice sessions. This way, the experience of all participants can be brought out and focused on the problem being discussed.

The third concept is *readiness to learn.* The main task of child education is to sequence the learning activities in a way that fits the developmental steps of the content. Adults, however, have already completed their basic education in reading, writing, speech, and so on, and their developmental tasks increasingly relate to the social roles that form their immediate concerns: working, living, family, recreational activities, and the like. In child education, the teacher decides on both the content to be learned and how and in what sequence learning will take place. In adult education, the learners themselves can help to identify what they wish to learn and the sequence of learning. The adult trainer acts as a resource person to help learners form interest groups to diagnose their learning needs.

The last concept is the *time perspective.* Education has been considered in terms of preparation for the future rather than preparation for the present. Thus, child education is the business of having students store up information for use on some far-off day; teachers present information neatly packaged so students can use it later. But in adult education, learning is problem-centered rather than subject-centered. Adult education is a process for defining problems and solving them for the present.

Staff Development

Education in hospitals includes programs for patients, their families, staff, and members of the general community. Education can be divided into two areas: staff development and patient education. Inservice education refers to the continuing education that seeks to improve staff members' knowledge of or ability to perform job-related tasks. Sometimes this is referred to as staff development, although the latter usually includes management training and other areas of staff enrichment such as assertiveness, counseling skills, and group process skills. Much of this staff development is done by the education department, but in this chapter, the focus is primarily on on-the-job training techniques and orientation. Patient education follows.

Orientation. Getting an employee started in the right way is important. Among other things, a well-planned orientation reduces the anxiety that new employees feel when beginning the job. In addition, socialization into the workplace contributes to unit effectiveness by reducing dissatisfaction, absenteeism, and turnover (see Chapters 13 and 16).

Orientation is a joint responsibility of both the hospital training staff and the nursing manager. In most institutions the new staff nurse will complete the hospital orientation program followed by an on-site orientation by the nurse manager or someone appointed to do this. There should be a clear understanding of the specific responsibilities of training and unit staff so that nothing is left to chance. The training staff should provide information involving matters that are organization-wide in nature and relevant to all new employees, such as information in regard to such things as the cafeteria, benefits, parking, or work hours. The nursing manager concentrates on those items unique to the employee's specific job.

New employees, as discussed in Chapter 13, often have unrealistically high expectations about the amount of challenge and responsibility they will find in their first job. Then, if they are assigned fairly undemanding, entry-level tasks, they will feel discouraged and disillusioned. The result is job dissatisfaction, turnover, and low productivity, so one function of orientation is to correct any unrealistic expectations. The nurse manager needs to outline very specifically what is expected of new employees and assure them that they will eventually be able to progress to more challenging tasks. Such *realistic job previews* should cover the informal or nonconcrete aspects of the job about which an employee could possibly have more unrealistic expectations than such concrete areas as the pay scale or hours.

Socialization of new employees can sometimes be very difficult because of the anxiety people feel when they first come on the job. They simply do not hear all of the information they are given; they spend a lot of energy attempting to integrate and interpret the information; and they consequently miss some information. One company experimented with incorporating a six-hour anxiety reduction session into its normal orientation period. The group did not have to work that first day, but were allowed to relax, sit back, and use that time to get acquainted with the organization and their new co-workers. This increased the learning rate of the new employees, increased productivity, and lowered absenteeism and tardiness (Knowles, 1970).

Since nurse managers are an extremely important part of the socialization process, everything that they expect of the new employee should be discussed openly and specifically. The new employee will adapt more rapidly to the new unit if this is done. Everything from standards of performance, attendance, how to treat the patients, to what to expect as far as feedback in performance appraisal, should be discussed.

Preceptor model. One method of orientation is to use the preceptor model to assist the new employee and the staff nurse. The preceptor model provides a means for orientation and socialization of the new nurse as well as providing a mechanism to recognize exceptionally competent staff nurses (May, 1980). Staff nurses who serve as preceptors are selected based on their clinical competence, organizational skills, ability to guide and direct others, and their concern for the effective orientation of new nurses. The primary goal is for the preceptor to assist the new nurse to acquire the necessary knowledge and skills so that he or she can function effectively on the division.

Preceptorships offer new nurses the advantage of an on-the-job training program tailored specifically to their needs. Staff nurses (preceptors) benefit by having an opportunity to sharpen their clinical skills, increasing their personal and professional satisfaction.

The new nurse will work closely with the preceptor for approximately three weeks, although the duration of the preceptorship may vary depending on the nurse's individual learning needs or the hospital's policies.

The preceptor's role is that of orientor, teacher, resource person, counselor, role model, and evaluator (Murphy & Hammerstad, 1981). The primary function of the preceptor's role is to orient the new nurse to the unit. This includes proper socialization of the new nurse within the group as well as familiarizing her with unit functions. The preceptor teaches any procedures which are unfamiliar and helps the new nurse develop any necessary skills. The preceptor acts as a resource person on matters of division functions as well as policies and procedures.

New nurses may need to utilize their preceptors as counselors as they make their transition to the unit. If new nurses experience discrepancy between their educational preparation or their expectations and the realities of working in the unit, the preceptor's role as counselor can prove invaluable in helping them cope with "reality shock."

The preceptor also serves as a staff nurse role model; the new nurse will learn not only actual work-related tasks, but will also observe the preceptor to learn how to set priorities, problem solve and make decisions, manage time, delegate tasks, and interact with others (Murphy & Hammerstad, 1981). In addition, the preceptor evaluates the new nurse's performance and provides both verbal and written feedback to encourage development.

The department of education plays an integral role in the preceptor concept. The education staff provide the new nurse an initial orientation, familiarization with the hospital and the general policies and procedures before beginning work with the preceptor.

The education personnel also provide the necessary training for staff nurses to become preceptors. The department of education's function is to teach the staff nurse the role of a preceptor, the principles of adult education applicable to training needs, how to teach necessary skills, how to plan as well as evaluate teaching and learning objectives, and how to provide both formal and informal feedback. Thus, the education department assists the staff nurse in acquiring the necessary knowledge and skills to effectively train new nurses.

Staff development methods.   Staff development can be divided into internal (on the unit) and external (off the unit) sources. Internal sources include on-the-job training, workshops for the unit nurses, and inservice programs. External sources are formal workshops presented by a training and education department within the hospital and all training activities done outside the hospital, including college courses, conferences, and continuing education workshops.

It simply is not feasible to discuss the relative merits of the many training methods available but, based on the concepts of social learning theory, a model to evaluate the different training programs can be developed. For effective adult education, we need at minimum: (a) presentation of the material, (b) practice of the material, and (c) feedback about that practice.

There must be opportunity for practice of the desired terminal behaviors and feedback about it. For instance, reading about or listening to a lecture about some clinical skill represents presentation of material, but it does not include practice of that skill. Or, if one showed workers how to perform that skill, had them practice it, and then walked away, there would be no feedback. All three elements are essential.

The most widely used training method is *on-the-job training*. This often includes assigning new employees to experienced nurses, preceptors, or the nurse manager. The trainee is expected to learn the job by observing the experienced employee (preceptor) and by performing the actual tasks under supervision.

On-the-job training has several positive features, one of which is its cost-effectiveness. Trainees learn effectively while providing some of the necessary nursing services. Moreover, it reduces the need for outside training facilities and reliance on professional trainers. Transfer of training is not an issue because the learning occurs on the actual job. However, on-the-job training often fails because it has not been formalized, and the on-the-job trainer does not know how to utilize learning theory. As a result, presentation, practice, or feedback may be neglected.

Wexley and Latham make several suggestions for implementing effective on-the-job training programs:

1. Employees who function as trainers must be convinced that training new employees in no way jeopardizes their own job security, pay level, seniority, or status.

2. Individuals serving as trainers should realize that this added responsibility will be instrumental in attaining other rewards for them.

3. Trainers and trainees should be carefully paired so as to minimize any differences in background, language, personality, attitudes, or age that may inhibit communication and understanding.

4. Trainers should be selected on the basis of their ability to teach and their desire to take on this added responsibility.

5. Staff nurses chosen as trainers should be carefully trained in the proper methods of instruction.

6. It must be made clear to employees serving as trainers that their new assignment is by no means a chance to get away from their own jobs or "take a vacation."

7. Trainees should be rotated to different trainers to compensate for weaker instruction by some trainers and to expose each trainee to the specific know-how of various staff nurses or education department trainers.

8. The nurse manager must realize that the efficiency of the unit may be reduced when on-the-job training occurs.

9. The trainer and nurse manager must realize the importance of close supervision of the trainee to prevent any major mistakes and the learning of incorrect procedures.

10. On-the-job training should be used in conjunction with other training approaches. Obviously, the skill learning derived on the job should include theoretical as well as practice knowledge; for example, a knowledge of fluid and electrolyte balance is essential to nurses administering intravenous fluids (Wexley & Latham, 1981).

Figure 14–6 lists the key behaviors for on-the-job training, which include the "basic three" of presenting the material, allowing the employee

Figure 14–6   Key Behaviors in On-the-Job Training

1. In writing, outline each step of the task to be taught.
2. Explain the objectives of the task to the employee.
3. Show the employee how to do it (without talking).
4. Explain key points (write them down if they are complex).
5. Let the employee watch you do it again.
6. Let the employee do the simple parts of the task (optional).
7. Help the employee do the whole task (watch and give feedback).
8. Let the employee do the whole task (give feedback when task is finished).
9. Praise the employee for doing the task correctly.

Adapted from Decker, P. J. *Health Care Management Microtraining.* Decker & Associates, 1983. Used with permission.

Figure 14—7 Job Breakdown Sheet for Training Purposes

Department _____ Job _____

Breakdown Made By _____ Date _____

Important Steps (What to Do) A logical segment of the operation, when something happens to advance the work	**Key Points (How to Do It)** Anything that may: Make or break the job; Injure the worker; Make the job easier to do

to practice the skill, and providing feedback about that practice. These behaviors also incorporate most of the elements of learning theory discussed earlier in this chapter. Figure 14–7 shows a form on which the trainers can write down the actual steps of the task and any key points to be made about those steps before beginning the training.

Audiovisual techniques. With the increased size of hospitals, rapid technological advances, and the number of people requiring training, there is always an attempt to make instructions more efficient and accelerate the learning process. Many organizations have therefore begun to use such audiovisual techniques as films, closed circuit television, audio tapes, videotape recordings, computer-assisted instruction, and interactive video training. These methods allow an instructor's message to be given in a uniform manner on several occasions or at several locations at one time and be reused often. They can enhance the instructor's presentation as well as reduce the need for an instructor to present every detail.

Audiovisual materials can be used in almost every training and development situation, ranging from orientation to more complex uses. However, a film or videocassette is a teaching aid, not an educational program in itself; there still must be practice and feedback. Audiovisual methods can be effective if they are encompassed within a well-developed program rather than made a substitute for such a program.

Their use should be considered, first, when there is a need to illustrate certain procedures or with any kind of behavioral demonstration; second, when there is a need to expose trainees to events not easily demonstrable in live presentations; third, when the training is organization-wide and is far too costly for the trainer to travel from place to place or assemble everyone in one location; and fourth, when audiovisual training is supplemented with live lecture, discussion, and/or practice.

Good audiovisual materials need to be adequately introduced. Viewers need to be told what to look for and what they will be seeing. Follow-up discussion is very important and, if the audiovisual is used as a demonstration, then practice and feedback need to be part of the training program. Remember, audiovisuals are not intended to stand alone in training, even though they are often misused in that manner. They should be carefully selected, adequately introduced, and followed up with adequate discussion, practice, and feedback.

The reader is referred to Wexley and Latham (1981) or Breckon (1982) for further information on training methods.

EVALUATION

Few issues in the training field create as much controversy or discussion as the word "evaluation." Trainers will always agree on the *need* for sound appraisal of training programs, but rarely agree on the best method of evaluation and rarely do empirical evaluation. Typically, a program is reviewed at the corporate level and if it looks good the organization uses it. The same programs are used again and again. Sometimes the trainees are asked how they liked it, but the program continues until someone in a position of authority decides that it is no longer useful or no longer works or, more commonly, attendance decreases. All of this is done on the basis of opinions and judgments. Rarely are training programs evaluated in such a way that one can determine whether they have caused a change in behavior or in some organizational variable. Most evaluation is done at the end of the program with questionnaires, which provide very little information on whether the trainees learned anything or if they will carry it through to the job. If one is going to put the money and time into developing a training program (and billions of dollars are spent in this area), then one should also put money and time into evaluation to determine whether the program is actually doing what it was intended to do and then to take action based on the evaluations.

This leads to the question, "Why evaluate?" One reason to evaluate is to improve the program, to identify elements of it that need to be improved. Another reason for evaluation is to justify staff and budget allocations. If there are objective data to prove that a training program does have a positive effect on day-to-day operating problems, rarely will money be cut from the training program budget. With effective evaluation of cost-effective training, the program will continue to be funded.

Despite its value, evaluation may still remain an absent ingredient. A major reason is the difficulty and cost of designing sound evaluation tools. Another reason is that the trainer may not be interested in evaluating; there is no vested interest in doing so. Additionally, many trainers lack the skills in experimental designs related to field settings that are required for organizational training evaluation. In short, unless an organization is committed to truly finding out whether its training programs work or do not work, evaluation is not going to be done. This is regrettable, because it all too often results in the continuation of ineffective programs and the cancellation or misuse of effective ones.

Evaluative Criteria

Given the commitment, interest, and skills to do evaluation, however, a program's effectiveness can be evaluated in terms of four criteria: *trainee reaction, learning, behavior change,* and/or *organizational impact. Trainee reaction* is usually ascertained through a questionnaire completed at the end of a program. The questionnaire may contain questions concerning the program's content, the trainer, the trainer's objectives, the methods used, physical facilities, meals, and other facilities. The specific reactions that the organization wants to know about should be decided upon before the training and included in any questionnaire; irrelevant data should not be gathered.

Favorable trainee reactions to a program do not guarantee that learning has taken place or that behavior has changed as a result of the training program. Nevertheless, trainee reactions are important because: (a) reports of positive reactions help ensure organizational support for a program; (b) trainee reactions can be used to assess the training; and (c) reaction data indicate whether or not the trainees like the program.

Learning criteria assess the knowledge—the facts and figures—learned in the training program. Knowledge is typically measured by paper and pencil tests that can include true-false, multiple choice, fill in the blank, matching, and essay type questions.

But the acquisition of knowledge is not enough. Was that knowledge converted into *behavioral change*? One of the biggest problems is that training does not necessarily transfer from the classroom to the job—often because trainees were taught the theory and principles of the technique, but never learned how to translate this into behavior on the job. There is a big difference between the two, as evidenced by the many training programs that teach factual material through lecture. A person going through such a training program may cognitively remember the material, but not have any new behavior to use on the job. A test at the end of such a program may prove that the training does, in fact, increase learning; if behavior is not measured after the program (or on the job), however, one does not know if the training program affects behavior or if it will help new behavior transfer to the job. The transfer of learning from classroom to job is critical, and measuring behavioral criteria is therefore very important in the business of teaching new skills.

The objectives of many training programs can be expressed in terms of some end result for the organization such as reduced turnover, fewer grievances, reduced absenteeism, increased quality of care, and fewer accidents. These are usually expressed in quantified data and can be easily tied to dollars.

It is often difficult to determine whether changes in such areas can be unequivocally attributed to the training program or to other variables in the organization such as changes in competitiveness or management, increased pay, new equipment, better selection, or changes of some other kind. In evaluating, one must take particular care in deciding on the length of data collection, the unit of analysis, randomization, and other experimental design issues to be able to rule out the effect of these variables. The most important criteria for measuring results are those that are closely related to the key training behaviors. Despite all of the difficulties in collecting and analyzing such data, the trainer should attempt to collect cost-related measures, as they give evidence to management that training efforts do have an effect on organizational effectiveness.

Figure 14–8 is an analysis form for assessing the cost-effectiveness of proposed programs. The first two items are simply the program name and description, and the next three look at implementation and predicted outcomes. The fifth item calls for identifiable benefits in terms of dollars.

Figure 14—8 Cost-Effectiveness Analysis Form

---

1. Program name:

2. Description: Legally Required: ☐ yes ☐ no

3. Ease of implementation and any special requirements:

4. Expected economic benefits:

5. Total identifiable benefits:

	Potential revenue impact($) ×	Probability of occurrence (0–1.0) =	Probable gross benefit($)
1.			
2.			
3.			
4.			
5.			
Total			

6. Total identifiable costs:

	Potential revenue cost($) ×	Probability of use (0–1.0) =	Probable cost($)
1. Trainer time			
2. Training time			
3. Training facilities			
4. Meals/coffee, snacks			
5. Line personnel time			
6.			
7.			
8.			
Total			

Figure 14—8 *(continued)*

7. Intangible costs and benefits:

8. Economic risks:

Consequences of not acting:

9. Assumptions and other considerations:

The sixth item is concerned with tangible costs; these are simply subtracted from the benefits to calculate probable net benefit/cost. The next two items consider intangible benefits and economic risks, while the last item covers any assumptions and other considerations that need to be calculated into this analysis. This form can be used to determine the probable dollar benefit to an organization conducting a training program; however, one should review Cascio (1982) to examine techniques to calculate human resource outcomes in terms of dollars.

Another consideration in determination of cost-effectiveness is the direct meeting costs, especially for off-site meetings. For the most part, off-site meetings are not needed in behavioral training, but they are often used. Cascio discusses a method of calculating these costs, as shown in Figure 14–9 (Cascio, 1982). This form can be used to calculate the cost of off- versus on-site programs. It can also be used to determine how time should be spent during the training days and whether increasing or shortening training hours will in fact change the cost of the training program.

PATIENT EDUCATION

A number of factors have converged to bring health teaching into prominence. The increasing effort in recent years to maintain health rather than just treat disease has enlarged the amount of knowledge people need and has demanded a change in attitudes about health and health care systems. Shortened hospital stays with early ambulation require preparation of the patient for convalescence at home. Long-term illnesses and disabilities have also increased, so that both patient and family need additional infor-

Figure 14–9 Cost Breakdown for an Off-Site Management Meeting

	Total Costs	Cost Per Participant Per Day
A. Development of programs (figured on an annual basis)		
1. Training department overhead		
2. Training staff salaries		
3. Use of outside consultants		
4. Equipment and materials for meeting (films, supplies, workbooks)	$100,000	$100 [1]
B. Participant cost (figured on an annual basis)		
1. Salaries and benefits of participants (figured for average participant)	$20,000	
2. Capital investment in participants (based on an average of various industries from *Fortune* magazine)	$25,000 $ 45,000	190.68 [2]
C. Delivery of one meeting of 20 persons		
1. Facility costs		
a. Sleeping rooms	1,000	
b. Three meals daily	800	
c. Coffee breaks	60	
d. Misc. tips, telephone	200	
e. Reception	200 2,260	56.50 [3]
2. Meeting charges		
a. Room rental		
b. A/V rental		
c. Secretarial services		
3. Transportation to the meeting	2,500	62.50 [4]

Summary: Total Per Day Per Person Cost

A. Development of programs	$	100
B. Participant cost		190
C. Delivery of one meeting (hotel and transportation)		119
Total	$	409

Note: Meeting duration: two full days. Number of attendees: 20 people. These costs do not reflect a figure for the productive time lost of the people in the program. If that cost were added—and it would be realistic to do so—the above cost would increase dramatically.

[1] To determine per day cost, divide $100,000 by number of meeting days held per year (10). Then divide answer ($10,000) by total number of management people (100) attending all programs = $100 per day of a meeting.

[2] To determine per day cost, divide total of $45,000 by 236 (average number of working days in a year) = $190.68 per day of work year.

[3] To determine per day, per person cost, divide group total ($2,260) by number of participants (20) and then divide resulting figure ($133) by number of meeting days (2) = $56.50 per day.

[4] To determine per day, per person cost, divide group total ($2,500) by number of people and then divide resulting figure ($125) by number of meeting days (2) = $62.50 per day.

Source: Adapted from W. J. McKeon. "How to Determine Off-Site Meeting Costs." *Training and Development Journal,* May 1981, p. 117. American Society of Training and Development. Reprinted with permission.

mation to assist them in adjusting to daily life. The increase in malpractice suits has also caused an increase in patient education. (If it can be established that hospitals and medical staff did not fully inform patients about what they were consenting to, liability may be established.) Finally, the need to control health care costs has led to increased patient teaching. This is especially important in these days of prospective reimbursement.

The Joint Commission for Accreditation of Hospitals (JCAH) has detailed the need for patient education, and policy statements from both the American Medical Association and the American Hospital Association (AHA) have indicated hospitals' responsibility for educating patients. The AHA's 1982 statement says:

A hospital has a responsibility to provide patient education services as an integral part of high quality cost effective care. Patient education services should enable patients and their families and friends when appropriate to make informed decisions about their health; to manage their illness; and to implement follow up care at home. Effective and efficient patient education services require planning and coordination, and responsibility for such planning and coordination should be assigned. The hospital should also provide the necessary staff and financial resources.

Nurse managers have several responsibilities in relation to patient education—first, to ensure that their staffs are prepared to function in this area. Nurse managers must document what is being done by their staffs and assess their quality of teaching, both written and oral. They must also be aware of hospital-wide programming to avoid duplication of efforts, and must serve on patient education committees, especially in their clinical specialties, to assist with program planning to meet the needs of their specific patients. They must identify both individual and general needs within their units, coordinate the patient education activities therein, and delegate responsibility to others. The staff must be provided with patient teaching skills and educational opportunities for their development.

Nurse managers may either do the patient teaching themselves, have staff nurses do it, ask the education department to assist the staff to develop the necessary skills, or utilize the group classes or video presentations being held on a hospital-wide basis. Methods of delivery vary and may be either one-to-one or group teaching. Printed materials are helpful to patient and family, and effective audiovisual materials contribute to patient learning. The latter are most effective when they augment teaching done by individuals. No teaching tool can replace the personal, nurse-patient interaction.

Often staff nurses place a high value on patient teaching, yet feel unprepared to teach. Most commonly, they feel they have a lack of content knowledge, of teaching experience, of skill in teaching techniques, or a lack of time. The nurse manager must correct these perceived deficiencies, and a good start would be to suggest that staff nurses read Redman (1980) and Corkadeel and McGlashan (1983). Patient education must go on at all times and at any location where effective learning can take place. It can be done while the nurse is caring for the patient at the bedside, during lab tests, in the hallway, and through watching television. It can be done by anyone in the hospital: any staff nurse, any nurse manager, a patient educator, or a specialized trainer.

Barriers to Teaching

A patient teaching program, even though it may utilize all of the activities in a learning process, may not always be successful. Certain factors can limit its effectiveness, and one must plan appropriate steps to minimize these barriers.

The first is *lack of priority*. If patient teaching is not given top priority by either the nurses or the institution, then it will probably not take place, even though opportunities for teaching are present. Specific ingredients essential in establishing patient education as a priority are: (a) development of a philosophy for patient education by the organization and by nurses; (b) commitment from hospital administration for support of patient education in terms of allocation of time, budget, and staffing; (c) inclusion of accountability for patient teaching as a component of performance evaluation; (d) rewards for doing it and sanctions for not doing it; and (e) provision of reinforcement and recognition for teaching efforts and accomplishments.

The second barrier is *lack of time*. Most nurses say they do not have enough time for patient teaching, often due to a heavy work load or inadequate staffing. It is important to foster the idea that patient education is not a 30-minute block of time specifically set aside to teach the patient. Questions can be answered and information given at any time the nurse is giving care.

The third barrier is *lack of communication*. Each of the staff members involved in a patient's care need to know about the latter's learning needs. This can be communicated through documentation of teaching in the patient's chart. The fourth barrier is an individual nurse's *lack of knowledge*; accompanying this is usually *lack of confidence* in ability to teach a patient. Consequently, content review is important for staff nurses and can be offered through patient education inservice programs or attendance at training sessions, workshops, and other continuing education programs.

The fifth barrier is *lack of training skill*: nurses need to know how to teach in order to be effective in patient education; with this knowledge, they will also be more likely to teach. The skill to teach involves specific skills, including interpersonal sensitivity, the ability to communicate, and specific knowledge about how people learn. Corkadeel and McGlashan have identified the specific patient teaching skills required of staff nurses as developing trust and rapport; recognizing and anticipating needs; assessing readiness to learn; developing and implementing teaching strategies; evaluating progress; and documenting and communicating (Corkadeel & McGlashan, 1983).

The sixth barrier to patient education is *lack of family involvement* in the teaching activities. The seventh barrier is *lack of continuity*. Again, many personnel interact daily with the patient and his family and may confuse them with different interpretations of facts and material. It is helpful if a detailed teaching record is maintained. The eighth barrier is *poor motivation*, on the patient's part, to learn. This can come from low self-esteem, a crowded schedule, lack of trust in and rapport with the staff, or fear. The ninth barrier is *the patient's physical condition*. Patients often cannot attend to the learning because they are weak or in pain.

The final barrier is the patient's *psychosocial adaptation to illness*, which may affect his motivation to learn. Readiness to learn differs at the various stages of the adaptation process.

A major way to promote patient teaching is to assemble a patient education planning group. This should: (a) help counteract physician resistance, to the extent that physicians are included in the planning group; (b) help develop a philosophy of patient education; (c) define staff expectations regarding patient teaching; and (d) build staff nurse knowledge of the learning process, including teaching skills as well as role clarification, nurse-patient rapport, content review, learning needs/assessment, assessment of readiness to learn, teaching strategies, and documentation.

The Hospital Education and Training Department

An excellent resource for patient education in the hospital is the education and training department, whose services can be used to increase the nursing staff's teaching skills and competencies. Such a department can offer courses, workshops, inservice and other patient education programs to improve the quality of patient teaching and promote consistency of information disseminated to patients. Often the patient education coordinator position is located within this department.

Having a hospital-wide coordinator of patient education is a national trend; among the reasons are the need for cost-effective programs; avoidance of duplication of efforts in program development and implementation; and centralization of planning, directing, and evaluating patient education programs. The patient education coordinator should be sought out for information, support, and assistance with any patient education situations or problems arising within the nursing units. Instructors within this department are also educational resources for the nurse manager.

In addition to the involvement in the preceptor program, the department of education interacts with nursing service by providing a variety of continuing education programs for nursing staff. The continuing education process begins with new employee orientation, by introducing the nurse to hospital policy and procedure, basic nursing skills, and CPR certification. On-going courses, workshops, and inservices conducted by the department of education provide current knowledge and skills to increase clinical competencies and ensure quality patient care. Department of education instructors provide consultation and facilitation services to each nursing division. The services help to identify and assess specific problems or unmet needs of individual nursing divisions.

Record Keeping and Evaluation

All hospitals and health education programs must keep records of patient education—records that can have a direct impact on any liability suit initiated by patients. Liability is usually based on negligence. Patients' records are written accounts of what happened to them while in the hospital. They are admissible in court and can be subpoenaed; therefore, they should be complete and accurate. Entries should be made when teaching occurs, and each entry should be dated and signed. They should never be erased, even if incorrect, because the erasures may look like an attempt at concealment. If these basic procedures are followed, liability can usually be reduced.

A variety of educational records can be kept, including the referral forms used when patients are billed specifically for an educational program. Standing orders for educational programs may also be included in a patient's record. So should an intake interview that may include information about a patient's educational needs. It is important to document what has been taught to patients and their families, including whether or not comprehension or competency on the patient's part has been demonstrated. This can be ascertained by observing the patient, asking direct questions, and discussing specifics with the patient. However, the ability to verbalize an understanding of a concept is not definitive and does not necessarily indicate that a person has developed a certain skill.

There have been a number of recent developments relating to patient education and staff development. One is further concentration of interest in the behavioral aspects of health and continuing use of the behavioral sciences. This simply recognizes that life style and behaviors are important determinants of health and illness.

Self-care is also developing as a philosophical position. It aims at giving an individual more tools to manage his own health and regulate his bodily processes. From the health care institution's viewpoint, it is a delegation of responsibility to patients and families for kinds of care formerly provided by health care professionals. It is essential, however, that patients and their families be taught the skills and knowledge necessary for such care.

SUMMARY

- There is always a need for staff and patient education. This education should be based on adult learning principles.

- Most hospitals have specialized training personnel but the nurse manager also has a role in both staff and patient education.

- The basic training function parallels that of nursing: assessment of training needs, planning, implementation, and evaluation.

- Three questions need to be answered in assessment: (a) Can the trainee do what is required? (b) If not, is it due to lack of skill or lack of motivation? and, (c) If it is lack of skill, is training a present employee a more cost-effective intervention than hiring a person already prepared with the skill?

- There are many principles of learning that must be built into any training program: (a) Is the trainee ready to learn? (b) Is the trainee motivated to learn? (c) Are practice opportunities properly provided? (d) Is transfer of training facilitated? (e) Is there too much material provided to learn at one time? (f) Is feedback provided? and, (g) Is the program formulated for adults?

- Staff development includes orientation, formalized education, and on-the-job instruction.

- Although done infrequently, evaluation should be carried out following training intervention to validate the success of the intervention. Criteria for such evaluation include trainee reaction to the program, learning achieved, behavior change, and organizational result.

- Patient education has increased because of the emphasis on maintaining health, shortened hospital stays, JCAH and AHA policy statements, and government funding changes (DRGs).

- Barriers to teaching include lack of patient education as a priority, lack of time, lack of communication between care givers, lack of knowledge, lack of training skill, lack of family involvement, and patient motivation.

- Educational records include billing records, standing orders, staff educational records, and results.

BIBLIOGRAPHY

Bandura, A. (1977). *Social learning theory.* Englewood Cliffs, NJ: Prentice-Hall.

Breckon, D. J. (1982). *Hospital health education.* Rockville, MD: Aspen.

Cascio, W. F. (1982). *Costing human resources: The financial impact of behavior in organizations.* Boston, MA: Kent.

Corkadeel, L. and McGlashan, R. (1983). A practical approach to patient teaching. *The Journal of Continuing Education in Nursing, 14*:9–15.

Craig, R. L. (editor). (1976). *Training and development handbook.* New York: McGraw-Hill.

Crate, M. A. (1965). Nursing functions in adaption to chronic illness. *American Journal of Nursing, 65*:72–76.

Decker, P. J. and Nathan, B. (1985). *Behavior modeling training: Theory and applications.* New York: Praeger Scientific Publishing.

Ellis, H. C. (1965). *The transfer of learning.* New York: MacMillan.

Goldstein, I. L. (1974). *Training: Program development and evaluation.* Monterey, CA.: Brooks/Cole.

Hall, D. T. (1976). *Careers in organizations.* Santa Monica, CA: Goodyear.

Knowles, M. S. (1970). *The modern practice of adult education.* New York: Association Press.

Marx, R. D. (1982). Relapse prevention for management training. *Academy of Management Review, 7*(3):433–441.

May, L. (1980). Clinical preceptors for new nurses. *American Journal of Nursing, 80*: 1824–1826.

Murphy, M. L. and Hammerstad, S. M. (1981). Preparing a staff nurse for precepting. *Nurse Educator,* (September–October).

Redman, B. K. (1980). *The process of patient teaching in nursing.* St. Louis: Mosby.

Shaw, M. E, Corsini, R. J., Blake, R. R. and Mouton, J. S. (1980). *Role playing,* Univ. Assoc.

Wexley, K. N. and Latham, G. P. (1981). *Developing and training human resources in organizations.* Glenview, IL: Scott Foresman.

THE PERFORMANCE APPRAISAL process includes day-by-day supervisor–subordinate interactions (coaching, counseling, disciplining); written documentation (recording critical incidents, completing the performance review form); the formal performance appraisal interview and follow-up with coaching and/or discipline as indicated. The main objective of this chapter is to provide a better understanding of the factors that go into and affect the entire performance appraisal process.

If a group of nurse managers were asked to list the things they liked least about their jobs, "doing performance appraisals" would probably be near the top of their lists; most managers dislike doing performance reviews. If the same group of nurses were asked why they disliked doing reviews, they would very likely submit a laundry list of reasons ("You can't evaluate nursing performance." "The form we use is lousy." "Nurses are professionals—they don't need to be evaluated." "If you give someone a low rating, it hurts his or her future performance." or "I don't have enough information to rate accurately."). Partly because of such reasons, people who do appraisals generally spend little time on them and tend to rate everyone highly.

But what about the subordinate's—say, the staff nurse's —perspective on performance appraisal? You might think back to your own most recent performance review and reflect on three questions: How prepared was the person who did the appraisal? How accurate was the feedback you received? Did the session help you improve your performance? If your answers are: "Not very prepared, not very accurate, and didn't help me improve," then your comments are typical of most persons whose performance is appraised.

None of this, however, should be construed as a recommendation to do away with performance appraisals altogether. Instead, this chapter is intended to provide the information that will help nurse managers do a better job of performance appraisals. Before getting into the specific "nuts and bolts" of doing appraisals, however, one must first understand the numerous factors that affect the way appraisals are done.

ASSUMPTIONS

This chapter is based on six underlying assumptions:

1. *One of the major reasons for doing performance reviews is to help employees improve their future performance.* Thus, performance reviews should be future-oriented.

2. *The performance appraisal process is a difficult one but one can become more skilled at it.* That is, appraisers can become more accurate in their ratings and more professional in giving constructive feedback.

3. *Very few persons like the performance appraisal form they are required to use.* The form "takes too long to complete," "is ambiguous," "requires me to make judgments which I lack data to make," and so on.

4. *In order to be effective in doing the formal, year-end review, one must carry out the day-to-day aspects of the performance appraisal process.*

5. *Supervisors always evaluate their employees' performance.* The question is whether the evaluation is written and fed back to the employee.

6. *The prescriptions given in this chapter will not work for approximately 5% of employees.* In fact, nothing works for this 5%. Possibly these individuals suffered severe head trauma at an early age, watched too many hours of Saturday morning cartoons, or were born on another planet. Whatever the reason, the focus here will be on the 95% of employees on whom these prescriptions will have a positive effect.

USES OF PERFORMANCE APPRAISAL

Performance appraisals can be the basis on which administrative decisions are made for salary increases, promotion decisions, transfers, demotions, terminations, and the like (Heneman et al., 1983). Ideally, accurate performance appraisal information allows an organization to tie rewards to performance. Performance appraisals are also used for employee development. That is, after a thorough review of an employee's performance, the supervisor and employee may jointly develop action plans to help that individual improve through such developmental activities as formal training, academic course work, or simple on-the-job coaching.

A final reason for doing performance reviews concerns Equal Employment Opportunity Law (Title VII, Age Discrimination in Employment Act). Performance appraisals and the decisions, such as termination, that are based on the appraisals, are covered by several federal and state laws. Numerous employees have successfully sued organizations about employment decisions that were based on questionable performance appraisal results.

Regardless of the purposes for which an organization uses performance appraisals, however, the appraisal must accurately reflect the individual's actual job performance. If the performance ratings are inaccurate, an inferior employee may be promoted, another employee may not receive needed training, or there may not be a tie between performance and rewards. Any of these may lessen employee motivation or the hospital may be sued and lose a costly lawsuit. Evaluations must be accurate.

PERFORMANCE APPRAISAL AND THE LAW

Since the passage of Title VII of the Civil Rights Act of 1964, the courts have addressed numerous employment decisions for promotions, terminations, and compensation in which performance appraisals have played an important role (Latham & Wexley, 1980). In many of these cases, the courts have ruled the employment decision to be illegal because the organization's performance appraisal system was in some way unsound. Although one can never be certain that a performance appraisal system is legally defensible, there are a number of steps which, if followed, help ensure that the procedures will be nondiscriminatory. Some of these steps may be beyond the control of the nurse manager—for example, determining the type of performance appraisal form used. However, there are some guidelines an organization or the person doing the appraisal can follow to decrease the likelihood of a discrimination finding or other legal difficulties.

1. The appraisal should be in writing and carried out at least once a year.

2. The performance appraisal information should be shared with the employee and the employee should have the opportunity to respond in writing.

3. There should be a mechanism by which an employee can appeal the results of the performance appraisal.

4. The supervisor should have adequate opportunity to observe the employee's job performance. If adequate contact is lacking (e.g., the appraiser and the appraisee work different shifts), then appraisal information should be gathered from other sources.

5. Notes (critical incidents) on the employee's performance should be kept during the entire evaluation period. These notes should be shared with the employee during the course of the evaluation period.

6. The evaluators should be trained how to carry out the performance appraisal process (e.g., what is reasonable job performance, how to complete the form, how to carry out the feedback interview).

7. Insofar as possible, the performance appraisal should be behaviorally based (focusing on what the person did) rather than trait-based (focusing on personality characteristics such as initiative, attitude, etc.) (Carroll & Schneier, 1982).

PERFORMANCE MEASUREMENT ISSUES

Although nurse managers may not have formal input into the type of performance appraisal instrument used in their institution, an understanding of some fundamental issues is important in order to fully understand the variety of forces that affect the way one does appraisals. Specifically, it is important to understand the philosophy that underlies the performance appraisal system as well as the general focus of the system.

Evaluation Philosophy

First, are the evaluations absolute or comparative in nature? Most evaluation systems are based on absolute judgment; that is, in appraising a staff nurse, the nurse manager evaluates the nurse against an internal standard of performance. This internal standard reflects what the manager perceives as reasonable and acceptable performance for a staff nurse. When evaluations are absolute in nature, it is possible for all nurses to be judged as exceeding the standard for acceptable performance. Alternatively, it is possible that all nurses are seen as just meeting or falling below the standard. In other words, the ratings are entirely dependent upon the judgment of the nurse manager.

In contrast, evaluations based on comparative judgment require the nurse manager to rate subordinates by comparing them with one another; that is, how a nurse is evaluated will depend on the level of performance of her or his peers. A teacher who grades on a curve is making evaluations based on comparative judgment. Thus, comparative judgments are based on the relative standing among employees. Since evaluation systems of this nature call for the nurse manager to differentiate among those rated (not all nurses can receive high ratings), it is not surprising that most nurse managers prefer to make ratings which are based on absolute judgment. Examples of items based on the two kinds of judgment are presented in Figure 15–1.

Components to Be Evaluated

Nurses engage in a variety of job-related activities. In order to reflect this multidimensional nature of the nurse's job, the performance appraisal form usually requires the nurse manager to rate on several different performance dimensions such as initiative, job knowledge, and the ability to work well with others. In developing a performance appraisal device, an organization can focus on employee traits, results, behaviors, or some combination thereof (Latham & Wexley, 1980). The specific focus of the form will affect the whole appraisal process.

Traits/personal characteristics. Most performance appraisal systems focus on personal traits and characteristics—for example, stability, or the ability to handle stress (Carroll & Schneier, 1982). Typically, the nurse manager is asked to rate staff nurses on each trait, and she or he does so largely by means of absolute judgments. The reason that most performance appraisal systems focus on traits is probably cost; trait-oriented appraisal instruments are inexpensive to develop and can be used for a wide variety of positions.

In recent years, however, there has been a gradual shift away from trait-oriented systems, primarily because of legal problems. In a number of cases, for instance, trait rating scores have been found to be lower for minorities and women than for white males. When such "adverse impact" is found, the institution must demonstrate the validity (job relatedness) of the appraisal ratings—a sometimes difficult thing to do since, in most court cases, trait ratings have not been found to be job-related (Klasson,

Figure 15—1   Sample Items Based on Absolute and Comparative Judgment

	Fails to meet (1) Performance Standard	Does Not Quite Meet (2) Performance Standard	Meets Performance (3) Standard	Exceeds Performance (4) Standard	Far Exceeds (5) Performance Standard
Absolute Judgment Items "Rate each staff nurse based on what you consider satisfactory performance."					
1. Initiative					
2. Dependability					
3. Job knowledge					
4. Adherence to hospital policies					

	Bottom 10% of All Staff Nurses	Next 20%	Middle 40% of All Staff Nurses	Next 20%	Top 10% of All Staff Nurses
Comparative Judgment Items "Rate each staff nurse you supervise by comparing him/her with the others you supervise."					
1. Initiative					
2. Dependability					
3. Appearance					
4. Proper utilization of time					

Thompson & Luben, 1980). Thus, the organization has been found guilty of illegal discrimination.

Another reason for the shift away from exclusive reliance on trait ratings is their lack of applicability to employee growth and development. In most health care institutions, a major reason for performance appraisals is to help the employee improve. However, because most trait rating dimensions are somewhat ambiguous (what precisely is meant by "initiative," for instance?), trait-oriented systems are of little use in helping an employee develop, nor do they tell a staff nurse what to do differently in the future.

Results. All organizations, even nonprofit health care institutions, need to be concerned with the so-called bottom line. If a hospital has a 20% occupancy rate, a 60% staff absenteeism rate, or dozens of pending malpractice suits, its future is in jeopardy. In recent years, top management has therefore turned to appraisal of some employees on the basis of the results they produce. Although an in-depth discussion of such results-oriented appraisal systems appears later in this chapter, some of the pros and cons of evaluating health care personnel on this basis are appropriate here.

In theory, a results-oriented appraisal system is ideal. Employees know in advance what results they are supposed to accomplish. These objectives are quantifiable, objective, and easily measured. Unfortunately, in practice, it is not easy to come up with easily measured, concrete objectives for most health care jobs. For example, some aspects of a staff nurse's job—providing a high quality of patient care, for instance—are not easily quantified. Other aspects may be easily quantified, such as the average number of minutes before answering a patient's call button, but not worth the cost of measuring them. In addition, a results-oriented system is of little help in staff development; telling someone that he or she didn't accomplish a goal doesn't tell that person how to accomplish it in the future. In sum, although a results-oriented appraisal system has a number of positive attributes, total reliance on such a system is impractical (Rakich, Longest & O'Donovan, 1977; Rowland & Rowland, 1980).

Behavioral criteria. In recent years, many health care institutions have moved to behavior-oriented performance appraisal systems rather than focusing on vague traits, which may cause legal problems, or difficult-to-measure results. Behavior-oriented systems focus on what the employee actually does, as exemplified in Figure 15–2. Such a system gives new employees specific information on how they are expected to behave, is less likely to lead to legal problems, and the behavioral focus facilitates employee development. The major drawback of a behavior-oriented appraisal system is that it is relatively time consuming to develop and is tied to only one job or a narrow range of jobs. For example, the behavioral items presented in Figure 15–2 were developed by interview-

Figure 15—2   Behavior-Oriented Performance Appraisal Items for the Job of Staff Nurse

	Outstanding (5)	Above Average (4)	Average (3)	Needs Improvement (2)	Unacceptable (1)
1. Reorders medication as needed.					
2. Communicates information from physician's rounds to nursing personnel.					
3. Keeps nurse manager or charge nurse informed of changes in patient's condition.					
4. Reports faulty equipment and safety hazards and follows up to see that appropriate action has been taken.					
5. Reviews and clarifies physician's orders before the physician leaves unit.					
6. Communicates pertinent patient information at the change of shift.					

ing a number of staff nurses and their immediate supervisors. Unlike more general trait dimensions (see Figure 15–1), these items would only be applicable to staff nurses.

Combination of criteria.   As health care institutions have become more concerned with employee productivity in the last few years, some have developed appraisal systems that combine the types of criteria that have just been discussed. For example, each employee has a few major objectives that he or she is expected to accomplish. However, in addition to being evaluated on whether these results were attained, individuals are also evaluated in terms of both general personal characteristics as well as behaviorally specific criteria.

SPECIFIC EVALUATION METHODS

Traditional Rating Scales

By far the most commonly used performance appraisal format is the traditional rating scale, which focuses primarily on personal characteristics/traits. According to Heneman, Schwab, Fossum, and Dyer, the traditional rating scale has the following characteristics.

1. Several performance dimensions are generated. Normally these dimensions (e.g., "dependability") are not based on a job analysis; instead, they are generated arbitrarily.

2. The performance dimensions are general in nature. Thus, they can be applied to a wide variety of jobs. In fact, one often finds that an organization uses the same rating scales for all employees in the organization.

3. The performance dimensions are equally weighted in arriving at an overall performance appraisal score. No dimension is seen as more important than any other dimension.

4. Absolute judgment standards are the basis on which ratings are made. Thus, identical behavior on the part of individuals may get a different score simply because different supervisors have different ideas of what satisfactory performance is (Heneman et al., 1983).

In filling out a traditional rating scale, the appraiser is required to reflect on the employee's performance over the entire evaluation period (usually 12 months) and rate the individual against the rater's internal standard of performance. A common complaint about such scales is that either the performance dimension (e.g., "leadership") is irrelevant to the job in question or that the appraisers do not know exactly what is meant by the dimension. Such complaints arise because one appraisal form is being used across a variety of jobs and because the performance dimensions are not tied to concrete behaviors.

Essay Evaluation

With the essay technique of evaluation, the nurse manager is required to describe the employee's performance over the entire evaluation period by writing a narrative that details the strengths and weaknesses of the individual being appraised. If done correctly, this approach can provide a good deal of valuable data for discussion in the appraisal interview. If used alone, however, an essay evaluation is subject to a number of constraints that limit its effectiveness.

For example, essay evaluations can be time consuming, they depend upon appraisers' ability to express themselves in writing, and they can be difficult to defend in court because comments made by appraisers may not be closely tied to actual job performance. Such evaluations are more useful when they are not used alone but in combination with other evaluation formats *and* when they are based on notes taken by the manager during the entire course of the evaluation period.

Forced Distribution Evaluation

The forced distribution approach to performance appraisal is similar to grading on a curve. The manager is required to rate employees in a fixed manner (see the comparative judgment items in Figure 15–1). For example, if the rating scale has five categories, the manager may be required to spread employees' ratings equally over the five categories. Since this technique constrains the rater, most evaluators don't like it. One hears such complaints as: "I have two exceptional employees but this system allows me to put only one of them in the highest category"; "I don't have an employee who deserves to be rated in the lowest category."

Because of this general dislike, forced distribution systems are not commonly used. In those instances where they are used, it is probably because managers were previously giving all of their employees high ratings.

Behavior-Oriented Rating Scales

As noted earlier, focusing on specific behavior in appraising performance has tremendous advantages: new employees have specific information on how they should behave, and legal problems are less common.

Although there are several varieties of behavior-oriented rating scales, they have a number of things in common and are developed as follows:

1. Groups of workers (generally individuals doing the job and their immediate supervisors) who are very familiar with the target job provide written examples (so-called "critical incidents") of superior and inferior job behaviors.

2. Critical incidents that are similar in theme are grouped together and these behavioral groupings (performance dimensions) are labelled— for example, "direct patient care," or "nurse-physician interactions."

3. Complex statistical procedures are used to arrive at a subset of the original pool of critical incidents. These procedures eliminate items that do not clearly reflect the performance dimension into which they were grouped, overlap other critical incidents, or are poorly worded.

In view of the way that behavior-oriented rating scales are developed, it is apparent that (a) such appraisal measures can be used only for one job or a cluster of very similar jobs; and (b) they are somewhat time consuming and therefore expensive to develop. For these reasons, behavior-oriented systems are generally developed where there are a large number of individuals doing the same job—such as staff nurses.

An advantage of these scales is the fact that because job incumbents and their supervisors actually develop the appraisal instrument, they have faith in the system and are motivated to use it.

Management by Objectives

Whereas the other approaches to performance evaluation focus on an employee's personal characteristics or behavior, management by objectives (MBO) focuses on the results the employee accomplishes. Although there are many variations of this technique, basically MBO involves two steps.

First, a set of work objectives is established for the employee to accomplish during some future time frame. These objectives can be developed either by the employee's supervisor and given to the employee, or the supervisor and the subordinate can mutually develop a set of objectives for the subordinate. Each performance objective should be defined in concrete, quantifiable terms and have a specific time frame; for example, one objective may need to be accomplished in one month, while another may take 12 months. In setting objectives, it is important that the employee perceive them as challenging yet reachable. (See Chapter 9 on goal setting theory.)

The second step in MBO involves the actual evaluation of the employee's performance. At this time, the supervisor and employee meet and focus on how well the employee has accomplished her or his objectives.

Although an MBO system can be excellent for evaluating some jobs, this system is often not used in hospitals, primarily because it is difficult to set challenging, clear, quantifiable goals for health care jobs where tasks are based on variable patient needs. For more detail on MBO, readers are referred to Chapter 3, as well as the books by Latham & Wexley (1980), and Carroll & Schneier (1982).

WHO EVALUATES?

In most institutions, an employee's immediate superior evaluates her or his performance. After all, the superior is very familiar with a subordinate's work and thus is best able to evaluate it. In some work settings, however, the immediate supervisor may not have enough information to accurately evaluate an individual's performance, but completes the performance evaluation form anyway. Obviously, an evaluation based on inadequate information is likely to be somewhat vague and inaccurate.

Two alternatives are available in this situation. First, the supervisor can seek performance-related information from other sources—the employee's co-workers, patients, or other supervisors, for instance—who are familiar with the person being evaluated. The supervisor weighs this additional information, integrates it with her or his own judgment, and does the evaluation.

The second alternative involves a more formal use of other sources. In a few institutions an individual is formally evaluated by a committee that includes supervisors, peers, and the individual's subordinates. To arrive at a final performance rating, such a committee also seeks information from the employee (nurse) and his or her clients (patients). Formal use of these nontraditional sources is infrequent, however, and there are several factors that can interfere with the accuracy of such evaluations.

For example, in the instance of the individual's peers, personal friendship can lead to inflated evaluations. The latter may also result when subordinate ratings are used without the subordinates being completely anonymous. To reduce this tendency, the individuals providing evaluation information should not be identified, and they should be asked to provide several specific examples of behavior upon which they base their judgments. Not surprisingly, self-evaluations may also be inflated, especially if the rating information is used to determine salary increases or promotion decisions.

POTENTIAL PROBLEMS

No matter what type of appraisal device is used, problems that can lessen the accuracy of the performance rating can arise. This, in turn, limits the usefulness of the performance review. For example, if a performance rating can be shown to be inaccurate, it will be difficult to defend it in court.

Leniency Error

Many nurse managers tend to overrate their staff nurses' performance; this is called leniency error. For example, a nurse manager may rate every one of her or his ten staff nurses as "above average." Although numerous reasons are given for inflated ratings ("I want my nurses to like me," "It's difficult to justify giving someone a low rating"), this does not lessen the severe problems that leniency error can create for both the manager and the health care institution. For example, giving a mediocre nurse lenient ratings makes it difficult to turn around later and take some corrective action such as disciplining or demoting the person (Boncarosky, 1979).

Leniency error also tends to have a demoralizing effect on one's best staff nurses, because *they* would have ratings higher than those of the others if it had not been for leniency on the part of their nurse manager. In effect, leniency error is viewed positively by the poorer nurses and negatively by the better nurses.

Recency Error

Another difficulty is the length of the time over which behavior is evaluated—in most institutions, a 12-month period. Evaluating employee performance over such an extended period of time, particularly if one supervises more than two or three individuals, is a difficult cognitive task. Typically, the evaluator recalls recent performance and tends to forget more distant events. Thus, the performance rating reflects what the employee has contributed lately rather than over the entire evaluation period. This is called "recency error" and can create both legal and motivational problems.

Legally, if a disgruntled employee can demonstrate that an evaluation that supposedly reflects 12 months actually reflects performance over only the last two to three months, an institution will have great difficulty defending the validity of the appraisal process. In terms of motivation, recency error demonstrates to all employees that they need only perform at a high level near the time of their performance review. In such situations, employees are highly motivated (e.g., asking their supervisor for more work) just prior to their performance appraisal but considerably less motivated as soon as their appraisals are completed.

As with leniency error, recency error benefits the poorly performing individual. Nurses who perform excellently year round may receive ratings similar to those of mediocre nurses who "spurt" as their evaluation time approaches. Fortunately, there is a simple procedure (recording "noteworthy behaviors," to be discussed later), that greatly lessens the impact of recency error.

Halo Error

Sometimes an appraiser fails to differentiate among the various performance dimensions (e.g., job knowledge, communication skills) when evaluating an employee and assigns ratings on the basis of an overall impression, positive or negative, of the employee. Thus, some employees are rated high, others may be rated average, and a few are rated below average on all dimensions. This is referred to as "halo error."

Sometimes what looks like halo error is actually accuracy. If a nurse is excellent, average, or poor on all performance dimensions, she or he deserves to be rated accordingly; this is not halo error, but a factual rating. In most instances, however, employees have uneven strengths and weaknesses. Thus, it should be relatively uncommon for an employee to receive the same rating on all performance dimensions. Although halo error is less common and troublesome than leniency and recency error, it still can lead to erroneous feedback (Beer, 1981).

Ambiguous Evaluation Standards

Most appraisal forms use rating scales that include such words as "outstanding," "excellent," "above average," "satisfactory," "adequate," or "needs improvement." But different evaluators attach different meanings to these words, giving rise to what has been labelled the "evaluation standards problem." The best way to reduce ambiguity about these standards is for a group of nurse managers to arrive at a consensus of what is meant by each one—e.g., "outstanding" patient care—through discussion. When agreement is reached, this information on what each standard reflects should be communicated to those being evaluated.

Written Comments Problem

Almost all performance appraisal forms provide spaces for written comments by the evaluator. The wise appraiser can use the "comments" space to justify in detail her or his ratings, comment on the employee's potential for promotion, discuss developmental activities for the employee in the coming year, put the ratings in context (e.g., to note that, although the evaluation form is for 12 months, the appraiser has only been the person's superior for the past three months), and so on. Unfortunately, few nurse managers use this valuable space appropriately; in fact, the spaces for written comments are often left blank. Or the comments may be few in number, general in nature ("Ms. Jones is conscientious," "Mrs. Thompson has a poor attitude"), focus totally on what the individual did poorly, or reflect only recent performance.

Many nurse managers, unfortunately, wait until the end of the evaluation period to do their appraisals and write their comments; this makes for a difficult, time-consuming task. Small wonder, then, that what few comments there are will be vague, negative in nature, and reflect recent events. Regular note-taking can lessen these written comments problems.

IMPROVING APPRAISAL ACCURACY

For an appraisal to serve a useful purpose, it needs to encompass all facets of job performance and be free from rater error. Although the effort to achieve total accuracy in evaluations is much like the search for the Holy Grail, there are ways to approach accuracy as closely as possible or more closely than in the past.

Appraiser Ability

Accurate evaluation of an individual's performance involves several components. First, the evaluator must know what behavior is called for by the job description. Second, the rater must have observed the employee's performance over the course of the evaluation period and be able to recall it. Third, he or she must know how to use the appraisal form and understand what is meant by each performance dimension such as "initiative." To the extent that any of these components is lacking, the evaluator's ability to rate accurately is constrained.

An appraiser's ability to rate can, however, be improved. An institution can develop detailed job descriptions and share them with the rater. Or the latter can be given greater opportunity to observe an employee's behavior, directly or indirectly. For example, other supervisors can provide information on an employee's performance when the immediate supervisor is not present. Raters can be encouraged to take notes on employees' behavior to facilitate recall. Lastly, supervisors can be made more knowledgeable concerning how to use the appraisal form through brief training sessions.

Formal training programs help to increase appraiser ability. Although the content of such programs varies, typically programs are designed to (a) make raters aware of the various types of rating errors, on the assumption that awareness may reduce the error tendency; (b) improve raters' observational skills; and (c) improve their skill in carrying out the performance appraisal interview. More specific information on ways to improve the observational skills and interviewing skills will be presented later in this chapter.

Appraiser Motivation

It is fallacious to assume that all managers are motivated to appraise their subordinates accurately. Motivation is discussed more fully in Chapter 9, but a brief examination of appraiser motivation is merited here.

Nurse managers have a multitude of tasks to perform, often immediately. Not surprisingly, then, performance appraisals are often viewed as something that "can be done later." Further, many managers do not perceive appraisals as a particularly important task, and some question the need for them at all. This is especially true if everyone receives the same percentage salary increase. So, if a nurse manager is to be motivated to do appraisals well, then some rewards are in order.

A nurse manager may take a dim view of and spend little time on appraisals for various reasons. The institution may not reward the individual for doing a good job; the nurse manager's superior spends little time on the manager's own appraisal, thus sending the message that appraisals aren't important; and if the nurse manager gives low ratings to a poor employee, the manager's superior may overrule her or him and raise the ratings. In short, and in many health care institutions, the environment may actually dampen appraiser motivation rather than stimulate it.

Given these reasons for not spending much time on appraisals, it is fairly obvious how one can enhance appraiser motivation. First of all, nurse managers need to be rewarded for doing a conscientious appraising job; this should be mentioned in their own reviews. In addition, nurse managers' superiors need to be good role models for the appraising function. And finally, insofar as possible, nurse managers should be able to reward those staff nurses they rate highly. Pay increases should not be across the board, layoffs should not be based on seniority, and promotions should be tied to superior performance.

DOCUMENTING PERFORMANCE

Appraising another person's performance can be a difficult job. The nurse manager is required to reflect on a staff nurse's performance over a considerable period of time (usually 12 months) and then accurately evaluate it. Inasmuch as many nurse managers have several individuals to evaluate, it is not surprising that they frequently forget what an individual did several months ago; they may actually confuse one employee's performance with another's. A useful mechanism for fighting such memory problems is the use of critical incidents: reports of behaviors that are out of the ordinary, in either a positive or negative direction.

Noteworthy Behaviors

The behaviors are recorded on a form or index card with space for four items: name of employee, date of incident, a brief description of the incident, and the nurse manager's report of action taken (see Figure 15–3). Index cards are usually preferred to the page-sized forms, as the cards can be easily carried and do not tear.

Recording noteworthy behavior as it occurs is bound to increase the accuracy of the year-end performance appraisal ratings. Although this type of note-taking may sound simple and straightforward, a nurse manager can still run into problems—timing, for instance, or personal misgivings about this kind of recording.

For instance, the best time to write critical incidents is just after the incident occurs, with the actual note focusing on specific behaviors, not an interpretation of them. For example, not "Ms. Hudson was rude," but "Ms. Hudson referred to the patient as lazy." The nurse manager decides what is noteworthy behavior. In some departments, it may be coming to work on time; in others, it may be coming to work late. Once a noteworthy behavior has been recorded, this should be made known to the indi-

Figure 15—3 Example of Critical Incidents

1. Name of employee   *Cindy Siegler*

2. Date of incident   4/2/87

3. Description   *I overheard Cindy discussing a patient's lack of personal hygiene in our coffee shop. She referred to the patient by name and spoke loud enough to be heard by people at other tables.*

4. Comments   *Her action was unprofessional. She could have caused embarrassment for both the patient and the hospital. I spoke with her concerning this matter.*

vidual by the nurse manager in private. If the behavior is positive, this provides an opportunity for the nurse manager to praise the subordinate; if the behavior is considered in some way undesirable, the nurse manager may need to coach the employee.

Many nurse managers are uncomfortable about recording behaviors because they see themselves as spies lurking around the unit attempting to catch someone. What they need to remember is that this note-taking will enable them to evaluate the individual more fairly, objectively, and accurately over a 12-month period. Without such notes, recency error creeps in.

Because most nurse managers are extremely busy, they sometimes question whether note-taking is time well spent, but such recording is not actually a time-consuming process. The average note takes less than two minutes to write. If one writes notes during the gaps in one's day—for instance, while waiting for a meeting to start or one's party to come to the telephone—little, if any, productive time is used. In the long run, such recording over the course of the year actually saves the nurse manager time when the appraisal is due. It also facilitates dealing with problems when they first occur and are small.

A key factor in effectively using these critical incident notations is how nurse managers introduce them to their subordinates. Managers need to keep in mind two important facts: (a) the primary reason for taking such notes is to improve the accuracy of the performance review; and (b) when something new is introduced, many people react negatively to it. Managers should be open and candid about the first fact, admitting that they cannot remember every event associated with every employee and telling employees that these notes will make possible more accurate evaluations. Even then, employees will still be suspicious about this new procedure. It helps if the first note on any employee can be about a desirable work behavior, even if the manager has to "stretch" a bit to find one. In this way, an employee's first contact with noteworthy behaviors will be positive.

Based on the experience of institutions that have formally introduced the use of noteworthy behaviors, nurse managers tend to make three types of mistakes. Some managers, for instance, fail to make notes specific and behavior-oriented; rather, they record that the nurse was "careless" or "difficult to supervise." A second mistake concerns the tone of the notes, with some managers recording only undesirable behavior. The third error is a nurse manager's failure to inform the nurse at the time that a note has been written.

Each of these errors can undermine the effectiveness of the process. If the notes are vague, the nurse may not know specifically what she or he is doing wrong and therefore does not know how to improve. If only poor performance is noted, employees will resent the system and the manager. If the manager does not share notes as they are written, the employee may react emotionally when confronted with them at the time of the evaluation. In sum, any nurse manager who is considering the use of this powerful note-taking procedure needs to take the process seriously and to use it as it is designed.

By increasing the accuracy of the performance review, written notes also diminish the likelihood of lawsuits. And, if a lawsuit is brought, written notes are very persuasive evidence in court. Sharing the notes with employees throughout the evaluation period also improves the communication flow between supervisor and employee; the latter is regularly told what is considered noteworthy behavior. Finally, written notes also give the manager considerable confidence when it comes time to complete the evaluation form and carry out the appraisal interview. She or he will be less prone to leniency and recency error and can feel confident about the accuracy of the rating. Not only does the nurse manager feel professional, but the staff nurse shares that perception. In fact, it is typically found that with the use of noteworthy behavior recordings, the performance appraisal interview focuses mainly on how the employee can improve next year rather than on how he or she was rated last year. Thus, the tone of the interview is constructive rather than argumentative.

Different employees will react in different ways to the use of notes. Good employees will react positively. Although nurse managers will record both what is done well and what is done poorly, good employees will have more positive than negative notes and therefore benefit from the notes. Poorer employees, in contrast, do not react well to notes being taken. Whereas once they would rely on the poor memory of the nurse manager as well as on a leniency tendency to produce inflated ratings, note-taking is likely to result in more accurate and therefore lower ratings. The negative reaction of poor employees, however, tends not to be a lasting one. Generally, the poor performers will either leave the organization or, upon discovering that they no longer can get away with mediocre behavior, their performance will actually improve.

THE PERFORMANCE APPRAISAL INTERVIEW

An accurate evaluation is the first prerequisite for an effective performance appraisal, but never think that when the form is filled out the job is finished. As stated earlier, one of the prime reasons for doing the appraisal is to help the employee improve, and the performance appraisal interview is a primary vehicle for employee development (Moore & Simendinger, 1976).

Preparing for the Interview

In preparing for the performance appraisal interview, the nurse manager must keep in mind what she or he wants to accomplish, remembering that if the evaluation is accurate and is perceived as such by the employee, then the latter will accept it as a basis for both rewards and future development. More specifically, in order to motivate employees, rewards need to be seen as linked to performance, and the performance appraisal interview is the key to this linkage. In the interview the nurse manager needs to establish that performance has been carefully assessed and that, when merited, rewards will be forthcoming. Developmental activities also need to be derived from an accurate evaluation. For example, if a person is rated as "poor" in "delegation skills," any effort to remedy this deficiency must stem from his or her acceptance of the fact that the rating is accurate.

Nurse managers should anticipate potential disagreement with some of their ratings. Most nurses, like most people in general, see themselves as above-average performers. They tend to forget their mistakes and recall their accomplishments. Besides, it is easy to rationalize away those instances where performance was substandard ("I forgot, but with this heavy workload, what do you expect?"). In addition, because many staff nurses may previously have had poor experiences with the evaluation process, nurse managers should expect that staff nurses will lack confidence in the whole appraisal process.

A key step for making the appraisal interview go well is proper planning. The interview should be set up in advance—preferably, with at least two days notice. The interview generally takes 20 to 30 minutes, although this will vary with the degree to which the manager and the nurse have talked regularly during the year.

In preparing for the interview, the nurse manager should have specific examples of behavior to support the ratings. Such documentation is particularly important for performance areas in which an individual receives low ratings. In addition, the manager should try to anticipate how the staff nurse will react to the appraisal. For example, will she or he challenge the ratings? By anticipating such a reaction, one can often deal with it effectively with such statements as "Before I made my ratings, I talked with two other nurse managers to make sure my standards were reasonable."

It is also critical that the interview take place in a setting which is private and relatively free from interruptions; this will enable a frank, indepth conversation. Although it is difficult to limit interruptions in the hospital setting, choosing the meeting time carefully will help. A nurse manager can perhaps schedule the meeting at a time when another nurse manager or assistant nurse manager can cover for her or him or at a time when interruptions are least likely to occur. The important thing to remember is that a poor setting will limit the usefulness of the interview. No one wants weaknesses discussed in public. Similarly, interruptions will destroy the flow of the conversation.

The Interview

The interview is most likely to go well if the nurse manager has written and shared noteworthy behaviors throughout the evaluation period. This means that the staff nurse will already have a pretty good idea of how she or he is likely to be rated and of what behavior led to the rating. If the manager has not kept notes throughout the year, it is very important that she or he recall numerous specific examples of behavior, both positive and negative, to support the ratings.

Nurse managers should try to establish a problem-solving climate for the interview, with the major focus on how manager and staff nurse can work together to improve the nurse's performance in the coming year. However, establishing such an improvement-oriented climate is easier said than done. If the climate is to be a constructive one, the manager needs to be aware that every employee has a tolerance level for criticism; beyond that point, defensiveness sets in. Thus, in reviewing an individual's past performance, one should emphasize only a few areas—preferably, no more than three—that need immediate improvement.

Unfortunately, evaluators often tend to exceed an employee's tolerance level, particularly if the performance has been mediocre. Typically, the nurse manager will come up with an extensive list of behaviors needing improvement, and the staff nurse gradually moves from a constructive frame of mind ("I need to work on that") after one or two criticisms are raised, to a destructive perspective ("She doesn't like me," "He's nitpicking," or "How can I get even") as the list of criticisms continues.

Key Behaviors

The use of a set of key behaviors, as listed in Figure 15–4, can greatly improve the way appraisal interviews are carried out. Each of these points will be elaborated upon here, numbered to correspond with the listing.

1. Many individuals are nervous at the start of the appraisal interview, especially new employees for whom this is a first evaluation, or those who have not received frequent performance feedback from the nurse manager throughout the evaluation period. So, to facilitate two-way communication during the interview, the nurse manager needs to find some way to put the staff nurse at ease. Some managers rely on small talk, such as discussing the weather or families. Others begin the interview by giving an overview of the type of information that was used in making the performance ratings—for example, "In preparing for this review, I relied

---

Figure 15–4 Key Behaviors: Performance Reviews

1. Put the person at ease.

2. Make it clear that the purpose of the performance review is to help the employee to do the best possible job.

3. Review the ratings with the employee, citing specific examples of behavior that resulted in a particular rating.

4. Ask for the employee's feelings about the ratings and listen, accept, and respond to them.

5. Together decide on specific ways in which performance areas can be strengthened. Write the resulting plans on paper.

6. Set a follow-up date.

7. Express your confidence in the employee.

Taken from Decker, P. J. *Healthcare Management Microtraining.* Copyright 1982 by Phillip J. Decker. Used with permission.

heavily on the notes I had taken and shared with you throughout the year." There really is no one best way to break the tension, but the manager can experiment with various approaches.

2. The next thing the nurse manager should do is clearly state that the purpose of the interview is to help the employee do the best possible job in the coming year. This improvement-oriented theme should be conveyed at the beginning of the interview.

3. The supervisor should go through the ratings one by one with the employee and provide a number of specific examples of behavior that led to each rating. Some nurse managers mistakenly use only behavioral examples to support low ratings, but this can cause problems. First of all, subordinates are more likely to become defensive because the entire focus is on problem areas. Furthermore, if no attention is paid to the nurse's good performance in certain areas, she or he may pay less attention to those areas in the future. Nor should the rater rush through the ratings. By taking up each one systematically and providing behavioral examples, the nurse manager projects an image of being prepared and of being a professional. This is important for getting the staff nurse to accept the ratings and act on them.

4. Next, the manager needs to draw out the staff nurse's reactions to the ratings—more specifically, to ask for the employee's feelings about the ratings and listen, accept, and respond to them. Of the seven key behaviors for performance reviews, nurse managers seem to have the most difficulty with this one. But, to carry out this phase of the interview effectively, the manager must have confidence in the accuracy of her or his ratings.

When asked to express their feelings, individuals who have received low ratings will frequently question the rater's judgment ("Don't you think your standards are a little high?"). The manager whose judgment has been questioned then tends to become defensive, cutting off the employee's remarks and arguing for the rating in question. Being cut off sends a contradictory message to the employee. He or she was asked for reactions but, when they were given, the supervisor did not want to hear them. Thus, the nurse manager should anticipate that ratings will be challenged and must truly want to hear the reactions to them.

After having listened, the manager should accept and respond to the staff nurse's feelings, conveying that she or he has heard what the individual has said (e.g., paraphrase some of the comments) and accept it as the individual's opinion ("I understand your view"). In addition, the nurse manager may want to clarify what has been said ("You misunderstood what I said about your patient care skills," "I do not understand why you feel your 'initiative' rating is too low. Could you cite specific behavior to justify a higher rating?"). In sum, the nurse manager wants a candid, two-way conversation and needs to know exactly how the subordinate feels.

5. The focus of the interview then shifts entirely to the future. Together the nurse manager and staff nurse decide on specific ways in which

performance can be strengthened, and the resulting plans are written down. Because of the possibility of defensiveness and the tolerance level for criticism, only one or two performance areas needing improvement should be addressed—ideally, the ones that present the most problems.

The first step in planning for improved performance is for the nurse manager to ask the staff nurse for his or her ideas on how performance can be improved. After hearing these, the nurse manager can add her or his own ideas. Such performance planning must be related to specific behavior. In some cases, not only will staff nurses be expected to do things in a different manner (e.g., "Will refer to a patient as Mr., Mrs., or Ms. unless specifically told otherwise") but supervisors may also be expected to change their behaviors (e.g., "Will post changes in hospital policy on bulletin board before enforcing them") (Moore & Simendinger, 1976).

6. After having agreed on specific ways to strengthen performance, the nurse manager should set a follow-up date for a subsequent meeting—usually, four to six weeks after the appraisal interview. At this later meeting, the nurse manager provides specific feedback on the nurse's recent performance. This meeting also gives the manager and nurse the opportunity to discuss any problems they have encountered in attempting to carry out their agreed-upon performance plans. In most cases, this follow-up session is quite positive in tone. With one or two areas to work on and a specific date on which the staff nurse will be accountable and on which feedback will be given, the nurse's performance usually improves dramatically. Thus, the follow-up provides the nurse manager with an opportunity to praise the nurse.

7. The final key behavior—expressing confidence in the employee—is simple but often overlooked. It is nevertheless important that the manager indicate her or his confidence that improvement will be forthcoming.

Although it has been suggested that no more than three problem areas should be addressed in the appraisal interview, the question of when to work on other problem areas can legitimately be raised. The answer is: later in the year. For example, a nurse manager decides to focus on only one performance area in the appraisal interview, specific ways for improving deficiencies in this area are developed and written down, a follow-up meeting takes place one month later, and performance in the targeted area has improved dramatically. At the follow-up meeting, the manager praises the staff nurse and encourages him or her to continue the excellent performance.

Then, one or two weeks after the follow-up session, the manager meets again with the staff nurse, this time raising a second area which needs attention. As before, specific ways to improve the deficiency are developed and written down and another follow-up meeting is scheduled.

In short, performance deficiencies are not ignored, they are merely temporarily overlooked. The experienced nurse manager knows such deficiencies can only be effectively dealt with in the manner outlined above.

DAY-TO-DAY COACHING

As must be apparent by now, performance appraisals represent a year-long process of recording and sharing noteworthy behaviors, and an essential element in this process is day-to-day coaching by the nurse manager. As with the performance appraisal interview, certain key behaviors (Figure 15–5) have been found to be quite effective for structuring nurse manager-staff nurse coaching interactions. Again, they will be discussed in their listed sequence but first, a word about preparation is in order.

Before entering into a coaching session, the nurse manager (the coach) should spend at least a few minutes preparing for the interaction. The goal of the meeting is to eliminate, or at least lessen, a performance problem such as excessive absenteeism or frequent personal phone calls. The manager should try to anticipate how the employee will react (e.g., "Everybody gets personal phone calls"), in order to formulate an appropriate response (e.g., "I am going to talk to each person about this problem"). Problems should be dealt with when they are small or first occur. In general, coaching sessions should last no more than five to ten minutes.

1. The first key behavior in coaching is to state the problem in behavioral terms: for example, "Mr. Jones's medication was not given on time this morning."

2. Then the supervisor should tie the problem to the functioning of the organization, professional standards, and/or to the person's self-interest: for example, "The hospital could be sued; you could be terminated." This is an important but often overlooked first step, since one

---

Figure 15–5 Key Behaviors: Coaching*

---

1. State the problem in behavioral terms; immediately focus on the problem, do not attack the person.

2. Tie problem to organizational and/or personal consequences.

3. Ask employee why the behavior occurred. Try to bring the reasons for the problem into the open.

4. Ask for suggestions on how to solve the problem. Listen openly. Discuss the employee's ideas or, if none are offered, lead the employee to your own preferred solution by asking if it has been tried.

5. Agree on steps each of you will take to solve the problem. Write them down. If appropriate: Ask for employee's commitment to the above steps.

6. Agree on and record a specific follow-up date.

---

*Always prepare before the meeting

Taken from Decker, P. J. *Healthcare Management Microtraining*. Copyright 1982 by Phillip J. Decker. Used with permission.

cannot take for granted that the employee knows why the behavior is a problem. After all, if persons are expected to act in a specific way, then they need to understand why the behavior is important and to be rewarded when it has improved.

3. Having stated the problem behavior, the nurse manager needs to explore the reasons for the problem, never jumping to any conclusions of his or her own but asking the staff nurse what caused the problem behavior. After the staff nurse has done so, the manager decides how to proceed with the coaching session. If the problem was caused by ignorance—for instance, lack of familiarity with hospital policy—the manager may simply inform the nurse of the appropriate behavior and end the coaching session.

4. For most problems, however, the nurse manager should ask the employee for his or her suggestions and discuss ideas on how to solve the problem. In many cases, the employee knows best how to solve the problem and is more likely to be committed to the solution if it is his or her own. It is nearly always better to encourage employees to solve their own problems, but this does not mean that managers cannot supplement with their own suggestions for ways to improve.

It is essential for managers to listen openly. They need to fully understand their subordinates' perspectives in order to coach them successfully.

5. How formal should the coaching session be? If the problem is minor and a first-time occurrence, the nurse manager may simply state what actions will be taken to solve the problem and end the meeting. In most cases, however, the nurse manager and staff nurse should agree on steps each will take to solve the problem, and these should be written down for later reference. The steps should be specific and behavioral.

6. Finally, the nurse manager should arrange for a follow-up meeting at which time the staff nurse will receive performance feedback.

It is possible that a staff nurse may bring up personal problems as a cause of his or her work problems. The coaching session then verges on becoming a counseling session, and the manager must be aware of his or her abilities in this area; most nursing supervisors are not trained in marriage counseling, individual therapy, or drug or alcohol rehabilitation, for instance. In other words, nurse managers must be cognizant of their limitations as counselors. When personal problems are raised, they should convey their concern and willingness to work with employees to get help for the problems. In most cases, nurse managers will not be the direct source of the help but rather will seek out other, appropriate sources. It is most important that nurse managers do not themselves delve into potential personal problems (e.g., "Are there problems at home that I should know about?") unless staff nurses raise them. The employee's personal life is not the manager's business.

DISCIPLINING EMPLOYEES

Most managers—and nurses are no exception—dread having to discipline a subordinate. There will nevertheless be occasions when this discipline is necessary, usually when a hospital rule or regulation has been violated, thereby jeopardizing patient safety, the quality of care, or the rights of others. It may lessen the dread of the disciplinary process to remember that its primary function is not to punish the guilty party but rather to encourage that party and others to behave appropriately at work (Boncarosky, 1979).

When faced with a disciplinary situation, the nurse manager should maintain close contact with the hospital's personnel department and nursing service, discussing the situation with them and obtaining approval before taking any disciplinary action. This close coordination between nurse manager and administration is essential to guarantee that any disciplinary action is administered in a fair and legally defensible manner.

To further ensure fairness, rules and regulations must be clearly communicated; a system of progressive penalties must be developed; and an appeals process must be available. In order to enforce a rule or regulation, employees need to be kept informed of them, preferably in writing.

If a rule is violated, penalties should be progressive. For minor violations—smoking in an unauthorized area, for instance—penalties may progress from an oral warning; to a written one placed in the employee's personnel folder; to a suspension; and, ultimately, to termination. For major rule violations (e.g., theft of hospital property), initial penalties should be more severe (e.g., immediate suspension). An appeals process should be built into the disciplinary procedure to ensure that discipline is carried out in a fair, consistent manner. In some hospitals, penalties are appealed to a higher-level manager. Other institutions may have an appeals board composed of individuals representing a cross section of jobs in the hospital.

Here are some guidelines for effective discipline:

1. Get the facts before acting.

2. Do not act while angry.

3. Do not suddenly tighten your enforcement of rules.

4. Do not apply penalties inconsistently.

5. Discipline in private.

6. Make the offense clear. Specify what is appropriate behavior.

7. Get the other side of the story.

8. Do not let the disciplining become personal.

Figure 15—6   Key Behaviors in Discipline*

1. Define the problem in terms of lack of improvement since the previous discussion.

2. Ask for and openly listen to reasons for the continued behavior.

3. Explain why the behavior cannot continue.

4. If disciplinary action is called for, indicate what action you must take and why.

5. Agree on specific steps to be taken to solve problem (write them down).

6. Set a follow-up date and outline further steps to be taken if the problem is not corrected.

7. Assure the employee of your interest in helping him/her to succeed.

---

*Always prepare before the meeting

Taken from Decker, P. J. *Healthcare Management Microtraining*. Copyright 1982 by Phillip J. Decker. Used with permission.

9. Do not back down when you are right.

10. Stay in touch with personnel. (Boncarosky, 1979)

As with performance appraisal interviewing and coaching, key behaviors (Figure 15–6) have also been developed for carrying out the disciplinary process. Inasmuch as these closely parallel the key behaviors for coaching, they do not need further discussion here.

SOME RULES OF THUMB

Thus far, techniques and guidelines for successful performance reviews have been systematically set forth, but there remain some additional suggestions—they might be called "tips"—that derive from practical experience. So here, in conclusion, are some "rules of thumb."

Go beyond the form.   Too often evaluators blame a "poor" form as their excuse for doing a poor job of evaluating their subordinates. But, no matter how inadequate the appraisal form, nurse managers can go beyond it. They can focus on behavior even if the form doesn't require it, set goals even if no other supervisor does, and use noteworthy behaviors as a managerial tool. In short, nurse managers should do the best job of managing that they can and not let the form handicap them.

Postpone the appraisal interview if necessary.   Once the appraisal interview begins, there appears to be some natural law of management that the session must be completed in the allotted time, whether or not the session is going well or has degenerated into name calling. Managers forget that the goal of the interview is not merely to get employees' signatures on the appraisal form but rather to encourage them to improve their performance in the coming year. So, if the interview is not going well, it should be discontinued until a later time. Such postponement allows both the manager and the subordinate time to reflect on what has transpired as well as to calm down.

In postponing the meeting, the manager should not assign blame ("If you're going to act like this, let's postpone the meeting"), but adopt a more positive approach ("This meeting isn't going the way I hoped it would; I'd like to postpone it to give us some time to collect our thoughts"). Most managers who have used this technique find that the second session, which generally takes place a day or two later, goes much better.

Don't be afraid to change an inaccurate rating. New managers often ask: "Should I change a rating if an employee challenges it?" They fear that by changing a rating they will be admitting an error or that other ratings will then be challenged. This practical rule of thumb may help: If the rating is inaccurate, change it—but *never* during the interview. Rather, if an employee challenges a rating and the manager believes she or he has a case, the manager should tell the person that he or she wants some time to think about it and will get back to the employee later.

This is a logical and sensible thing to do. If managers do a careful job of evaluating performance, they should make few inaccurate ratings. But no one is perfect and, on rare occasions, managers may err. When such an error occurs, it should be corrected. Most employees respect a manager who admits a mistake and corrects it. And managers, by allowing themselves some time to reflect on their ratings, free themselves from the pressure to make snap judgments.

SUMMARY

- Doing performance appraisals is one of the most difficult and one of the most important nurse manager activities.

- Accurate appraisal provides a sound basis for both administrative decisions (e.g., salary increases, promotion decisions) and employee development.

- Poorly done performance reviews can result in legal problems.

- There are a variety of different performance evaluation methods (e.g., rating scales, essay evaluation). It is possible to do an effective job of evaluating employees no matter what system/method is used.

- Most supervisors are subject to leniency and recency errors.

- In order to improve the accuracy of evaluations, we need to improve the evaluator's ability and/or motivation to rate accurately.

- Keeping a record of "Noteworthy Behaviors" can greatly improve the way a nurse manager does performance reviews.

- Preparation is essential for doing effective appraisal interviews.

- Following performance appraisal interview key behaviors will enhance the value of this meeting.

- Day-to-day coaching is a critical component of the appraisal process.

- If disciplining an employee is necessary, following established guidelines and key behaviors will increase managerial effectiveness.

BIBLIOGRAPHY

Beer, M. (1981). Performance appraisal: Dilemmas and possibilities. *Organizational dynamics*, (Spring): 24.

Boncarosky, L. D. (1979). Guidelines to corrective discipline. *Personnel J*, (October): 698.

Brucks, A. (1985). Performance appraisal: Evaluating the evaluation. *The Healthcare Supervisor*, 3(4): 17–30.

Carroll, S. J., and Schneier, C. F. (1982). *Performance appraisal and review systems*. Glenview, IL: Scott, Foresman.

Ganong, J., and Ganong, W. (1983). *Performance appraisal for productivity: The nurse manager's handbook*. Gaithersburg, MD: Aspen Systems Corporation.

Heneman, H. G., Schwab, D. P., Fossum, J. A., and Dyer, L. D. (1983). *Personnel/human resource management*. Homewood, IL: Irwin.

Kjervik, D. K. (1984). Progressive discipline in nursing: Arbitrators' decisions. *J Nurs Adm*, (April) 14(4): 34.

Klasson, C. R., Thompson, D. E., and Luben, G. I. (1980). How defensible is your performance appraisal system? *Personnel Adm*, (December) 25(12): 77.

Lachman, V. (1984). Increasing productivity through performance evaluation. *J Nurs Adm*, 14(12): 7–14.

Latham, G. P., and Wexley, K. N. (1980). *Increasing productivity through performance appraisal*. Reading, MA: Addison-Wesley.

Meyers, S. (1983). *Procedural instructions for the performance and development review*. Evanston, IL: Evanston Hospital Corp.

Moore, T., and Simendinger, F. (1976). Evaluating is a two-way street. *Superv Nurs* (June).

Rakich, J., Longest, B. B., and O'Donovan, T. (1977). *Managing health care organizations*. Philadelphia: Saunders.

Rowland, H. S., and Rowland, B. I. (1980). *Nursing administration handbook*. Germantown, MD: Aspen Systems Corporation.

16

Understanding and Effectively Managing Absenteeism and Turnover

HISTORICALLY, HEALTH CARE institutions have had serious problems with excessive employee absenteeism and turnover. In this chapter, these two so-called withdrawal behaviors will be examined. The chapter will cover reasons why these costly behaviors occur, the possible adverse and desirable consequences of absenteeism and turnover, and proven mechanisms for controlling them. Several of the themes developed in Chapter 9, on motivating staff, will also be stressed in this chapter. Because many of the causes and consequences of absenteeism are quite different from those of turnover, these two withdrawal behaviors will be examined individually. The overall purpose of the chapter is to offer insight into what can be done to increase employee attendance and retention, the counterparts of absenteeism and turnover. The chapter has a "proactive" (action-oriented) emphasis. Rather than merely trying to live with absenteeism and turnover problems, nurse managers can utilize a variety of strategies for actively managing these withdrawal behaviors.

ABSENTEEISM

In order to provide high quality patient care, adequate personnel must be available to staff the health care unit. If staff nurses are absent, the patient suffers either directly or indirectly. For example, a staff shortage can lead to patient care being rushed and, therefore, of poorer quality. Or, if a nurse works a double shift to cover for an absent co-worker, the added cost of the overtime is ultimately passed on to the patient. Dealing with such staff absenteeism is an important aspect of the nurse manager's job.

Although it is not possible to estimate precisely the extent or cost of nurses being absent from work, it is well established that absenteeism in health care institutions is both pervasive and expensive. Recent surveys (e.g., Bureau of National Affairs, 1985) suggest that health care employees have one of the highest absenteeism rates of any employee group. Based on an average of the surveys conducted by the Bureau of National Affairs in the 1980s, the yearly absenteeism rate for health care employees is approximately 6.5 days. Including the cost of the absent nurse's salary and fringe benefits as well as the cost of absent nurse's replacement, the cost of a day of absenteeism has been estimated at over $175. Multiplying these two figures yields an absenteeism cost estimate of over $1100 per nurse per year. Although one can quibble over the precision of this estimate (e.g., the Ontario Department of Labor suggests the cost of absenteeism may be as high as three times the absent employee's salary), it seems reasonable to conclude that the annual absenteeism cost per nurse per year falls between $800 and $1400.

However, the costs of absenteeism go beyond its effects on patient care and dollar costs. Absenteeism can have a detrimental effect on the work lives of the other staff nurses. In some cases, they may have to work shorthanded; they are expected to cover the unit despite their missing colleagues. Working shorthanded, especially for an extended period of time, can create both physical and mental strain. These nurses may be forced to skip breaks, hurry through meals, work extended hours, abbreviate their interactions with patients, pass up continuing education workshops offered by the hospital, cancel scheduled nonwork activities, and so on. Even if temporary replacements are called in, the work flow of the hospital unit will still be disrupted. For example, standard hospital procedure will need to be explained to replacement or agency nurses. And, generally, these temporary nurses will be given the easier cases to handle because the administration and nursing staff lack confidence in their ability.

Given these as well as other undesirable effects of absenteeism, it is not surprising that absenteeism has drawn a good deal of attention in the health care field. For the nurse manager, the question is, "What, if anything, can I do to lessen our recurrent absenteeism problem?" But, before one can suggest ways to "manage" absenteeism, one must understand its causes. In the following section, a useful model for understanding nurse absenteeism and, conversely, nurse attendance is presented.

A Model of Employee Attendance

In attempting to understand employee absenteeism, it is important to distinguish between "voluntary" and "involuntary" absenteeism. For example, not coming to work in order to finish one's income tax would be seen as voluntary absenteeism (i.e., absenteeism that is largely within the employee's control). In contrast, taking a sick day to recover from food poisoning would be considered involuntary absenteeism (i.e., largely outside of the employee's control). Although this voluntary/involuntary distinction seems reasonable in theory, in practice it is often difficult to distinguish between these two categories due to a lack of accurate information (i.e., few employees will admit to abusing sick leave).

Some organizations try to distinguish between voluntary and involuntary absenteeism by the way they measure absenteeism. Traditionally, health care institutions have measured absenteeism in terms of "total time lost" (i.e., the number of scheduled days an employee misses). Given that one long illness can drastically affect this absenteeism index, it is clearly not a good measure of voluntary absenteeism. In contrast, "absence frequence" (i.e., the total number of distinct absence periods regardless of their duration) is somewhat insensitive to one long illness. Therefore, absence frequency has been used as an indirect estimate of voluntary absenteeism.

This distinction between absence frequency and total time lost also makes sense to nurse managers. For example, an individual who missed seven Mondays in a row would have seven absence frequency periods as well as seven total days absent. In contrast, an individual who missed seven consecutive days of work would have one absence frequency period but seven total days lost. Intuitively, it seems likely that the first individual was much more prone to being absent voluntarily than the second individual. In fact, based on statistical analysis of absenteeism records, Breaugh (1981) demonstrated that managers' performance appraisal ratings of their employees' absenteeism/attendance were much more closely related to absence frequency periods than to total days lost. Thus, it appears managers really do consider the pattern of the absences more than simply the number of days lost.

Although there are many models of attendance/absenteeism behavior, a model developed by Steers and Rhodes (Figure 16–1) is particularly useful for the practicing manager (Steers & Rhodes, 1978). In this chapter, only those aspects of the model that are particularly germane to the nurse manager are discussed. According to the model, an employee's attendance at work is largely a function of two variables: the individual's *ability to attend* and *motivation to attend*.

As can be seen in Figure 16–1, Steers and Rhodes posit that an employee's ability to attend is affected by such factors as illness, accidents, family responsibilities, and transportation problems. Most man-

Figure 16–1   Major Influences on Employee Attendance

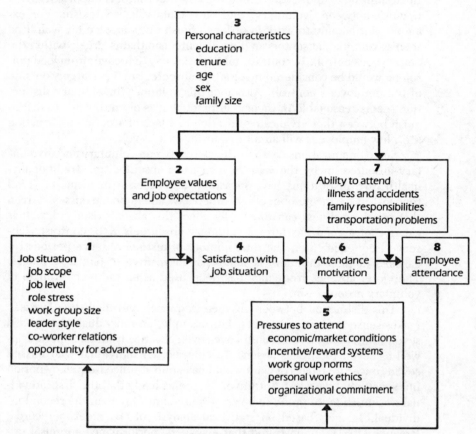

Adapted from Steers, R. M., and Rhodes, S. R. Major influences on employee attendance: A process model. *J Appl Psychol*, 1978, 63:391–407.

agers see ability to attend as corresponding closely to involuntary absenteeism.* Ability to attend is seen as influenced by a number of personal characteristics (Steers & Rhodes, 1984). For example, for many married couples, the woman takes primary responsibility for child care. It is not

---

*In examining the model, it is important to keep in mind that in practice some distinctions may on occasion be fuzzy. Although the model should be a helpful tool for managers, it clearly simplifies the reality of the workplace. For example, determining whether staying home because of a sore back should be classified as due to an inability to attend as opposed to lack of motivation to attend asks for information that the nurse manager may not possess (e.g., how bad was the back?). Despite such occasional difficulties, the Steers and Rhodes model offers a powerful framework for understanding what factors influence employee attendance/absenteeism.

surprising therefore that studies have shown that working women with young children may have less ability to attend work than others. In a similar vein, it has been shown that those with larger families (i.e., with a greater likelihood of family problems arising) are less able to attend (Muchinsky, 1977).

Employee motivation to attend is seen as directly affected by two factors: satisfaction with the job situation (all important aspects of the job) and pressures to attend. Employees who are satisfied with the important aspects of their job are seen as more likely to be motivated to attend work than those who are less satisfied. According to the model, the individual will be satisfied with the job situation to the extent that characteristics of the job are congruent with her or his values and expectations.

Several aspects of the job situation are hypothesized to have an important effect on satisfaction with the job. Many of these aspects are covered in detail in other chapters of this text. Among the major factors seen as influencing an employee's satisfaction with her or his job situation are: the leadership style of the employee's supervisor (see Chapter 10 on leadership skills), one's job scope (i.e., the extent to which one's job is "enriched"; see Chapter 9 on motivating staff), the degree of role stress one encounters (see Chapter 22 on dealing with conflict and Chapter 24 on working with higher management), co-worker relations (see Chapter 8 on communication skills and Chapter 22 on dealing with conflict), and opportunity for upward mobility (see Chapter 9 on motivating staff).

In terms of *employee values and job expectations* and their effect on satisfaction with the job situation, the importance attached to these varies with each individual. For example, some staff nurses may desire a job situation that affords promotion potential; others may not. Similarly, some nurses may be greatly disturbed by a somewhat authoritarian supervisor while others may not be overly affected by this type of supervisor. Thus, in order for a nurse manager to influence satisfaction with the job situation, she or he must attempt to get congruence between the job situation attributes and the employee's values and expectations. In attempting to arrive at such a "fit," the nurse manager can focus on changing the job situation and/or the type of nurse that is hired (see Chapter 13 on recruiting and selecting staff). Both of these strategies will be discussed in more detail shortly.

The other major factor seen as influencing a worker's attendance motivation is the *pressure to attend work*. Several factors can pressure (motivate) an employee to attend work, even if the job itself is not perceived as attractive: economic conditions, a personal work ethic, work group norms, organizational commitment, and an organizational incentive system that rewards attendance and/or applies sanctions for not attending. For example, during times of high unemployment, Steers and Rhodes (1984) suggest there is increased pressure to maintain a good attendance record out of fear of losing one's job. Recent research (Johns, 1984) has demonstrated the important influence that group norms, either pro- or anti-absenteeism, can have on attendance behavior. In the next section, on controlling absenteeism, these various ways of increasing the pressure on the employee to attend will be systematically discussed.

Three considerations are important in relation to the Steers and Rhodes model. First, for maximum employee attendance, both ability and motivation to attend must be present. Second, a number of empirical studies support the basic elements of the model (Steers & Rhodes, 1984). Finally, the model should provide a useful framework for nurse managers as they attempt to understand why staff nurses are absent and what they might do about it. In the following section, several variables in the Steers and Rhodes model will be addressed in more detail.

Controlling Absenteeism

The Steers and Rhodes model is useful not only for understanding why absenteeism occurs but also for developing potential strategies for controlling it. Some of the causes of absenteeism, however, such as transportation difficulties or child care problems, may be beyond the control of nurse managers. Their goal, then, should be to do what they can—either directly, in interactions with staff nurses, or indirectly, by attempting to get the health care institution to change policies that may currently be rewarding absenteeism. Overall, one wants to create a climate that discourages the abuse of sick days. However, one must be careful that steps taken do not go so far as to discourage the legitimate use of sick leave. Clearly, one does not want sick nurses coming to work and exposing patients and co-workers.

Although the Steers and Rhodes model makes clear several possible factors that can result in absenteeism problems, it is important for nurse managers to systematically diagnose the key factors leading to absenteeism in their units. In doing so, they may need to gather information from several sources, including subordinates, the personnel department, other nurse managers, and higher level supervisors. In investigating (i.e., in attemping to make sense of) absenteeism, studying absence patterns can be particularly informative. Among the questions a study of absenteeism data can answer are: (a) Is absenteeism equally distributed across staff nurses? (b) In comparison to other units in your hospital, does your unit have a high absenteeism rate? (c) Are most absences short (one or two days) or long in duration? (d) Does the absenteeism have a consistent pattern (e.g., occur predominantly on Mondays? before holidays? shortly before a person quits?). The usefulness of answering these questions will become clearer as we discuss specific strategies for controlling absenteeism.

After reflecting on the factors that affect the ability of staff nurses to attend, most nurse managers conclude there is nothing they can do to influence this key variable. This may be an overly pessimistic reaction. While there may be little that a nurse manager can directly do to affect ability to attend, there may be several things the health care institution can do. For example, to lessen child care problems, the hospital could set up or sponsor a child care center. Milkovich and Gomez (1976) have demonstrated that the presence of day-care facilities was inversely related to absenteeism. To lessen transportation problems, the health care institution could provide shuttle buses or coordinate car pools. To reduce illness, health fairs, exercise programs, and stress reduction classes can be offered (Latham & Napier, 1984). Nurse managers should attempt to influence their hospital to consider offering some of these possible actions. Such influence attempts are more likely to be successful if other nurse managers, and, conceivably, other managers throughout the hospital coordinate their actions.

In addition to these institutional actions, the nurse manager, through coaching, may be able to influence a staff nurse's ability to attend. For example, through discussions with a staff nurse, the nurse manager may develop a plan for reducing illness or solving child care problems. The nurse manager's own creativity can expand the list of such actions. Chapter 15, on performance appraisal, discusses coaching in more detail.

Clearly, the best way for nurse managers to control absenteeism is by affecting the staff's motivation to attend. Again based on the Steers and Rhodes model, nurse managers need to affect both employees' satisfaction with their job situation as well as the pressure to attend that the employee feels. The satisfaction level can be enhanced in several ways. For instance, when possible, the staff nurse's job may be "enriched" by adding greater responsibility, autonomy, or more challenging tasks. In Chapter 9, on motivating staff, specific suggestions for enriching a job are delineated. In addition, the nurse manager can attempt to reduce job stress (e.g., provide more timely and more concrete information), build group cohesiveness (e.g., encourage socializing outside of work), enhance advancement opportunities (e.g., provide developmental experiences so that your best employees are promotable), and improve co-worker relations (e.g., to the extent possible, consider co-worker compatibility when scheduling work and creating work teams). Finally, one must not overlook the effect of job expectations on job satisfaction. Numerous studies have shown that individuals who enter into a job with unrealistically high expectations will be dissatisfied (Premack & Wanous, 1985). Thus, nurse managers can affect staff nurse job satisfaction, and ultimately attendance motivation, by providing realistic job previews before hiring (see Chapter 13 on recruiting and selecting staff). Given that the aforementioned strategies (e.g., reducing stress, providing realistic job previews) for influencing motivation to attend have been addressed in detail in other chapters in this book, they will not be discussed further in this section.

If the manager's diagnosis of the situation suggests that pressure to attend or lack thereof is a key factor underlying absenteeism, then there are several actions that can be taken to enhance attendance motivation.

The most powerful of these may be to change the hospital's absenteeism policy (more will be said about this shortly), but other actions the nurse manager may pursue are: clarifying the rewards for good attendance; encouraging an attendance-oriented work group norm; fostering a personal work ethic; and developing greater nurse commitment to the job, the work unit, the supervisor, and the hospital. In short, the nurse manager wants to establish a climate in which attendance is seen as important.

A key mechanism for focusing attention on the importance of good attendance is the employee performance appraisal. The simple fact of measuring something and discussing it tends to convey importance. In every performance appraisal, the nurse manager should discuss the staff nurse's attendance record and communicate the importance of said attendance (e.g., its impact on patient care, co-workers). If merit pay is available, this motivational tool should be used to reward good attendance behavior. In fulfilling her or his leadership role, it is important that the nurse manager always remember that she or he is a model. Nothing communicates the importance of good attendance better than the manager's own behavior. Beyond communicating the importance of attendance during the performance review and by her or his own behavior, the nurse manager regularly needs to "sell" the importance of good attendance. Sometimes this can be done in a group setting (e.g., a regular staff meeting); other times a one-on-one conversation is more appropriate. In a group setting, the nurse manager can emphasize absenteeism costs (most employees have no idea of the expenses incurred in replacing an absent employee), the impact on patient care, the hardship created on co-workers, etc. In private conversations with problem employees, in addition to the preceding themes, the nurse manager may want to raise the potential for future discipline (if none is yet called for) and the impact of excessive absenteeism on merit pay, advancement opportunities, etc. In addition to these supervisory activities, peer pressure should be brought to bear, if possible, on absence-prone individuals. For example, having a co-worker discuss with the absent employee the hardships she or he has caused is more effective than if the supervisor indirectly conveys the difficulties created. In sum, by using a variety of communication strategies, the nurse manager wants to communicate clearly the problems created for all concerned by employee absenteeism.

Absenteeism Policies

In most hospitals, the formal absenteeism policy may actually hinder the nurse manager's efforts to reduce absenteeism. Although absenteeism policies differ slightly, in most health care institutions employees accrue paid sick days—typically, one paid sick day for every month employed. Unused sick days accrue across time to some maximum number, generally 40–60 days. Although such a policy may seem reasonable, it may actually be rewarding unwanted behavior. For example, once an individual has reached the maximum limit (e.g., 60 days), she or he simply loses additional unused sick days (e.g., there is no reward for not using them). Such a policy also encourages absenteeism on the part of employees who know they will be leaving the organization (e.g., those about to retire, change jobs, go back to school). Knowing they will receive nothing for unused sick leave, exiting employees tend to use up their allotment of paid sick days prior to leaving.

Recently, a few progressive hospitals have taken a close look at their absenteeism policies and realized they have not been rewarding (motivating) good attendance behavior. In attempting to reward attendance, these organizations have taken a variety of different tacks. For example, incorporating the motivational principles outlined in Chapter 9, some hospitals have allowed sick days to accumulate without an upper limit. Then, when an employee leaves the institution, she or he is paid for sick days that have not been used—typically, one-half day's pay for each unused sick day. Retiring employees may be allowed to add unused sick days to days worked, enabling retirement at an earlier date. Panyan and McGregor (1976) examined the effectiveness of paying (e.g., $10) for each unused sick day and found over a 35% drop in absenteeism the first year. Over the next three years, absenteeism averaged less than 50% of the rate prior to this new policy.

As hospitals have gradually come to realize that employees will use sick days for carrying out personal business, another innovative approach for managing absenteeism, substituting "personal days" or extra vacation days for unused sick days, has been tried. The problem arising with not giving personal days is twofold. Employees are "forced" to lie (i.e., say they are sick when they are not) to carry out what they see as legitimate activities (e.g., closing on a house, attending a conference with their child's teacher). In addition, their manager has no warning and therefore has difficulty covering for the "sick" employee. By substituting personal days for sick days, the employee no longer has to lie and the nurse manager now has time to plan for a replacement. In moving to a policy that incorporates the use of personal days, a hospital will typically allocate 9 paid sick days and 3 personal days per year instead of 12 paid sick days. With the availability of personal days, an individual can inform the nurse manager in advance of the need for a personal day off, and the two of them can determine which day is best. In a recent study, Schlotzhauer and Rosse (1985) examined the effects of allowing hospital employees to convert unused sick leave to either additional vacation days or pay. They reported that absenteeism fell 32% as a result of this attendance incentive.

Although uncommon, a few organizations have experimented with special financial incentives such as cash bonuses or other prizes as a reward for good attendance. Some hospitals have actually established lotteries for rewarding good attendance, where one's chances of winning the lottery are tied to one's attendance record. For example, Stephens and Burroughs (1978) designed two incentive systems for six nursing units in a hospital. In the first system, individuals were eligible for the lottery ($20 for every 20 employees eligible) if they had no unscheduled absences for a three-week period. In the second system, to be eligible nurses had to be at work on eight randomly chosen, unannounced days over three weeks. Stephens and Burroughs found both incentive systems to be equally effective, with the incentive being linked to a drop in absenteeism of over 40%.

Obviously, changing the hospital's paid sick leave policy is beyond the responsibility of the nurse manager. However, a concerted effort by an organized group of nurse managers can be very effective in getting the personnel department to initiate such changes. Simply stated, the innovations that have been discussed reward good attendance. Considering the high costs of absenteeism, these changes can be quite cost-effective.

Although we have not dwelled on using discipline (see Chapter 15) to reduce excessive absenteeism, such a strategy obviously has a place. Most hospitals have formal policies concerning how much absenteeism is allowable. Once this limit is reached, prescribed disciplinary steps are carried out. In performing her or his role, it is important that the nurse manager follow the discipline policy carefully. The major reason we have not emphasized the use of discipline as a strategy for reducing absenteeism is that its effectiveness is limited. Most hospital discipline policies take effect only after several days have been missed. Not surprisingly, most employees know what this critical number of days is and are careful not to exceed it. In effect, the nurse manager is left with an absenteeism problem but not one she is able to address through the use of discipline.

A Systems Perspective

Although in this chapter numerous strategies for improving employee attendance have been discussed, it should be made clear that with regard to absenteeism there are no panaceas. The nurse manager is cautioned to avoid a "quick fix" approach at all costs. Rather, what is needed is a systems perspective. The nurse manager (and the personnel department) needs to view absenteeism within the context of the whole work environment. One obvious first question is: Is there an absenteeism problem? As has already been discussed, one should never have a goal of zero absenteeism. Not only is such a goal unrealistic (it will discredit the nurse manager), but it can ultimately lead to sick nurses coming to work. If, after comparing the absenteeism in one's unit to other relevant comparison data (e.g., rates in other units, other hospitals, other industries) the nurse manager perceives an absenteeism problem, then she or he should attempt to get a better understanding of why the absenteeism is occurring. Such an investigation can involve conversations with various parties (e.g., higher-level supervisors, absence-prone nurse) as well as an examination of absence patterns (e.g., does most absenteeism occur in the month before an employee quits?). Based on the results of such an investigation, the nurse manager should have a better understanding of how to attempt to manage absenteeism.

As has been noted throughout this chapter, many of the nurse management activities addressed in other chapters are relevant to the control of absenteeism. For example, in recruiting employees, the use of a realistic job preview should increase the congruence between job characteristics and employee values and expectations. Similarly, basing merit pay and advancement opportunities on performance appraisal ratings (part of which is based on employee attendance) will motivate better attendance behavior. We have also stressed the importance of leadership skills in getting the hospital to make major shifts in policy in order to lessen absenteeism (e.g., the establishment of child care facilities, providing payment for unused sick days). In closing, it is important to address two specific issues (i.e., the use of personal characteristics and past behavior) relevant to employee selection. Although personal characteristics (e.g., marital status, child care responsibility) have been linked to higher absenteeism rates, for legal reasons (see Chapter 13), the nurse manager should not base a hiring decision on such personal characteristics. Simply stated, it is difficult to argue that every individual within a category (e.g., married females with children) is likely to be absence-prone. On the other hand, the past behavior of the individual job candidate is particularly useful information. Several authors (e.g., Breaugh, 1981) have demonstrated that absenteeism tendencies tend to be quite consistent over time. Although the reasons why some individuals have been shown to have a higher level of absenteeism year after year are unclear (e.g., some people may be more susceptible to illness, others may have less of a work ethic), it is quite acceptable to use one's past behavior as a predictor of future behavior. Given the consistency of absenteeism behavior, nurse managers, in making hiring decisions, should seek prior absenteeism information. An applicant's previous absenteeism record can often be acquired by means of written or telephone reference checks.

In summary, a multitude of factors affect employee attendance. Some of these are beyond the control of nurse managers, but others can be directly or indirectly influenced. The goal of the nurse manager should be to do what is possible to alleviate this serious employee problem.

TURNOVER

Although turnover rates differ among health care institutions, it is widely accepted that the field of health care, and in particular nursing, has one of the highest turnover rates in the United States. In the 1980s, the yearly turnover rate in health care institutions has averaged between 18% and

25%, according to the Bureau of National Affairs (e.g., Bureau of National Affairs, 1985). Although an annual turnover rate in the 20% range is remarkable in and of itself, it is truly astounding in view of the depressed economic conditions in the United States during much of this time.

As with absenteeism, it is difficult to estimate the actual dollar costs of nursing turnover. However, given the numerous expenses incurred in hiring a new nurse (e.g., recruitment, selection, orientation, on-the-job training) and temporarily replacing a nurse who quits or is fired (e.g., paying other nurses to work overtime or filling the vacancy with a temporary replacement), the costs must certainly exceed the estimated turnover cost of $2800 for a bank teller (Premack & Wanous, 1985).

Clearly, nursing turnover is an expensive phenomenon that needs to be better understood and more effectively controlled. To facilitate such understanding and control, it is important that turnover be both clearly defined ("the cessation of membership in an organization by an individual who received monetary compensation from that organization") and differentiated (Mobley, 1982). For too long, turnover has been thought of in simplistic terms and seen as universally "bad." Such a primitive view of turnover is not helpful to the nurse manager as she or he attempts to deal with this costly and pervasive phenomenon. Rather, varieties of turnover need to be differentiated: Did the individual leave of his or her own accord (voluntary turnover) or was the person "asked" to leave (involuntary turnover)? Was the departing individual's performance exceptional (dysfunctional turnover) or mediocre (functional turnover)? Will the departed nurse be easy or difficult to replace? Questions such as these have only recently been asked by health care institutions. Yet, until they are answered, it is difficult to establish whether the institution truly has a turnover "problem" and, if so, what can be done about it.

The discussion in this section will focus mainly on voluntary turnover. If the health care institution finds a significant amount of involuntary turnover (i.e., the organization terminating employees), then it needs to carefully examine the way it recruits, selects, trains, and motivates employees. These topics have been addressed in detail in other chapters in this book. If the organization finds it is laying off employees because of over-hiring, it needs to carefully assess its personnel planning strategy. Although important, this complex topic is beyond the scope of this chapter (the interested reader is referred to Heneman et al., 1986).

Measurement Issues

As with absenteeism, before a nurse manager can hope to "manage" turnover, an understanding of the causes of turnover is critical. However, in order to arrive at such an understanding, the nurse manager must appreciate the complexity of many of the measurement issues involved in studying turnover. In studying turnover, one of the first questions that needs to be answered is, Was the turnover voluntary or involuntary? Although this may seem like an easy question to answer (i.e., did the nurse quit?), it often isn't. For example, some employees are given a chance to resign prior to being terminated. Thus, the question becomes, If a nurse quits prior to being terminated, is this voluntary or involuntary turnover? To add to the complexity, although a given nurse manager may know that a staff nurse was pressured into quitting to keep her record "clean," the personnel department may not have this information. Thus, if turnover studies are conducted in the future, the situation described above is likely to be categorized as voluntary turnover. Beyond the complexity of determining if turnover was voluntary or involuntary, two other measurement-related issues (i.e., determining the reasons for turnover and determining whether or not it was functional) also need to be addressed.

Traditionally, health care institutions have attempted to determine the reason(s) for voluntary turnover through two sources. Generally, the exiting employee's immediate supervisor is asked why the employee is leaving. In addition, it is traditional that an "exit interview" with the departing employee be conducted by someone in the personnel department. Although such an approach for determining the cause of voluntary turnover is certainly straightforward, the validity of such an approach has been questioned. For example, Hinrichs (1975) has shown that the reasons given by departing employees in their exit interviews differ greatly from their responses to anonymous questionnaires completed several months after leaving the organization. Hinrichs argues persuasively that, since future employers often ask for reference information from prior employers, exiting employees provide "safe" responses (e.g., a better opportunity came along) during the exit interview so as not to jeopardize future job opportunities. In summarizing his results, Hinrichs found it was rare for departing employees to say anything negative about the organization they were leaving or about their immediate supervisor. Although this tendency of departing employees to make safe responses is certainly understandable, it makes it more difficult to determine why turnover is occurring. In attempting to gather more veridical information, a health care institution may need to utilize questionnaires that are sent to former employees several months after they have terminated employment. These former employees will need to be assured that their responses will be confidential, will in no way affect their personnel files, and will be used only in establishing the cause of past employee turnover. Another way to attempt to discover the cause of nurse turnover is through the use of interviews with the former employee's co-workers. Often, former co-workers know why an employee left, and, given the right circumstances (e.g., their remarks will be confidential; they trust the personnel department representative), these co-workers will be willing to discuss the cause.

In evaluating the overall impact of an employee leaving, a useful distinction is to think of turnover as being either functional or dysfunctional

(Dalton, Krackhardt & Porter, 1981) for the institution. For example, losing a nurse who is an excellent performer will be a greater loss to the hospital than losing one who is a mediocre performer. Similarly, if a nurse can be easily replaced, the costs to the hospital are less than if she or he is hard to replace. Thus, the nurse manager needs to be most concerned about turnover when the nurses who are leaving are of high quality and difficult to replace (i.e., dysfunctional turnover). In contrast, if poorly performing nurses who can be easily replaced quit, the hospital may actually benefit from the turnover (i.e., experience functional turnover). Recently, Dalton and Todor (1982) have added additional complexity to this functional/dysfunctional turnover distinction. By utilizing actual payroll records, they have shown that, in assessing the costs and benefits of voluntary turnover, one also needs to be sensitive to a "hard dollar" criterion. For example, Dalton and Todor demonstrated the importance of examining whether the departing employee had a vested pension as well as the dollar savings that might result because of the difference between the departing employee's salary and the replacement employee's starting salary.

Our purpose in summarizing the work of Dalton and his colleagues was not to overwhelm the reader with information but rather to provide a sense of the perspective that is necessary to better understand the costs and benefits·of voluntary turnover. Nurse managers need to destroy the myth that all turnover is bad and replace it with an appreciation of the numerous factors that should be involved in determining whether turnover is a problem meriting attention. In the section that follows, we will briefly discuss many of the numerous factors that should be considered in making such a determination.

Consequences of Turnover

In discussing the consequences of turnover, writers have traditionally focused on the costs to the organization (e.g., hiring expenses). Although turnover obviously often does involve real costs to the organization, this traditional perspective is too narrow. Turnover not only can have a negative effect on the hospital, it also can have an undesirable effect on patients, co-workers, etc. And, as discussed above, voluntary turnover is not always undesirable. Anyone with work experience can remember some individual (e.g., co-worker, subordinate, supervisor) whose departure would have significantly improved the organization's functioning. Simply stated, in evaluating the consequences of turnover, the nurse manager (and the hospital) must remember that voluntary turnover can have costs and/or benefits attached to it. In addition, it should be recalled that what may be seen as a desirable departure by some (e.g., the nurse manager) may be viewed as a loss by others (e.g., a subset of co-workers).

Whether or not turnover is seen as functional or dysfunctional, there still are direct costs to the hospital in replacing a nurse. Figure 16–2 rep-

Figure 16–2 Model for Measurement of Human Resource Replacement Costs

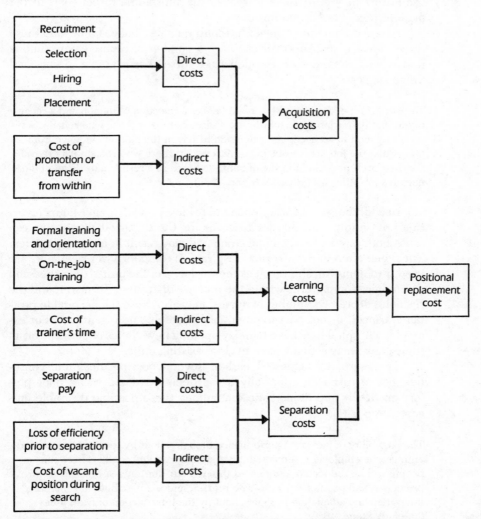

Source: Flamholtz, E. G. *Human Resource Accounting* (Encino, CA: Dickenson, 1974). Reprinted by permission of Dr. Eric G. Flamholtz.

resents a model of the possible replacement costs of an individual who has left the organization. Replacement cost is made up of direct and indirect costs related to acquisition of a new person, that person's learning the job, and the separation costs of the person leaving. (For a more detailed presentation of the factors and respective costs involved in employee separation and replacement, the interested reader is referred to Cascio's *Costing*

Human Resources [1982].) One need not attach dollar values to each of the factors in Figure 16–2 to realize the substantial direct costs to the organization of employee turnover.

However, nursing turnover has consequences that go far beyond these direct dollar costs. Turnover can have a number of repercussions among nurses who worked with the departed nurse. For example, Steers and Stone suggest:

Turnover can be interpreted by co-workers as a rejection of the job and a recognition that better job opportunities exist elsewhere. For those who remain, ways must be found to reconcile their decision to stay in the light of evidence from others that the job may not be good. As a result, those who remain may reevaluate their present position in the organization and, as a result, may develop more negative job attitudes (Steers & Stone, 1982).

In addition, nurses who remain may have to work longer hours (overtime) or simply work harder to cover for the departed nurse; this can cause both physical and mental strain and may result in more departures. Thus, one often finds a "turnover spiral." If temporary replacements are used, problems can still result as the workflow of the unit is disturbed and communication patterns within the unit are disrupted. Turnover, and the resultant decreased number of nurses, may also cause the hospital to postpone, cancel, or not pursue potentially profitable new ventures. For example, a hospital may have to delay opening new clinics or services or, in some cases, may actually have to close existing units.

There are, as suggested earlier, several possible desirable consequences of turnover, especially if the departed nurse was a poor performer. Steers and Stone state that among these possible desirable outcomes are:

The possibility of increased performance brought about by recently trained and enthusiastic employees, the possibility that long-running conflicts between people will be reduced or eliminated through attrition, increased chances for promotion and transfer for those who remain, and the possibility for increased innovation and adaptation brought about by the introduction of fresh ideas (Steers & Stone, 1982).

To this list of desirable consequences could be added three additional outcomes: the opportunity for overtime (i.e., some nurses desire voluntary overtime as a way to increase wages), the stimulation of needed policy changes (i.e., as a result of losing a "star performer" an organization may be stimulated to change a problematic policy), and the avoidance of layoffs (i.e., natural attrition may lessen or eliminate the need for forced reduction of staff during times of economic recession).

Although a detailed discussion of the consequences of turnover is beyond the scope of this chapter, the abbreviated discussion provided should make clear the numerous issues that need to be considered in attempting to determine whether a given turnover rate actually is a "turnover problem." (For a more detailed coverage of the consequences of turnover, the reader is referred to Mobley's *Employee Turnover: Causes, Consequences, and Control* [1982].) If the nurse manager decides that she or he has a turnover problem, then action should be initiated. The turnover model (see Figure 16–3) introduced in the next section should be a useful vehicle for helping the nurse manager diagnose the cause of voluntary turnover and, subsequently, actively manage it (e.g., attempt to reduce the turnover rate, influence who is resigning).

A Model of Employee Turnover

Numerous models have been developed to explain the employee turnover process. Each has its relative strengths and weaknesses (e.g., March & Simon, 1958; Mobley, 1982; Price & Mueller, 1981; Steers & Mowday, 1981). However, a model presented in Figure 16–3 is particularly useful for the nurse manager. This model, which is a modification of the one developed by March and Simon, is not unduly complex, yet it portrays the major factors that affect voluntary turnover. Emphasis will be placed on those aspects of the model that are particularly important for nurse managers.

Figure 16–3   A Model of Voluntary Employee Turnover

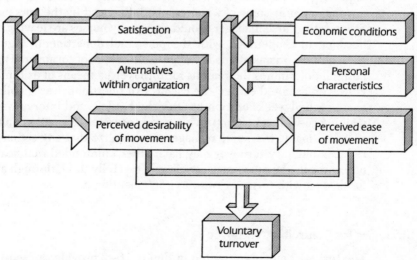

Source: Modified from J. G. March, and H. A. Simon, *Organizations* (New York: John Wiley & Sons, 1958), 90–106. Copyright 1958 John Wiley & Sons, Inc. Reprinted by permission.

According to the model, voluntary turnover is a direct function of a nurse's perceptions of both the *ease* and the *desirability* of leaving the hospital. Perceived ease of movement depends on the nurse's personal characteristics (e.g., education, area of specialization, age, marital status, number of contacts at other health care institutions, and ownership of a car) as well as economic conditions (e.g., number of job openings at other hospitals, non–health care institutions hiring nurses for nonnursing positions).

As with ease of movement, perceptions of the desirability of movement can be affected by several factors. Two important ones are the existence of job alternatives within the health care institution and the nurse's level of satisfaction. To the degree a nurse perceives that there are other work opportunities (positions) within the hospital, voluntary turnover should be reduced. That is, a nurse may be able to leave her current position within the hospital by means of a lateral transfer, promotion, or demotion. For example, if a nurse is having problems with one of her or his co-workers, the nurse may be able to transfer to a new unit. To some degree, the nurse manager can influence such alternative job opportunities as a way of reducing voluntary turnover.

Job satisfaction also has an effect on perceived desirability of movement. A number of studies have shown that the greater the satisfaction level, the lower the probability of the individual quitting. Job satisfaction involves various facets of the work environment, including relationships with the nurse manager, other staff nurses, nurse aides, patients, and physicians, as well as the shift worked (e.g., day vs. evening, rotating vs. fixed) and one's compensation level.

In dealing with turnover, nurse managers need to be aware of three important considerations. First, voluntary turnover can be caused by several factors, only some of which can be influenced by the nurse manager. Second, the nurse manager should assess why nurses are leaving; this may be done in cooperation with the personnel department. Figure 16–4 presents one organization's list of possible causes of turnover. Typically, a hospital determines the reasons for turnover by means of exit interviews. However, as noted earlier, the use of "exit questionnaires" (mailed to the nurse several weeks or months after she has left) and interviews with remaining co-workers often provide more accurate information on turnover causes. Finally, the nurse manager must realize that any action taken to reduce voluntary turnover may have other unintended ramifications. In other words, the nurse manager should carefully think through a strategy for dealing with turnover prior to implementing it.

Strategies for Controlling Turnover

The turnover model presented in Figure 16–3 provides a useful organizing framework for deriving strategies for controlling turnover. The nurse manager's goal should be to do what is within her or his direct and indirect

Figure 16—4 Categories of Reason for Turnover

Dissatisfaction:

Wages—amount
Wages—equity
Benefits
Hours or shift
Working conditions
Supervision—technical
Supervision—personal
Co-workers
Job security
Job meaningfulness
Use of skills and abilities
Career opportunities
Policies and rules
Other: _____

Living Conditions:

Housing
Transportation
Child care
Health care facilities
Leisure activities
Physical environment
Social environment
Education opportunities
Other: _____

Personal:

Spouse transferred
To be married
Illness or death in family
Personal illness
Personal injury
Pregnancy

Alternatives:

Returning to school
Military service
Government service
Starting own business
Similar job: same industry
Similar job: other industry
Different job: other industry
Voluntary early retirement
Voluntary transfer to subsidiary
(loss of seniority)
New position:
    Organization
    Position
    Location
    Earnings

Organization Initiated:

Resignation in lieu of dismissal
Violation of rules, policy
Unsatisfactory probation period
Attendance
Performance
Layoff
Layoff: downgrade refused
Layoff: transfer refused
End of temporary employment

Other:

Transfer to: _____
Leave of absence from: _____
On loan to: _____
Retirement
Death

From Mobley, W. H.: *Employee Turnover: Causes, Consequences, and Control.* Addison-Wesley, Reading, Mass., 1982, p. 38.

control to reduce dysfunctional voluntary turnover. (As discussed earlier, a nurse manager may actually welcome functional turnover—a poor nurse quitting.) Direct measures of control include those in which the nurse manager exerts influence directly, as in her interactions with her staff. Indirect turnover control measures include the nurse manager's participation with others (e.g., other nurse managers, other department heads) in changing institutional policies or procedures.

From the model depicted in Figure 16–3, it is obvious that if the nurse manager wants to decrease voluntary turnover, she can focus on decreasing staff nurse perceptions of desirability of movement or ease of movement. Each of these variables is in turn affected by other variables. Concerning perceived ease of movement, there is relatively little the nurse manager or the hospital can do to influence economic conditions (e.g., whether other hospitals are hiring). Therefore, attention should be focused on personal characteristics. For example, a nurse manager in co-ordination with the personnel department may be able to develop a pro-file of a "long-tenure" staff nurse and subsequently rely on this profile in making hiring decisions. Although a detailed discussion of how to develop a profile for selecting such long-term nurses is beyond the scope of this chapter (see Chapter 13), a logical predictor would be a nurse's previous turnover record. In fact, recently the author was able to document that tenure on one's previous job was an excellent predictor of how long one stayed in his or her next position.

Although a nurse manager's potential for influencing perceived ease of movement is somewhat limited, a nurse manager can have a substantial impact upon the desirability of movement. For example, she can facilitate (or hinder) movement within the health care institution. Thus, if a staff nurse is "burnt out" from working on a radiation/oncology floor, one op-tion is to allow a transfer to another unit. Unfortunately, many nurse man-agers will often hinder or even prohibit such a transfer (particularly if the potential transferee is an excellent performer); she or he does not want to lose a good nurse. However, this perspective is shortsighted. If the staff nurse cannot transfer to another unit (intraorganizational mobility), she or he will often leave the hospital entirely (interorganizational mobility). Nurse managers must realize that facilitating transfers within the hospital is essential.

Job satisfaction can be influenced by the nurse manager both directly and indirectly by such actions as providing a realistic job preview (see Chapter 13), enriching or redesigning the staff nurse's job (see Chapter 9), facilitating upward and downward communication (see Chapter 8), linking rewards and performance (Chapter 15), developing work group cohesive-ness (see Chapter 10), helping resolve interpersonal conflicts (see Chap-ters 22 and 23), and providing training and educational opportunities (see Chapter 14).

A Systems Perspective

Both absenteeism and turnover are employee withdrawal behaviors. Both behaviors allow an employee to leave the workplace, one temporarily and one permanently. In many cases, these withdrawal behaviors share a common cause: job dissatisfaction. Given this common cause, it is not sur-prising that many of the effective strategies for reducing absenteeism (e.g., providing child care, using realistic job previews, improving super-visory behavior, coordinating car pools, offering stress management workshops, using past behavior as a selection factor) will also have a positive effect on turnover. Therefore, in this section we quickly cover themes that have already been discussed vis-a-vis absenteeism and emphasize issues that are somewhat unique to turnover.

As with absenteeism, in dealing with turnover the nurse manager must avoid the temptation to look for a quick fix. There are no panaceas. In addition, the nurse manager must be cognizant that what appears to be a simple change (e.g., trying to enrich the job of a high performing nurse) may not be. For example, providing additional duties to enrich a nurse's job may lead to complaints of favoritism from other nurses or from the personnel department worrying about assigning duties not outlined in the job description. Such potential difficulties should not cause the nurse manager to revert back to "status quo" behavior. Rather, the nurse manager needs to anticipate such potential problems and deal with them (e.g., be able to justify the differential treatment through the use of performance appraisal data; have the affected nurse agree to the additional duties in writing).

As has already been discussed, in actively managing turnover the nurse manager wants to create an environment that rewards nurse performance. Obviously, this calls for careful attention being given to the performance appraisal process (e.g., careful documentation) and, when possible, the use of merit pay. However, the nurse manager should go beyond the use of money. Simply stated, the nurse manager wants to do everything in her power to reward top performing nurses for their efforts. Such a performance-oriented climate will increase the likelihood of functional turnover (i.e., of a poorly performing, easily replaced nurse quitting) and decrease the probability of dysfunctional turnover. To be effective, the nurse manager needs to view things in terms of what is good for the hospital, not just herself. For example, the nurse manager may need to allow a star performer to transfer to another unit rather than risk the loss of this individual to another health care institution (although many nurse managers do not think of it, if every nurse manager facilitated transfers, each would be as likely to gain a star performer as to lose one).

A particularly important area for the nurse manager to be concerned about is work scheduling (i.e., fixed vs. rotating shifts, flexible work hours, job sharing). This area is important not only because of its relationship to voluntary turnover, but also because of its frequent linkage to unionization attempts (it should not be surprising that working conditions that lead to turnover can also motivate interest in unionization). For example, in a recent *Wall Street Journal* article (February 3, 1987) it was reported that approximately 10% of all registered nurses are unionized and that two key causes of this unionization are staff shortages and rotating work schedules. In another recent *Wall Street Journal* article (January 27, 1987), the use of flexible work schedules and job sharing as ways to recruit and retain nurses at Children's Hospital in Stanford, California, was de-

scribed. Over 90% of the 200 nurses there worked nontraditional schedules. According to the hospital's nursing director, these innovative work
schedules have had positive impacts on both nurse recruitment and retention. Although going to work schedules that are seen as more advantageous by staff nurses (i.e., fixed shifts, flexible hours, job sharing) obviously involves costs (e.g., coordination time, paperwork), such schedules
also provide clear benefits. Most nurses prefer fixed shifts. If possible,
nurses also prefer flexible hours. And, for many child-rearing nurses, job
sharing is a perfect way to remain in health care and, at the same time,
fulfill parental responsibilities. Before implementing such innovative
work schedules, considerable planning (e.g., cost-benefits analysis) clearly
needs to take place. Unfortunately, many health care institutions, even
those that are having trouble recruiting and retaining nurses, simply dis-
miss such schedules out of hand. As with a number of the strategies for
reducing turnover and absenteeism discussed in this chapter, a single
nurse manager is unlikely to be able to change a hospital's policy concerning work schedules. However, if several managers coordinate their efforts,
change is more likely to occur. To increase the likelihood of a successful
influence attempt, the group of managers may need to build a persuasive
case (e.g., document the success of job sharing at other hospitals, cost out
the possible financial gain—often part-time nurses are paid at a lower rate
and do not receive pension benefits).

In closing this section, it should be reiterated that sometimes a nurse
manager may simply need to adapt to a high turnover rate. Even if this is
the case, the nurse manager may be able to lessen potential problems by
doing two things. First, the nurse manager may want to "manage" beliefs
about why a nurse left. Sometimes, the reason is unclear and the hospital
grapevine will often provide an inaccurate and a less than attractive reason from the hospital's perspective (e.g., she left for $1.05 more an hour at
a competitor hospital). Secondly, the nurse manager may be able to provide the personnel department with her or his preferred list of replacement workers. For example, a health care organization the author has
worked with keeps an up-to-date list of former employees who will fill in
on an occasional basis. Such former employees are more familiar with organizational procedures and thus can handle things more efficiently.

In summary, as with absenteeism, in managing turnover the nurse
manager wants to do everything she can to lessen the problem. Sometimes this will involve coordinating her or his efforts with other managers
in order to change hospital policy. The strategies outlined in this chapter
have been shown to be effective in reducing turnover. However, not all
are equally applicable to all situations. As a manager, the nurse must be
able to analyze situational factors and determine what is appropriate for
her particular set of circumstances. For example, flexible work hours may
be suitable for a clinic but not for an around-the-clock operation. By being
creative, nurse managers not only can reduce the overall turnover rate,

but they can also have an influence on which nurses leave by providing incentives for the exceptional nurses to stay and by doing less to retain mediocre nurses.

SUMMARY

- Historically, health care institutions have had serious problems with excessive employee absenteeism and turnover. Fortunately, there is much the nurse manager can do to actively manage their occurrence.

- Annual absenteeism costs per nurse can range between $800 and $1400.

- Steers and Rhodes present a model of attendance behavior that is particularly useful for the nurse manager. It suggests absenteeism is a direct function of an individual's ability and motivation to attend.

- A nurse manager can influence absenteeism through such techniques as coaching, changing organizational policies, encouraging peer group pressure, and setting an example.

- In attempting to deal with an absenteeism problem, it is important that the nurse manager have a systems perspective, investigate why the absenteeism is occurring, and communicate to both staff nurses and the personnel department the problems absenteeism creates.

- Turnover averages between 18% and 25% in the health care industry.

- Consequences of turnover are many: lost productivity, especially if high performers leave; increased training costs; the cost of temporary replacements and/or overtime for remaining nurses; and lower quality patient care.

- It is important to determine if turnover is functional or dysfunctional.

- In order to effectively manage turnover, the nurse manager must understand the underlying causes. March and Simon provide a useful model for doing such.

BIBLIOGRAPHY

Beyers, M. et al. (1983). Results of the nursing personnel survey. Part 2: R.N. vacancies and turnover. *J Nurs Adm*, (May) *13*(5): 26.

Breaugh, J. A. (1981). Predicting absenteeism from prior absenteeism and work attitudes. *J Appl Psychol*, *66*:555–560.

Bureau of National Affairs. (1985). *Bulletin to management*. Washington, DC, (March).

Cascio, W. (1982). *Costing human resources*. Boston: Kent Publishing.

Dalton, D., Krackhardt, D., and Porter, L. (1981). Functional turnover. *J Appl Psychol*, *66*:716–721.

Dalton, D., and Todor, W. (1982). Turnover: A lucrative hard dollar criterion. *Acad Mngmt Rev*, 7:212–218.

Decker, P. J., Moore, R. C., and Sullivan, E. (1982). How hospitals can solve the nursing shortage. *Hospital Health Services Administration*, 27(6): 12.

Heneman, H., Schwab, D., Fossum, J., and Dyer, L. (1986). *Personnel/human resource management*. Homewood, IL: Irwin.

Hinrichs, J. (1975). Measurement of reasons for resignation of professionals: Questionnaire versus company and consultant interviews. *J Appl Psychol*, 60:530–532.

Johns, G. (1984). Unresolved issues in the study and management of absenteeism from work. In: *Absenteeism*. Goodman, P., Atkin, R., and associates (editors). San Francisco: Jossey-Bass.

Latham, G., and Napier, N. (1984). Practical ways to increase employee attendance. In: *Absenteeism*. Goodman, P., Atkin, R., and associates (editors). San Francisco: Jossey-Bass.

March, J., and Simon, H. (1958). *Organizations*. New York: Wiley.

Milkovich, G., and Gomez, L. (1976). Day care and selected employee work behaviors. *Acad Mngmt J*, 19:111–115.

Mobley, W. (1982). *Employee turnover: Causes, consequences, and control*. Reading, MA: Addison-Wesley.

Muchinsky, P. (1977). Employee absenteeism: A review of the literature. *J Voc Behavior*, 10:316–340.

Panyan, S., and McGregor, M. (1976). How to implement a proactive incentive plan: A field study. *Personnel Journal*, 55:460–463.

Premack, S., and Wanous, J. (1985). A meta-analysis of realistic job preview experiments. *J Appl Psychol*, 70:706–719.

Price, J., and Mueller, C. (1981). A causal model of turnover for nurses. *Acad Mngmt J*, 24:543–565.

Saddler, J. (1987). Labor letter column. *Wall Street Journal*, (February 3): 1.

Schlotzhauer, D., and Rosse, J. (1985). A five-year study of a positive incentive absence control program. *Personnel Psychology*, 38:575–585.

Steers, R., and Mowday, R. (1981). Employee turnover in organizations. In: *Research in organizational behavior*. Cummings, L., and Staw, B. (editors). Greenwich, CT: JAI Press.

Steers, R., and Rhodes, S. (1984). Knowledge and speculation about absenteeism. In: *Absenteeism*. Goodman, P., Atkin, R., and associates (editors). San Francisco: Jossey-Bass.

Steers, R., and Rhodes, S. (1978). Major influences on employee attendance: A process model. *J Appl Psychol*, 63:391–407.

Steers, R., and Stone, T. (1982). Organizational exit. In: *Personnel management*. Rowland, K., and Ferris, G. (editors). Boston: Allyn and Bacon.

Stephens, T., and Burroughs, W. (1978). An application of operant conditioning to absenteeism in a hospital setting. *J Appl Psychol*, 63:518–521.

Sullivan, E., and Decker, P. J. (1984). Solving the nursing shortage: Drawing nurses back to the hospital. *The Health Care Supervisor*, 2:79.

Trost, C. (1987). Labor letter column. *Wall Street Journal*, (January 27): 1.

17

Nursing Associations and Collective Bargaining

FOR THE PAST several decades, the U.S. economy has begun to shift from a goods producing economy to a service producing economy. Unionization has tended to follow this trend, and more and more service employees have become unionized. Collective bargaining in the health care industry can be traced back to the 1920s in the San Francisco area; not until the late 1970s, however, did it reach significant proportions.

National labor law initially excluded most hospital employees. The Wagner Act (298 U.S. 238), passed in 1935 and now the prevailing U.S. labor law, excluded public employees, so all state and local hospitals operated by governmental units were exempt from coverage. The Wagner Act did not specifically exclude private/nonprofit hospitals; in fact, the National Labor Relations Board (NLRB), which is charged with enforcing the Wagner Act, initially claimed jurisdiction over these institutions. In 1947, however, the Taft-Hartley amendment to the Wagner Act did exempt private, nonprofit health care facilities from federal collective bargaining laws (Public Law 101, 80th Congress, June 23, 1947). Furthermore, the NLRB declined to exert jurisdiction over proprietary (privately owned, for profit) hospitals until 1967. But in 1974 the Wagner Act was amended again and the Taft-Hartley exclusion was lifted so that federal labor legislation was extended to private, nonprofit hospitals, nursing homes, health maintenance organizations, health clinics, and other health care institutions in addition to all proprietary health care facilities.

The 1974 health care amendments were not enacted without reason. The health care industry now employs more than five million people. As an economic activity, health care has increased enormously. From 1947 to 1974, hospitals became very complex organizations, and rising expenditures far exceeded inflation in most years. Also, in spite of technological advances, health care has remained very labor-intensive and rapid growth has brought with it a host of employee relations problems. Large-scale operations have tended to breed interprofessional tensions and rivalries. The pay of many health care employees has lagged behind that received by comparably educated groups in other industrial sectors.

In addition, the basic structure of the health care industry has changed over these years. Charity activities within hospitals have declined at the same rate as third-party benefit systems have expanded. Medicare and Medicaid insurance coverage has become institutionalized. Consequently, Congress had begun to view health care as "just another business." Furthermore, the argument that private/nonprofit health care facilities ought to be immune from collective bargaining because the burden of wage increases may be passed on to "sick" patients did not hold up under institutionalized payments (Luttman, 1982). Consequently, Congress enacted the 1974 amendments to include health care employees under U.S. labor law.

HEALTH CARE LABOR RELATIONS

Any hospital owned and operated by a nongovernmental agency is now subject to jurisdiction under U.S. labor law. However, a major question remains, "What is a private/nonprofit hospital?" Frequently, hospitals are operated by private organizations, but public agencies own the assets. NLRB rulings seem to indicate that the body which employs and directs the management, rather than the owner of the physical assets of the facility, determines whether or not a health care facility comes under the NLRB's jurisdiction. Consequently, if a private organization is responsible for day-to-day operations, the hospital is covered by U.S. labor law.

The Service Employees International Union, the National Union of Hospital and Health Care Employees, and the American Nurses' Association and its constituent state nurses' associations are the major organizations recognized as collective bargaining agents. Nurses are also represented by other organizations as shown in Figure 17–1. At least 125,000 to 130,000 of the nurses in the U.S. are covered by some kind of labor contract, and between 1970 and 1976, the number of employed professional nurses covered by contracts grew at an annual rate of about 14%

Figure 17—1 Unions Representing Health Care Workers

Name	Total Membership (Approx.)	Registered Nurses Represented (Approx.)
American Federation of Government Employees, AFL-CIO	265,506	7,000
American Federation of State, County, and Municipal Employees, AFL-CIO	963,764	6,000
American Federation of Teachers, AFL-CIO	568,359	5,000
American Nurses' Association	162,000*	120,000**
Communication Workers of America, AFL-CIO	530,000	1,000
National Education Association	1,600,000	3,000 (public school nurses)
National Union of Hospital and Health Care Employees (District 1199) of Retail, Wholesale, and Department Store Union, AFL-CIO	115,000	15,000
Service Employees International Union, AFL-CIO	625,000	12,000
United Food and Commercial Workers International Union, AFL-CIO	1,235,500	1,000

*Members of state constituent associations

**Members and nonmembers in SNA bargaining units

From *Collective Bargaining and the Nursing Profession,* published by the American Nurses' Association, 1983. Used with permission.

(Dilts & Deitsch, 1977). Researchers who have examined union activity in hospitals predict that unions will continue to grow in representation of hospital employees and that the number of occupational groups represented will also increase (Becker, Sloan & Steinwald, 1982). However, unionization overall in America is declining.

The Wagner and Taft-Hartley Acts were enacted 11 years apart but are now combined into the Labor Management Relations Act of 1947. (For text of these laws, see the appendices of Taylor and Whitney [1983], or the text of the Wagner Act.) The Wagner Act was pro-labor and the Taft-Hartley Act was pro-administration. The Wagner Act, as amended, establishes the National Labor Relations Board, which consists of five members appointed by the president and confirmed by the senate. This board administers all the provisions of the law.

Section 7 is the heart of the original Wagner Act and reads:

Employees shall have the right to self organization, to form, join, or assist labor organizations, to bargain collectively through representatives of their own choosing, and to engage in other concerted activities for the purpose of collective bargaining or other mutual aid or protection, and shall also have the right to refrain from any or all of such activities except to the extent that such right may be affected by an agreement requiring membership in a labor organization as a condition of employment as authorized in Section 8(a)(3) (Wagner Act, 298 U.S. 238, 1935).

This section indicates that all employees covered by the act shall have the right to join a union or not as they wish unless they are covered by a closed shop agreement, which requires union membership as a condition of employment, or a union shop agreement, which requires union membership after employment (i.e., 60 days after hire). The former is only found in the construction industry, where the latter is common.

Section 8 of the Wagner Act, as amended, specifies actions of employers and unions that are considered unfair labor practices. For employers these are: (a) assisting or dominating any labor organization; (b) discriminating in hiring, assigning, or other terms of employment on the basis of union membership; (c) penalizing or discriminating against an employee for charging an employer with a violation of the act; and (d) refusing to bargain in good faith with the union over issues of wages, hours, and conditions of employment.

The union unfair labor practice provisions are: (a) unions may not coerce employees in the exercise of their Section 7 rights; (b) unions cannot demand or require that an employer violate anything in the act; (c) unions cannot engage in or encourage individuals to strike or to refuse to handle some type of product where the object is to accomplish any of the following: to cease handling nonunion products, force an employer to bargain with an uncertified labor organization, require excessive initiation fees, force an employer to pay for services not rendered, or picket to force recognition; and finally, (d) unions must bargain in good faith with management over wages, hours, and conditions of employment. "Good faith" has a precise definition because of numerous NLRB rulings, but, basically it means that if one party proposes, the other counterproposes. (See Allen and Keavenly [1983:258–261] for a discussion of good faith bargaining. This is also a good reference for all labor law issues.)

Special Bargaining Issues for Hospitals

The 1974 health care amendments stipulate fairly special procedural regulations for health care in order to minimize the prospect of work interruptions and harm to patients. They provide an institution that may be facing a strike, the lead time required to make alternate arrangements for the care of patients or residents. For example, in most labor situations, it is relatively easy for internal union organizers to have access to employees. In hospitals, however, this is not the case. In 1976, the NLRB held that a no-solicitation rule prohibiting union organizing activities from any area of the hospital where patient contact was possible was overly broad. On appeal, however, the Tenth Circuit Court reversed the NLRB and held that the needs of patients outweigh the organizing rights of employees. So employees or organizers may be banned from organizing in any area to which patients or residents may have access. Passive activities, however, like wearing union membership pins, are approved.

There are also different requirements in negotiations where health care facilities are involved. The party wishing to change the terms of an existing contract is obliged to notify the other party, in writing, within 90 days and not less than 60 days prior to the expiration date of the agreement. Neither party may strike or lock out until this 90-day period has elapsed or the contract has expired, whichever is later. Consequently, there is considerable time for the hospital to make alternate arrangements before any strike.

Until 1984, the NLRB held that bargaining units in hospitals would be structured along occupational lines. Although there had been attempts to place registered nurses in mixed units with other categories of hospital personnel before 1984, the nurses usually ended up in a separate bargaining unit. Technical employees, including licensed practical nurses, X-ray technicians, and laboratory technicians, tended to be grouped into a distinct unit, as did maintenance and service employees, and office and clerical employees. Physicians, when organized, were also in a separate professional unit.

In 1984, the NLRB ruled that maintenance employees at Memphis' St. Francis Hospital could not organize a separate unit. Up to 1984, the NLRB had used a traditional "community of interest" test for determining bargaining units and had allowed up to seven separate units in hospitals, including one for RNs. The St. Francis case meant that only one or two (professional and nonprofessional) units would be allowed in health care institutions.

In March 1987, however, the U.S. Court of Appeals for the District of Columbia reversed the NLRB's St. Francis decision and remanded the case back to the NLRB for further consideration. This decision, if accepted by the NLRB, may return the process of organizing units in hospitals to one similar to that which existed before 1984.

In many states with health care bargaining laws, there is a history of multiemployer bargaining in the hospital industry—for instance, a state or regional hospital association bargaining for several organizational employers. The reverse also holds true: a union bargaining agent will sometimes represent workers in several different institutions—for example, the nurses in one city's municipal hospitals. There is evidence to believe that the NLRB will allow this multiemployer bargaining to continue (Dilts & Deitsch, 1977).

About 23% of all hospitals have one or more organized employee groups (Fossum, 1982). Unionization seems to be more prevalent in large cities, in larger hospitals, in federally controlled hospitals, and in hospitals located in the Northeast and West. Fewer religious or proprietary hospitals are organized. Fewer nurses than other health care employees are unionized.

Effect of Unionization in Health Care

Numerous studies have attempted to measure the effects of health care unionism on wages, employment, and ultimately on costs (Fossum, 1982; Davey, Bognanno & Estenson, 1982). One study found that the annual salary of registered nurses is from 4% to 7% higher for those nurses represented by a bargaining agent; another study showed slightly less than 7% (Link & Landon, 1975). However, unionization tends to be geographically specific, and wages in the Northeast and California (where nurses are more heavily unionized) are higher regardless of unionization. In terms of total compensation, aggregating across unionized hospital occupations, the union to nonunion differential is about 8%.

Given the relative wage gains that seem to be brought about by hospital unionization, the next question is whether there is a relative reduction in the numbers of workers under contract who are employed. There is evidence supporting a reduction, but it is quite modest. Since traditionally it was easy to pass costs on to patients, a significant decrease in employment of the higher cost unionized employees was not evident. Today, with hospitals receiving fixed fees (due to DRGs) for services, it is impossible to imagine that they would not meet their costs by reducing staff numbers in response to increased cost per staff member. Also, hospitals do substitute among occupational work groups in response to relative wage changes among them. Studies have shown that where LPNs have unionized and their wages have gone up faster than RNs, there tends to be an increase in the proportion of RNs in nursing service (Dilts & Deitsch, 1977).

There are few studies showing the impact of unionization on hospital costs. One study has shown that unionization may increase relative average costs per patient day in a short-term general hospital by about 3.8% (Miller, Becker & Krinsky, 1979). However, with only a single study, this can only be an estimate. It is highly likely that a certain amount of the cost of unionization is passed on to patients, a certain amount is made up by lesser employment of higher wage employees, and that possibly there is some increase in RN efficiency because of certain work rules demanded in union contracts—for instance, how long "breaks" last. Consequently, the costs and benefits of collective bargaining probably are almost equal.

WHY INDIVIDUALS JOIN UNIONS

Research has shown that union membership tends to increase in periods of prosperity and decrease during depressions. This also seems to have been the pattern in the early days of American trade unions. Unionism apparently follows money in that workers attempt to get what they believe is their fair share of the organization's income. Obviously, workers also want to protect job security and have decent working conditions. Many craft unions were formed, for instance, in response to the Industrial Revolution, because products could then be produced by cheaper labor with machinery. And, as the U.S. economy moved from the "labor-intensive" shop to the "capital-intensive" factory, artisans and craftsmen formed unions to try to control production in the market.

However, capital-intensive factories have decreased the need for skilled labor and increased employment of unskilled or semiskilled labor. Industrial workers have tended to organize simply to keep their jobs because they can be replaced so easily. Industrial workers and professional workers, however, tend to react to employer pressure differently because their work entails different modes of production and management relationships. Industrial (semiskilled) workers, in order to pressure an organization, must shut down production by preventing workers from entering the factory. In contrast, craft and professional (skilled) workers may simply withhold their labor collectively to shut down production.

A health care organization is not greatly different from any other industrial organization. It is labor-intensive, and most health care workers work in large, impersonal, capital-intensive organizations. This creates a dependency relationship, because the worker must rely on the organization for both a job and a living wage. An authority relationship is created in the work place, giving the employer control over the workers' job security, tenure, and wages. Organization by the worker therefore presents a credible threat to the employer; it tends to equalize the economic relationship and rationalize the employment relationship.

In essence, the worker attempts to control the labor market so the organization cannot purchase labor without paying a certain minimum wage, asking the union to supply that labor, or both. The union wants to guarantee job security and income while negotiating rules and procedures against arbitrary employer actions. Collective rather than individual bargaining increases the strength of the individual worker. The essence of unionism in this country is that collective action increases workers' bargaining power so that job security and wages can be negotiated to a much higher level than the free market (without this counterforce against employers) would pay for that relative amount of labor.

Professional associations act much like craft unions in that they attempt to control the requirements for entry to—and thus the numbers

entering—the profession. State licensing laws and educational requirements for professionals help control the market.

In the United States people also join unions because, due to many
union job agreements, they have little choice. There may be a union shop
clause, which means that employers may hire whom they please but,
within a specified period (usually 30–60 days), the new employee must
join the union and maintain his or her membership or face discharge.
Most individuals in the United States join unions because of a union shop
contract; however, this is not prevalent in health care, where most union
membership is voluntary.

NURSES, UNIONS, AND PROFESSIONAL ASSOCIATIONS

Many people believe that collective bargaining is a new movement in
nursing, but the fact is that nurses have been concerned with their economic and general welfare for some time. In 1893, nursing leaders established their first organization, The American Society of Superintendents
of Training Schools for Nurses, one of whose purposes was a commitment
to promote the general welfare of nurses (Miller, 1980). The Nurses' Associated Alumnae of the United States and Canada was formed four years
later to provide a national association for all nurses rather than just those
interested in education. This association became the American Nurses'
Association (ANA) in 1911.

In the early 1900s, working conditions and salaries for nurses were
extremely poor. The nation was in a general economic depression and the
health care system reflected the lack of growth found in other sectors of
the economy. Nurses' working conditions were abysmal: long hours, no
fringe benefits, and substandard wages. Just prior to the collapse of the
economy in 1929, some nurses began to recognize that protest and collective action were necessary if the conditions of the nurse were to improve.
In 1928, ANA incorporated into its legislative policy specific references to
the general welfare, health, and education of nurses.

In 1945, Shirley Titus, then the executive director of the California
Nurses' Association, chaired a committee to study the employment conditions of nurses; as a result of the findings of this committee, ANA adopted
what was called the Economic Security Program. However, just as this
program began to make progress, ANA adopted a no-strike policy in
1950—a policy that was rescinded some years later. At the time, though,
this position, along with the passage of the Taft-Hartley Act in 1947, which
excluded nonprofit hospitals from any legal obligation to bargain with
their employees, left the nurses with virtually no power to bring about
change in their working conditions or salaries. The only options available
were work stoppages, mass resignations, informational picketing, or indi-

vidually leaving a work situation. None of these activities, however, was very influential in bettering the situation of the nurse in general.

In 1974, the health care amendments referred to earlier made it possible for nurses to use legal sanctions if necessary to ensure bargaining related to conditions of employment. Since the passage of these amendments, many state nurses' associations (SNAs) have qualified as legal bargaining agents for nurses. In addition, ANA changed its structure in 1982 to become a federation of state nurses' associations—a change that has rendered the state associations more direct representation of their member nurses. It remains to be seen how this structured change will affect nurses' collective bargaining activities. Many unions, including the Teamsters, the Meatpackers, and the American Federation of Teachers, are also seeking to organize nurses in the work place. In 1980, Barbara Nichols, then ANA president, stated that the ANA "currently represents more registered nurses for collective bargaining purposes than all other labor organizations combined" (Nichols, 1980).

Collective bargaining looks increasingly attractive to nurses because of their growing frustration about the inability to practice nursing as they believe it should be practiced, to influence their working conditions, or gain improved personnel policies and benefits. The National Commission on Nursing, after an extensive literature review and public hearings, found that nurses are meeting this frustration in several ways: they leave nursing, they seek another position in the same or different health care agency, they endure their present position, or they seek some form of collective action by joining a union or seeking to have a state nurses' association represent them (National Commission on Nursing, 1983). Historically, the use of the SNA as a bargaining agent has been a very divisive issue among nurses within the professional organization and among employing agencies. Some nurses believe that the professional organization should not serve as a labor organization, that this dualism represents a conflict of professional purposes and standards. Others believe that there is no conflict, that the promotion of nurses' economic security and general welfare is a major responsibility of the organization. This conflict continues to be a major issue dividing ANA members.

Another major difficulty in the representation of nurses by SNAs is the conflict regarding membership of supervisory personnel in the association. In other words, how can a nurse manager or supervisor who is helping administer a union contract belong to the same organization that serves as bargaining agent for the nurses who are her subordinates? An apparent conflict exists over the nurse manager's divided loyalty. Proponents of SNAs as collective bargaining agents suggest that collective bargaining is only one responsibility of the professional organization and that nurses in administration *can* belong to the same organization. Opponents argue otherwise. Some nurses in administrative positions have resigned from their professional association, either because of their disapproval of the association acting as a bargaining agent or because of its effect on them as administrators.

Adding to this dilemma is the fact that people often change positions over time—from nurse manager to staff nurse, for instance—as they "drop out" to have a baby, go back to school, or just to take some time off. Although they held management positions in the past, they may return as staff nurses.

A few SNAs have been charged with violating federal labor laws because association board members have held hospital administrative positions. However, the NLRB has consistently ruled that associations are *not* in violation of labor law when these board members are "insulated" from labor relations activities. When they are not "insulated," and thus control finances of the organization and give local units collective bargaining advice, federal appeals courts have ruled that those associations *are* in violation of federal labor law (Lorenz, 1982). Furthermore, where there is a clear conflict of interest the NLRB has revoked the SNA's certification as sole agent (NLRB v. North Shore Univ. Hosp., 724 F.2nd, 269, 2nd Cir., 1983, 259 NLRB 852). This creates a dilemma for SNAs which, in following this NLRB ruling, may be in violation of ANA membership rules when they change their by-laws excluding administrators from holding office in the organization. In summary, NLRB and federal appeals decisions have upheld the supervisory nurse's right to belong to the professional association so long as she does not participate in the administration of any aspect of the organization that assists collective bargaining activities.

Hunt (1979) has detailed step-by-step instructions for management when employees are attempting to organize.

THE NURSE MANAGER'S ROLE

The nurse manager in a hospital where the nurses are organized and the parties have negotiated a contract participates in administering the union contract in several ways. The contract will always specify wages, hours, and working conditions; it may specify other items such as union security (e.g., dues deducted from pay checks) and grievance procedures. Most of these items will be handled by the personnel office. The nurse manager, however, actively helps administer the grievance procedures. Besides issues relating to discipline (discussed in Chapter 15), this entails handling grievances at the first and second steps of the grievance procedure.

Grievances can usually be classified as: (a) caused by misunderstanding; (b) caused by intentional contract violations; or (c) caused by symptomatic problems outside the scope of the labor agreement. Grievances caused by a misunderstanding usually stem from circumstances surrounding the grievance, a lack of familiarity with the contract, or an inadequate labor agreement. Self-interest is the usual motivation for using the grievance procedure in an attempt to protect one's perceived, contractual rights. This type of grievance is inevitable even in the most mature, efficient labor/management team. Intentional violation of a contract usually is an effort to capitalize on ambiguous contract language or past practice. Symptomatic grievances are the most difficult to identify and prevent. These grievances are simply a means for the employee to show dissatisfaction or frustration and have three basic causes: (a) personal problems; (b) union politics; and (c) unfavorable contract language. This category describes grievances that stem from the human element in the management/labor relationship.

Any grievance procedure used will be negotiated and clearly described in the labor agreement. Most likely, it will contain a series of progressive steps and time limits for submission/resolution of grievances.

The Grievance Process: An Example

The employee talks informally with her or his direct supervisor, usually as soon as possible after the incident has occurred. A representative of the bargaining agent is allowed to be present. The following steps comprise the typical grievance process:

Step 1. If the grievance is not adjusted in the informal discussion, a written request for the next step is given to the immediate supervisor within 10 workdays. A written response must be received within 5 workdays. The employee, supervisor, and agent will be present for any discussion.

Step 2. If the response to Step 1 is not satisfactory, a written appeal may be submitted within 10 workdays to the director of nursing or her designee. The employee, agent, grievance chairperson, and the director of nursing or designee can be present for discussion. Again, written response will be provided in 5 workdays subsequent to these meetings. In most bargaining units the positions of agent and grievance chairpersons are separated. Generally, the grievance chairperson is an officer in the bargaining unit.

Step 3. The employee, agent, grievance chairperson, director of nursing, and director of personnel meet for discussions. The 10- and 5-day time limits for appeal and answer are again observed.

Step 4. This final step is arbitration, which is invoked when no solution suggested is acceptable. An arbitrator who is a neutral third party is selected and is present at these meetings. The submission of a grievance may be required in 15 days after Step 3 is completed.

Often a statement included in each of the steps states that if the time limits are not observed by one party, the grievance may be considered resolved and further action barred. The contract also usually specifies how an arbitrator is selected.

Beletz offers some suggestions that may be helpful in handling grievances:

1. The objective of the grievance procedure is not to achieve conquest. You do have to work with one another after resolution of the grievance, so treat each other with courtesy and respect.

2. Don't threaten or bluff. On the other hand, this is not an unheard of tactic. Some people use it all the time. If you have investigated properly, you will be able to spot this strategy.

3. Don't withhold facts or information relating to the grievance. This rule is implicit to good faith in bargaining.

4. *Do not*, whatever your position, exhibit internal disagreements or disputes. Both the bargaining unit and the management team must present a solid front when faced with one another.

5. Expediency is a must; delaying tactics serve only to heighten emotions. However, allow time for consideration of all of the facts.

6. Don't blame the other side for taking advantage of your mistakes. Learn from them and don't repeat them the next time.

7. Stay objective. Emotionalism usually leads to further problems.

8. Evaluate and anticipate the other party's position and possible response. The implementation of decisions or the filing of grievances may require planned strategy.

9. Utilize all the resources available. Seek guidance from those higher in administrative positions.

10. Never refuse to meet with the grievant's representatives. The right to representation is one of the advantages of being under the auspices of a collective bargaining unit.

11. The bargaining unit representative, though in a unique position, is not immune from reprimand or discipline. When not involved in bargaining unit activities, the agent is an employee, responsible to the rules and regulations of the institution and the employer has the right to a full day's work and an acceptable level of performance. However, while handling grievances, the employee/agent is not really considered an employee. She or he is considered the representative and advocate of the employee who filed the grievance.

12. On occasion, discussions in settling grievances become quite heated and emotional. Neither party has to tolerate personal abuse. The

meeting should be adjourned and rescheduled at a time when the talks can continue on a more objective level.

13. Whether one is a supervisor or an agent, when first contacted regarding a grievance, the grievance may be denied based on the feeling that none of the aforementioned violations have occurred. This does not limit the employee from pursuance of the grievance and seeking redress at the next step in the procedure.

14. One should not submit to emotional appeals as to what is fair. The contract is the sole determinant of what is fair; if necessary, a neutral third party will be utilized to interpret the contract. What one person considers fair may not necessarily be seen in the same light by the other.

15. Be prepared to give or take acceptable compromises and alternative solutions within the framework of the contract, no matter which party suggests them.

16. Know the strengths and weaknesses of the issue for either side.

17. Integral to bargaining are solutions that may also accommodate future changes and needs. Therefore, one must think ahead.

18. Pat formulas do not settle grievances or solve problems. A formula would negate the needed judgment and flexibility that are so necessary to grievance handling.

19. Know where your bottom line is for compromise.

20. Observe the time limits. If you do not, the bargaining unit may lose the right to continue the grievance to the next level or both the bargaining unit and management may lose in an eventual arbitration.

21. It is wise to remember that once a grievance is filed, it may chain-react and almost any imaginable outcome may end up as the solution. However, a carefully written grievance should obviate this possible outcome.

22. When adjusting a grievance, knowledge is very important. As with any interaction between people, one's statement is colored by one's temperament and is interpreted by the other party in accordance with his or her own temperament.

23. Gloating over a "win" is human; just remember that you may "lose" the next one; don't become overconfident.

24. One of the most important points in grievance handling is being a good detective. Get all the facts and information, witnesses, and documentation. Find out whether any similar situation ever occurred and what the decision was (Beletz, 1977).

The grievance hearing. In actually hearing the grievance in an informal hearing, remember these key behaviors, as set forth by Trotta:

1. Put the grievant at ease. Do not interrupt or disagree with her or him. Let the grievant have her or his say.

2. Listen openly and carefully. Search for what the employer is trying to say. Take notes.

3. Discuss the problem with her or him calmly and with an open mind. Avoid arguments, avoid antagonizing the employee, and avoid the urge to win. Negotiate.

4. Get her or his story straight. Get all the facts. Ask logical questions to clarify doubtful points. Distinguish between fact and opinion.

5. Consider the grievant's viewpoint. Do not assume she or he is automatically wrong.

6. Avoid snap judgment. Do not jump to conclusions. But be willing to admit mistakes.

7. Make an equitable decision, then give it to the grievant promptly. Do not pass the buck (Trotta, 1976).

SUMMARY

- The 1974 health care amendments to the Wagner Act bring health care employees under U.S. labor law. This also includes public-owned hospitals administered by a private firm.

- Several unions and state nursing associations represent nurses.

- The Wagner Act defines the rights of individuals in collective bargaining, outlines union/hospital unfair labor practices, establishes the NLRB, and provides for remedies.

- Collective bargaining is different in health care in order to provide protection for patients or residents. Most bargaining units are structured along occupational lines.

- The effects of unionization on health care costs have been negligible. There is little research showing effects on nurses and nursing practice.

- Nursing units often act like craft unions. State associations often represent nurses. This causes conflict because the association then has contact with labor and administration.

- The nurse manager's major responsibility in collective bargaining is to help administer the contract. Hints are provided to help handle grievances.

BIBLIOGRAPHY

Allen, R. E., and Keavenly, T. J. (1983). *Contemporary labor relations.* Reading, MA: Addison-Wesley.

Becker, E. R., Sloan, F. A., and Steinwald, B. (1982). Union activity in hospitals: Past, present and future. *Health Care Financing Review, 3:4* and 11.

Beletz, E. (1977). Some pointers for grievance handlers. *Superv Nurs,* (August) 8:56.

Davey, H. W., Bognanno, M. F., and Estenson, D. L. (1982). *Contemporary collective bargaining,* 4th ed. Englewood Cliffs: Prentice-Hall.

Dilts, D. A., and Deitsch, C. R. (1977). *Labor relations.* New York: Macmillan. P. 334.

Fossum, J. A. (1982). *Labor relations,* 2nd ed. Dallas: Business Pub.

Henry, K. H. (1984). *The health care supervisor's legal guide.* Rockville, MD: Aspen Publications.

Hunt, J. W. (1979). *Employer's guide to labor relations.* Washington, DC: Bureau of National Affairs.

Link, C. R., and Landon, J. H. (1975). Monopsony and union power in the market for nurses. *South Exon J, 41*(4): 644.

Lorenz, F. J. (1982). Nursing administration and undivided loyalty. *Nurs Adm Quart, 6*(2): 67.

Luttman, P. (1982). Collective bargaining and professionalism: Incompatible ideologies? *Nurs Adm Quart,* (Winter) 6:21.

Miller, R. U. (1980). Collective bargaining: A nurse dilemma. *AORN J, 31*(7): 1195.

Miller, R. U., Becker, B. E., and Krinksy, E. B. (1979). *The impact of collective bargaining on hospitals.* New York: Praeger.

National Commission on Nursing (1983). Summary Report and Recommendations. Chicago: American Hospital Association, April.

Nichols, B. (1980). Belonging to your professional organization: A commitment to personal growth and professional development. Imprint (October), 27(4): 18. American Nurses' Assoc.

NLRB vs. North Shore University Hospital; 724 F.2nd, 269; 2nd Cir., 1983, 259 NLRB 852.

Public Law 101, 80th Congress, June 23, 1947.

Sain, T. R. (1984). Effects of unionization. *Nurs Mngmt,* (January) 15(1): 43.

Sargis, N. M. (1985). Collective bargaining: Serving the common good in a crisis. *Nurs Mngmt, 16*(2): 123–127.

Taylor, B. J., and Whitney, F. *Labor relations law.* Englewood Cliffs, NJ: Prentice-Hall.

Trotta, M. S. (1976). *Handling grievance: A guide for management and labor.* Washington, DC: Bureau of National Affairs.

Wagner Act, 298 U.S. 238, 1935.

Labor Relations
in Canadian Nursing

NURSE MANAGERS IN Canada, because of the nature of labor relations in that country, need ever-increasing knowledge and skill in the administration of nurses' collective agreements. In other countries, where collective bargaining by nurses is less common or is conducted within differing frameworks, the Canadian experience may provide a helpful perspective from which to view emerging trends.

The chapter begins with a discussion of the legal framework for labor relations. The evolution of collective bargaining and labor action by nurses in Canada is presented from a historical perspective. The structure of the collective bargaining process and dispute resolution are then described.

The discussion of management rights and responsibilities toward unionized workers focuses on the first-line nurse manager.

LEGAL FRAMEWORK

Labor statutes provide the framework for labor relations and collective bargaining and, in a liberal democratic country such as Canada, generally reflect popular attitudes toward the union movement. One purpose served by labor legislation is to identify the obligations of unions and management toward one another. Another purpose is to protect the rights of all parties concerned, including the general public as represented by the state. Labor legislation is designed to provide both management and labor with certain legal procedures and "weapons" that can be employed to structure their relationships to one another as collective agreements are negotiated and administered.

In Canada, collective bargaining rights are extended to all but a very few workers. Although there are differences among provinces, the exceptions generally include certain professionals, employees whose work is of a confidential nature, and employees whose work is defined as managerial. Public sector employees, such as civil servants, teachers, and nurses, were granted most of the same collective bargaining rights, including the right to strike, as private sector employees in the wake of changing public attitudes and enabling legislation in the late 1960s and early 1970s (Muir, 1974). Certain essential service workers such as police officers and fire fighters are usually not permitted to strike and are required to settle their disputes by compulsory arbitration. Overall, in Canada the proportion of unionized workers in the work force is slightly higher than in the United States; for example, in 1980, 37.6% of the work force (exclusive of agricultural workers) in Canada were members of unions, compared to 24.7% in the United States (Wood & Kumar, 1982).

Under the Canadian constitution, the regulation of employer-employee relations falls primarily within provincial jurisdiction. However, federal government employees, territorial workers, and workers in certain industries that cross provincial and national boundaries are entitled to bargain collectively under federal labor laws. Canada consists of ten provinces and two territories. These are governed by eleven sets of labor laws: one federal, and ten provincial. Despite this diversity, the legislation is relatively similar across Canada, having been modeled originally after labor legislation in the United States as discussed in the previous chapter.

There are some major differences, however, between the U.S. and Canadian approaches to labor legislation. Carter (1982) has identified four. These are: (a) the certification process; (b) strike restrictions; (c) compulsory grievance arbitration; and (d) recognition of the right to union security. Each of these has implications for the first-line nurse manager.

Certification

The certification process is a mechanism that gives the union legal status and the rights accorded by labor legislation. Additionally, it ensures that only one union is authorized to represent a certain group of employees. To obtain exclusive bargaining rights for nurses, a trade union must apply to the appropriate labor relations board, providing evidence that it represents the majority of a group of employed nurses. The trade union could be any one of a variety of organizations—for example, a professional nursing association, an exclusive "craft" union for nurses, or an industry-wide employees' union. In the United States, employee vote is used to establish that a trade union is truly authorized by the group of employees it claims to represent. In Canada, such elections are the exception, rather than the rule. Moreover, the employer is prohibited from attempting to dissuade employees from joining unions. A union may submit a complaint of unfair labor practice to the labor board should the employer attempt to interfere in the union organization process.

Labor boards are official tribunals specifically established to administer the labor laws. They are empowered to oversee all aspects of labor relations, including approval of applications for certification and assisting parties in the resolution of disputes. The labor boards generally consist of equal numbers of union and management representatives, and government appointees.

A union can also obtain collective bargaining rights by seeking voluntary recognition as a bargaining agent from the employer or employer's association. The rights of nurses to engage in collective bargaining are unrestricted. However, like many of their colleagues in the United States, Canadian nurses have been disinclined to obtain assistance from or to join established trade unions, preferring to work through their professional associations or, more recently, to establish independent unions.

Strike Restrictions

Strikes are generally regarded as the ultimate economic sanction that can be exercised by a union. Although strikes are legally permitted as a means of bringing pressure on an employer to make concessions at the bargaining table, various legal restrictions control the use of the strike weapon in Canada. Strikes are not allowed for the purpose of gaining recognition as a bargaining agent. With the exception of the province of Saskatchewan, strikes are not allowed while a collective agreement is in effect. Strikes may be used during the process of negotiating a contract, but certain mediation and conciliation procedures must usually be followed first. A strike vote must be taken before a union is entitled to strike, and a formal notice of strike must be given to the employer.

At present, strikes by hospital workers are permitted in all provinces except Prince Edward Island, Newfoundland, Ontario, and Alberta. Collective bargaining impasses in these three provinces must ultimately be settled through the process of compulsory arbitration. There have been three province-wide strikes by hospital nurses since 1977 in Alberta. However, in June 1983, the Progressive Conservative government amended the labor laws to prohibit strikes by all hospital workers in the province. In Ontario, strikes by hospital workers have been outlawed since 1965. Public health nurses are entitled to strike, however. On one occasion, public health nurses went on strike to back up their demand for compulsory arbitration for the resolution of interest disputes.

Compulsory Grievance Arbitration

Because strikes are illegal if held during the lifetime of a collective agreement (except in Saskatchewan), the parties must make provision for the peaceful resolution of disputes that arise out of the interpretation, administration, or alleged violation of the agreement. The labor statutes usually provide mandatory provision for arbitration should the agreement fail to include such a procedure. If the parties cannot settle a dispute about a grievance, they may jointly appoint a single arbitrator or separately appoint nominees to a tribunal consisting of a union representative, a management representative, and a neutral chairman chosen jointly by the two nominees. The decision of a majority of the arbitration board is binding on the parties.

Appeals may be lodged through the courts by either party when there has been an error at law, when the arbitration board has exceeded its jurisdiction, and in certain other circumstances. The powers of the arbitration board are usually specified in the legislation; in general, an arbitrator may not modify the provision of a collective agreement. He may, however, be entitled to reduce the severity of a disciplinary penalty imposed on a grievant.

Union Security

Unions in Canada are permitted to bargain for their own financial security and, accordingly, nursing unions have negotiated what is known as the Rand Formula into their contracts. This ensures that all nurses who benefit directly from the provisions of the collective agreement must contribute union dues through payroll deduction, irrespective of their involvement in union activities or their willingness to consider themselves union members. The Rand Formula ensures a continuous and predictable income for the union. This feature of labor relations differs significantly from the United States system in which some jurisdictions have introduced right-to-work laws, curtailing the ability of unions to negotiate union security clauses.

HISTORICAL REVIEW OF COLLECTIVE BARGAINING BY CANADIAN NURSES

The Canadian Nurses' Association (CNA) accepted the principle of collective bargaining in 1944, the same year in which the Canadian government introduced its influential Wartime Labor Relations Regulations (Carter, 1982). At that time, the prevailing method for influencing the terms and conditions of employment consisted of the circulation of recommended salaries and personnel policies by provincial nursing associations to their members and to employers. This proved ineffectual because the recommended terms and conditions of employment were not binding on anyone; while other hospital workers resorted to collective bargaining in increasing numbers, the salaries for registered nurses barely kept ahead of salaries for nursing assistants and nursing orderlies. Even so, it was more than 20 years after the CNA took its stand on collective bargaining that the major thrust towards large-scale union organization in nursing occurred.

The first Canadian nursing union seems to have been l'Association des Gardes-Malades Catholiques Licenciées, established in the city of Quebec in 1927, evidently as a result of attempts by the clergy to restrict hospital nursing to Roman Catholic nurses (Michaud, 1980). Nineteen years later (1946), on the other side of the country, the Registered Nurses' Association of British Columbia was granted recognition as a bargaining agent under the provincial Labor Relations Act and began a very active and effective collective bargaining program for its members (Cormick, 1969).

Another nine years elapsed before any further event of much significance took place. Then, in 1965, in the Province of Alberta, the Calgary General Hospital Staff Nurses' Association obtained certification under provincial legislation and signed its first collective agreement with its hospital board. The Alberta Association of Registered Nurses had by this time hired an employment relations officer to assist the membership in forming staff nurse associations in hospitals and health agencies and to provide educational programming in labor relations and collective bargaining. All other provincial nursing associations soon followed suit, as part of a broader social movement in which employees in the public sector accepted collective bargaining as a respectable method of improving their socioeconomic status.

The diversity of provincial legislation and the reluctance of nurses and their professional associations to obtain certification as trade unions led to the use of a variety of forms of collective bargaining. For instance, several provincial nursing associations entered into procedural agreements with provincial hospital associations, obtaining voluntary recognition as bargaining agents and negotiating terms and conditions of employment on a province-wide basis. The appropriateness of the professional nursing association serving as a bargaining agent, however, was debated from the earliest days of collective bargaining by nurses. Many of the officers of provincial nursing associations were drawn from the ranks of nursing management and, from the perspective of a labor relations board, both the bargaining unit and the bargaining agent were very probably dominated by the "employer." Paradoxically, in many cases, the nursing leaders were responsible for steering their professional nursing associations towards collective bargaining, even though they themselves were ineligible for membership in the collective bargaining unit according to the law.

Relationships Between Professional Association and Nurses' Unions

A legal challenge to the composition of the professional nursing association as bargaining agent came eventually in the Province of Saskatchewan when another union, the Service Employees International Union, objected to the certification of a local affiliate of the Saskatchewan Registered Nurses' Association on the grounds that it was "company dominated." The battle was fought all the way to the Supreme Court of Canada, which in 1973 upheld the decision of the Saskatchewan Labor Relations Board to deny certification to the professional association (News, 1973).

Nursing associations in other provinces, assuming that similar legal challenges would be launched, immediately began to modify their constitutions and bylaws to establish semiautonomous collective bargaining subdivisions within their organizational frameworks. The emergence of autonomous socioeconomic subdivisions of the professional nursing associations proved to be an interim phase in the evolution of collective bargaining in the nursing profession in Canada. Gradually, one after another, the staff nurse divisions of the professional associations broke away to become full-fledged nursing unions devoted exclusively to labor relations activities. Members of staff nurse divisions became union members in every sense of the word, and were thus obliged to pay union dues as well as professional association fees. (A unique situation now exists in Ontario where the affairs of the nursing profession are distributed among three associations: the Ontario Nurses' Association [the union], the Registered Nurses' Association of Ontario [the professional association], and the Ontario College of Nurses [the registration and disciplinary body].)

The development of independent nursing unions that are unaffiliated with the trade union movement has been a very distinctive feature in the Canadian nursing profession, indicating the importance to nurses of remaining in full control of their own socioeconomic affairs. Today each province has both a professional nursing association and a nursing union, with the exception of Prince Edward Island, where the professional association remains the collective bargaining agent for registered nurses. In the Province of Quebec nurses are represented by a diversity of unions. There are unions composed of French-speaking and bilingual nurses and even an association of middle management nurses who have limited negotiating power. Nurses in Quebec are also represented by other unions having a broad spectrum of health care workers among their members.

Relationships between professional associations and unions in the various provinces are maintained through the establishment of liaison committees for the purpose of discussing issues of mutual interest. A recent development was the founding of the National Federation of Nurses' Unions in 1981. This federation currently consists of one federal and six provincial unions representing 25,000 nurses. The larger provincial nursing unions (i.e., those in British Columbia, Alberta, Ontario, and Quebec) have not as yet joined the federation. Of the 161,000 practicing nurses in Canada, 105,000, or 65%, are now unionized (Rowsell, 1983).

DISPUTES RESOLUTION AND EMERGING ISSUES

Historically, the use of the strike weapon to back up socioeconomic demands was not acceptable to nurses. The Canadian Nurses' Association established its official position on the matter of strikes in 1946 in a resolution that opposed strikes by nurses at any time or for any reason. This position was held until 1972 when the resolution was rescinded (Mussallem, 1977). The idea of allowing economic self-interest to interrupt services to clients appears, in some respects, inconsistent with the goals and values of any helping profession. However, the number of professional groups using industrial relations strategies has grown considerably in the past two decades. The realities of fluctuating economics and the increasing political sophistication among women may account for nurses' changing attitudes toward strike action.

The first legal strike by Canadian nurses occurred in 1966, when some 3000 nurses joined 29,500 other hospital workers in a 20-day strike against 139 hospitals in the Province of Quebec (News, 1966). Since then, there have been legal strikes by nurses in almost every province. In many of these situations, striking nurses have enjoyed significant public support. Nevertheless, governments have usually intervened in interest disputes that have placed the health and safety of patients at risk.

Grievance arbitration was described earlier in this chapter as a process which provides for the assistance of a third party in resolving disputes that arise from the interpretation, administration, or alleged violation of an existing collective agreement. Grievance arbitration has been invoked by nurses in a variety of circumstances and is often the mechanism which clarifies the application of a particular clause in the provincial collective agreement at the local level. Precedents set in grievance arbitrations may pave the way for the achievement of certain goals at the bargaining table. For example, contracts at one time generally allowed dismissal of an employee during the probationary period without recourse to the grievance procedure. The general stance of unions was that the employer should always be required to demonstrate cause for dismissal, even during the probationary period, and that all employees should, therefore, have access to grievance procedures. Historically, the unions' stance on this issue was not reflected in current collective agreements. However, unions made repeated efforts to establish precedent in this area by bringing probationary dismissals to grievance. If an arbitrator can be convinced of the merits of an individual situation in which a probationary employee was unfairly treated, the arbitration ruling may establish the precedent for future rulings on the same issue. Today, consequently, most employers must show "reasonable cause" for dismissal during the probationary period.

Professional Responsibility Committees

When certain management practices give rise to recurring union concerns, trends may be set through grievance arbitration. For example, in one case the validity of professional nursing judgment was tested against the employer's judgment in determining safe work loads in an intensive care unit (Sklar, 1979). In this instance, the management position was upheld. In general, determination of work load, staffing, and staff/patient ratios is management's right. On this point arbitrators have upheld the employer, unless the latter has negotiated the right away.

In other instances, however, nurses have successfully demonstrated that the province-wide structure of collective bargaining does not solve the problem of effective management–union communications at the institutional level. Although the grievance procedure specifies the steps to be taken in the event of contract administration disputes, nurses wanted a mechanism for direct consultation and discussion with management on a regular basis. Their major reason for insisting upon such a mechanism has been concern about nonmonetary issues such as the appropriateness of work loads and patient assignments. Professional responsibility committees have therefore become a major bargaining issue.

Not surprisingly, management tried to resist such efforts of nursing unions as representing one more example of the erosion of its right to direct the work force. Nurses persevered, however, and the requirements to establish professional responsibility committees for the purpose of discussing patient care concerns were eventually negotiated into a number of Canadian nurses' contracts. In Ontario nurses have negotiated into their contracts the right to refer unresolved professional responsibility issues to an external adjudication panel of expert nurses. Although the panel of expert nurses has had authority to investigate the circumstances and to make recommendations, employers have not, so far, been obliged to act on such recommendations. However, developments in this area illustrate how the use of power by nurses' unions may have a positive effect on the allocation of resources to and within nursing departments.

STRUCTURE OF COLLECTIVE BARGAINING

The "bargaining agent" which is authorized at the stage of certification is one of two major participants in the collective bargaining process. The agent may be the local collective bargaining unit of nurses, in which case collective bargaining occurs face-to-face at the local level with members of the hospital or health agency board. The chief advantage of collective bargaining at this level is the opportunity it affords for nurses to discuss directly with their employers specific problems relative to their employment relationship. Local issues pertaining to the administration of the contract, as well as concerns related to patient care and clinical practice, can all be brought to the attention of the board and appropriate solutions negotiated.

While this model of collective bargaining allows nurses to govern their own negotiations at the local level, maximizing their perception of control over working conditions, a major problem is that local union executives often lack the special skills and knowledge required to conduct successful labor negotiations. Hence, the common practice is for groups of local nurses' bargaining units to be represented at the negotiating table by one common bargaining agent. Joining together in this way to negotiate terms and conditions of employment has led to province-wide bargaining and has significantly increased the power of nurses at the bargaining table.

The second major participant in the collective bargaining process is the employer, as represented by the hospital or public health agency board. In the same way that local bargaining units have joined together for the purpose of collective bargaining, hospital and health agency boards have formed associations at regional and provincial levels to negotiate with nurses on behalf of their respective groups. A province-wide employers' association appoints a negotiating team whose membership is made up of trustees, administrators, personnel managers, and, in the case of contract talks with nurses, directors of nursing. This team is then authorized to negotiate a new agreement and sign a memorandum of settlement that must then be ratified by the respective principals.

Historically, provincial bargaining has been considered advantageous to management because it allows all member institutions to be represented by expert negotiators, thus reducing duplication of effort and costs. Uniform terms and conditions of employment for nurses, in addition to their obvious administrative advantages, allow even the very small hospitals to compete in the recruitment process for staff nurses.

There are certain advantages and disadvantages to the provincial bargaining model. By virtue of their province-wide base of support, each of the two parties can be very powerful, since a strike, lockout, or arbitration settlement will probably affect all union locals or health agencies represented by the two negotiating teams. But, when provincial bargaining teams from both parties meet at the negotiating table, represented by their respective labor relations specialists and/or legal counsel, it is inevitable that some stereotyping and generalization will occur. This may inflame or stalemate the need to maintain day-to-day, face-to-face relationships with one another prior to or after the bargaining process. It may also lead to increased costs attributable to the negotiating process and its outcomes. However, province-wide bargaining may serve to deflect animosity from the local hospital to the larger association and hence preserve a better relationship at the local level.

An inherent difficulty with the provincial bargaining model is that since most hospitals and health care agencies are funded by government, they may not be aware of their funding base for the coming year as negotiations take place. The negotiating team of the provincial hospital association is therefore to some extent negotiating on behalf of government as well as of member agencies. The government is indirectly one of the participants in public sector labor relations, or the "ghost" at the bargaining table. Some critics of this approach argue that negotiations should be taking place directly between government and nurses, as is the case with physicians and some other professionals, since the ability of the negotiating team to make commitments on behalf of government and member agencies is limited. Other disadvantages are the domination of large over small hospitals in decision making, and the fact that employment provisions appropriate for large hospitals are not always appropriate for small ones, and vice-versa.

In recent years, as certain types of health care agencies have become more specialized or highly differentiated, other disadvantages of province-wide bargaining have been acknowledged. The most obvious is perhaps the problem of finding terminology and contract provisions that can work equally well in small rural hospitals or complex tertiary care centers. It has been suggested that the salaries, benefits, and working conditions of nurses have lagged behind those of many other occupational groups. This may be because nurses have remained independent of trade unions in their labor activities so that, in some cases, precedents that have been established for other workers have not been applied to nurses' collective agreements and arbitration settlements.

Dispute Resolution Procedures

When collective bargaining breaks down due to an impasse in negotiations, the parties usually exhaust a series of mediation or conciliation procedures before resorting to final dispute resolution strategies. In provinces where strikes by hospital workers are prohibited, impasses in negotiations are referred to independent boards for compulsory binding arbitration.

In the majority of provinces in Canada, nurses may use the strike weapon to bring pressure on their employers to concede to their demands. If the employer considers these demands excessive or damaging to the economic viability of the institution, it, too, has recourse to an economic sanction: to lock out employees and to close the institutions. In practice, hospitals have been loathe to lock out employees in contract disputes.

However, public health agency boards have been known on occasion to lock out their public health nurses. Clearly, public health nurses do not enjoy the same kind of bargaining power as their hospital colleagues. When public health nurses withdraw their services, there is no immediate threat to the health and safety of the public served. Therefore, public health nurses have generally preferred to solve their collective bargaining disputes by compulsory arbitration.

The major effect of a strike is its interference with the revenue-producing capabilities of an organization. Within publicly funded health care agencies in Canada, the revenue-producing function is less obvious than in the private sector but still important. Since the major source of revenue is government funding, which usually continues during a strike, withdrawal of nursing services may actually spare the agency an embarrassing operating deficit or at least allow it to accumulate surplus funds.

ROLE OF THE NURSE MANAGER

Until recently, most first-line nurse managers were "in-scope" employees: that is, they were entitled to be members of the nurses' union and were covered by the collective agreement. Following increases in the numbers of labor disputes and implementation of decentralized nursing facilities, however, the roles of first-line nurse managers in many agencies were expanded to include responsibility for discretionary management functions such as budgeting, hiring, and employee discipline. Widespread recognition of the managerial requirements on nursing units has led to the exclusion of first-line nurse managers from many bargaining units.

The first-line nurse manager, whether in- or out-of-scope, is in a position to significantly influence the labor relations climate in her own unit and in the institution as a whole. Since she may still be or has recently been a union member herself, she may feel a considerable amount of empathy and identification with the concerns and positions of her staff as union members. On the other hand, she may have sought a management position in a conscious effort to dissociate herself from union activity. As an individual, she is entitled to her own opinions and feelings about the existence of the union and the "rightness" or "wrongness" of its positions on various issues. However, in accepting a position as a first-line manager, she has also accepted certain obligations to her employer and to her staff. In her leadership role, she will be expected to take a stand in situations where the demands or behavior of staff members may have a detrimental effect on the patients for whom she is responsible. She must be thoroughly familiar with the collective agreement and with the limits and extent of her own role in employee discipline as it is specified in the policies of the organization.

Her rights and obligations as a member of the management team are elaborated upon in her job description and are derived, in part, from the "management rights" clauses in the collective agreement. She must thoroughly understand these rights and responsibilities if she is to provide effective leadership. She must understand the rights of her employees as they are enshrined in labor and human rights legislation as well as in the collective agreement. Failure to do so could result in a loss of leadership credibility and a high incidence of grievance behavior.

The task of management is to lead and direct the employees within an organization so that the objectives of the organization can be achieved. Where no collective agreements exist, the rights of management and its responsibilities to individual employees are those that exist in common law. Where the employer and a bargaining agent have signed a collective agreement, the requirements for management to direct the work force, establish job descriptions and performance standards, and maintain discipline in order to achieve its organizational objectives are acknowledged in a "management rights" clause.

The rights of management are balanced and limited by the collective agreement and by labor legislation prohibiting unfair labor practice. Unfair labor practice is defined within the labor legislation and includes such things as interference with the right of eligible employees to become unionized, refusal to allow an employee to be represented by the appropriate union official in discussions with the employer, and certain other arbitrary actions by the employer that may unduly influence the outcome in a labor relations situation.

The first-line nurse manager is responsible for the quality of patient care and the work behavior and performance of her staff. Whether she hires her own staff and is expected to initiate disciplinary action, or whether she makes recommendations in these matters, the first-line nurse manager is in a position of potential conflict with members of the bargaining unit. She will be expected to document all critical incidents for review with her supervisor. On some occasions she must take immediate action to see that an employee whose behavior is dangerous, uncontrolled, or insubordinate is suspended and leaves the premises immediately.

The courses of action she chooses, whether immediate or long-range, can be critical if such disciplinary actions give rise to employee grievances and proceed to grievance arbitration. Dealing with a grievance that proceeds to arbitration can be costly, not only in financial terms, but also in terms of working relationships and morale on the nursing unit. It can also be a test of leadership ability and personal strength for the first-line nurse manager, who must continue to respect the rights of her staff and maintain courteous and effective communication with them so that patient care and other activities in the nursing unit can continue.

During grievances and negotiations, and prior to or following a strike, there may be unique tensions in the working environment that arise from the roles which the first-line manager and her unionized staff are expected to play. At such times, it is critically important for the nurse manager to understand the rights of her employees and her own management rights. For example, she is entitled to insist that employees refrain from discussion of personal matters or union business during their working time. However, she is not in a position to interfere with their attendance at union meetings during lunch or coffee breaks (the employee's own time) or after working hours. She is obligated to recognize the appropriate roles and functions of duly elected or appointed union officials, but she is entitled to prevent them from interfering with patient care and other essential activities on the nursing unit.

Labor relations is a specialized area, and many of the management skills it requires must be learned over a period of time under the guidance of a superior and with the help of labor relations specialists who are available in most organizations. It is vital that the first-line nurse manager familiarize herself with the legislation relevant to her professional and managerial responsibilities. A thorough understanding of the collective agreement and related organizational policies and procedures is also essential. Networking and mentor relationships with experienced nursing managers can be a valuable source of information and support as the first-line nurse manager applies new knowledge and skill and as she experiences the anxiety and ambivalence that characterizes most instances of employee discipline or labor action. The expertise of labor relations specialists and the support of senior administration within the organization are resources that should be available to assist the nurse manager in her role in employee relations.

SUMMARY

- Labor relations in Canadian nursing differs significantly from relations in the United States, with most nurses belonging to collective bargaining units.

- There is a wide variety in union organization, activity, and law in various Canadian provinces.

- A union becomes the legal representative of a group of employees by the process of certification granted by a labor relations board.

- Unions that represent nurses may be the professional association or an independent union organization. Nurses may belong to both organizations.

- First-line nurse managers function at the interface between senior management and employees. This places them in a unique position to improve the organizational climate through their knowledge, skill, tolerance, and integrity.

- The nurse manager who has developed excellent interpersonal skills, particularly in the areas of nondefensive and assertive communication, has an excellent base upon which to build specialized labor relations skills.

- The manager's most important contribution to both her own employees and superiors lies in the maintenance of professional nursing standards and organizational policies and procedures that provide a framework for the safety of clients as well as legal protection for workers.

BIBLIOGRAPHY

Carter, D. D. (1982). Collective bargaining legislation in Canada. In: *Union-management relations in Canda*. Anderson, J., and Gunderson, M. (editors). Don Mills, Ont: Addison-Wesley.

Cormick, G. W. (1969). The collective bargaining experience of Canadian registered nurses. *Labor Law Journal*, 20(10): 670.

Michaud, A. (1980). The evolution of nurses' unions vis-à-vis professional associations. Unpublished paper presented to the Annual Meeting of the Canadian Nurses' Associations, Vancouver, June 24.

Muir, J. D. (1974). Canada's experience with the right of public employees to strike. In: *Contemporary issues in Canadian personnel administration*. Jain, H. C. (editor). Scarborough, Ont: Prentice-Hall of Canada.

Mussallem, H. K. (1977). Nursing and political action. In: *Issues in Canadian nursing*. LaSor, B., and Elliott, M. S. (editors). Scarborough, Ont: Prentice-Hall of Canada. P. 169.

News. (1966). *Can Nurs*, 62(9): 7.

News. (1973). *Can Nurs*, 69(8): 9, 12.

Rowsell, G. (1983). Personal communication. Labor Relations Dept., Canadian Nurses' Assoc.

Sklar, C. L. (1979). Sinners or saints? The legal perspective. (2 parts.) *Can Nurs*, 75(10): 14 and 75(11): 16.

Wood, W. D., and Kumar, P. (editors). (1982). *The current industrial relations scene in Canada 1982*. Kingston, Ont: Queen's University.

5

BASIC
SURVIVAL SKILLS

THE ECONOMIC CLIMATE for the future of health care is uncertain, and with competition for funds increasing, financial resources are becoming scarce. Since the nursing department budget can account for as much as half of a hospital's total expenses, there continues to be significant pressure on this department to increase efficiency and effectiveness. For nursing to respond to the pressures and the uncertainty, nurse managers at all levels must become proficient in the budgeting process. Many nurse managers, though already familiar with this process, have not developed the skills necessary to project costs based on current and anticipated needs. The monitoring aspects of budget control are even less well understood. Yet, it is the nurse manager on the unit level who is in the best position to predict trends in census and acuity, as well as supply and equipment needs. The purpose of this chapter is to present the conceptual framework of budgeting, to relate the resources necessary to provide patient care to the dollars required to sustain it. Examples will be presented to facilitate understanding this relationship.

Budgeting is the process of planning and controlling future operations by comparing actual results with planned expectations. A budget is a detailed plan that communicates these expectations and serves as the basis for comparing them to actual results. As such, it can never be definite or absolute. The budget shows how resources will be acquired and used over some specific time interval; its purpose is to allow management to project activities into the future so that the objectives of the organization are coordinated and met. It also helps to ensure that the resources necessary to achieve these objectives are available at the appropriate time or that operations are carried out within the resources available. Lastly, a budget helps management control the resources expended.

Budgeting is performed by business, government, and individuals. In fact, nearly everyone budgets, even though he or she may not identify the process as such. A budget, in fact, may exist only in an individual's mind, but it is nonetheless a budget. Anyone who has planned how to pay a particular bill at some time in the future, say, six months, has a budget. Although it is very simplistic, that plan accomplishes the essential budget functions. One now knows how much of a resource (money) is needed and when (in six months) it is needed. Note that the "when" is just as important as the "how much." The money has to be available at the right time.

PLANNING AND CONTROL

A budget helps management plan and control the distribution of resources within the organization.

Planning

Planning involves reviewing the established goals and objectives of the nursing unit, the nursing department, and the hospital for the next fiscal year. Financial projections are then developed. A budget forces managers to look into the future and may thus help them identify problems and take corrective steps before the problem becomes unmanageable. Budgeting moves the budget, organizational or individual, from a haphazard reaction method of management to a formal, controlled method. With a budget, the manager spends less time reacting to unanticipated problems and more time on productive endeavors.

As part of the budgeting process, planning has two additional advantages: improved communication and functional coordination.

Communication. Operating budgets are prepared for the entire organization, yielding the master budget, and therefore all levels of management are involved and the organization's goals are communicated to them. The process of compiling, reviewing, and revising data for the budget opens up lines of communication between subordinates and superiors and among managers of those departments whose operations are related and interdependent.

Coordination. Without a coordinated budget system, each department may operate without regard to what any other department is doing or to the organization's objectives. Obviously, this lack of coordination results in inefficiency and increasing costs. The operating budget becomes the master plan of action for the entire organization, reflecting the coordinated efforts of all levels of management. This helps the organization operate smoothly and efficiently so that particular goals and objectives are met.

Control

Not only is a budget a planning tool to help management establish future objectives and decide how they are to be achieved, it is also a tool to control what is going on. Control involves the steps taken by management to ensure that the objectives are met and that all parts of the organization are working in a manner consistent with organizational policies. Controlling is the process of comparing actual results with the results projected in the budget. By measuring the differences between the projected and the actual results, management is better able to make modifications and corrections. Controlling, then, depends on planning. Without a plan, there is no way to compare actual versus planned or anticipated performance. A responsibility summary is a formal document generated by the finance department, showing budgetary expectations, actual results, and the difference (see Figure 19–1). The difference between budget and actual performance is called a variance.

It is unlikely that the projected and actual results will be the same. Some variance is to be expected, and management will decide how much variance will be tolerated. For example, anything under 4% or $500 is acceptable, thus management would examine only variances over that percentage or dollar amount.

BUDGETARY CONCEPTS AND CONSIDERATIONS

Responsibility Accounting

The basis for budgeting is the concept of responsibility accounting; that is, each manager's performance is judged by how well those items directly under his or her control are managed. To judge a manager's performance in this way, the costs and revenues over which he or she has control must be carefully scrutinized and classified. The effect of responsibility ac-

Figure 19–1   Example of a Form in Which Monthly Expenditures for an Area of Responsibility Are Logged and Sent to the Nurse Manager for Review

Units of Service (Patient Days)		Current Month Actual			Current Month Budget			YTD Actual	YTD Budget
NAT CLS	**Account Description**	Current Month			Year-to-Date			Average Unit Cost		
		Ac-tual	Bud-get	Vari-ance	Ac-tual	Bud-get	Vari-ance	Ac-tual	Bud-get	Vari-ance
100	Inpatient Revenue									
10	Management									
20	Technician & Specialist									
30	Registered Nurses									
40	Licensed Vocational Nurses									
50	Aides & Orderlies									
60	Clerical									
90	Other Salaries									
100	Paid Vacation									
110	Paid Holiday									
120	Paid Sick Leave									
180	FICA Tax									
250	Other Professional Fees									
320	Sutures and Surgical Needles									
330	Surgical Packs									
340	Surgical Supplies									
370	IV Solutions									
380	Other Medical Care Materials & Supplies									
390	Cleaning Supplies									
400	Office Supplies									
410	Employee Wearing Apparel									
420	Instrument & Minor Equipt.									
430	Other Minor Equipt.									
440	Laboratory Supplies									
450	Repairs & Maintenance									
460	Purchased Services									
470	Dues and Subscriptions									
500	Rentals									
510	Outside Education & Travel									
520	Other Expenses									
	Total Direct Expenses									

counting is to personalize the accounting system; this is essential to effective planning and control.

Responsibility accounting is based on three premises: (a) that costs can be organized according to levels of management responsibility;

Figure 19–2 Variance Report

Cost Center _____
Month _____ Year _____

	Current Month Actual	Current Month Budget	$ Difference ( )	% Difference ( )
UNITS OF SERVICE				
Revenue (100)				
Expense (Nat. Class)				
Salaries (10,20,30,40, 50,60,90)				
Benefits (100,110,120)				
Other Professional Fees (250)				
SUB-TOTAL				
Medical Supplies (320,330, 340,370,380,440)				
Non-Med. Supplies (390,400)				
Employee Wearing Apparel (410)				
Equipment (420,430)				
Repairs & Maint. (450)				
Purchased Services (460)				
Rentals (500)				
Dues & Subscript. (470)				
Outside Education & Travel (510)				
Other Expenses (520)				
TOTAL EXPENSE				

Explanation of all variances in excess of ± __4% & $500.00__
Use brackets () to indicate unfavorable variances.

Adapted from Children's Hospital, Los Angeles, Dept. of Nursing.

(b) that the costs that are charged to a manager be controllable at that level of management; and (c) that timely budget data can be generated as a basis for evaluating performance.

A formalized system to ensure accountability to budgetary controls is shown in Figure 19–2. This form can be completed monthly by nurse managers using information obtained from the responsibility summary. Thus, variances are justified and necessary modifications in future expenses can be made.

Motivational Aspects

When used properly, the budget can be an effective way to motivate employees. Thus, the most effective budgets are those that the employees help to develop; such a process helps ensure that the budgets represent fair standards for evaluating employees' work. Also, job satisfaction can result from achieving the goals and objectives of the organization set forth in the budget. In contrast, an improperly developed or administered budget can cause friction among the employees and management.

For the budgeting process to be a motivational tool, management must recognize that the budget is not perfect. In other words, if the actual results do not match the projected ones, this does not necessarily represent poor performance by the employees. Management may have made mistakes in judgment and prediction, and not all circumstances can be foreseen. Therefore, changes and modifications are sometimes necessary. Top management is responsible for communicating the proper attitude toward the budget to lower levels of management. The budget is a tool and, to be effective, it must not be viewed as infallible. The budget should be used as a positive instrument to aid in establishing operating goals, measuring operating results, and isolating areas that need extra attention. Administration of a budget program requires a great deal of insight and sensitivity from management. Lower-level managers will not respect the budget if they believe that top management is not committed to it or is using it to intimidate. The ultimate objective must be to develop an awareness that the budget is designed to be a positive aid in achieving both individual and institutional goals.

Budget Period

The planning horizon for budgeting may vary from a year or less to many years, depending on the objectives and the uncertainties involved. Budgets covering the acquisition of land, buildings, and equipment have longtime horizons and may extend 5, 10, or 20 years or more into the future. Obviously, such budgets will not be as detailed as one set up for only a year hence.

Nursing unit budgets are usually developed to cover the one-year period that corresponds to the organization's fiscal year. Most organizations will then divide the one-year budget into four quarters and each quarter into the separate three months. The near-term figures can generally be projected with considerable accuracy.

Continuous or perceptual budgets are being used increasingly often.

These are budgets that add one month in the future as the month just ended is dropped, so there are always 12 months of budget data before management. Continuous budgets are desirable because they compel managers to think specifically about the coming 12 months. Thus, it stabilizes the planning horizon.

Zero-Base Budgeting

Zero-base budgeting is a budgeting process that requires managers to start from zero budget levels every year; it has been given a good deal of attention. Managers are required to justify all costs as though they were being initiated for the first time. No cost is viewed as continuing into the future. Traditionally, proposed budgets have been justified on an incremental basis; that is, the manager starts with last year's budget and adds to or subtracts from it according to projected needs, objectives, and the inflation rate or consumer price index.

This latter system can reward a manager for overutilizing dollars since next year's budget is based on last year's figures, allowing adjustments in units of service. It can also penalize prudent managers who do not use all allocated dollars within the months preceding the development of the next fiscal year's budget.

Zero-base budgeting, in contrast, attempts to get back to such basic questions as why does this activity or department exist and what should be its goals and objectives. It requires that established programs maintain their productivity. Although zero-base budgeting requires much time and is costly, in some situations its use is justified.

Flexible Budgeting

Flexible budgets allow management to adapt to changes in activities and unplanned costs once the fiscal year has begun. Patient census, activity mix, and the use of supplies can change suddenly in today's economic environment. Expenses based on a fixed patient census will not reflect true productivity. A flexible budget takes into account actual costs of personnel and supplies per unit of service and compares that to the actual units of service. Variance results are then compared against a flex standard rather than a budgeted one. For example, let's look at total supplies used on one nursing unit for one month:

Supplies	Actual	Budget	Variance
	$2300	$2400	$100

Suppose the supply budget had been based on 600 patient days. Actually, the nursing unit had 550 patient days for the month. In a flexible budgeting system, it is important to know the cost of supplies per patient day. If

$4.00 per patient per day was the calculated average supply expense ($2400 ÷ 600), then the example would be as follows:

Supplies	Actual	Budget	Flex Budget	Variance
	$2300	$2400	$2200	($100)

In this example, supply costs were $100 over budget. Flexible budgets like other budgetary systems require the manager to investigate negative variances. A higher than normal patient acuity and/or an excessive utilization of a high cost item are two examples of when expenditures over budget may be justifiable.

The Operating Budget

The operating budget tells management how much money it will cost to maintain the routine operations of the organization during the fiscal year. Each nursing unit generates an operating budget that combines requirements for personnel, benefits, supplies, and other items necessary to operate the unit, which is defined as a cost center. A cost center is the smallest functional unit that generates costs within the organization. Cost centers may be revenue producing, such as laboratory and radiology, or non–revenue producing, such as environmental services and administration. Each nursing unit is usually considered a cost center. In all but a few hospitals nursing is not directly reimbursed for its services. Nursing service costs are within the room rate.

Formulation of the operating budget should begin several months before the beginning of the next fiscal year in order to provide sufficient data and time for planning.

Units of Service

Nearly all hospital budgets are derived in some way and to some extent from the forecast of patient occupancy rates, acuity levels, or some other activity standard. A unit of service is the budgetary concept on which expenses are based. Environmental service departments use square footage; the dietary department uses meals served, the emergency room uses patient visits, labor and delivery uses numbers of deliveries, and nursing care units use patient days. Patient days reflect the number of days that any one patient is in the hospital. Thus, a census of 20 patients per day for 365 days would equal 7300 patient days a year. If this forecast is significantly inaccurate, budgets based on it will also be significantly inaccurate. If the variance is too large, the usefulness of the budget and the entire budgeting process is undermined.

Capital Expenditure Budget

The capital expenditure budget is established to fund the purchase of major equipment or architectural renovations. It is a planning process that should occur throughout the fiscal year and culminate at budget preparation time. Each nurse manager should keep a chronological list of all capital items purchased. Reference to the dates of purchase will help in replacement planning, as equipment wears out.

Each institution will have its own definition of capital, but there are usually two common criteria: The item must be above a certain cost and have a life expectancy greater than a set time period. For example, a hospital may define capital as any item that costs over $500 or has an expected life of greater than one year. Some institutions also define a capital purchase as two or more items of the same specifications that together exceed a fixed dollar amount. (For example, one bedside chair = $250. The unit will purchase two chairs under the capital budget for a cost of $500.)

Capital items are usually requested on forms designed for that purpose (see Figure 19–3). Included in the capital request are cost estimates of installation, delivery charges, and service contracts. The justification for each item should be well documented. The purchasing and accounting department can help the nurse manager obtain information about depreciation time span, salvage value, age of equipment, and the like. This data, coupled with clinical information, aids in the preparation of the request. Since institutions usually set aside a fixed amount for total capital purchases, a well-documented request helps the decision maker determine need.

Other aspects of the operation such as personnel or supply budgets must be considered. For example, if monitoring equipment is being requested, the cost of EKG paper and electrodes should be determined, documented, and included in the supply budget. Likewise, the need for additional personnel to operate the new equipment, training of personnel already on hand, or possibly, the need for additional nursing hours per patient day should be quantified, documented, and included.

Capital expenditure budgets can be difficult to develop due to rapid changes in technology; however, by working closely with the medical staff and nursing staff, and keeping current with the changes and future trends, nurse managers can be most effective in anticipating capital needs.

SUPPLY AND EXPENSE BUDGET

The supply and expense budget funds the noncapital equipment and supplies needed to operate a nursing unit: It includes such items as medical-surgical supplies, pharmacy items, and paper and office supplies, in addi-

Figure 19—3 Capital Item Request Form

Priority Listing #

1. Department ___Nursing___

   Location _____

2. Cost Center Title _____

3. Cost Center Number ___6062___

4. _5 Physiologic Monitor (ECG & Respiratory)_
   Request Title and Quantity

5. _78833B_
   Model No., Type, Catalog No., Size, etc.

6. _Hewlett-Packard_
   Potential Vendor, Tel. No. or Vendor Location
   (Alternate Vendor, if Available)

JUSTIFICATION:

Current monitors are constantly down for repair.

This model is outdated and has been phased out.

With the type of patients that are admitted to this

unit, we need a more sophisticated and reliable

system to monitor continuously the cardiac and

respiratory status of sick infants. This is phase II

of the planning for replacement in a systematic

approach. We have 12 more monitors to be

replaced over the next 3 years.

_____

_____

If more space is needed, please turn over.

PURCHASING'S COMMENT	ELECTRONIC/ENG'S COMMENT

BUDGET USE ONLY

Budget Request #_____

Equipment Cost $_____

R & C Cost $_____

Total Cost $_____

Estimated:

7. Equipment Cost ___$5,705.70 ea × 5 = $28,000___

8. R & C Cost _____

9. Tax ___$1,854.35___

10. Freight _____

11. UL Approval _____

12. Other _____

13. Total Costs ___$30,682.35 + freight___

14. Related New Operating Costs:
   a. Salaries
      (No. of FTE) _____
   b. Non-Wage
      Supplies _____
      Repair & Maint. _____

15. Reason for Request:

   [X] Patient Care

   [ ] Non-Patient

   [X] Replacement of Equipment
       Specify ID # _F-13-576, F13-577,_
       F13-575, F13-584, F13-580

   [ ] Enhancement of Existing Equip.

   [ ] Comply with Statutory Mandate

   [ ] Expanding or New Program

   [ ] Will Increase Revenue or Cut
       Expenses

   [ ] Other _____

16. Funding source, if any, other than hospital
    funds:
    1. Grant/Account #_____
    2. Contract/Account #_____
    3. Special Fund #_____
    4. Other/Account #_____

17. Projected Month of Purchase _____

18. Person to Contact _____
    (please print)

Date	Exten.	Division Head
Date	Exten.	Department Head

tion to other operating expenses such as rentals, maintenance costs, and service contracts.

An essential tool used in developing this budget is a report or statement of expenses. Such a statement, if prepared at the end of each accounting period (usually a month), should include the amount budgeted, the amount actually spent, and a year-to-date total. This information should be available for each expense category, such as medical-surgical supplies or pharmacy, and for the unit total, as shown previously in Figure 19–2.

The first step in developing the supply budget is to analyze the previous expense statements to determine any trends that could be significant in forecasting for the coming year. Changes in supply requirements or utilization can result from volume changes, a change in patient mix, a change in the type of patients, a new piece of equipment, or change in procedure. Of course, such changes can occur for numerous other reasons as well; these need to be considered on a unit-by-unit basis and quantified as accurately as possible.

Supply budgets also need to be adjusted for inflationary impact, and adjustment guidelines are usually provided by the purchasing department. For instance, the purchasing department may predict a 5% increase in all pharmacy costs and a 4% increase in all other categories.

To budget for the next year, assuming no major changes (e.g., in census, acuity, or new services) would require only an adjustment for inflation. Using the pharmacy expense (medical supplies) as an example, we will calculate the amount to be budgeted, assuming 5% for inflation. Thus the pharmacy expenses for the first six months were $2370 or $395 per month; for the coming year, we should budget $395 per month plus 4% more, which would be $415 per month.

As another example, assume the same six-month expense report; however, now it is anticipated that due to the purchase of new equipment, additional EKG paper and electrodes will be required. The cost of paper and electrodes is estimated to be an additional $180 per month in the medical-surgical supply expense account, and the inflationary impact is expected to be 4%. For the first six months of this year, the expenses for medical-surgical supplies were $17,982 or $2997 per month. To plan for additional supplies, we should budget the previous $2997 per month plus $180 plus 4%, which would yield $3117 per month.

Nurse managers must be familiar with expense account categories and the items in each one so that current expenses can be properly analyzed and the impact of future changes can be accurately predicted.

Monitoring the Supply and Expense Budget

The supply and expense budget is monitored in much the same way as the personnel budget, using monthly expense statements as the tool. Again, the first step is to determine whether there are significant variances and, if so, to determine the cause so that corrective action can be taken.

In determining causes for variations, the activity level of the unit should be examined for any relationship to the variance. For example, if a variance in supply costs is due to increased use of an item because of an unanticipated increase in census, there is a legitimate reason for the variance and corrective action may not be indicated. However, if the variance is due to improper utilization of supplies, then a plan to correct the situation should be developed. From time to time the nurse manager may find it necessary to make staff aware of budget overruns and ask for their assistance in conserving supplies and equipment. The important thing is to evaluate the situation carefully so appropriate steps, if indicated, may be taken.

Reports received from the accounting department should include information about all supplies received from the in-house ordering systems and those received from out-of-hospital purchases. Supply costs should be shown and the nurse manager can then determine if appropriate charges to the unit's cost center were made. The nurse manager must have a clear understanding of those charges that are patient charge items and those that are unit charges. Some hospitals charge the nursing unit for patient charge items that are used by the unit but accidentally not charged to the patient. The nurse manager must then develop a mechanism for tracking "lost charges."

PERSONNEL BUDGET

The personnel budget (also referred to as the salary or manpower budget) is an especially important part of the budgeting process. It can account for as much as 90% of the total nursing service budget. It includes the salaries of all nursing staff, as well as compensation for such things as vacation time, sick leave, holidays, overtime, differentials, merit increases, and orientation and education time. Nurse managers at the unit level are the best sources for determining staffing requirements. Staffing requests should be developed with as much objective information as is available.

Relevant Components

When computing the personnel budget, one must take into consideration the following significant factors:

1. Units of service

2. Mix in patient acuity

3. Required hours of nursing care

4. Fixed and variable staffing

5. Technological changes

6. Changes in medical practice

7. Regulatory requirements

8. Support services

9. Plans for the next year

Units of service. Personnel budget needs are based initially on the projected units of service. This projection is usually made by the hospital's financial department in collaboration with the department of nursing. The bed capacity of a nursing unit as well as the actual rate of occupancy should be considered. These data should be analyzed for any identifiable trends or patterns. As a general rule, if the occupancy rate is 90% or greater, the census can probably be considered fairly stable, with relatively little variation from day to day. However, the lower the occupancy rate, the greater the possibility for daily variation, which then creates the need to look more closely for patterns or trends.

Consider, for example, a 30-bed nursing unit with a 65% occupancy rate. In this case, it would be important to know if the census is evenly distributed over the time period or if there are discernible patterns or fluctuations. The distribution can be fairly equal, with a census of 19–20 patients per day, or there could be a very high census on weekdays with a very low census on weekends. Such a distribution of patient population will affect significantly the staffing patterns and the personnel budget.

Mix in patient acuity. The acuity levels of the various patients on the unit at any given time must also be considered. A patient classification system is a valuable tool in measuring the complexity of care needed by patients and in categorizing patients according to the level of care required over a specified period of time. Such systems can be beneficial in objectively defining staffing needs and supporting staffing requests. While a nurse manager can probably predict staffing needs fairly accurately with subjective data, it is difficult to support staffing and budgetary needs without objective evidence. Thus, it becomes important to base future personnel requirements on the amount of nursing care that patients actually need, rather than the amount of care actually provided. In situations of understaffing, patients do not receive the required hours of nursing care. Unless data reflect the hours indicated as well as the actual hours provided, labor projections will be false.

Classification systems will vary for different nursing areas. Numerous patient classification systems are available today, ranging from the simplest to very comprehensive management information systems. All of these, however, should enable classification of patients according to the level of nursing care required, not on time actually spent delivering the care. Tools must minimize subjectivity and demonstrate validity and reliability if they are to accurately predict nursing work load.

Required hours of nursing care. The first step in calculating staffing need for a given unit is to predict patient days by level of acuity. This information can be obtained from the census information and patient classification data. Assume, for instance, a 30-bed medical-surgical unit with an average census of 26 patients per day per month. On the basis of trend analysis, the average daily patient distribution is budgeted from historical data and may be displayed in this manner.

Level of care (from lowest acuity [I] to highest [IV])	Number of patients per day
I	5
II	15
III	4
IV	2
	26

The next step is to determine the hours of nursing care required for this particular mix of patients on the basis of an (assumed) patient classification system that utilizes the following standard hours of care needed by each patient for each acuity level:

Level	Hours per patient day
I	5.0
II	6.4
III	8.0
IV	12.0

To determine the daily hours of nursing care required, multiply the number of patients of each type by the standard hours of care required.

Standard Labor Hours Budget
(For the period January 1 through December 31)

Classification	Patients per day	Hours per patient day	Hours of care per 24 hours
Level I	5	5.0	25
Level II	15	6.4	96
Level III	4	8.0	32
Level IV	2	12.0	24
Total	26		177

Thus, given a stable patient census and mix, the direct hours of nursing care per patient day would be 6.80:

Total hours of care required in 24-hour period ÷ Average daily census

or

$$177 \div 26 = 6.80$$

Fixed and variable staffing.   Fixed staffing does not change as volume changes. The nurse manager, clinical nurse specialist, nurse educator, unit secretaries, monitor technicians, and a charge nurse on each shift are examples of individuals that may be needed regardless of the patient census and/or acuity.

Direct care givers, which include registered nurses, licensed vocational nurses, and nurses aides, are examples of individuals whose numbers will vary depending on the census.

Technological changes.   Changes in technology that could affect the number or type of personnel required should be considered. For example, an intensive care unit that is about to purchase more sophisticated monitoring equipment may need additional staff due to the increased complexity of care; or, if the unit does not have enough registered nurses to manage the new equipment, an increase in their numbers should be considered when the staffing pattern and resulting budget are developed.

Changes in medical practice.   Changes in medical practice may create needs for different types of personnel, for additional personnel, or for a change in personnel mix. A significant increase in the use of hyperalimentation, for example, might increase the nursing care and staff requirements significantly. Also important is whether the ratio of RNs to support personnel is appropriate to provide the type of care required with hyperalimentation. The development of a home hyperalimentation program would require increased patient care hours and may necessitate hiring a clinical nurse specialist as program coordinator.

Regulatory requirements.   The complexity of health care services provided to patients, the increasing acuity of hospitalized patients, and the growing recognition that quality of care affects outcomes has resulted in increasing attention to nursing requirement regulations for hospitals. The Joint Commission on Accreditation for hospitals and various state guidelines often explain the number and/or level of nursing personnel required on specific units.

Support services.   Support services such as environmental services, dietary services, radiology, and the laboratory should be considered with regard to the level of support they are now providing, how that support affects staffing levels, and whether any changes in these services are anticipated.

Plans for the next year. To accurately predict staffing requirements, institutional, nursing department, and nursing unit goals for the coming year should be set first. These should include, at least, projections of activity level and any new programs or services.

Careful evaluation of these factors is the key to realistic planning. Such evaluation enables an accurate forecast to be made for the coming year, and this, in turn, is essential in developing staffing and budgetary requirements. The director or vice-president of nursing is an essential resource at hospital budget sessions; the director can identify the impact of these areas on nursing's overall budgetary needs for patient care.

Staffing Patterns

Using the recommended hours of care as a guideline, nurse managers can distribute those hours over all shifts by developing a staffing pattern. In addition to the previously mentioned relevant components of a personnel budget, factors should be considered such as personnel mix, hours of work, distribution of work load, and delivery system.

Personnel mix. Personnel mix includes the number of personnel currently available at each skill level (RN, LVN, or aide), as well as the skill level recommended due to patient acuity.

Hours of work. Whether 8-hour, 10-hour, 12-hour, or other flexible scheduling is used, work shifts will affect the staffing pattern, as well as the number of personnel needed.

Distribution of work load. The nurse manager must analyze the work load distribution over the three shifts and determine how the staffing should be distributed. This decision-making process needs to be individualized to particular patient requirements. Two possible alternatives are: (a) 35% of the staff allocated to all three shifts; or (b) 45% on days, 30% on evenings, and 25% on nights. The key is flexibility. Things can change from month to month or shift to shift. Initial projections merely serve as a guide.

Delivery system. The method of delivering care—primary, team, or functional nursing—will also affect the staffing patterns.

Position Control

The position control is the list of approved labor positions for the department. The positions are displayed by category of personnel (e.g., nurse manager, RN, LVN) as well as the number of full-time equivalents (FTE). An FTE is a full-time position that can be equated to 40 hours of work per week or 80 hours per pay period. In institutions where nurses work 12-hour shifts, 72 hours per pay period may constitute one FTE.

An FTE is the equivalent of 2080 paid hours per year (40 hours per week × 52 weeks per year = 2080 hours). For a 36-hour workweek, one FTE = 1872 paid hours (36 × 52 = 1872). Paid hours include productive time (hours actually worked) plus nonproductive time (vacation, holiday, sick). The amount of nonproductive time actually built into each FTE varies with each organization. For purposes of budgeting, the nonproductive time is an expense that must be covered by additional paid productive hours.

The FTE budget.   Using a hypothetical 26-bed unit where all staff work 8-hour shifts, the number of variable nursing staff needed on duty for 24 hours can be determined in the following manner.

The required nursing hours were determined to be 177 hours per 24 hours. Thus, 177 ÷ 8-hour shifts = 22.12, the variable FTEs required per day. Since each nurse works 8 hours a day, 5 days per week, additional FTEs (over 22.12) will be required to cover days off:

177 × 365 (days per year) = 64,605 (paid hours required in 1 year)
64,605 ÷ 2080 = 31.06 FTEs (required for the personnel budget)

For a nursing unit staffed totally by nurses who work 72 hours per pay period on 12-hour shifts, the FTEs required would be higher:

64,605 (total required hours) ÷ 1872 (paid hours) = 34.51 FTEs

The fixed positions required for the nursing unit are added into the overall position control. Since fixed positions are not usually replaced when off, each position is simply budgeted as 1.0 FTE.

Once unit staffing requirements have been determined, the required FTEs need to be compared to the available resources. When FTEs needed do not match the position control either by available numbers or necessary mix, the nurse manager considers budget requests for new positions.

Differentials and Overtime

The budget for differentials for evenings and nights is calculated by multiplying the hours by the differential rate. For example, based on an average daily census of 26, a nursing unit needing four RNs each on evenings and nights would multiply the differential rate on each shift by 8 and then multiply that number by 4:

Evening differential = $1 per hour
$1 per hour × 8 hours per shift = $8 per shift per nurse
$8 × 4 nurses = $32 per day additional needed budget dollars
$32 × 365 days a year = $11,680 a year

Night differential = $2 per hour
$2 × 8 hrs = $16 per shift per nurse

$16 × 4 nurses = $64 per day additional needed budget dollars
$64 × 365 days = $23,360 a year

Evening differential = $11,680
Night differential = $23,360
Total additional budget dollars for differential = $35,040

An overtime budget is established to cover situations that cannot be anticipated, such as fluctuations in work load or temporary shortages of staff due to illness or other reasons. Overtime should be calculated by determining the historical average number of hours of overtime worked and multiplying by one-and-one-half times the hourly rate. Thus, if the average number of overtime hours is expected to be 8 hours per week, the overtime rate is $18 or $12 × 1.5. The weekly overtime costs would then be $126, and the annual cost would be $6552.

When trends are used to predict overtime, nurse managers should consider whether the amount of overtime used in the past was really justified and whether the level predicted is really appropriate. It may be possible to reduce overtime by adjusting the staffing schedule.

Nursing units on 12-hour shifts need to account for the last 4 hours of each shift as overtime dollars. Whether this figure is accounted for within the overtime dollar figures, as well as within the overall salary projections, will depend on the institution.

Benefits

To complete the personnel budget, benefits are figured as a percentage of the average yearly salary. In most institutions, vacation pay, holiday pay, sick leave, insurance premiums, workman's compensation, and any other benefits, such as life insurance or child care, usually average around 23% to 33%.

At this point, accumulation of data for the personnel budget should be complete. In summary, the first step is to project the activity for the coming year in terms of patient days and acuity of illness. The daily hours of care required for the projected mix of patients are then calculated by using the standard hours of care. A staffing pattern is then developed, and the required variable and fixed FTEs are determined. The final steps include calculating differentials, overtime, and indirect labor costs.

Monitoring the Personnel Budget

Constant monitoring is necessary to ensure that expenses remain within the projected budgetary limits. This calls for the use of monthly expense statements, which include the amount budgeted for the month, the amount actually spent, and year-to-date information. Figure 19–4 illustrates such a statement.

Figure 19—4 Monthly Personnel Expense Statement

Expense	Current Month—June			Year-to-Date (6 Months)		
	Actual	Budget	Variance	Actual	Budget	Variance
Management	3,200	4,000	800	22,200	24,000	1,800
Technician &						
Specialist	2,855	2,855	0	15,421	17,130	1,709
Registered Nurses	57,911	53,974	(3937)	179,479	181,929	2,450
Licensed Vocational						
Nurses	4,321	7,058	2,737	17,166	26,559	9,393
Aides & Orderlies	0.00	0.00		0.00	0.00	
Clerical	3,813	3,650	(163)	22,420	21,900	(520)
Total	72,100	71,537	(563)	256,686	271,518	14,832

The monthly report should be analyzed for significant variances. The causes for variances should then be determined and corrective action should be taken where indicated. In most cases, it is acceptable to be underbudget unless the dollar amount is significant—this might indicate improper planning.

The areas of variance that require most effort in problem identification are those that are overbudget where the variance is significant. To be significant means to be over some percentage set by management, say 5%. In Figure 19–4, for instance, the RN salaries are significantly overbudget, and the reason for the variance should be explored carefully. Some questions to ask are: Was the patient activity during the period at the expected level or greater? Were the hours actually worked the number planned? Were the salaries as anticipated? And were unworked hours, vacation, sick time, holiday pay, and so on as expected? The important point to determine is whether the variations were due to inappropriate planning or to unanticipated activity that was beyond control.

As stated earlier, personnel costs represent the major portion of the total nursing service budget, and this requires that significant attention be paid to managing human resources. Lack of attention to this fact can affect the personnel budget indirectly or directly: indirectly, through such factors as high turnover rates or high sick-leave time; directly, by poor scheduling techniques or improper monitoring and use of overtime.

SUMMARY

- Budgeting is the process of planning future operations and controlling operations by comparing actual results with planned expectations.

- A budget is a detailed plan used to communicate these expectations and serve as the basis for comparing them to actual results.

- The master budget represents a series of interrelated budgets for all activities of the organization.

- Planning and control are two separate functions of the budget.

- Planning involves establishing future goals and objectives and the steps necessary to achieve those goals.

- Controlling is the process of comparing actual results with planned or budgeted results. By measuring these differences, management is better able to make modifications and corrections.

- A total unit budget includes a personnel budget, a supply and expense budget, and a capital expenditure budget.

- The personnel budget is influenced by patient census, activity levels, technological changes, and changes in medical practice and clinical service.

- A unit personnel budget can be developed by: (a) predicting patient days by level of activity; (b) determining hours of nursing care required for this patient mix; (c) distributing hours required over all shifts; (d) developing a staffing pattern considering personnel mix available; and (e) converting hours of care to actual costs.

BIBLIOGRAPHY

Arndt, C., and Huckabay, L. M. D. (1975). *Nursing administration: Theory for practice with a systems approach.* St. Louis: C. V. Mosby.

Cleland, V. (1982). Relating nursing staff quality to patient needs. *J Nurs Adm, 12*:32.

Dale, R., and Mable, R. J. (1983). Nursing classification system: Foundation for personnel planning and control. *J Nurs Adm, 13*:10.

Donovan, H. M. (1975). *Nursing service administration: Managing the enterprise.* St. Louis: C. V. Mosby.

Finkler, S. A. (1984). *Budgeting concepts for nurse managers.* Orlando, FL: Grune and Stratton.

Hillestad, E. A. (1983). Budgeting: Functional or dysfunctional? *Nurs Econ*, (November/December) *1*(3): 199.

Huttmann, B. (1984). Selling your budget. *RN, 47*:25.

Kirby, K. K., and Wiczai, L. J. (1985). Implementing and monitoring variable staffing. *Nurs Econ*, (July/August) 3(4): 216–222.

Knight-Sheen, J. P. (1983). *The Medrec calculator: A new way to plan for nurse staffing.* San Antonio, TX: Medrec.

McLane, A. M. (1987). Classification of nursing diagnosis. In: *Proceedings of the seventh conference.* St. Louis: C. V. Mosby.

Rotkovitch, R. (1981). The nursing director's role in money management. *J Nurs Adm, 11*(11, 12): 13.

Stevens, B. J. (1980). *The nurse as executive.* 2nd ed. Wakefield, MA: Contemporary Pub.

Stevens, B. J. (1981). What is the executive's role in budgeting for her department? *J Nurs Adm, 11*:22.

Strasen, L. (1987). *Key business skills for nurse managers.* Philadelphia: J. B. Lippincott.

Using Computers in Health Care

USES OF COMPUTERS IN NURSING

The acceptance of computers in nursing has paralleled that in the business community. Most hospitals, like most businesses, were introduced to computers by financial systems, such as patient billing and payroll. Hospital administrators generally accepted such systems because they facilitated the handling of enormous amounts of paperwork, thereby decreasing the confusion and delay associated with the billing process. In other words, systems were chosen initially because they could expedite the filing of insurance claims, reduce lost charges, and improve the cash flow of the hospital.

The move toward using computers in the delivery of patient care came more slowly. In this case, it was difficult to justify such a move because the benefits of a computerized system were intangible and because many health care professionals were against the change. In addition, appropriate systems were usually neither available nor, if available, as dependable as necessary. Further, as with any technological change, the evaluation and acceptance processes were slow. Now, however, computers are being used both directly in nursing and in applications that affect nursing. (For information about computers, see Appendix E, Computer Basics.)

Patient Monitoring

One of the first applications of computers in patient care was in patient monitoring. At the present time almost all coronary and intensive care units do some type of computer monitoring of patient's vital signs, cardiac output, and blood gas changes (Curtin, 1982), and the extent of the applications is increasing. For example, in some hospitals, computers are used to regulate the isolette temperature while taking into consideration an infant's temperature and the air of the isolette (Endo, 1981). Other computer systems monitor the vital signs of infants to alert nurses to changes in the heart or respiration rate of infants. Finally, some systems track premature infants with respiratory distress syndrome by measuring the stiffness of the lung and lung volumes and alerting the nurses' station when a change occurs (Dolcourt & Harris, 1982).

The primary functions of such systems are to record the progress of the patient and alert the nurse when a significant change occurs. While some computer-monitoring systems record the patient's progress on paper, many (see Figure 20–1) also transmit the information to monitors at the nursing station. Where there are such monitors, the computer may print a notice on the monitor to alert the nurse when a change occurs. Otherwise (or in addition), the computer will sound an alarm.

In addition, computers are used as early warning signals. For example, labor rooms in most hospitals have computers that monitor the progress of both the mother and the child during all stages of labor. These computers record not only progress through the labor process, but also the respiratory and heart rate data of the infant to determine how he or she is responding to that progress. Generally, the record is made on paper and is also transmitted automatically to monitors at the nursing station so that nurses can easily track the labor process.

With the recent advances in their capabilities, computers have become more valuable in patient monitoring (Squire, 1982; Edwards, 1982). Not only are they able to assimilate information from the patient continuously and to detect changes, they can also help analyze data and even interpret it. While almost all current systems simply provide this information to a health professional for action, some equipment has been developed that not only detects undesirable trends, but also automatically administers medication appropriate to the problem.

Such developments facilitate the nurse's efforts to handle unexpected or poorly defined problems. However, these developments also present challenges. It is crucial that the nurse manager, by developing training programs, help the staff become skilled in the use of computer equip-

Figure 20–1   Patient Monitoring

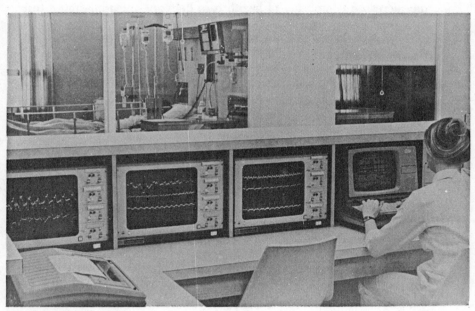

From Honeywell, Inc.

ment. If the nurses are not trained in its usage, the highly technical monitoring equipment will not provide the intended efficiencies. However, the nurse manager must provide more than training in the technical aspects of the equipment. She must, in addition, provide support so the staff nurses feel comfortable with the equipment; if the nurses are not comfortable with the equipment, their anxiety may frighten or demoralize the patient, and the intended increase in quality of care will not be achieved.

In addition, the nurse manager needs to be sure that the use of computers does not dehumanize care. That is, she needs to monitor computer use by staff nurses to ensure that they rely on the equipment as an aid to the nursing function, not as a replacement for the interpersonal aspects of patient care. These aspects are the essence of nursing care and are essential, because not everything that is relevant to know about a patient appears on a monitor, and equipment can break.

Patient Histories and Medical Records

The patient chart is a tool intended not only to identify and record important attributes of a patient's condition, but also to provide an account of the care given. The need for an orderly summary of the care that is provided to the patient and his or her reactions to care were identified as early as the mid-nineteenth century (Nightingale, 1946:6). Today, with the increased complexity of health care delivery, including more tests, protocols, and procedures, the quantity of information in that medical chart has exploded. In most noncomputerized systems, each time new data are recorded, they are entered as independent events. This results in a sequential listing of events, not the integrated description of the patient's responses necessary for the delivery of professional health care. The patient's problems and symptoms are likely to be randomly scattered throughout the protocol descriptions, test results, and nursing notes. Because it is often difficult to locate and integrate them, their cumulative implications are often underevaluated or missed. Furthermore, the pressures of legal liabilities, quality assurance investigations, audits, and research have mandated more attention to patient records.

Computerization makes the increased information easier to use. In most systems, the computer is able to rearrange data from the chart in any form that would be useful to the health care professional. For example, using a computer, a nurse could isolate and examine the history of symptoms that a patient experienced during a stay (or even, in some cases, in a previous stay). Or, the nurse could investigate the effects of specified regimens on a particular symptom by relying on those same sorting and summarizing capabilities of the computer.

Such a system eliminates the expense of time and energy associated with assimilating and summarizing the data that are necessary for the development of care plans. With a computer, the nurse does not need to waste valuable time on searching through the chart or Kardex system for information or on summarizing that information. Instead, she just strikes a few keys on the terminal and the information is almost instantly available. This capability can be particularly valuable when a patient's records from previous hospital stays are also relevant.

Care plans can be developed more easily with a computer. First, because the system provides standard screens with standard choices, nurses can be more efficient in recording their observations and developing appropriate plans. Having the possible options in front of them while they are involved in these processes not only simplifies the process, it reduces the likelihood that some factor might inadvertently be left unrecorded. An example of a nursing assessment menu is shown in Figure 20–2. Second, because information from ancillary departments and some monitoring equipment is sent to the nursing station automatically, the nurse is made aware of changes that require her intervention as soon as possible; this allows her to change the care plan without delay. Third, computerization allows for some analyses (most notably the sorting of information in the patient record) to be done by the computer. This means that the nurse can have available the necessary information to help in the development of the care plans. Further, as noted earlier, because she can isolate the

Figure 20–2 Nursing Assessment Menu

Page Nos. for Nursing Orders
Basic Care
1. General Hygiene—excluding Facial Hygiene.
2. Facial Hygiene.
3. Pressure Area & Sore Care.
4. Aids for Relief of Pressure.
5. Position.
6. Mobility.
7. Intake—Diet.
8. Intake—Fluids.
9. Observation Charts.
10. Observations.
13. Recordings.

Tests
20. Urine Tests (Ward).
21. Urine Tests (Laboratory).
22. Tests—Excretary (except urine) & Blood.
26. Swabs & Aspirates.
28. Biopsies.
30. X-Ray Investigations.
35. Investigations—excluding X-rays.
39. Bovey Day Cases.

Treatments
40. Alimentary Canal—Upper.
41. Cardiac Therapy.
42. Dialysis.
43. Genito-Urinary Tract—Catheters.
44. Urology.
45. Genito-Urinary Tract—excluding Catheters.
47. Infusion Therapy.

48. Intestinal Tract.
50. Orthopaedic—Traction.
51. Orthopaedic—Plaster.
52. Orthopaedic—Exercise & Appliances.
53. Ear, Nose & Throat.
55. Radiotherapy—Oncology.
56. Respiratory Tract—Inhalations.
57. Respiratory Tract—excluding Inhalations.
58. Skin—Topical Applications.
59. Skin—Non Topical.
60. Bandages.
61. Clips, Sutures, Clamp & Rod.
63. Drains.
64. Dressings.
66. Packs.
67. Operation or Investigation.
69. Treatments & Applications—Hot & Cold.

Miscellaneous
70. Patient/Relative Tuition.
71. Patient/Relative Appointments, etc.
72. Therapy, Clinics, Visits & Domiciliary Services.
73. Transfer & Transport.
74. Handicaps, etc.
75. Special Precautions.
76. Reminders to Nurse in Charge.
77. ⎫ Nursing Problems (Printed on Care
78. ⎭ Plans).
79. Sensitive Problems (Not printed on Care Plans).

Astbury, C. Nursing care plans: Aspects of computer use in nurse-to-nurse communication. In: *Medinfo-83 Seminars*. Fokkens, O. et al. (editors). © IFIP-IMIA; North-Holland (1983).

necessary information, she or he can identify trends or peculiarities more easily. Examples of care plans are shown in Figures 20–3 and 20–4.

Computerized recordkeeping also improves the usability of patient information (Keliher, 1975). For example, it allows for greater continuity of patient information. If computers are used in an emergency medical system, information about rescue squad reports, patient symptoms, laboratory data, treatment outcomes, and demographic data can be easily traced from the first intervention. This facilitates continuous patient monitoring, communication with diagnostic centers, and consolidation of large databases.

Figure 20–3 Nursing Care Plan

CARE PLAN

4436-02 MYERS MARTHA R   24Y BROWN JC   08-03--PAGE 1 END
CUR DIAG: ABDOMINAL PAIN   PT CLASS: 02
       MED INFO:

SURGERY:
SURGERY DATE/TIME: DAYS-SAY 06   POST-OP   POST-PARTUM
ALLERGIES FOOD: CITRUS FRUITS AND MILK PRODUCTS
ALLERGIES MED/OTHER:
PATIENT PROBLEM: HEARING IMPAIRMENT—USES HEARING AID   ISOLATION:

PROCEDURES-TESTS		08	09	10	11	12	13	14	15
0011	GB SERIES—RULE OUT GALLSTONES	ONCE	X							
A	NO SMOKING DURING PREP	CONT								
B	DELAY DIET AND FLUIDS EXCEPT SMALL AMTS OF H2O WITH NECESSARY PO MEDS	SFT 3 & 1								
ACTIVITY/MISCELLANEOUS										
0002	BLOOD PRESSURE BID	BID		X						
	PT CARE SUPPORTIVE ASSISTANCE	CONT								
A	SELF PERSONAL HYGIENE & FEEDING	CONT								
A003	LOW FAT DIET	CMEALS	X					X		
NURSING PROBLEMS/NURSING ACTION										
A002	PROBLEM 1—UPPER RT ABD PAIN	CONT								
A	OBSERVE AND REPORT TYPE OF PAIN, ONSET, DURATION, CONSTANCY AND SEVERITY	CONT								
B	OFFER PAIN MEDICATION PRN AS ORDERED	PRN								
C	RECORD RESULT OF MEDICATION	CONT								
LONG AND SHORT-TERM GOALS										
A004	SHORT-TERM GOAL—REASONABLE RELIEF FROM PAIN AND NAUSEA	CONT								
SOCIO-PSYCHOLOGICAL NEEDS										
A007	ANXIETY DUE TO IMPENDING TESTS ENCOURAGE VERBALIZATION OF FEELINGS	CONT								
TEACHING PLANS										
A006	EXPLAIN ALL TESTS AND TEST PREPARATIONS	ONCE	X							
NURSING OBSERVATIONS										

                   VISIT CONDITION   SHIFT
4436-02 MYERS MARTHA R   K36752   RV   G   WED 08-03 --   1

Computerizing the patient chart has other benefits for nursing (Muirhead, 1982; Romano, McCormick & McNeely, 1982). For example, nurses' notes can be recorded more easily, since most notations can be selected from a menu with preprogrammed entries. The nurse simply types the code or presses the appropriate button to indicate her choice. In other systems, physicians enter their own notes, including diagnoses and protocols, directly into the computer, thereby saving valuable nursing time that might otherwise be spent transcribing the physicians' notes. Further,

Figure 20—4 An Example of a Care Plan Summary When a Patient Is Discharged from an ICU Equipped with a HELP System

```
              CURRENT NURSING CARE PLAN              CRARRY, LARRY NMI          6001200
                    05/29/1985   10:51                  TEST

  1. ALTERED VENTILATION/OXYGENATION   TIME INITIATED: 04/17/1985 20:56   LAST UPDATED: 05/28/1985 15:29

      RELATED TO (CAUSES):                    ACTIONS:
        1 PNEUMONIA                             1 RECORD CHARACTER/FREQUENCY/EFFECTIVENESS OF COUGH
                                                2 INCENTIVE SPIROMETRY: Q2H
      OUTCOMES:                                 3 ENCOURAGE AMPLE FLUID INTAKE
        1 RESPIRATIONS REGULAR/UNLABORED        4 ELIMINATE RESPIRATORY IRRITANTS
        2 CHEST CLEAR PER CXR/AUSCULTATION      5 USE NASAL CANNULA WITH 24 FT TUBING
        3 ARGS XXX FOR PT ON RA OR SUPP 02
        4 INDEPENDENTLY HANDLES SECRETIONS    ROUTINE ACTIONS:
                                                1 ASSESS/RECORD BREATH SOUNDS Q8H & PRN
                                                2 EVALUATE RESP PATTERN/EFFORT Q8H & PRN
                                                3 TCD8 Q4H & PRN
                                                4 MONITOR & REPORT S/S HYPOXIA
                                                5 MONITOR ARGS & REPORT ARNL VALUES FOR PATIENT
                                                6 CHECK ADEQUACY & RATE OF O2 FLOW Q SHIFT & PRN
                                                7 CHECK POSITION OF O2 CANNULA/MASK Q SHIFT & PRN
                                                8 CHECK EARS/NARES FOR BREAKDOWN FROM O2 ADMINISTRATION

  4. ALTERED LOC/IMPAIRED NEUROLOGICAL STATE  TIME INITIATED: 05/24/1985 11:35   LAST UPDATED: 05/28/1985 16:26

      RELATED TO (CAUSES):                    ACTIONS:
        1 HYPOXIA/ISCHEMIA                      1 MONITOR FOR CHANGES IN LOC/PERSONALITY
                                                2 RESTRAIN AS NECESSARY TO PREVENT INJURY
      OUTCOMES:                                 3 DECREASE EXTERNAL STIMULI
        1. WITHOUT NEUROLOGICAL DEFICIT
        2 ORIENTED TO PERSON/PLACE/TIME       ROUTINE ACTIONS:
                                                1 ASSESS/RECORD ORIENTATION
                                                2 EVALUATE SENSATION & MOVEMENT OF EXTREMITIES
                                                3 EVALUATE RESPIRATORY PATTERN
                                                4 NOTIFY MD STAT OF ANY CHANGE IN NEURO STATUS
                                                5 ORIENT PATIENT TO TIME/PLACE/SITUATION
                                                6 SIDE RAILS UP AT ALL TIMES

 10. PT/FAMILY ANXIETY & UNIQUE PROBLEMS  TIME INITIATED: 04/17/1985 20:58   LAST UPDATED: 05/28/1985 16:28

      RELATED TO (CAUSES):                    ACTIONS:
        1 INFORMATIONAL NEEDS                   1 REDUCE ENVIRONMENTAL STIMULI AS MUCH AS POSSIBLE
        2 HOSPITAL ADMISSION                    2 PLAN/PROVIDE UNINTERRUPTED PERIODS OF REST
        3 PSYCHOSIS
                                              ROUTINE ACTIONS:
      OUTCOMES:                                 1 KEEP CALL LIGHT WITHIN EASY REACH
        1 PT COOPERATIVE WITH RX REGIMEN        2 ASSURE PATIENT OF NURSE ACCESSIBILITY
        2 S/O UNDERSTANDS DX/RX/PROGNOSIS       3 TEACH/REVIEW DIAGNOSIS & RELATED S/S
        3 OPTIMAL COMFORT                       4 TEACH/REVIEW PT/SO INPATIENT TREATMENT REGIMEN
                                                5 KEEP PT/SO INFORMED OF PROGRESS & CHANGES IN THERAPY
                                                6 INVOLVE PT IN PLANNING CARE/SET SHORT-TERM REALISTIC GOALS

  LAST NURSE TO UPDATE CARE PLAN: KLINGLE, CONNIE J      05/28/1985 16:28      6001200
  ///////////////////////////////////////////TEMPORARY REPORT—DISCARD WHEN UPDATED ///////////////////////
```

Figure 20–4 *(continued)*

```
NURSING CARE PLAN HISTORY      MCC      HF      PRO            369      W5      05/29/1985 10:49

    9. IMMOBILITY/IMPAIRED MUSCULO-SKELETAL FUNCTION                              TIME INITIATED: 05/25/1985 20:49
                                                                                  TIME RESOLVED: 05/29/1985 10:48

        A. RELATED TO (CAUSE) (BT – ET #) :
           1. FRACTURES          (05/25 – 05/29)
           2. PROLONGED BEDREST          (05/25 – 05/29)
           3. COMMENT:DVT RIGHT LEG          (05/25 – 5/29)

        B. ACTIONS (BT – ET #):
           1. POSITIONING: ELEVATE RIGHT LEG ON PILLOWS          (05/25 – 05/29)
           2. TEACH/REVIEW S/S WHICH REQUIRE MEDICAL ATTENTION          (05/25 – 05/29)

        C. ROUTINE ACTIONS (BT – ET #):
           1. CHECK/RECORD MOVEMENT/STRENGTH/SENSATION OF EXTREMITIES          (05/25 – 05/25)
           2. EVALUATE/RECORD RANGE OF MOTION Q SHIFT & PRN          (05/25 – 05/2))
           3. CHECK FOR/RECORD SKIN DISCOLORATION/BREAKDOWN/IRRITATION          (05/25 – 05/29)
           4. EVALUATE/RECORD ADEQUACY OF PERIPHERAL CIRCULATION Q SHIFT          (05/25 – 05/29)
           5. MONITOR FOR S/S THROMBOPHLEBITIS          (05/25 – 05/29)
           6. MASSAGE BONY PROMINENCES/PRESSURE AREAS PRN          (05/25 – 05/29)
           7. TURN & REPOSITION Q2H & PRN          (05/25 – 05/25)
           8. MAINTAIN PROPER BODY ALIGNMENT          (05/25 – 05/29)
           9. ASSIST WITH XXXX PRN          (05/25 – 05/29)
          10. EVALUATE & RECORD ACTIVITY TOLERANCE          (05/25 – 05/29)
          11. TEACH/REVIEW PT/SO INPATIENT TREATMENT REGIMEN          (05/25 – 05/29)

        D. EXPECTED OUTCOMES (BT – ET #):
           1. SKIN INTACT/NO BREAKDOWN          (05/25 – 05/29)
           2. BOWEL FUNCTION XXX FOR PATIENT          (05/25 – 05/29)
           3. OPTIMAL COMFORT          (05/25 – 05/29)


   12. ALTERED HEMATOLOGIC/COAGULATION STATUS   TIME INITIATED: 05/25/1985 20:44   TIME RESOLVED: 05/29/1985 10:48

        A. RELATED TO (CAUSE) (BT – ET #) :
           1. ANTICOAGULANT THERAPY          (05/25 – 05/29)

        B. ACTIONS (BT – ET #):
           1. USE INFUSION PUMP FOR CONTINUOUS HEPARIN DRIP          (05/25 – 05/29)
           2. TEACH/REVIEW ANTICOAGULANT REGIMEN/PRECAUTIONS          (05/25 – 05/29)
           3. TEACH/REVIEW S/S REQUIRING MEDICAL ATTENTION          (05/25 – 05/29)

        C. ROUTINE ACTIONS (BT – ET #):
           1. HANDLE PT GENTLY AT ALL TIMES          (05/25 – 05/25)
           2. CONTINUOUSLY MONITOR FOR S/S BLEEDING          (05/25 – 05/25)
           3. ASSESS/RECORD TEMP, COLOR, SENSATION OF FINGERS & TOES          (05/25 – 05/29)
           4. HEMATEST ALL URINE & EMESIS/GUAIAC ALL STOOLS          (05/25 – 05/29)
           5. OBSERVE FOR PETECHIAE/CONTUSIONS          (05/25 – 05/25)
           6. OBSERVE FOR BLEEDING GUMS OR MUCOUS MEMBRANES          (05/25 – 05/25)
           7. MONITOR ARTERIAL/VENIPUNCTURE & INJECTION SITES FOR BLEEDING          (05/25 – 05/29)
           8. CAUTIOUS MOUTH CARE WITH SOFT BRUSH OR SWABS          (05/25 – 05/25)
           9. SHAVING WITH ELECTRIC RAZOR ONLY          (05/25 – 05/25)
          10. MONITOR PERTINENT LAB: _____          (05/25 – 05/29)
          11. TEACH/REVIEW PT/SO INPATIENT REGIMEN          (05/25 – 05/25)

        D. EXPECTED OUTCOMES (BT – ET #):
           1. PT WITHIN THERAPEUTIC RANGE          (05/25 – 05/29)
           2. PT/SO UNDERSTAND HOSPITAL ROUTINE          (05/25 – 05/29)

   XX. RN'S INITIATING/CHANGING CARE PLAN FOR THIS PATIENT
           1. KLINGLE, CONNIE J          05/25
           2. PFN   , SHE J          05/25
```

Cengiz, M., Ranzenberger, J., Johnson, D., et al. Design and implementation of computerized nursing care plans. In: *Proceedings of the Seventh Annual Symposium on Computer Applications in Medical Care.* Dayhoff, R. (editor). Silver Spring, MD: IEEE Computer Society Press, 1983.

these instructions may be printed to the appropriate nursing station and to all relevant ancillary departments to alert staff to patients' needs. The usefulness of such systems, of course, depends on the system's flexibility as well as on the nurses' abilities to use the system. The latter, of course, presents another challenge for the nurse manager's training program.

Computerization also facilitates communication among nurses, especially between shifts. Most important in this regard is the fact that patient care plans become uniform and easily readable, thus reducing the possibility of ambiguity in instructions or observations. Further, because a report for each patient is updated at the beginning of a shift and printed out, the nurses have a good means for communicating needs and concerns between shifts.

The computerized chart also has implications for nursing audits, since the system has the capability of summarizing data in any desirable form. For example, a report including information about the interventions of a particular nurse can be examined easily with regard to different types of patients, on different shifts, and with regard to different criteria.

The computer also facilitates the nursing audit function in that it forces nurses to indicate their interventions more clearly than is typically done on the traditional chart. Handwritten nurses' notes are generally lengthy narratives that follow no standard format. Often they are illegible, inconsistent, full of trivia, or so brief that they are meaningless, thereby making them difficult to use, control, or audit. Computerized systems tend to force better documentation since they require nurses to choose from a specified set of options for their basic documentation and because the system reminds them if documentation is not provided. This not only makes the auditing function easier, it also solves the problems created by fear of litigation (Schifiliti, Bonasoro & Thompson, 1986).

Provision of Care

Computers are also being used to help nurses provide care to the patients. For example, computers are being used to monitor and, in some cases, control the intake and output systems to which patients might be connected. Jelliffe et al. (1983) describe the use of computers to calculate the rate at which IVs drip and to monitor and regulate that drip rate. In addition, computers are being used to regulate the pressure, volume, and flow rate of ventilators to ensure that they deliver adequate volumes of gas. Further applications include the control of fluid resuscitation, anesthesia, serum glucose levels, and arterial pressure.

Computers are also being used to help educate the patient regarding his or her health needs (Sinclair, 1985). Some systems help the nurse to explain post-hospitalization procedures to patients. Others provide interactive programs designed to help the patient increase his or her own awareness of good health habits. Some, such as PLATO STAYWELL, actually help the patient change behaviors involving weight control, smoking, or exercise—changes that are necessary for post-hospitalization care (and general good health).

Computers are increasingly being used to assist in surgery. For example, computers assist in arteriography and angiography, and participate in autotransfusion during open heart and vascular surgery. In addition, computers are being used to maintain intraocular pressure during eye surgery. They are used as well to facilitate diagnostic procedures or reconstructive surgery (Paquet, 1982).

Computerization can help the nurse evaluate symptoms. For example, one system, COMMES (Creighton On-Line Multiple Modular Expert System), acts as a professional consultant to which a nurse can turn if she is unable to interpret symptoms or if she wants help in developing care plans. This system provides the same information as a professional who is totally up to date and who never forgets (Ryan, 1985). Other systems recommend care plans based on nursing diagnoses (Oryn, 1985).

Scheduling and Staffing

Scheduling is one of the nurse manager's most frustrating and least fulfilling activities. No matter how much effort she puts into juggling the resources and policies to determine working hours, she is not likely to arrive at a stable schedule or, according to nurses, one that is both flexible and fair. The problem in developing a schedule is that there is generally too much information for one person to handle. However, the computer's specialty is just that: handling a lot of information systematically; that makes it a natural to help in the scheduling function.

The first step in developing a schedule, of course, is to analyze the need for nursing care in a particular unit. This step is, in part, dictated by hospital standards. It is also influenced by the current and expected demands for various types of nursing personnel occasioned by the patient mix of the unit. The computer can help in determining this latter requirement. The computer can determine each patient's current nursing needs by screening his or her record for assessment indicators and determining the illness acuity. This needs analysis can be helpful not only for the specific time period for which the schedule is being created, but also for long-term staffing. That is, by analyzing the historical needs per type of patient as well as needs determined by patient mix, the nurse manager can better estimate how many of what types of nurses are needed to handle the expected load of the unit (Miller, Pierskalla & Rath, 1976). (See Chapter 19 for more on classification systems to determine nursing care requirements.)

If the hospital's computer does not include historical data, then such information must be entered as input by the nurse manager (see Figure

ure 20-5 Weekly Staff Requirements

Unit Number _____

	S	M	T	W	T	F	S

Staffing Categories

(Administrators include head nurse and assistant head nurses)

Min. # administrators (SUP) shift 1 (beg 7am)
Desired # administrators (SUP) shift 1
Min. # administrators (SUP) shift 2 (beg 3pm)
Desired # administrators (SUP) shift 2
Min. # administrators (SUP) shift 3 (beg 11pm)
Desired # administrators (SUP) shift 3

(Exclude head nurse and assistant head
nurse in R.N. counts)

Min. # R.N. staff shift 1 (beg 7am)
Desired # R.N. staff shift 1
Min. # R.N. staff shift 2 (beg 3pm)
Desired # R.N. staff shift 2
Min. # R.N. staff shift 3 (beg 11pm)
Desired # R.N. staff shift 3

Min. # L.P.N. staff shift 1 (beg 7am)
Desired # L.P.N. staff shift 1
Min. # L.P.N. staff shift 2 (beg 3pm)
Desired # L.P.N. staff shift 2
Min. # L.P.N. staff shift 3 (beg 11pm)
Desired # L.P.N. staff shift 3

Staffing Categories (con't.)

Min. # aide staff shift 1 (beg 7am)
Desired # aide staff shift 1
Min. # aide staff shift 2 (beg 3pm)
Desired # aide staff shift 2
Min. # aide staff shift 3 (beg 11pm)
Desired # aide staff shift 3

Min. # secretaries shift 1 (beg 7am)
Desired # secretaries shift 1
Min. # secretaries shift 2 (beg 3pm)
Desired # secretaries shift 2
Min. # secretaries shift 3 (beg 11pm)
Desired # secretaries shift 3

Minimum Requirements for Skill Categories in Combination

Min. # SUP + R.N.'s shift 1 (beg 7am)
Min. # SUP + R.N.'s shift 2 (beg 3pm)
Min. # SUP + R.N.'s shift 3 (beg 11pm)

Min. # SUP + R.N. + L.P.N.'s shift 1 (beg 7am)
Min. # SUP + R.N. + L.P.N.'s shift 2 (beg 3pm)
Min. # SUP + R.N. + L.P.N.'s shift 3 (beg 11pm)

Min. # SUP + R.N. + L.P.N. + aides shift 1 (beg 7am)
Min. # SUP + R.N. + L.P.N. + aides shift 2 (beg 3pm)
Min. # SUP + R.N. + L.P.N. + aides shift 3 (beg 11pm)

From Smith, L. Douglas and A. Wiggins "A Computer-Based Nurse Scheduling System" Computer and Operations Research, p. 195–212. Pergamon Press, Ltd, 1977.

Figure 20–6 Prototype

Employee Data Form for Shift Scheduling

1. Name ___Blank, L.___   2. Employee Number _____10886_____

3. Classification _____1_____ (1-head nurse, 2-assistant head, 3-RN, 4-LPN, 5-NA/ORD, 6-Sec.)

4. Unit Number _____215_____

Number of Shifts to be Assigned Weekly:
5. Minimum __3__   6. Desired __5__   7. Maximum __6__

8. Number of weekends can work between weekends off _____1_____

Length of work stretch (consec. days):
9. Min. (usually 2) __2__   10. Max. (usually 6) __6__

11. Shift Rankings (1: beg.—7 am; 2: beg.—3 pm; 3: beg.—11 pm)
(If hired for straight shifts, specify first choice only)
First Choice __1__   Second Choice __3__   Third Choice __2__

12. Allocate 10 aversion points among choices of shift (aversion points must *increase* in value from 1st to 2nd to 3rd choice—let first choice aversion be 9999 if on straight shifts).
First Choice   Second Choice   Third Choice
Aversion __0__   Aversion __5__   Aversion __5__

13. Indicate preference for the first day off in a week prior to a weekend off. (2=Mon.; 3=Tues.; 4=Wed.; 5=Thurs.; 6=Fri.)

First Choice	Second Choice	Third Choice	Fourth Choice	Fifth Choice
__2__	__3__	__4__	__6__	__5__

14. Indicate preference for the second day off in a week following a weekend off.

First Choice	Second Choice	Third Choice	Fourth Choice	Fifth Choice
__6__	__2__	__4__	__3__	__5__

15. Indicate preference for day-off pairs midweek. [Usual alternatives are (2,3), (3,4), (4,5), (5,6), (2,5), (2,6), (3,6).]
First Choice Pair _3_,_4_ ; Second Choice _2_,_3_ ; Third Choice _4_,_5_ ; Fourth Choice _5_,_6_ ;
Fifth Choice _2_,_6_ ; Sixth Choice _3_,_6_ ; Seventh Choice _2_,_5_ .

16. Cumulative number of holidays due __0__

17. Cumulative number of vacation days due __0__

18. Current value of shift aversion index __5.__

19. Current value of day-off aversion index __2.__

20. Number of times shifts worked to date:
Shift 1 __0__   Shift 2 __0__   Shift 3 __0__

21. Shift worked on last day of previous month __1__

22. Number of weekends worked since last weekend off __1__

23. Last day off previous week __6__

24. Remarks:

Adapted from Smith, L. Douglas, and Wiggins, A. A Computer-Based Nurse Scheduling System.
Computer and Operations Research, 195–212. Copyright 1977, Pergamon Press, Ltd., 1977.

20–5). Once the accumulated work load needs have been established, the computer can consider the actual scheduling question. A nurse manager would use the nursing needs, the hospital policies in regard to nurse scheduling, and the numbers and qualifications of available staff as input to the system. Many systems have additional flexibility and can accept information about the preferences of nurses and their past schedules or performance to help obtain a schedule that meets not only the requirements, but also the preferences of the nursing staff (see Figure 20–6).

Once given these data, the computer, much like a nurse manager, juggles the demands of the unit against the supply of nursing personnel for that unit. One difference between the approach that the computer and the nurse manager use is that the computer can consider all possible options and their value before choosing a given schedule. Further, the computer is impartial and can weigh many more factors at any given time than can the nurse manager.

An example of a schedule that might result from computer evaluation of the staffing needs is shown in Figure 20–7. It obviously looks very much like one prepared by hand. This may be the final schedule, or, if the system has not been able to consider staff preferences and other qualitative factors, it can be considered a good starting point for building a schedule.

The nurse manager does not need to rely on the capabilities of the hospital's computer to perform these tasks. There are some relatively low cost microcomputer packages, such as "Recommended Staffing" and "Daily Report," that provide help in setting staffing levels. Further, packages such as MONA (MOdular Nursing Administrator), also available for the microcomputer, help in creating schedules that meet staffing needs and are sensitive to staff preferences.

In summary, it is advantageous to use computers for scheduling functions. Nurses are often more satisfied with their schedule, primarily because they perceive that they are being treated more fairly. Also, unlike most nurse managers, the computer can easily balance all the necessary information for even the largest of units (Smith & Bird, 1979; Smith, Wiggins & Bird, 1979). Further, because the computer can consider the needs for personnel beyond any one unit, it can evaluate opportunities for sharing personnel with other units to improve the overall efficiency of nursing coverage. Finally, the computer can handle the complexities associated with flextime and split shifts that are almost impossible to consider by hand; this capability can make the unit a more desirable working place (Fitzpatrick, Farrell & Richter-Zeunick, 1987).

Training and Evaluation

Computerized instruction can be an invaluable tool for nurse managers who need either to transmit new information to their staff or to review acquired information (Sweeney, O'Malley & Freeman, 1982). For ex-

Figure 20–7 Schedule Results

Schedule for Period Beginning June 10 1973

	10 Su	11 Mo	12 Tu	13 We	14 Th	15 Fr	16 Sa	17 Su	18 Mo	19 Tu	20 We	21 Th	22 Fr	23 Sa	24 Su	25 Mo	26 Tu	27 We	28 Th	29 Fr	30 Sa	1 Su	2 Mo	3 Tu	4 We	5 Th	6 Fr	7 Sa	Ro/%n	WE	RG	RM	*W
1. Hale	D	D	D		D	D	D			D	D	D		D	D	D	D		D	D	D		D	D	D		D	D		50	0	0	28
2. Collins	D		D	D	D	D		D	D	D		D	D	D		D	D	D		D	D	D	D	D	D	D			50	0	0	12
3. Smith	N	–	–	–		N	N	N	N	N	N	N			N	N	N		N	N	N	N	N	N		N	N		51	0	0	28
4. Palmer	N	N			N	N	N	N	B		–	–	–	–	–		N	N	N	N	N		N	N	N	N			0	0	28
5. Jones	N	N	N					N	N			N	N	N	N	N		*	*	*	*	N	N						51	40	40	28
6. Peabody	DE	D		E	E	E	E		E	E		D	D	D	D		D	D		D	D	D	D		D	D	D	*	26	48	5	5	28
7. Penna	DN	N	N		D	D	D	*	–	–	C		N	N	N	N		N	D	D	D	D		D	D	D		D	D	27	48	5	5	28
8. Clark	DN	*	–	–	–	–	–	*	D	D	D		N	N	N		D	D	D	D		D	D	D	D		D	D		23	50	12	12	28
9. Cunkle	DR	D		N	N	D	D		D	D	D	D		D	D		E	C	C	C		E	E	E	E		D	27/10	50	0	0	28
10. Myers	DR		D	D	D	D		N	N	D	D		D	D		D	D	E	E		E	E	E	E		D	D		28/9	50	0	0	28
11. Hill	DR		D	D	D		D	E	E	E		D	D	D		D	C	C	C		N	D	D	D		N	25/10	51	0	0	28		
12. Andrews	E	E	E		E	E	E	*	*	–	E	E		E	E	E	E		E	E	E		*	*	E	E	E		E	E	50	10	10	28
13. Sutherland	E	E	E	E		E	E	*	*	–	E	E	E		E	E	E	E		E	E		*	*	H	–	–	–		*	51	35	35	28
14. Levine	E		E	E	E	E		E	E	E		E	E	E		E		E	E	E		E	E	E	E		E	E		50	0	0	28
15. Anderson	D		D	D	D		D	D	D		D	D	D	D		D	D	D	D		D	D		D	D		D	D		53	0	0	8
16. Green	DE		D	D	D	D	D		D	D		E	E	E	E		D	D	D	D		D	D		E	E	E		27	51	0	5	28
17. Majors	N		N	N	N	N	N		–	–	–	–		*	*	–		N	N	N	N		N	N	N	N			6	6	28	
18. Greenberg	DE	D	E	E		D	D	*	*	B	–		D	D	D	D		C	C	C		E	E		D	D	D		25	50	13	13	28
19. Waxman	DR		D	D	D		D	D	D	N	N	N		N		D	E	E		D	D	D	D		D	D	D		26/10	50	0	0	28
20. Hagen	DE	D	D	D		E	E		D	D	D	D	*		–	*	*	*		D	D	D		D	E	E		D	24	51	11	11	28
21. Pearlman	DE	E		D	D	D	D		*	D	D	D		D	D	E	E		D	D	D		D	D		D	D	D	23	50	5	6	28
22. Wilson	DE		D	D	D	D		E	E	E	E		D	D	D	D		D	D		*	D	D	D	D		E	25	51	5	5	28
23. Grycz	E		E	E	E	E	*	E	E	E	*		E	E	E		E	E	E	E		*	E	E	E	*		E	E	E	50	5	5	28
24. Rapley	E	E	E	E		E			E		E	E	E	E	E		E	E		E	E	E	*		E	E	E		50	0	0	28
25. James	E			E			E	E	E									E	E	E	E								50	0	0	28
26. McCarry	N	N	N			N	N	N	N			N	N	N	N				N	N	N	N			N	N			0	0	28	
27. Barkan	N	N	N	N	N	N		N	N	N	N	N		N	N	N	N	N		N	N	N	N	N			N	N	0	0	28	
28. Downing	N			N	N	N	N	N		N	N	N	N	N		N	N	N	N	N		N	N	N	N				0	0	28	
29. Gammer	D			D	D	D	D	D		D	D	D	D		D	D	D	D	D		D	D	D	P	D				0	0	28	
30. Mitchell	D	D	D	D	D			D	D	D	D	D		D	D	D	D	D		D	D	D	D						0	0	28	
31. Liary	E		E		E		E		E		E	E		E		E	E			E		E	E		E	E	E		0	0	28	
32. Santos	E		E	E	E	E		E	E	E	E		E	E	E	E		E	E	E	E		E	E	E	E			0	0	28	

RNS

	10	11	12	13	14	15	16	17	18	19	20	21	22	23	24	25	26	27	28	29	30	1	2	3	4	5	6	7
Nite	2	2	2	2	2	2	2	2	2	2	2	3	2	2	2	2	2	2	2	2	2	2	2	2	2	2	2	2
Day	3	6	5	6	6	6	4	3	6	5	6	6	3	3	6	7+6	5	5	4	4	7+6	6	6	6	3			
Even	2	3	3	3	4	3	2	2	3	3	3	3	3	3	3	3	3	3	2	2	3	4	3	3	3	2		

RN+LPN

	10	11	12	13	14	15	16	17	18	19	20	21	22	23	24	25	26	27	28	29	30	1	2	3	4	5	6	7
Nite	2	3	3	3	3	3	3	3	3	3	3	2	3	3	3	3	2	2	3	3	3	3	3	2				
Day	5	9	9	9	9	10+5	5	8	7	7	7	8	6	5	9	9	8	8	9	5	9	9	9	9	10+6			
Even	4	6	6	5	6	5	4	4	6	5	5	6	5	4	5	6	5	5	5	4	6	6	5	6	5	4		

TOTAL

	10	11	12	13	14	15	16	17	18	19	20	21	22	23	24	25	26	27	28	29	30	1	2	3	4	5	6	7
Nite	4	5	5	5	5	4	4	5	5	5	5	4	4	5	5	5	5	4	4	5	5	5	5	4				
Day	6	10	11	11	11	6	6	9	9	9	9	6	10	11	10	10	6	6	10	11	11	11	7					
Even	4	7	7	7	7	5	4	7	6	7	7	5	5	7	6	7	6	7	5	4	7	7	7	7	5			

* REQUEST;   – VACATION;   C HOSPITAL BUSINESS;   B BIRTHDAY;   H HOLIDAY OFF

From Warner, Michael (1976) "Scheduling Nursing Personnel According to Nursing Preference—A Mathematical Programming Approach." *Operations Research*, p. 642–56. Operations Research Society of America. No further reproduction permitted without the consent of the copyright owner.

ample, computer-aided instruction (CAI) has been used in such areas as postoperative nursing care, diagnosis of myocardial infarctions, heredity/genetics, maternity nursing, and introductory pharmacology. These systems provide text, graphics, and automation to make the material easier to understand. Further, because of its interactive nature, CAI allows the student to receive immediate feedback and to proceed at her or his own speed.

With the proliferation of microcomputers came increasing opportunities for interactive systems that facilitate the teaching and practicing of nursing functions. Such technology allows the nurse to practice a wide range of skills, such as the calculation of fractional medication dosage, without jeopardy to the patient. Furthermore, the technology provides a variety of modes, from programmed learning to graphic simulations of nursing situations. One system, for example, provides a self-learning program on the physical assessment and clinical interpretation of arterial pulses. Another system helps nurses become proficient in calculating drug dosages by providing pharmacological information and simple mathematical formulas as references, as well as problems (with explanations) on which the students can practice.

Other systems provide realistic situations on which the nurse can practice. For example, one provides descriptions of ICU patients whom the nurse must evaluate and for whom she must select a course of action; the system responds with an evaluation of those choices. Another system simulates three hours of postoperative care with which the nurse must interact at 15-minute intervals; evaluations are made of her performance.

New packages are becoming available for nursing education at a rapid pace. A good summary of over 90 packages (and ordering information), from clinical simulations of postoperative care of a child to help with medical terms can be found in Saba and McCormick (1986:366–386). More information about currently available systems can be found in the "Software Exchange" section of *Computers in Nursing*. If nurses do not find what they need there, however, they can still take advantage of this new technology because many companies are now marketing CAI "shells," such as NEMAS (Nursing Education Module Authoring System) for use by nursing professionals. These shells can help the nurse manager develop her own software to use for training. Once the nurse manager communicates the intention of the CAI, the content of the information about which the training is intended to communicate, and the mode that she would like to use, the shell devises a training package to meet her needs. The form of this communication with the computer varies from choices of options available to actual programming of procedures and drawing of graphics. As with other software products for the microcomputer, these shells are becoming more sophisticated, easier to use, and less expensive over time. Further, literature in which individuals explain how they developed a package and provide guidelines for others is increasing as well (see, for example, Thiele [1986]).

However they are created, these computerized instructional systems can be an asset to the nurse manager. The advantages lie primarily in their flexibility in allowing learners to proceed at their own pace, their infinite patience in repeating material for individual users, and their nonjudgmental approach to instruction. Programs for remedial training can spare the learner anxiety and embarrassment and liberate instructors from tedious, time-consuming sessions. Further, as the amount of nursing information continues to explode, computerized instructional packages will help everyone keep pace, and computerized databases of nursing information will provide a ready source of instructional material. Finally, computers will allow more effective dissemination of information to nurses in remote areas who might not have continuing education or inservice programs available.

The nurse manager cannot, however, rely on the computer to fulfill all of her or his instructional responsibilities. There will continue to be a need for human-to-human interaction in the learning process. Further, even if some of the training can be done with a computer, there will always be a need for supervision and feedback when the nurse implements new skills in the work setting. Nevertheless, using the computer to teach the initial concepts and skills allows the instructor or manager more time for individual instruction and for helping nurses gain proficiency with a skill.

INDIRECT APPLICATIONS TO NURSING

Pharmacy, Laboratory, and Radiology Systems

While the major benefits to nursing of a computerized system are the reduction in time spent doing paperwork and the associated increase in time available for professional nursing functions, computers are also helpful when nursing is interfacing with support units such as pharmacy, laboratory, and radiology (Johnston et al., 1976). Computers can increase the effectiveness of the interface between nursing and these units by making the communications clearer and more uniform, and can increase the efficiency of the interface by reducing the amount of time spent in this function.

For example, in many hospitals, nurses are responsible for recordkeeping related to medication orders and administration; in smaller hospitals they might also be responsible for dosage preparation and medication inventory. A computerized system can help in the recordkeeping and can be used to request medication from the pharmacy (see Figure 20–8).

The nurse's interface with such systems varies. In one system, pharmacy personnel collect and use carbon copies of physicians' medication orders; they input the information into the system. Then, at regular intervals, the pharmacy makes the requested medication available to the nurses for administration. The only paperwork necessary for the nurse is to complete a form that is returned to the pharmacy indicating that the medication has been administered or, if not, why not. All other recordkeeping is done on the computer at the pharmacy.

If the charts are computerized, the orders to the pharmacy are placed automatically when the physician enters instructions. Alternatively, the nurse might simply enter the information on a terminal at the nursing station.

Whatever the form of input to the system, computerized pharmacy systems allow for better auditing of medication (Freibrun, 1976; Long, 1982). For example, on some systems, when a medication order is input into the system, it is accompanied by diagnosis, allergy information, and demographic data. This information is automatically checked to ensure

Figure 20–8   Nursing/Pharmacy Interfaces

```
■       P H A R M A C Y   A C T I V E   O R D E R   P R O F I L E  07-30--- 1200
PATIENT NAME                 AGE  SEX  NSTA  ROOM-BED   PATIENT-ID   WEIGHT      SURG DT/TM

▶MYERS MARTHA R          ◀24Y   F    4C    4436-02     803254      110 LB
  ALLERGIES-FOOD:       CITRUS FRUITS AND MILK PRODUCTS
▶ALLERGIES-MED/OTHER:PENICILLIN
  PATIENT PROBLEMS:     HEARING IMPAIRMENT-USES HEARING AID
CURRENT DIAG: POSSIBLE CHOLECYSTOLITHIASIS                          MED INFO:

ORDER  PROC   RT  FREQUENCY   START DT/TM  LAST DT/TM  DOSAGE  ORDERING DOCTOR
0015   14652 ▶IM  Q4HPRN      07-29 1400               50MG    BROWN J C
       ▶DRAMAMINE            50.000MG/1ML INJECTION
DIMENHYDRINATE                SEAPLE
0016   17854 ▶IM  Q4HPRN      07-29 1400   08-01 1400  50MG    BROWN J C
       ▶DEMEROL              50.000MG/1ML INJECTION
       MEPERIDINE HYDROCHLORIDE           XXXXX




                                                                   Page 1
```

(a) Obtaining medication information from a pharmacy profile.

BHIS (Unisys)

```
■          P H A R M A C Y   I V   O R D E R   E N T R Y      07-29---1030
PATIENT NAME             PTID/RMBD    ORDERING DOCTOR
MYERS MARTHA R           4436-02      BROWN J C                     SURG:
CURR DIAG: POSSIBLE CHOLECYSTOLITHIASIS                  MED INFO:

▶024    SOLUTION—SELECT ONE FROM BASE SOLUTIONS BELOW OR ENTER OTHER SOLUTION
▶14     VOLUME 1 = 1000CC   2 = 500CC  3 = 250CC  4 = 100CC  OTHER ▶      ◀
                   ENTER X BESIDE ADDITIVES TO INCLUDE IN ORDER
                        ▶****** A D D I T I V E S ******◀
  ▶ ◀ KCL 40 MEQ                    ▶ ◀ AMINOPHYLLIN 500 MG
  ▶ ◀ BERROCA-C 500 4 CC            ▶ ◀ KEFLIN 10M
  ▶ ◀ BERROCA-C 2 CC               ▶ ◀ SODIUM PENICILLIN C 5 MG
  ▶ ◀ MVI CONCEN 5 CC              ▶ ◀ ADDITIONAL ADDITIVES
                        ▶****** B A S E   S O L U T I O N ******◀
01 = 5% DEX & 2% SOD CHL           11 = 50% DEX INJ
02 = 5% DEX INJ                    12 = 5% DEX EL-LYTE #75
03 = 5% DEX & .45% SOD CHL         13 = 5% DEX/ASCOR-B-SOL
04 = 5% DEX IN LACT RING INJ       14 = 2.5% DEX & .45% SOD CHL
05 = LACTATED RINGERS INJ          15 = AMMON CHL IN W 2.14%
06 = SOD CHL INJ .9                16 = 10% DEX & .9% SOD CHL
07 = 10% INV SUGAR IN ELECT 2      17 = SODIUM LACTATE INJ
08 = DEX & .9% SOD CHL             18 = 5% SOD BICARBONATE
09 = 5% DEX EL-LYTE #48            19 = 6% SOD BICARBONATE
10 = 10% DEX INJ                   OTHER=▶
                                                                   Page 1
```

(b) Entering medication orders.

BHIS (Unisys)

that the medication ordered will not conflict with other medication or with treatments or individual characteristics contraindicating use, such as age. Further, the nurse or pharmacist can double-check the appropriateness of medication for a particular diagnosis.

The computer also creates an easily accessible record of medication patterns and reasons for failure to maintain those patterns. For example, in some systems, the nurse receives medication prepackaged for each patient and must return the package after the medication has been administered. If the medication was not given, the nurse must state those reasons on the package. These packages, when returned to the pharmacy, provide data to be used as input into the pharmacy system. These data can be accessed easily for evaluating a particular patient, all patients in a particular unit, all patients in a particular diagnostic category, or all patients receiving that medication. More important, these summaries can be provided in a matter of minutes.

Further, when medications are prepared for a unit, an accompanying list, categorized by patient is provided to the nursing station. In some systems, this list may include dosage information as well as cautions for the administration of the medication and possible or expected reactions of the patient to the medication. In other systems, the computer sends a reminder that medications are due at a given time; it also sends a "late" reminder if a record of medication administration is not received when it should be.

Computerized systems can be designed to include as part of the pharmacy system a "library" of drug information that can be reviewed to determine the expected side effects of medication, drug interactions (especially synergistic ones), and associated nursing requirements. Or, the nursing unit may have a stand-alone system, such as "Nursing Pharmacology," on which they can check the compatibility of drug interactions, drug dosages, time infusion rates, etc. Such systems can also prepare instructions for patients when they leave the hospital, including the purpose for each drug, its possible side effects, appropriate dietary or activity instructions, and effects that should be reported to the physician.

Laboratory and radiology systems have similar advantages from the nursing perspective (Grams, 1977). Entering an order into the patient's chart automatically alerts the appropriate unit to schedule a test. Once the test has been scheduled, some systems will send a pretest regimen for the patient or reminders of schedules to the nursing station. In many cases, these studies are analyzed by a computer and the results are routed immediately to the nursing station, entered into the patient's chart, and summarized for review by the nurse and physician.

Such computerized systems tend to decrease errors because they have better and more systematic checks than manual operations, they reduce the amount of nursing time spent away from patient care, and they reduce the amount of waste due to errors. However, they can also have some disadvantages, which need the attention of the nurse manager. The most significant problem is how the nurses react when the computer is not available for use. Many nurses, even those who were at the hospital before computerization, forget the necessary procedures for ordering medication, X-rays, and tests without the computer. Since computer failures are a reality in all organizations, the nurse manager must prepare the staff for handling this situation. Furthermore, she must ensure that appropriate regimens are being followed even if, because of computer failure, nurses are not able to receive "reminders."

The second problem associated with these systems with which the nurse manager must cope is more subtle: it is the absence of human interaction between the unit and other units on a regular basis. Sometimes, smoothly operating systems exist because people can relate to people in the other unit on a one-to-one basis. If all the communications are electronic, then those relationships and the value they add to the system are lost. Thus, if such relationships are necessary for operations, the nurse manager must foster them in other ways.

Supplies and Materials Management

Nurse managers and materials managers frequently clash because the former contend that supplies are not available when needed while the latter contend that too many supplies are not being used or kept in inventory. The resulting conflict stems from the perspectives of the two positions. The nurse manager's responsibility is to ensure that the supplies necessary for high quality care are available; she, therefore, perceives the shortage costs as the highest priority in determining an inventory policy. Materials managers, on the other hand, are responsible for the total cost of supplies, including holding and transaction costs in addition to the costs of shortages; these managers, therefore, are concerned about economy in purchasing and minimizing costs for holding unused items in inventory. Obviously a "good" inventory policy is one that can be understood by all parties involved. Once again, the computer, with its almost limitless capability for weighing many factors simultaneously, organizing data, and preparing reports can be an effective tool for resolving conflict between the two perspectives.

A computerized inventory system has two purposes: (a) to generate efficient inventory policies that could be considered for implementation and (b) to maintain control over how supplies are being used. To meet these goals, the system must be able to keep accurate records of the supplies being used in each unit as well as to determine when to place an order for more supplies. Obviously, these goals require the system to maintain records that go beyond how much inventory is available at any given time. The system must also be able to forecast usage of supplies, determine the time at which reordering should occur, and determine the total amount of an item that should be ordered at any given time. Furthermore, the system must be able to analyze each item or group of items separately to determine if different ordering policies are warranted for different supplies.

Most systems for supplies and materials management have the capacity to examine each product separately, maintain records of available supplies, and determine when new orders should be placed (Housley, 1974; Klein, 1979). Further, in each of the systems, the materials manager or the nurse manager can set a "safety stock" level, that is, the amount of supplies that should be available in case of emergency or if an order is not delivered on time.

The differences among systems center on how the forecasting of future demand is computed and on how the removal of products from inventory is controlled and audited. Some systems require that demand be input by the nurse manager; she must make an educated guess on what the patient mix will be over time and what supplies are warranted for that mix. In other systems, demand is computed on the assumption that the same usage of supplies that was observed in the most recent similar period will continue over some future period. The remainder of the systems have a forecasting component that analyzes trends in past usage of supplies for a particular mix of patients at a particular time of year and bases the forecast on the assumption that these conditions will continue.

Similarly, packages differ on how the requests for items are entered into the system and on how much control there is over reporting of items on that system. For example, in some systems, the nurse manager completes an inventory request form that is forwarded to the materials manager who will provide the materials and enter the information into the computer system. On more sophisticated systems, the nurse manager would simply type a request for supplies into the terminal; the request would then automatically be forwarded to the materials management department for action.

The second system enables greater control over the inventory. It limits the number of people with authority to order items by assigning codes to authorized individuals and allowing access to order particular items only to those individuals. This makes it possible to keep track of who ordered a specific item, when it was ordered, and for what unit. On the other hand, the first system has more flexibility in terms of who may order supplies. More important, however, because items need not be entered into the system before requests are filled, this activity might be delayed, records might be lost, and control may not be maintained. Thus, although it may take more time if the system is not well designed, it is easier to set up an audit trail (to find where an error is) in the second system that will maintain appropriate records. Such a system not only minimizes unauthorized use of supplies but also develops an historical database for the study of usage trends.

COMPLETE HOSPITAL INFORMATION SYSTEM

Each of the applications previously identified, as well as some others, can be used independently. However, computerization is more effective when an integrated system is in place through which the various units might communicate (Valentino, 1974; Slack, 1981). An integrated system such as this is referred to as a hospital information system (HIS) or a medical information system (MIS).

The specifics of what is meant by the term differ depending on what level of system is implemented. The lowest level of HIS is primarily a financial tracking system, whereby computers are used to record admissions and discharges of patients, and to compute bills. Typical systems have terminals in admissions and in the billing departments; more sophisticated systems also have terminals at the nursing stations, through which admissions can inform the nurses that patients are being admitted or transferred to their floor and through which nurses can record services rendered.

The next level of HIS retains records of patient progress as well as facilitates interaction between the nursing station and ancillary departments. Computers can be used not only to record protocols for and responses of the patients, but also to save these data for future evaluation. Furthermore, the HIS can be used to request tests and to receive the results from the tests.

The highest level of HIS allows all of the previous possibilities plus uses the computer to analyze trends in patient response and to develop care plans. This last level is referred to as a total hospital information system. The benefits of such a system will be illustrated by showing how information about a typical patient flows through the system (see Figure 20–9).

When a patient enters the hospital (let us assume that it is a man), his registration information is entered into the system. If the patient was previously hospitalized, the information from that stay can be retrieved, verified, and updated with any information that has changed since the previous registration. After admission, the physician's orders are entered into the system by ward clerks or directly by the physician. Requisitions for tests, medications, and supplies will print automatically in the appropriate department. The physician or nurse will enter the patient assessment information, which will later lead to the patient care plan process.

After evaluation of the patient and after receiving the physician's orders, the nurse also will develop a care plan that she or the ward clerk can enter into the system. Requests for tests will automatically be sent to the appropriate departments. The laboratory automatically receives admission and order data from the HIS. If necessary, the laboratory sends the schedule for the test and necessary information about patient preparation to the nursing station. After the test, the technologist releases the results

Figure 20–9 Information Transfer in a Hospital Information System

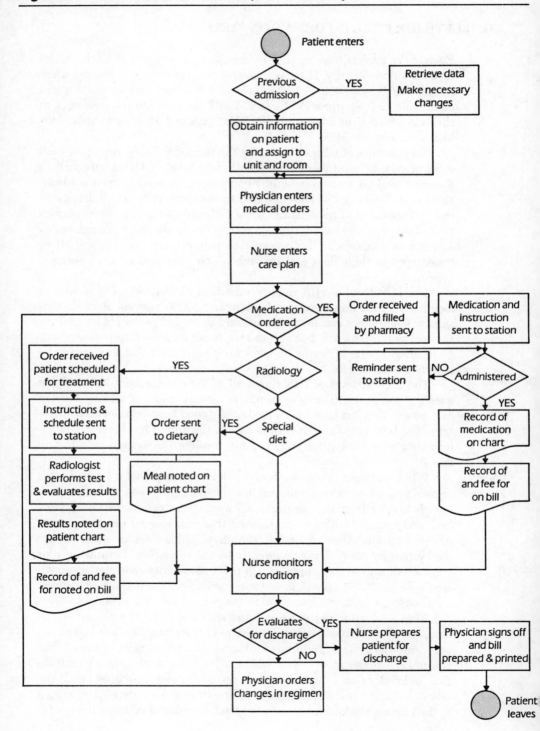

from the instruments to be available immediately for retrieval at any terminal. If the results are abnormal or the test was ordered "stat," the result will print automatically and an alarm on the printer will alert the nursing staff.

After the patient has been to radiology, stenographers will enter results from the radiologist's dictations. These can be reported by means of preformatted normal results or a free text format to summarize any deviations from normal. The radiologist reviews the preliminary results, noting any corrections, and then releases the result to the nursing unit. The radiology department receives a daily report of patients with outstanding orders and those whose tests were completed the previous day. This is all done automatically. As tests become available, they will be sent directly to the nursing station. This allows the nurse to evaluate results immediately and make any changes to the care plan.

The respiratory therapy department receives daily lists of patients with a respiratory therapy order from the nursing units. These lists are used as the basis for assigning therapists and rounds. The therapists chart their treatments and notes on a terminal. Their entries also create the charges associated with the treatments, which are then transferred to the financial system for billing.

The dietary department and the nursing units receive a diet list prior to each meal and a supplement list in the evening that reflects the patient's current diet and any information regarding special preparation for tests.

The pharmacy receives a requisition in the form of a label for each new order. A patient profile is printed daily, containing each patient's current medication orders plus other tests, orders, and patient information that require the pharmacist's attention. A medication due list is printed each hour at the nursing station to remind nurses to administer medications promptly. The nurse then charts the medications as "given" or "not given," time administered, and route of administration, along with any associated information such as an apical pulse or patient complaint. For medications that are not charted as given, a reminder notice will print automatically. Prior to each shift, the nursing unit receives a printout for each patient reflecting current orders, test preparation information, and nursing measures. In some units, the system will also be recording changes in the patient and will inform the nurse (through an alarm) of any change that needs her attention immediately.

At discharge, the physician can review the chart at a CRT, sign any phoned or verbal orders, and then enter the discharge summary information. All the charges associated with medications, tests, and treatment have been automatically captured and transferred to the financial system.

After the patient is discharged, all the information related to his admission is transferred to a magnetic tape. The database can be used by hospitals to determine the utilization of drugs, admissions by diagnosis, and statistics for strategic planning or research, or it can be used as patient history if the patient is readmitted.

Of course, this is only a sampling of the interactions that a nurse might have with an HIS. The example does, however, illustrate several important advantages for the nurse. First, HIS facilitates reading and understanding of both the physician's instructions and the nursing care plans. Since all entries use standard forms, the chart documents have a uniform format that makes them readable and clear. This reduces the ambiguity that often results from handwritten observations and instructions. Second, the system allows results from tests and radiology to be available to the nursing staff as soon as possible, thus reducing the delay that is often characteristic of manual systems and allowing the nurse to make changes in her care plans as early as possible. Third, it facilitates the discussion of patient care between shifts because care plans and test results are available in an easily followed format for consideration. Fourth, it provides reminders of care needs such as medication administration or special preparation for tests. Fifth, it facilitates the preparation of care reports. Finally, it improves the utility of the patient chart not only because of the previously stated advantages, but also because the computer itself can perform some analyses of the information in order to highlight abnormalities that need attention or peculiarities that arise in response to patient care.

Figure 20–10 illustrates the changes that would be experienced by

Figure 20–10 Comparison of Manual and Automated System

Manual	Automated
Physician order	Physician order
Check chart.	Check chart.
Stamp pharmacy request with patient plate.	Sign on to terminal.
Transcribe order to requisition.	Enter medication order via pharmacy pathway.
Telehone pharmacy regarding STAT. Have STAT request taken to pharmacy.	Requisition prints in pharmacy. New order prints on unit (bells on both printers ring because of STAT).
Fill out medication card or sheet. (Calculate schedule and stop time.)	Give copy of new order to nurse.
Add medication to patient Kardex.	
Tell nurse of STAT order.	

Problems	Solutions
1. Legibility	1. All reports legible
2. Number of forms handled on nursing unit	2. None used to enter order
3. Error potential on schedule calculated	3. Calculated automatically
4. Delay in pharmacy receiving request	4. Immediate notification

the staff as a result of conversion to an automated system. In the manual system, the nurse spends substantial time completing paperwork, waiting on the telephone, and running errands. With a computerized system she has only to enter the information on the terminal and all of the paperwork is completed and all orders are sent automatically (Cook & McDowell, 1975). Further, the total system eliminates problems in reading reports and delays in sending or receiving orders and decreases the errors made in calculations because the human interaction in these areas is minimized.

NONHOSPITAL SYSTEMS

Computers can be used in nursing outside of the hospital environment, such as in home health care. Historically, the use of computers in the non-hospital environment has followed the same pattern of use as that in hospitals. The early use was in the development of financial and accounting records through which the agency could track patients and employees as well as generate bills. For example, using computerization, agency directors were able to analyze the sources of patient referrals as well as the patterns of where patients were located. With this new information, agency directors were better able to determine how to improve the effectiveness and efficiency of their marketing strategies.

Over time, computerization has facilitated the management of staff as well. Schedules can be developed that will minimize the amount of time the nurse spends in nonnursing activities, thus maximizing the amount of time available for patient care. Also, with greater confidence in computers, managers have begun to use them to track nurses' performance, thereby allowing them to evaluate staff more fairly. This, in turn, has reduced the need for close monitoring; nurses often do not need to check in with their supervisors daily and so can spend more time with their patients.

More recently, computers have also been used by nurses in patient care. Nurses can keep uniform notes on patient changes, thus providing more reliable observation records and care plans. Based on these developments, nurses in home health care will probably soon be deriving the same benefits from computerized systems that nurses in hospitals do now. That is, nurses will have available a base of information for reference, the capability to communicate with other professionals, and access to extensive training packages.

SURVIVING WITH COMPUTERS

One purpose of a computerized system is to reduce the amount of paperwork done by nurses and thus facilitate patient care. The key to surviving with computers is to remember that fact.

The nurse's and nurse manager's jobs will change as a result of computerization. For example, the nurse manager will not need to dedicate as much attention to the scheduling function and hence will have more time and energy for improving the interworking relationships and the efficiency and the effectiveness of her unit, and for developing better educational programs for the unit staff. In short, the nurse and nurse manager will spend less time being clerks and more time being professional nurses.

The transition from a noncomputerized system to a computerized one will not be easy, however. The difficulty was, perhaps, best described by Machiavelli in 1513:

There is nothing more difficult to plan, more doubtful of success nor more dangerous to manage than the creation of a new system. For the initiator has the enmity of all who would profit by the preservation of the old system and merely lukewarm defenders of those who would gain by the new.

In other words, there generally will be a great deal of resistance to the introduction of computerization (or even to a new type of system or the addition of new capabilities). There are things the nurse manager can do, however, to make the adoption of and adaptation to computers easier for her unit. For example, Ward (1984) suggests there are three keys: (a) the development of a nursing manual, (b) the creation of computer classes for nurses, and (c) the creation of a user group. The manual is necessary, according to Ward, because the computer manual that comes with the system is generally too technical and not relevant to nurses. A manual written expressly for nurses will give them something to which to refer and hence make the nurses feel more secure about using the system. The second recommendation is to develop courses about the system for nurses. Based on her experience, Ward recommends that nurses attend these courses off-hours, but be paid at their regular rate. By having them off-hours, job conflicts are eliminated; by paying the regular rate, the likelihood of participation is increased. Finally, she recommends that a nursing users' group be established and meet regularly. This group could serve as a forum for discussion (and, one hopes, resolution) of problems or anxieties and perhaps also as a forum for generating ideas for enhancing the system to better meet the needs of nursing.

Gibson and Rose (1986) also suggest strategies for managing resistance to computerization. They too feel that making time for education for the nursing staff is crucial. Further, they recommend that the nurse manager market the concept before installation by highlighting the advantages of the system to her nurses; the greater the apparent advantage *before* the system appears, the more likely the advantage will be realized. Finally, they suggest that after the system is in place, the nurse manager provide time, where necessary, for additional tutelage for her nurses on how to work the system *and* time to allow nurses to handle frustrations over problems of transition.

Negative attitudes can occur at any time (not just during transition), and they can make the system far less valuable. If evidence suggests that a negative attitude has developed among the staff to the point of causing disruption, the nurse manager must address the problem. Her first step should be to determine the reason for the negative attitude. While there are some areas over which the nurse manager has no control, such as the fact that the computer system crashes at inopportune times, there are areas over which she does have control. These include: the adequacy of training; the adequacy of planning to avoid double work; the reluctance of staff to give up the manual procedures; the appropriateness of procedures for the unit; and past reluctance on the part of other nurse managers to use the system. Once the reason has been determined, it should be addressed directly. Not only will this help the nurses to adjust to the system, it will help the nurse manager's overall rapport with them.

Once the system has been adopted and accepted, there is a continuing challenge for the nurse manager: just as many nurses may need to change their view of the job to adapt to the changing technology, the computer will need to adapt to changes in personnel, policy, and demand. Information about changes that nurses see as necessary, however, must originate with nurses and nurse managers; when better alternatives exist, nurses must propose them, not just sit back and do things the same old way.

In one hospital, for example, a pharmacist designed a patient profile that replaced a standard resupply list included in the pharmacy module provided by the vendor. Although many hospitals had previously implemented the system successfully, he noticed a deficiency in it after examining the printouts received by nursing. The recommended change allowed the pharmacist to evaluate a patient's drug therapy considering all aspects of the patient's treatment. This change was made not only to the system in that hospital, but also in systems in other hospitals serviced by that vendor.

Several conditions will determine whether a recommended change is made. One condition is the flexibility that was built into the system initially. Although the flexibility to respond to innovation varies, most systems implemented since the mid-1970s allow for some hospital-defined options. Further, the likelihood of change is related to the cost effectiveness of the option itself. As in the early stages of design, if the effort needed to implement the change is not at least matched by the extra advantages it confers, it will not have much chance of being adopted. Finally, the likelihood of change will also be affected by the flexibility of the people in both the nursing and system development departments. If such flexibility is minimal, then better communications and interpersonal relations need to be established, as discussed in other chapters of this book.

CONCLUSIONS AND SUGGESTIONS

This is a transitional period for computerization in the health care field. What is common now was not even conceived of 15 years ago and was not available commercially even 5 years ago. And the trend is likely to continue into the future. On the horizon are increased networking of services and sharing of resources among hospitals. Such a situation will, of course, allow for greater efficiencies and for better service to small hospitals that might now be able to afford systems of their own. In addition, such networking could provide better recordkeeping and, hence, more informed care to patients. For example, in Stockholm, Sweden, an interactive regional health information system is in use at all 74 hospitals in the country. This system keeps information about recent examinations and tests that can be accessed by medical and nursing staff at any hospital in the region. Thus, the staff does not need to rely on the memory of the patient and still is able to have the most up-to-date information.

One should also expect better research capabilities because the computerized patient systems will readily provide data that have not been available previously. Hence, medical and nursing staff will have more opportunities to study care plans and medication to trace diseases and outcomes of treatment with large numbers of subjects (thereby increasing the validity of the findings).

Some hospitals are already experiencing patient interaction with the systems, especially with activities such as patient histories. One should certainly expect this to become more common.

One potentially exciting advancement is in the area of expert systems and intelligent decision support systems applied to the provision of health care. An expert system is software that simulates the behavior of a human expert by drawing upon a large base of information and a set of rules for evaluating that information; intelligent decision support systems appear to be more consultative than do expert systems because there is more interaction with the user. One of the first expert systems developed was MYCIN, a system that helps medical professionals select the appropriate antimicrobial therapy for hospital patients with certain infections. More recently, expert systems have been created to help nurses develop care plans and evaluate symptoms. While the future is quite uncertain in this area, the trends suggest that currently available expert systems will be used more widely in the future and that other systems that will aid nursing will become available. The potential is seemingly endless.

More information about computerized systems for hospitals can be obtained from the references at the end of this chapter; the articles describe many types of applications. In addition, surveys of computer usage and package availability are usually available from private consultants or firms.

Finally, there are the providers themselves; most large consulting

Figure 20—11 Vendors of Computerized Hospital Systems

A. R. Medical Management, Inc.
Burroughs Corp.
Compucare, Inc.
Computer Sciences Corp.
Computer Synergy, Inc.
Datacare, Inc.
Dynamic Controls Corp.
Electronic Data Systems Corp.
HBO and Company
Hewlett-Packard
IBM Corp.
McDonnell Douglas Automation Company
MJS Systems, Inc.
National Data Communications
NCR Corp.
Pentamation Enterprises, Inc.
Sentry Data, Inc.
Shared Medical Systems
Space Age Computer Systems, Inc.
Systems Associates, Inc.
Systems Management Company
Technicon Medical Information Systems
Whittaker Medicus

Adapted from Fedorowicz, Jane. (1983). Current trends in hospital information systems. TIMS/ ORSA Joint National Meeting, Chicago, April 25–27.

firms specializing in accounting have some group that develops software. Of these, Ernst and Whinney provides the greatest amount of tailored software. Other companies either specialize in providing hospital computing systems or have a division that provides such a service. A partial listing of vendors is shown in Figure 20–11. Like some accounting firms, these vendors provide a spectrum of systems: some provide only financial systems while others provide total hospital information systems. Finally, still other companies provide shared computer services—that is, companies that actually house the computer and sell time to the hospital. A partial listing of such systems can be found in Kuntz (1983).

SUMMARY

– Computers are used in hospitals for patient records and billing, as well as for nurses to use in patient monitoring and histories, scheduling, training, and evaluation. Computers also are used to order and record pharmacy supplies, laboratory tests, radiology orders, and supplies and materials management. The most effective use of computers, however, is a hospital information system (HIS), integrating all computer use in one system. In this system, all components can interact with each other.

- Learning to use computers is similar to learning nursing techniques. This includes acquiring a new vocabulary, learning what the equipment can do and how to operate it.

- Computers come in many sizes depending on their capabilities. It is essential that the computer selected can perform the functions needed in the job.

BIBLIOGRAPHY

Adams, R., and Duchene, P. (1985). Computerization of patient acuity and nursing care planning. *J Nurs Adm*, (April): 11–17.

Albrecht, C. A., and Lieske, A. M. (1985). Automating patient care planning. *Nurs Mngmt*, 17(7): 21–26.

Anne, A., Spyker, D., Edlich, L., and Attinger, E. (1981). A comprehensive information system for emergency medical services. In: *Proceedings of the fifth annual symposium on computer applications in medical care*. Heffernan, H. (editor). Silver Spring, MD: IEEE Press. P. 979.

Aybalajobi, F. (1979). Characteristics of the software for computer application in medicine. *Med Info*, 4:79.

Badura, F. K. (1980). Nurse acceptance of a computerized arrhythmia monitoring system. *Heart and Lung*, 9(6): 1044.

Bellinger, K., and Laden, J. (1985). Nurses use of general-purpose microcomputer software. *Nursing Outlook*, 33(1): 22–25.

Bronzino, J. D. (1982). *Computer applications for patient care*. Reading, MA: Addison-Wesley.

Cook, M., and McDowell, W. (1975). Changing to an automated information system. *Am J Nurs*, 75:46.

Curtin, L. L. (1982). Nursing: Patient care and computers. How they work together. *Nurs Mngmt*, 13:25.

Dolcourt, J., and Harris, T. (1982). Pulmonary function in critically-ill newborn infants: Measurement by microprocessor. In: *Proceedings of the sixth annual symposium on computer applications in medical care*. Blum, B. (editor). Silver Springs, MD: IEEE Press. P. 649.

Dornfest, S. I., and Kennedy, A. G. (1980). Small hospitals' computer usage will increase rapidly through 1983. *Modern Healthcare*, 10(2): 88.

Drazen, E. L. (1983). Planning for purchase and implementation of an automated hospital information system: A nursing perspective. *J Nurs Adm*, (September) 13(9): 9.

Edwards, L. (1982). Computer-assisted nursing care. *Am J Nurs*, 82(7): 1076.

Endo, A. (1981). Using computers in newborn intensive care settings. *Am J Nurs*, 81(5): 1336.

Fedorowicz, J. (1983). Current trends in hospital information systems. Paper presented at the TIMS/ORSA joint national meeting, Chicago, April 25–27.

Fitzpatrick, T., Farrell, L. Y., and Richter-Zeunick, M. (1987). An automated staff scheduling system that minimizes payroll costs and maximizes staff satisfaction. *Computers in Nursing*, 5(1): 10.

Freibrun, R. B. (1976). Operations analysis applied to a drug distribution system. *Am J Hosp Pharm*, 33:452.

Gibson, S. E., and Rose, M. A. (1986). Managing computer resistance. *Computers in Nursing,* 4(5): 201.

Grams, R. R. (1977). Progress toward a second generation laboratory information system. *J Med Syst,* 7(3): 263.

Grazman, T. E. (1983). Managing unit human resources: A microcomputer model. *Nurs Mngmt,* (July) 14(7): 18.

Grobe, S. J. (1984). *Computer primer' and resource guide for nurses.* Philadelphia: J. B. Lippincott.

Hassett, M., and Kennedy, M. A. (1986). Computers in nursing practice. *Kansas Nurse,* 61(1): 2–4, 9–11.

Housley, C. E. (1974). Provocative approaches to materials management. *Dimensions in Health Service,* 51:32.

Jelliffe, R., Shumitzky, A., D'Argenio, D., et al. (1983). Improved 2-compartment time share programs for adaptive control of digitoxin and digitoxin therapy. In: *Proceedings of the seventh annual symposium on computer applications in medical care.* Dayhoff, R. (editor). Silver Spring, MD: IEEE Computer Society Press. P. 231.

Johnston, S. V. et al. (1976). The doctor, the pharmacist, the computer and the nurse: The prescription, supply, distribution and administration of drugs in a hospital. *Med Info,* 1:133.

Keliher, P. (1975). The standardized form. *Superv Nurs,* 6:40.

Kiley, M., Halloran, E. J., and Weston, J. L. (1983). Computerized nursing information systems. *Nurs Mngmt,* (July) 14(7): 26.

Klein, B. (1979). MM teamwork with nursing cuts prosthesis inventory by 12%. *Hosp Purchasing Mngmt,* 4(2): 14.

Kuntz, E. F. (1983). Shared service activity might spurt in '83 after sluggish '82. *Mod Healthcare,* (August) 12:106.

Long, G. (1982). The effect of medication distribution systems on medication errors. *Nurs Res,* 31:182.

Miller, H. E., Pierskalla, W. P., and Rath, G. J. (1976). Nurse scheduling using mathematical programming. *Oper Res,* 24(5): 857.

Muirhead, R. (1982). Happening now: The decline and fall of paperwork. *RN,* 45:34.

Nightingale, F. (1946). *Notes on nursing: What it is and what it is not.* (Facsimile of 1859 edition). Philadelphia: J. B. Lippincott.

Nursing Administration Quarterly. (1986). 10(2). Entire issue is on computers in nursing administration.

Nursing Clinics of North America. (1985). Symposium on Computers in Nursing. (September) 20(3).

Oryn Publications. (1985). *Computerized nursing care planning.* Washington, D.C.

Paquet, J. (1982). OR computers: The future is today. *Today's OR Nurse,* 4(1): 10.

Piankian, R. A. (1978). Computer hardware: Operation, applications and problems. *J Nurs Adm,* 8:8.

Reed, D. E., and Lapenas, C. (1975). Data retrieval in the coronary care unit: Prospective vs. retrospective. *Med Care,* 13:1055.

Rees, R. L. (1978). Understanding computers. *Nurs Adm,* 8:4.

Romano, C., McCormick, K. A., and McNeely, L. D. (1982). Nursing documentation: A model for a computerized data base. *Adv Nurs Sci,* 4:43.

Romano, C., Ryan, L., Harris, J., Boykin, P., and Power, M. (1985). A decade of decisions. *Computers in Nursing,* 3(2): 64.

Ryan, S. A. (1985). An expert system for nursing practice: Clinical decision support. *Computers in Nursing,* 3(2): 77.

Saba, V. K., and McCormick, K. A. (1986). *Essentials of computers for nurses.* Philadelphia: J. B. Lippincott.

Schifiliti, C., Bonasoro, C. L., and Thompson, M. (1986). LOTUS 1-2-3: A quality assurance application for nursing practice, administration and staff development. *Computers in Nursing*, 4(5): 205.

Sinclair, V. (1985). The computer as a partner in health care instruction. *Computers in Nursing*, 3(5): 212.

Slack, P. (1981). SNIPPET: A computerized nursing information bank. *Nurs Times*, 77:656.

Smith, L. D., and Bird, D. A. (1979). Designing computer support for daily hospital staffing decisions. *Med Info*, 4(2): 69.

Smith, L. D., and Wiggins, A. (1977). A computer-based nurse scheduling system. *Computers and Operations Res*, 4(1): 195.

Smith, L. D., Wiggins, A., and Bird, D. (1979). Post implementation experience with computer-assisted nurse scheduling in a large hospital. *Infor*, 17(4): 809.

Soja, M. E., and Lentz, K. E. (1987). Development of a hospital-based computer users course for student nurses. *Computers in Nursing*, 5(1): 15.

Somers, J. B. (1979). Information systems: The process of development. *J Nurs Adm*, 9(1): 53.

Sorkin, J., and Bloomfield, D. A. (1982). Computers for critical care. *Heart and Lung*, 17:287.

Squire, P. (1982). Monitoring a sick pattern. *Nurs Mirror*, 20:154.

Summers, S. (1987). The nurse as an information manager. *Kansas Nurse*, 62(3): 2.

Sweeney, M. A., O'Malley, M., and Freeman, E. (1982). Development of a computer simulation to evaluate the clinical performance of nursing students. *J Nurs Ed*, 21(9): 28.

Thiele, J. (1986). The development of computer-assisted instruction for drug dosage calculations: A group endeavor. *Computers in Nursing*, 4(3): 114.

Thomas, A. M. (1985). Management information systems: Determining nurse manager requirements. *Nurs Mngmt*, 17(7): 23–26.

Valentino, H. N. (1974). Real-time HIS has medical uses. *Hospitals*, 48:54.

Viers, V. M. (1983). Introducing nurse to computer world. *Nurs Mngmt*, (July) 14(7): 24.

Ward, E. F. (1984). Implementing a computer system: A guide for nursing. *Computers in Nursing*, 2(5): 171.

Waterstradt, C. (1981). Computers: Bringing nursing service "on-line". *Nurs Mngmt*, 12:9.

Weaver, C. G., and Johnson, J. E. (1984). Nursing participation in computer vendor selection. *Computers in Nursing*, 2(2): 31.

Werley, H. H., and Grier, M. R. (Editors). (1981). *Nursing information systems*. New York: Springer.

Zielstorff, R. D. (Editor). (1980). *Computers in nursing*. Wakefield, MA: Nursing Resources.

Zielstorff, R. D. (1985). Cost effectiveness of computerization in nursing practice and administration. *J Nurs Adm*, (April): 22–26.

Zielstorff, R. D. (1976). Orienting personnel to automated systems. *J Nurs Adm*, 6:14.

Zielstorff, R. D. (1984). Why aren't there more significant automated nursing information systems? *J Nurs Adm*, (January) 14(1): 7.

Quality Assurance
and Risk Management

THE ACCOUNTABILITY OF health care institutions, physicians, and nurses has changed drastically in the past decade. This is due largely to the increased number of successfully litigated claims and the increased dollar amounts awarded in the settlements; and to the legislative and judicial decisions that have put responsibility for patient safety on health care providers, both individuals and institutions.

Several landmark decisions have had their impact on accountability. In a 1965 case, *Darling v. Charleston Community Memorial Hospital*, the Illinois Supreme Court found the hospital liable for the care of a young athlete whose leg was amputated following complications from a fracture.* The court found the hospital negligent in two areas: (a) by the nurses' failure to inform the physician or hospital regarding the onset of complications, and (b) by not protecting the patient from incompetence of the physician. Decisions in similar cases have been based on this precedent of corporate responsibility for providing a system to monitor patient

*211 N.E. 2d 53, 33 Ill. 2d, 326 (1965), cert. denied 383 U.S. 946, 16 L.Ed. 2d 209, 86 S.Ct. 1204 (1966).

care and to correct deficiencies in quality. In addition, hospitals and other not for profit institutions (including schools and churches) lost their charitable immunity through a Supreme Court decision in 1969. Since that time, hospitals have experienced a steady increase in litigation, insurance premiums, and dollar settlements.

Negligence, known as an "unintentional tort" in civil law, is the largest area of malpractice litigation. Hospitals sustain liability in two categories of negligence: custodial (environmental) and professional (Lanham & Orlikoff, 1981). *Custodial* negligence refers to environmental conditions that result in falls or other such injuries. Financial loss from custodial negligence is generally low, although the number of claims is high. *Professional* negligence refers to patient injury due to the quality of care given or the absence of care when it was indicated. According to a 1980 American Hospital Association publication, both types of negligence are preventable (Dixon et al., 1980).

As a consequence of increasing litigation, malpractice insurance premiums have skyrocketed, pushing hospital costs even higher. Some insurance carriers now require hospitals to develop risk management programs as a condition for coverage. On January 1, 1977, Florida became the first state with a law requiring hospitals, regardless of size or type, to have a program designed to reduce risks, including an incident review committee (Federation of American Hospitals manual, 1977). Then, on January 1, 1980, the Joint Commission on Accreditation of Hospitals' requirements for risk management and quality assurance went into effect.

A risk-free health care setting is impossible. Systematic action to reduce risks, however, is not only possible but essential. A risk management program must be established because the disturbing trends that have given rise to the hospital liability problem will persist and probably worsen. Rising insurance premiums, record settlements, rising patient expectations, less reluctance on the part of patients and their families to sue faceless institutions and rarely seen specialists, and more pressure for quality assurance are forces that are not going to go away.

As the cost of health care has escalated and as the federal government has become increasingly involved in paying for health care, there is increased pressure to ensure that services rendered are necessary and that services provided meet nationally recognized standards of care. Further, both the federal government and other third-party payers (insurance carriers) are insisting that services be provided at the lowest possbile cost. This is a change from prior times when any services needed were provided without much concern about the cost—the government or insurance company would pay after the cost had been incurred. Today, the prospective payment system demands that costs be contained within the DRG allotment and thus, quality, cost-effective care becomes essential.

Controlling costs is discussed in Chapter 4 on productivity, and in Chapter 19 on budgeting and resource allocation. This chapter will focus on assuring quality and managing risk.

QUALITY ASSURANCE

Accountability is operationalized by what is known in health care as quality assurance. Quality assurance describes all activities related to establishing, maintaining, and assuring high quality care for patients. It includes assessment of patient care and correction of problems identified.

Quality assurance can be voluntary or mandatory. Nursing practice that conforms to the ANA *Standards of Nursing Practice* is a voluntary form of quality assurance. When the institution meets the state board of health requirements, quality assurance is mandatory. (Theoretically, it is voluntary for hospitals to meet the JCAH standards for accreditation, but without accreditation they will not be reimbursed by third-party payers [Medicare, insurance carriers].)

Quality assurance is the method by which performance of care is evaluated for effectiveness. Standards for appropriate care are established and provide the basis upon which potential risk can be assessed. Then, measures taken to reduce that risk are begun. Quality assurance is the foundation of any risk management program.

Quality Assurance Process

Quality assurance is the systematic process of evaluating the quality of care given in a particular unit or institution. It involves: setting standards, determining criteria to meet those standards, evaluating how well the criteria have been met, making plans for change based on the evaluation, and following up on implementation for change.

Setting standards. The profession itself has designated generic standards of nursing practice (see Appendix A, the American Nurses' Association *Standards of Nursing Practice*). In addition to these general standards, each institution and each patient care unit must designate standards that are specific to the patient population served. These standards are the foundation upon which all other measures of quality assurance are based. An example of a standard is: Every patient will have a written care plan.

Determining criteria. After standards of performance are established, criteria must be determined that will indicate if the standards are being met and to what degree they are met. Just as with standards of care, criteria must be general as well as specific to the individual unit. One criterion to demonstrate that the standard regarding care plans for every patient are being met would be: A nursing care plan is developed and written by a registered nurse within 12 hours of admission. This criterion, then, provides a *measurable* indicator to evaluate performance.

Evaluating performance. Several methods can be used to evaluate performance. These include reviewing documented records, observing activities as they take place, examining patients, and interviewing patients, families, and staff. Records are the most commonly used source for evaluation because of the relative ease of their use but they are not as reliable as direct observations. It is quite possible to write in the patient's chart activities that were not done or to not record those things that were done. Further, the chart only indicates that care was provided; it does not demonstrate the quality of that care. In the previous example, records would be examined to determine if care plans were written on each patient within 12 hours of admission and, if so, that standards had been met. Other criteria would be used to measure the quality of the care plan, such as, "Every care plan will include patient education appropriate to the patient's medical diagnosis, nursing diagnosis, interventions planned, and discharge planning". Then, the care plan would be checked to see if it contained these components.

Making plans for change. Since no performance standards can be met perfectly at all times, quality assurance planning must include methods for correcting deficits. First, the unit and/or institution must determine how much deviation from the standard is acceptable before changes are made. If 45 out of 50 patients admitted have a care plan recorded within 12 hours of admission and the other 5 have recorded care plans within the next 6 hours, is this deviation acceptable? If not, then, how should this be corrected? Is the unit short-staffed? Have there been an unusually large number of admissions recently? Are a number of new graduates being oriented on the unit? Plans for correcting deficiencies in performance are the responsibility of the nurse manager and, after collecting all pertinent information about possible causes, the nurse manager should consult with staff and/or the supervisor and make plans for correcting the performance deficit.

Follow-up. Following up on how effective changes have been in improving performance is the final, but very necessary, step in the quality assurance process. Many times, quality assurance programs fall short of doing what it is they are designed to do—assure quality of care—because they only record performance and plan to improve it. If, in the example described, the nurse manager found that the next 50 patients had care plans recorded within 12 hours, then the performance had improved relative to that standard. If it had not improved, then another approach would need to be taken or, possibly, the criterion should be evaluated for appropriateness for that unit.

Monitoring Nursing Care

In addition to the individual patient care activities described, another component of quality assurance is the ongoing monitoring of nursing care. Several methods are used to monitor nursing care. These include: nursing audit, peer review, utilization review, and patient satisfaction.

Nursing audit.   A nursing audit can be retrospective or concurrent. A retrospective audit is conducted after a patient's discharge and involves examining records of a large number of cases. The patient's entire course of care is evaluated and comparisons made across cases. Recommendations for change can be made from the perspective of many patients with similar care problems and with the spectrum of care considered.

A concurrent audit is conducted during the patient's course of care; it examines the care being given to achieve a desirable outcome in the patient's health and evaluates the nursing care activities being provided. Changes can be made if they are indicated by patient outcomes.

Peer review.   Peer review occurs when practicing nurses determine the standards and criteria that indicate quality care and then assess performance against these. In this case, nurses are the "experts" at knowing what the indicators of quality care are and when such care has been provided. Their expertise is especially useful in complicated cases; sometimes more than one expert's opinion is used for comparisons.

Utilization review.   Utilization reviews are based on the appropriate allocation of resources and are mandated by the JCAH. Such a review is not specifically directed toward nursing care, but it may provide information on nursing practices that will require further investigation.

Patient satisfaction.   Most institutions have a method to determine patients' satisfaction with their care. The usual method is a questionnaire the patient is asked to fill out either before leaving the institution or after returning home. Although patient satisfaction is very important, standards of professional care are often not indicated due to the fact that the consumer's knowledge of expert care is limited. However, the patient is quite aware of receiving care in a timely fashion and of the many variables in the environment that contribute to recovery. Patient satisfaction should be used as one of several indicators of quality.

Once standards have been set, criteria established, and methods for evaluating adherence to the standards determined, the institution is prepared to examine its risk in relation to its accountability. Risk management programs in health care institutions involve two important areas: patient and/or family incident review, and employee and visitor safety. Since nursing is involved most with patient care, this chapter emphasizes a risk management incident program for patients, their families, or both.

A RISK MANAGEMENT PROGRAM

Risk management follows the current trend of adapting business strategies to hospital management; it is the hospital parallel to product liability prevention in industry. Risk management is a planned program of loss prevention and liability control. Its purpose is to identify, analyze, and evaluate risks, followed by a plan for reducing the frequency and severity of accidents and injuries. Risk management is a continuous daily program of detection, education, and intervention.

Risk management calls for a team approach involving all departments of the hospital. It must be a hospital-wide program with board of directors' approval and input from medicine, nursing, and other professional departments. Input from medicine and nursing is received through several mechanisms: annually, through review by the medical quality assurance committee or the policy procedure committee, and through the review by the medical and nursing administrative staff. The program must have high-level commitment, including that of the chief executive officer and the director of nursing service.

A risk management program includes the following activities:

1. *Identifying* potential risks for accident, injury, or financial loss. Formal and informal communication with all hospital departments and inspection of facilities are essential to identifying problem areas.

2. *Reviewing* present institution-wide monitoring systems (incident reports, audits, committee minutes, oral complaints, patient questionnaires), evaluating completeness, and determining additional systems needed to provide the factual data essential for risk management control.

3. *Analyzing* the frequency, severity, and causes of general categories and specific types of incidents causing injury or adverse outcomes to patients. To plan risk intervention strategies, estimating the possible loss associated with the various types of incidents is needed.

4. *Reviewing and appraising* safety and risk aspects of patient care procedures and new programs.

5. *Monitoring* laws and codes related to patient safety, consent, and care.

6. *Eliminating or reducing* risks as much as possible.

7. *Reviewing* the work of other committees to determine potential liability and recommend prevention or corrective action. Examples of such committees are infection; medical audit; safety/security; pharmacy; nursing audit; and productivity. In many hospitals the quality assurance and risk management committees and programs have been combined.

8. *Identifying* needs for patient, family, and personnel education suggested by all of the foregoing and implementing the appropriate educational program.

9. *Evaluating* the results of a risk management program.

10. *Providing* periodic reports to administration, medical staff, and the board of directors.

The establishment of a risk management program starts at the top. The hospital's board of directors directs the administrator to establish the program and commits the necessary resources. The administrator then appoints a risk management committee, whose members are responsible for the overall planning and decision making that are involved in risk management. However, for effective implementation, a risk manager should be appointed to manage the day-to-day operation of the program.

Membership on the risk management committee should be interdisciplinary, with representatives from medicine, nursing, medical records, legal counsel, education, and insurance claims. Typical members of a risk management committee would be:

1. A risk manager

2. Nursing representatives
   Nursing service administrator
   Nurse manager representative
   Staff nurse representative

3. Medical staff representatives

4. Related committee chairs
   Quality assurance
   Utilization review
   Infection control
   Pharmacy and therapeutics
   Operating room

5. Patient accounts representative

6. Legal counsel (ex-officio)

7. Others by invitation
   Education and training coordinator
   Insurance claims representative

The chairman can be any member of the committee. Typically, the chairman is a member of administration or the risk manager. The committee's purpose is to develop and promote appropriate measures to minimize risk to patients and hospital personnel and to carry out the risk management activities listed above. The committee develops risk management policies and guidelines for handling critical incidents. It establishes programs for increasing staff awareness, detection, education, and proper reporting of risk potential and incidents.

The Risk Manager

The risk manager administers the program and serves as the liaison between administration, the risk management committee, and other related hospital committees and departments. This person usually also serves as the liaison between insurance company representatives, hospital attorneys, and others. The risk manager should report to the chief administrator and should have a clearly defined role in the organizational structure of the institution.

There is no typical profile for risk managers. They come from a variety of backgrounds, including administration, law, nursing, former quality assurance coordinators, and former claims representatives from insurance companies. They need effective communicative skills, evaluative skills (such as those learned in research methodology), should be able to develop positive interpersonal relationships, and must exhibit leadership and team building skills.

The responsibilities of the risk manager include, but are not limited to, the following:

1. Schedules meetings and prepares agenda for risk management committee (if risk manager is the chairman; if not, helps with agenda).

2. Reviews incident reports daily; investigates as needed; takes action or refers to appropriate physician, nurse manager, or committee; follows up with patient and family as appropriate.

3. Monitors data collection mechanisms such as incident report summaries.

4. Visits periodically the patients and their families who are at high risk, since individual concern for patients is the single most effective way to reduce litigiousness. High risk patients include those on long-term care or ones with repeated admissions, transfers from intensive care to general units and vice-versa, night emergency room admissions, and postoperative patients.

5. Summarizes litigation on a periodic basis, including dollar outcome.

6. Prepares monthly incident report summary.

7. Develops, with help of risk management committee members, staff education programs.

The risk management organizational model shown in Figure 21–1 illustrates the relationship among units in a risk management program.

NURSING'S ROLE IN RISK MANAGEMENT

In the hospital setting, nursing is the one department involved in patient care 24 hours a day; nursing personnel are critical to the success of a risk management program. The chief nursing administrator must be com-

Figure 21–1 Risk Management Organization Model

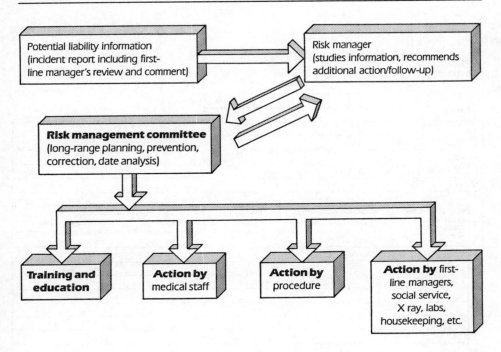

mitted to the program. His or her attitude will influence the staff and their participation. After all, it is the staff, with their daily patient contact, who actually implement a risk management program.

High risk areas in hospitals fall into five general categories: (a) medication errors; (b) complications from diagnostic or treatment procedures; (c) falls; (d) patient or family dissatisfaction with care; and (e) refusal of treatment or to sign consent for treatment. Nursing is involved in all areas, but the medical staff may be primarily responsible in cases involving refusal of treatment or of consent to treatment.

Medical records and incident reports serve to document hospital, nurse, and physician accountability. However, it has been estimated that for every reported incident, 35 are unreported. If records are faulty, inadequate, or omitted, the hospital is more likely to be sued and more likely to lose (Dixon et al., 1980). Incident reports are used to analyze the severity, frequency, and causes of incidents within the five risk categories. Such analysis serves as a basis for intervention.

Incident Reports

Accurate and comprehensive reporting on both the patient's chart and in the incident report is essential to protect the institution and the care givers from litigation. Incident reporting is most often the nurse's respon-

Figure 21—2 Incident Report Form

PATIENT INCIDENT REPORT

NUMBER	00520

PATIENT NAME							

ADDRESS							

P A T I E N T

HOSPITAL NO.	ROOM NO.	HOME PHONE NO.		AGE	SEX ☐M ☐F	DATE ADMITTED

REASON FOR HOSPITALIZATION ▶

ATTENDING PHYSICIAN   CHARGE/ PRIMARY NURSE ▶

LIST MEDICATIONS WITHIN LAST 6 HOURS, IF PERTINENT: ▶

ACTIVITY ORDERS	ADJUSTABLE BED HEIGHT	BEDRAILS	TYPE OF INCIDENT
☐ RESTRAINTS	☐YES ☐NO	☐UP	☐MEDICATION ☐PATIENT MOVEMENT
☐ BEDREST		☐DOWN	☐DIAGNOSTIC PROCEDURE ☐PATIENT/PARENT ATTITUDE
☐ UP c̄ ASSISTANCE	POSITION	☐NONE	☐PATIENT TREATMENT ☐MEDICO-LEGAL
☐ UP s̄ ASSISTANCE	☐HIGH ☐LOW		

I N C I D E N T   F A C T S

EXACT LOCATION OF INCIDENT: ▶

	DATE	TIME	SHIFT ☐DAY ☐EVE ☐NIGHT

DESCRIPTION BY PERSON PREPARING REPORT (use separate sheet if necessary) ▶

NAME OF PERSONS PRESENT AT TIME OF INCIDENT (include employees)	ADDRESS	PHONE

M E D I C A L

WAS PERSON INVOLVED EXAMINED BY A PHYSICIAN IN HOSPITAL? ☐YES ☐NO	DATE	TIME	WHERE

EXAMINING PHYSICIAN'S NAME ▶   ANY APPARENT INJURY ☐YES ☐NO   X-RAY ORDERED ☐YES ☐NO

SIGNATURE OF PERSON PREPARING REPORT X	TITLE	DATE

IMMEDIATE FOLLOW-UP ▶

FOLLOW-UP AT DISCHARGE ▶ (if pertinent)

X
(Signature)   PATIENT CARE MANAGER

Form No. 1036   Rev. 2/80

A form used by St. Louis Children's Hospital. Used by permission.

sibility. The reluctance to report incidents is usually due to fear of the consequences. This can be alleviated by two techniques: (a) staff education programs that emphasize objective reporting, omitting inflammatory words and judgmental statements; (b) a clear understanding that the purpose of the incident reporting process is for documentation and follow-up and that the report will not be used, under any circumstances, for disciplinary action.

A reportable incident should include any unexpected or unplanned occurrence that affects or could potentially affect a patient or family member. The report is only as effective as the form on which it is reported, so attention should be paid to the adequacy of the form as well as to the data it calls for (Duran, 1980). Figure 21–2 is a sample incident report form.

The suggested process of reporting incidents involves the following steps:

1. *Discovery.* Physicians, nurses, patients, families, or any hospital employee or volunteer may report actual or potential risk.

2. *Notification.* The risk manager receives the completed incident form within *24 hours* after the incident. A telephone call may be made earlier, to hasten follow-up in the event of a major incident.

3. *Investigation.* The risk manager or representative investigates the incident immediately.

4. *Consultation.* The manager consults with physician, risk management committee member, or both.

5. *Action.* The manager should clarify any misinformation to the patient or family, explaining exactly what happened. The patient should be referred to the appropriate source for help and for compensation for any needed service; the latter should be offered, if indicated.

6. *Record.* The manager should be sure that all records, including incident reports, follow-up, and action taken, if any, are filed in a central depository.

Some Examples

The following are some examples of actual events in the various risk categories.

Medication errors, including administration of intravenous fluids. It is a reportable incident when a medication or fluid is omitted, given to the wrong patient, given at the wrong time or in the wrong dosage, or given by the wrong route. Administration of the wrong medication or fluid is also reportable.

Patient A. Weight was transcribed wrong from emergency room sheet. Medication dose was calculated on incorrect weight; therefore, patient was given double the dose required. Error discovered after first dose and corrected. Second dose omitted.

Patient B. Tegretol dosage written in Medex as "Tegretol 100 mg chewable tab—50 mg p.o. B.I.D." Tegretol 100 mg given p.o. at 1400. Meds checked at 1430 and error noted. 50 mg Tegretol should have been given. Doctor notified. Second dose held.

Patient C. During rounds at 3:30 P.M. found D/5/ISO/M hanging. Order was D/5W. Fluids last checked at 2:00 P.M. Changed to correct fluid. Doctor notified.

Diagnostic procedure. Any incident occurring before, during, or after such procedures as blood sample stick, biopsy, X ray, lumbar puncture, or other invasive procedure is categorized as a diagnostic procedure incident.

Patient A. When I checked the IV site, I saw that it was red and swollen. For this reason, I discontinued the IV. When removing the tape, a small area of skin breakdown was noted where tape had been. There was also a small knot on the medial aspect of the left antecubital above the IV insertion site. Doctor notified. Wound dressed.

Patient B. When I was turning Mrs. Jones, she complained of a burning sensation. A rash was noted over both buttocks. Pad under patient heavily saturated. Changed bed linen and powder applied to patient's buttocks.

Medical-legal incident. If a patient or family refuses treatment as ordered and prescribed, or refuses to sign consents, the situation is categorized as a medical-legal incident.

Patient A. After a visit from a member of the clergy, patient indicated he was no longer in need of medical attention and asked to be discharged. Physician called. Doctor explained potential side effects if treatment were discontinued. Patient continued to ask for discharge. Doctor explained "against medical advice" (A.M.A.) form. Patient signed A.M.A. form and left at 1300 without medications.

Patient B. Patient refused to sign consent for bone marrow. States side effects not understood. Doctor reviewed reasons for test and side effects three different times. Doctor informed the patient that without consent he could not perform the test. Offered to call in another physician for second opinion. Patient agreed. After doctor left, patient signed consent, still indicating lack of understanding of the side effects.

Patient or family attitude toward care. When a patient or family indicate general dissatisfaction with care and the situation cannot be or has not been resolved, then an incident report is filed.

Patient A. Mother complained that she had found child saturated with urine every morning she arrived (around 0800). Explained to mother that diapers and linen are changed at 0600 when 0600 feedings and meds are given. Patient's back, buttocks, and perineal areas are free of skin breakdown. Parents continue to be distressed. Discussed with primary nurse.

Patient B. Mr. Smith obviously very angry. Greeted me at the door complaining that his wife had not been treated properly in our emergency room the night before. Waited to speak to someone from administration. Was unable to reach the administrator on call. Suggested Mr. Smith call administrator in the morning. Mr. Smith thanked me for my time and assured me that he would call the administrator the next day.

ROLE OF THE NURSE MANAGER

A risk management system allows the hospital to act on the root causes of liability claims. It identifies individuals, areas, and procedures that are deficient. It spots communication failures immediately and allows the hospital to remedy a breakdown before an angry patient or family files a claim. The nurse manager plays the key role in the success of any risk management program.

A patient incident or a patient's or family's expression of dissatisfaction regarding care not only indicates some slippage in quality of care, it also indicates potential liability. A distraught, dissatisfied, complaining patient is a high risk; and a satisfied patient or family is a low risk. A risk management or liability control program should therefore emphasize a personal approach. Many claims are filed because of a breakdown in communication between the health care provider and the patient. In many instances, after an incident or bad outcome, a quick, simple visit or call from a hospital representative to the patient or family can soothe tempers and clarify misinformation.

For instance, Stephanie's parents wrote a letter indicating that they discovered a needle sticking out of their child's foot about four days after discharge. The nurse manager called the mother to discuss Stephanie's present condition and follow-up. The mother informed her that Stephanie was fine and expressed pleasant surprise about the follow-up call. Although the nurse manager asked the mother to send her the piece of needle and (after consultation with administration), offered to make an appointment for Stephanie to be seen at no charge, she never heard from the mother again. A subsequent letter from the mother thanked the nurse manager for "caring."

David received an overdose of preoperative medication. The child suffered some ill effects and his surgery was cancelled and rescheduled for a later date. The nurse manager discussed with the parents what had happened and committed a staff member to observe the child closely until there was absolutely no possibility of his being in any danger. Several weeks later the family wrote a letter thanking the nursing staff for the care and special attention.

In both of these situations, prompt attention and care by the head nurse protected the patients involved and may have averted a potential liability claim. The important factors in these successful endings are obvious: recognition of the incident; quick follow-up and action; personal contact; and immediate restitution (where appropriate). It is estimated that 90% of patients' concerns can and should be handled at the unit level. When that first line of communication breaks down, however, the first-line manager needs a resource—usually the risk manager or nursing service administrator.

Key Behaviors

Handling a patient's or family member's complaints stemming from an incident can be very difficult. These confrontations are often highly emotional, and the patient or family member must be calmed down, yet satisfied. Sometimes just an opportunity to release the anger or emotion is all that is needed. Figure 21–3 shows a set of key behaviors that may be used to defuse a complaint from a patient or family member.

The first three key behaviors have to do with *listening* to the person so as to defuse the situation. Arguing or interrupting will only increase the person's anger or emotion. After the patient or family member has had his or her say, then an attempt can be made to solve the problem by asking what they expect in the form of a solution. The nurse manager or other hospital representative should then explain what can and cannot be done and try to negotiate with the injured party an agreement on a solution. It is important to be specific. Vague resolutions of problems may only lead to more problems later on if expectations for solution and timetable differ.

The nurse manager must also be sure that all incidents are properly documented. The documentation on the incident form should be detailed, including all the factors relating to the incident as demonstrated in

---

Figure 21–3 Key Behaviors for Handling Complaints

1. Listen openly.
2. Do not speak until the person has had his or her say.
3. Avoid reacting emotionally (don't get defensive).
4. Ask for his or her expectations about a solution to the problem.
5. Explain what you can and cannot do to solve the problem (if appropriate).
6. Agree on specific steps to be taken and specific deadlines.

Adapted from Decker, P. J. *Healthcare Management Microtraining.* Decker & Associates, St. Louis, 1982. Used with permission.

the previous examples. The documentation in the chart, however, should be only a statement of the *facts* and of the patient's physical response; no reference to the incident report or words like *error* or *inappropriate* should be used. When a patient receives 100 mg of Demerol instead of 50 mg as ordered, the proper documentation in the chart is, "100 mg of Demerol administered. Physician notified." The remainder of the documentation should include any reaction of the patient to the dosage such as "Patient's vital signs unchanged." If there is an untoward reaction, a follow-up note should be written in the chart, giving an update of the patient's status. A note related to the patient's reaction should be written as frequently as the status changes and should continue until the patient returns to his previous status.

Documentation

Documentation in the incident report form, however, should indicate all factors related to the incident. There is a section in Figure 21–2, for instance, asking for "immediate follow-up" and "follow-up at discharge." These sections are ordinarily completed by the nurse manager. Thus, in the case of the patient with tissue change around the IV site, the nurse manager's immediate follow-up included notifying the physician and caring for the skin around the IV. At the time of the patient's discharge, the entry in the "follow-up at discharge" space read as follows: "The space around the IV site is healing well. Mother given appointment to follow-up clinic in seven days to check site and healing process. Will report status at that time and continue follow-up as needed."

The chart must never be used as a tool for disciplinary comments or action or expressions of anger. Notes such as "Incident would never have occurred if Doctor X had written the correct order in the first place" or "This carelessness is inexcusable" are totally inappropriate and serve no meaningful purpose. Carelessness and incorrect orders do indeed cause errors and incidents, but the place to address and resolve these issues is in the risk management committee or in the nurse manager's office, not the patient chart.

A Caring Attitude

It is also the nurse manager who sets the tone on the unit that contributes to a safe and low risk environment. Situations that contribute to patient incidents and eventually legal problems are mistrust, misinformation, guilt (and thus the need to blame others), confusion, conflicting stories, and, ultimately, gross negligence. Except for gross negligence, the most common cause for legal action is an unfriendly, uncaring attitude on the part of hospital staff.

Compare, for instance, the very different outcomes for two similar, actual incidents. The report on *Patient A* read: "Upon the patient's return from X ray, it was noted that the skin around the IV site was very puffy from obvious leaking of dye into the tissue. After three days the skin sloughed." A note by the physician in the chart at discharge indicated that the patient would require plastic surgery in the future. No incident report was filed, however, nor was there any indication of any discussion with the patient. Six weeks after the patient's discharge the hospital received a letter from an attorney, indicating that an intent to sue had been initiated by the patient.

The report on *Patient B* was similar, to begin with: "IV infiltration in X ray." In this case, however, an incident report was filed as soon as the patient returned from X ray and it was noted that the dye had infused into the tissue. The nurse manager requested on the incident report that it be returned to her for follow-up. The risk manager was notified and returned the incident report to the nurse manager. The two of them then discussed going to the patient, along with the physician, to discuss the possibility of a slough and, if indicated, to provide the patient with appropriate referral and treatment. The nurse manager, the risk manager, and the physician did discuss the situation with the patient. Three days after the infusion, there was an indication of skin sloughing and the physician determined that plastic surgery might be required in the future. Arrangements for future treatment were made with the patient. The family took no legal action.

Analysis of these two incidents strongly suggests that it was the nurse manager's quick and appropriate action in the second case that made the difference in outcome. If an unfriendly, uncaring attitude is the cause of most legal suits, what are the implications for the nurse manager? Take the example of the mother who was distressed about her baby's condition each morning she arrived. If no personal response or follow-up had been made and the patient's treatment had not met the mother's expectations, her first reaction might have been, "This is another example of careless, sloppy care." But, when the situation is handled with personal follow-up, an opposite reaction can be expected. When the mother complained about the child's care, the staff nurse and the nurse manager, rather than being defensive, discussed the complaint and established a plan of action, including explanation of the nurse's routine, checking the baby immediately, and correcting the situation. Most important, the nurse changed the routine to accommodate the mother's concern.

When the man complained to the nurse manager that he did not think his wife had received appropriate care during the night, the nurse manager might very well have said, "That's not my problem. I didn't work last night." Instead, the manager indicated with whom he should discuss his problem and gave him that person's phone number. If the nurse had simply disclaimed responsibility, it would have added fuel to the man's anger, but, when his concerns were listened to and he was given an appropriate referral, his anger was dissipated.

The nurse manager might also be involved in other activities of the risk management program, such as determining staff educational needs and participating in programs designed to meet those needs, or in establishing protocols for classifying patients at risk—for example, for falls. Whatever activity is pursued in a risk management program, the nurse manager's participation is critical to its success.

EVALUATION OF RISK MANAGEMENT

Identifying and reducing risks involves close monitoring and analysis of incident reports. Incident reports that include statements of blame should be discussed. A risk management program needs support and participation from all staff. To elicit their commitment, the use of incident reports must be limited to risk reduction only. This policy must be emphasized and practiced.

A risk management program requires resources and, in times of budget reductions, it may be one of the first to be cut. However, risk management is directed toward reducing losses; it is a case of spending money to save it. Return on the investment takes time, however, and it is difficult to estimate what might have been lost. Comparison with past data is of course one way, but that is based on the premise that future loss can be assumed from past loss figures. Over time, a risk management program can be cost-effective as well as provide a safer environment for patients.

An additional benefit of a risk management program may be an increase in positive attitudes toward the institution on the part of both employees and the community. When implemented in a spirit of concern and responsibility, a risk management program can be a visible means of responding to patient needs. Hospitals, physicians, and nurses have had their share of negative press in the past—sometimes with good reason. The courts, insurance carriers, and legislative action have mandated that hospitals respond to patient demands. Risk management meets this obligation.

Risk management makes sense. It improves the quality of patient care and reduces liability claims. It represents the outstanding characteristic of health care professionals: care and concern for people. It provides the best care possible at the most reasonable cost.

SUMMARY

- Accountability in health care institutions has prompted the recent development of quality assurance and risk management programs.

- Quality assurance is the method by which performance of care is evaluated for effectiveness.

- A quality assurance program is the basis for managing risk.

- The key ingredients in a successful patient risk management program are an organized program of incident reporting; review and follow-up; a risk management program, including a risk manager and committee with well-defined objectives; nurse managers who support the risk management program; and, most important, a friendly, caring environment as perceived by the patient and his family.

- Steps in reporting incidents have been described, as well as suggested behaviors in handling a dissatisfied or angry patient and family. Differences between documenting on the incident form and the patient's chart were discussed.

- Risk management is a recent development and the literature is just beginning to be available. Some suggested reading in this area appears in the bibliography.

BIBLIOGRAPHY

American Nurses' Association. (1973). *Standards of nursing practice*. Kansas City, MO: American Nurses' Association.

Brooten, D. A., Hayman, L., and Naylors, M. D. (1978). *Leadership for change: A guide for the frustrated nurse*. Philadelphia: J. B. Lippincott.

Brown, B. L., Jr. (1979). *Risk management for hospitals: A practical approach*. Gaithersburg, MD: Aspen.

Decker, C. M. (1985). Quality assurance: Accent on monitoring. *Nurs Mngmt, 16*(11): 20–24.

Dixon, N. E. et al. (1980). *Quality, trending and management for the 80's: A hospital-wide quality assurance program*. Chicago: American Hospital Association.

Duran, G. S. (1980). On the scene: Risk management in health care. *Nurs Adm Quart*, 5:19.

Federation of American Hospitals. (1977). FAH manual outlines control programs on risk management for hospital use. *Review*, 10:17.

Kraus, G. P. (1986). *Health care risk management: Organization and claims administration*. Owings Mills, MD: National Health Publications.

Lanham, G. B., and Orlikoff, J. E. (1981). Full coverage of issues reflects importance of risk management. *Hospitals*, 55:165.

Monahan, M. L. (1987). Quality assurance and nursing. In: *Medical surgical nursing: Concepts and clinical practice*. Phipps, W., Long, B., and Woods, N. (editors). St. Louis: C. V. Mosby. Pp. 113–123.

Poteet, G. W. (1983). Risk management and nursing. *Nursing Clinics of North America, 18*(3): 457–465.

Ulrich, B., Fredin, N., and Cavouras, C. A. (1986). Assuring quality through a professional practice approach. *Nurs Econ, 4*(6): 277–287.

CONFLICT IS PRESENT in all aspects of life and in all organizations due to the complexity of organizational relationships, the interactions among the members of the organization, and their dependence on one another. The presence of conflict does not necessarily mean that a negative process is occurring. Conflict is neutral, but the results of conflict can be constructive or destructive. Poorly managed conflict can create distance and distrust among employees in an organization and lead to lowered productivity. Well-managed conflict can stimulate competition, identify legitimate differences within organizations, and serve as a powerful motivator.

This chapter discusses the phenomenon known as conflict, and presents a model of conflict and various conflict resolution techniques that are applicable to nursing. It is important for nurse managers to understand this process, the conditions that lead to conflict, and the means to resolve conflict in order for their units to perform effectively.

IMPORTANCE OF CONFLICT

Dealing with conflict has become increasingly important to administrators in health care institutions. This is in part due to the increasing complexity of delivering health care, the rising expectations of those delivering and receiving health care, the changing role of nurses, increased competition among health care institutions, pressure from Medicare, increased government regulations, and the threats posed by legal action.

Conflict is viewed as not only inevitable but as a natural condition and necessary if people and organizations are to change. Conflict is both functional and dysfunctional to individuals and organizations. Some of the positive and negative aspects of conflict are noted below.

Positive Aspects of Conflict

Even though conflict is inevitable in organizations, it does not have to be destructive to the organization. There can be many positive consequences of conflict. For one, it provides heightened sensitivity to problems. Conflict can serve as a stimulus in developing new facts or solutions; when there is disagreement about the choice of a solution to a problem, a novel solution is often discovered. Some conflict in organizations can be useful in that it can help deal with the cost vs. benefit issue facing every organization. For example, disagreements over patient care can cause the parties in conflict to become more aware of the trade-offs, especially costs vs. benefits, of a particular service or technique. Conflict helps people to recognize legitimate differences within an organization or profession and serves as a powerful motivator. In fact, conflict over the past 25 years has led to a number of positive changes both for nursing and the status of women (Brooten, Hayman & Naylors, 1978:18).

Negative Aspects of Conflict

Conflict can result in the conflict's being suppressed, which does not resolve the conflict and may cause severe consequences in the future. Conflict often leads to aggressive behavior on the part of those individuals or groups in conflict. For example, groups that are placed in "win-lose competition" have the tendency to increase the in-group/out-group bias between them (Sherif & Sherif, 1961) and to increase the evaluation of their own group while decreasing their evaluation of the other group, therefore making it very difficult for the groups to work together in the future.

Conflict can be very stressful to individuals. Individuals vary in their ability to adapt to conflict. The effects of conflicts on individuals and the resulting stresses will be discussed more fully in Chapter 23.

WHAT IS CONFLICT?

Conflict can be viewed from both a behavioral and a process standpoint. From a behavioral standpoint conflict is defined "as a perceived condition that exists between parties (e.g. individuals, groups, departments) in which one or more of the parties perceive (a) goal incompatibility and (b) some opportunity for interfering with the goal accomplishment of others" (Albanese, 1981:458). From a process standpoint conflict can be defined as what occurs when real or perceived differences exist in the goals, values, ideas, attitudes, beliefs, feelings, or actions of two or more parties (individuals or groups). Conflict exists when two or more mutually exclusive goals, values, ideas, attitudes, beliefs, feelings or actions occur:

1. Within one individual (intrapersonal)

2. Between two or more individuals (interpersonal)

3. Within one group (intragroup)

4. Between two or more groups (intergroup)

COMPETITION VS. CONFLICT

Conflict is not the same as competition. Competition has some of the elements of conflict in that goal attainment by one unit prevents the other unit from achieving its goals, but competition follows basic rules and is not typically associated with anger and hostility. Filley (1975:2) defines *competitive conflict* as a victory for one side at a loss for the other side. The process by which the conflict is resolved is determined by a set of rules. The goals of each side are mutually incompatible, but the emphasis is on winning, not the defeat or reduction of the opponent. When one side has clearly "won," the competition is terminated.

Disruptive conflict, on the other hand, does not follow any mutually acceptable set of rules and does not emphasize winning. The parties involved are engaged in activity to reduce, defeat, or eliminate the opponent. This type of conflict takes place in an environment charged with fear, anger, and stress. For example, an intern on night call may demonstrate disruptive conflict by refusing to answer pages, turning off the beeper, or by belittling nurses for calling with "minor" problems. Nurses react to this type of behavior with their own disruptive behavior; frequent, "by the book," middle-of-the-night phone calls to get back at the offending intern. A more subtle example of disruptive behavior would be a failure to extend minor work-saving courtesies to an unpopular intern. Disruptive conflict can, in unusual circumstances, result in irrational, disruptive, or violent behavior.

THE CONFLICT PROCESS MODEL

Filley's model of conflict resolution provides a generalized format for examining conflict behavior in relation to the nurse manager's job. This model provides a framework that will help explain how and why conflict occurs and, ultimately, how one can minimize conflict or resolve it with the least amount of negative aftermath.

Filley suggests that conflict and its resolution develop according to a specific process. This process begins with certain preexisting conditions (antecedent conditions). The parties are influenced by their feelings or perceptions about the situation (perceived or felt conflict), which initiates behavior (manifest behavior). The conflict is either resolved or suppressed (conflict resolution or suppression), and in the aftermath new attitudes and feelings between the parties evolve (see Figure 22–1).

Antecedent conditions are conditions that have been shown to exist in a conflict situation. These conditions are not necessarily the cause of con-

Figure 22–1   Conflict Process

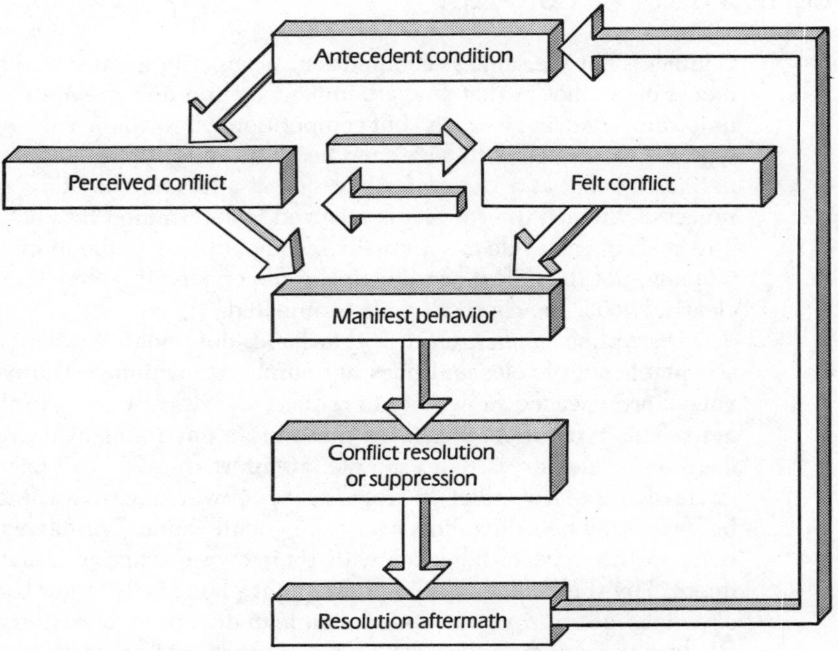

Adapted from Filley, A. C., House, R. J., and Kerr, S.: *Managerial Process and Organizational Behavior*. Copyright © 1976 by A. C. Filley, University of Wisconsin, Madison, Wisconsin. Reprinted by permission.

flict but have been associated with increased rates of conflict and may propel a situation toward conflict. For the nurse manager these include incompatible goals, differences in values and beliefs, task interdependencies (especially asymmetric dependencies where one department is dependent on the other but not vice-versa), unclear/ambiguous roles, competition for scarce resources, differentiation or distancing mechanisms, proximity, and unifying mechanisms.

Nature of Goals and Their Importance to Conflict

The most important antecedent condition to conflict is *incompatible goals*. As discussed in Chapter 3 goals are desired results toward which behavior is directed. Even though in health care institutions the common goal is achieving the highest quality patient care given the resources, conflict in goals is inevitable as individuals often view this from different perspectives. In addition, individuals and organizations have multiple goals that change over time. A health care organization may have specific goals to achieve the best possible care for the patient and control costs in order to stay within budget, while at the same time provide intrinsically satisfying jobs for its employees. These multiple goals will frequently conflict with each other, creating a situation in which decisions will have to be made regarding the relative priorities of these conflicting goals. This issue of priority setting can be one of the most difficult but at the same time important activities a health care administrator must face. Goals are also important because they become the basis by which resources are allocated in organizations and, therefore, are an important source (antecedent) of conflict in the organization.

Similarly, individuals experience goal conflicts due to multiple goals and the inability to achieve each goal. Individuals allocate scarce resources such as their time on the basis of the goal priority and, therefore, might achieve one goal at the expense of achieving others. It is the ability to interfere with goal attainment that is the source of conflict, whether it is because of multiple (and mutually incompatible) personal or departmental goals.

An example of goal conflict in nursing is the dichotomy between nursing education and nursing service. This issue can best be described as a conflict between groups with differing goals. Nursing education teaches the practice of nursing based on a conceptual foundation. Nurse managers who employ new graduates have criticized the lack of clinical experience in the educational program (Brooten, Hayman & Naylors, 1978:60). They want to hire nurses who will need a minimum of orientation and be able to function independently as quickly as possible.

Other Antecedent Conditions

Roles are defined as the expectations of each regarding one's own and others' behavior. *Unclear roles* occur when one or more parties have related responsibilities that are ambiguous or overlapping. The nurse manager might experience conflict in her responsibility as administrator versus her role as staff member. Similar to this are unclear or overlapping job descriptions or assignments. For example, there could be conflict over such mundane issues as the responsibility of the nurse versus transporters in sending a patient to another department or moving a patient from bed to chair.

Competition for scarce resources could be internal (among different units in the hospital) or external (among different hospitals). Internally, competition for resources could involve the assigning of staff from one unit to another or the stockpiling of supplies, such as linen or wheelchairs, by one unit. Externally, hospitals may compete for patients due to reduced occupancy rates. Recently, competition for resources has become a conflictive factor between nurses and physicians. Physicians have challenged the role of nurse practitioners, charging them with practicing medicine without a license, on the basis of legal interpretations of medical and nursing practice acts.* While these charges are publicly touted to promote patient care, many of the involved parties believe they really stem from economic concerns and are intended to reduce competition for health care services.

Differences in values and beliefs is a frequent contributor to conflict in health care institutions. Values and beliefs result from the socialization processes that individuals experience. Conflicts between physicians and nurses, or between nurses and administrators, or even between nurses with associate degrees versus diplomas versus baccalaureate degrees often come from differences in values and beliefs. The latter division raises conflict over which education is the best preparation for practice.

Task interdependency is a potential source of conflict in health care institutions. The three levels of functional interdependence are pooled interdependence, sequential interdependence, and reciprocal interdependence (Thompson, 1967). *Pooled interdependence* exists when units are relatively independent of each other—they are members of the same organization and draw their budgets and other resources from a common pool. An example in a health care unit might be the interaction between the finance department and the nursing department. Direct interaction seldom occurs, and managing the relationship between these units is not difficult. *Sequential interdependence* is where the output of one unit is the input of another unit, where the tasks of the first unit need to be performed before the second unit can perform its task. This is similar to

*Sermchief v. Gonzales, 660 S. W. 2d 683 (Mo. banc 1983), pp. 683–690.

the relationship between support groups such as admissions, discharge, and nursing. Functional nursing involves sequential interdependence. Sequential interdependence can become a particularly difficult situation when the dependent unit is of higher status—for example, when a nurse has to wait for housekeeping services. *Reciprocal interdependence* is where the output from each unit becomes the input of the other unit and vice-versa. The relationship between the nurse and the physician is typically reciprocal in nature, as are the relationships among shifts; among the LPN, NA, and the RN; and between units such as radiology and the medical-surgical unit. Team nursing and primary nursing are also examples of reciprocal interdependencies.

Distancing mechanisms or *differentiation* serve to divide a group's members into small distinct groups, thus increasing the chance for conflict. This tends to lead to a "we-they" distinction. Examples might be opposition between intensive care nurses and floor nurses, night versus day shifts, and nursing aides versus registered nurses. One of the more frequently seen examples is distancing between physicians and nurses. Differentiation among subunits is also due to differences in structure. Many of the administrative units are very bureaucratic in nature, nursing units are structured on a more professional basis, while the staff physicians have even a different structure, and the nonstaff physicians, who are entrepreneurs, are relatively independent from the health care unit.

Unifying mechanisms occur when a greater intimacy develops or when unity is sought. All nurse managers might be expected to reach consensus over an issue but experience internal conflict as they find themselves forced to accept a position as a group, while individually they may not be wholly committed to the group's position. The most classic example of a unifying mechanism is the relationship between husband and wife. As intimacy increases, issues arise that would not normally cause conflict in a casual relationship but do affect these closer relationships. A nurse manager's friendship with a staff member may lead to this type of conflict.

Conflict commonly seen in the health care environment is often *structural* conflict. This conflict evolves from the relationship between members of organizations. These relationships (superior to subordinate, peer to peer) provoke conflict due to inadequate communication, competition for resources, opposing interests, or a lack of shared perceptions or attitudes. A nurse manager (superior) stimulates conflict between herself and a staff member (subordinate) in reprimanding the staff member for some inappropriate act. If the nurse manager is unable to communicate to the staff member why the act was unacceptable, opposing interests develop and the conflict is sustained. In this situation, positional power is often imposed. Positional power refers to the authority that is inherent in a certain position—for example, the director of nursing service has greater positional power than a nurse manager.

Other Aspects of the Conflict Process

Perceived and felt conflict are parts of the conflict process that explain how conflict may occur when the parties involved view the situations or issues from differing perspectives or misunderstand each other's position, or when positions are based on limited knowledge. Perceived conflict refers to each party's perception of the other's position. It is a logical and impersonal set of conflicting conditions present between two or more parties. Felt conflict refers to the feelings of opposition within the relationship of two or more parties. It is characterized by mistrust, hostility, and fear.

To demonstrate how this process may work, consider this situation. Nurse manager Jones and surgeon Smith have worked together for years. They have mutual respect for each other's ability and skills and communicate frequently. When their subordinates clash, they are left with conflicting accounts of a situation where the only agreed-upon fact is that a patient received less than appropriate care. Now consider the same scenario if the nurse and doctor have never dealt with each other or if one feels that the other will not approach the problem constructively. In these situations, the attitudes and feelings of the nurse and doctor are critical.

In the first situation, because of their positive regard for each other's abilities, nurse and physician believe they can constructively solve the conflict. The nurse does not feel the physician will try to dominate, while the physician respects the nurse manager's managerial ability. With these preexisting attitudes, the physician and nurse can remain neutral while assisting their subordinates to solve the conflict. In the second situation, the nurse and physician may approach the situation differently. If each assumes the other will defend her or his subordinates at all costs, communication will be inhibited. The conflict is resolved by domination of the stronger person, either in personality or position. One wins; the other loses.

Manifest behavior is the action that results or what happens. Overt action may take the form of aggression, competition, debate, or problem solving. Covert action may be expressed by a variety of indirect tactics such as scapegoating, avoidance, or apathy.

The final stages of the conflict process are suppression or resolution and the resulting aftermath. *Suppression* occurs when one person or group defeats the other. Only the dominant side is committed to the agreement and the loser may or may not carry out the agreement. *Resolution* occurs when a mutually agreed-upon solution is arrived at, and both parties commit themselves to carry out the agreement. The optimal solution to conflictive situations is to manage the issues in a way that will lead to a solution wherein both parties see themselves as winners and the problem is defeated. This leaves an aftermath that will affect future relations and can influence feelings and attitudes. In the example of conflict between the nurse manager and the physician, consider the difference in the aftermath and how future issues would be approached if both parties felt positive about the outcome, as compared to future interactions if one or both parties felt they had lost.

GROUP PROCESSES

Groups are often a source of conflict in organizations. Understanding why groups form and how they influence behavior in organizations is important for a nurse manager. Whenever humans interact together in organizations, they are likely to form cohesive groups. Nurses are no exception. Often highly cohesive groups of nurses develop strong norms as to how nurses ought to behave. Cohesive groups are more likely to develop where there are shared values and beliefs, where individuals have similar goals and tasks, where individuals have to interact together to achieve these tasks, where there is proximity in both time and distance (i.e., they work in the same unit and on the same shift), and where they have specific needs that can be satisfied by the group. For example, groups provide a means of satisfying social needs and opportunities for interaction; provide an identity; provide protection from common enemies; provide a means of testing reality; and help to accomplish tasks that the individual cannot achieve alone. These groups are likely to develop strong norms that influence the behavior of the group members through enforcement by the group members. For example, Feldman (1984:48–49) states: "(1) Norms are likely to be enforced if they facilitate group survival. . . . (2) Norms are likely to be enforced if they simplify, or make predictable, what behavior is expected of group members. . . . (3) Norms are likely to be enforced if they help the group avoid embarrassing interpersonal problems. . . . (4) Norms are likely to be enforced if they express the central values of the group and clarify what is distinctive about the group's identity." These norms are often a source of either intragroup or intergroup conflict.

Intragroup Conflict

Intragroup conflict can occur when these group norms or standards are violated or changed. For example, in an organization undergoing decentralization, nurse managers might be expected to change in various ways, such as earning a bachelor's degree or wearing street clothes and a lab coat instead of a conventional uniform. This change might conflict with group norms and could stimulate internal conflict for nurse managers who have perceived themselves differently. Groups often develop norms relative to how hard a person is expected to work, making it more difficult for the nurse manager to influence productivity. Another potential intragroup conflict problem that a nurse manager must deal with would be the introduction of new members into a cohesive group. The nurse manager must make sure that the new members are accepted and made part of the group.

Intergroup Conflict

Intergroup conflict arises between groups with differing goals, the achievement of which by one group can occur only at the expense of the other. These types of conflicts can range from small day-to-day problems to broader issues. For example, administration's goal is to control salary expenses, while nursing's goal is to upgrade staffing with a resultant increase in salary costs. A smaller day-to-day issue might be when the radiology department wants patients sent to X ray in gowns without metal snaps on the sleeve because the snaps show on the film. Nursing staff prefer these snaps because they make it easier to change gowns on patients receiving intravenous fluids. Neither side wants the bother of changing gowns prior to X rays and believes the other should do this task.

Intraorganizational Conflict

Conflict between groups, departments, or divisions of an organization is often a consequence of the degree to which these units are differentiated from another. According to Lawrence and Lorsch (1967), differentiation between units may be due to differences in structure, time orientation, interpersonal orientation, or subenvironment orientation. For example, some units in hospitals such as food service and housekeeping tend to have more mechanistic structures, while financial services and accounting might have a bureaucratic structure, and units such as nursing will be structured on a more professional basis. In terms of time orientation, research units might have long-time orientations while the emergency room would be an example of a unit with a short-time orientation. Some units in a hospital such as personnel or public relations might have strong interpersonal orientations, while laboratories might have strong task orientations. The final dimension of differentiation is subenvironment orientation. Administrative units such as finance would have an orientation toward the economic environment, while units such as radiology would have a more technical or scientific subenvironment orientation.

The more differentiated units are the greater the potential for conflict, especially if these units must work together to perform their tasks or when one unit is highly dependent on the other unit. Similarly, there may be conflicts between staff units—those units providing support services— and line units—those units providing specific care and services to patients. The manner in which a health care institution is departmentalized or how units are physically located can be sources of conflicts. As noted before, resource allocations and different goals may also be sources of intra-organizational conflict.

COMMUNICATION PROBLEMS

Marriner (1979) identifies conflicts originating from senders (those initiating the communication—see Chapter 8), groups, and individuals. Sender conflict can be either intra- or intersender. Intrasender conflict occurs when one sender gives conflicting instructions to another—the director of nursing, for instance, demands that the floor be adequately staffed but forbids the use of paid overtime. Intersender conflict occurs when two conflicting messages are received from differing sources. This might occur when staff is encouraged by the risk manager to report medication errors, while the nurse manager follows up with discipline over the error. The nurse is caught between conflicting messages from two sources. The nurse is encouraged to "tell all" to help the hospital protect itself, but by doing so may be subjected to disciplinary action. In the case of a "not so serious error," the nurse may rationalize that the error did not cause any harm so why subject herself or himself to potential discipline just to report the error.

CONFLICT MANAGEMENT

The management of conflict is an important part of the nurse manager's job. A number of techniques can be used by the nurse manager to manage conflict. Some of these are more effective than others. One method of conflict management is suppression of the conflict. This could even include the elimination of one of the parties in the conflict through transfer or termination. The opposite of suppression is a form of conflict resolution that stresses harmony or a "don't rock the boat" attitude. One party is dominated by the other without resistance. In the past, nurses have been subordinate to physicians and were taught to follow physicians' orders without question.

Some of the other, less effective techniques for managing conflict include withdrawing, smoothing, avoiding, forcing, and competing, though each of these modes of response is useful in given situations. *Withdrawal* from the conflict simply removes at least one party, thereby making it impossible to resolve the situation. The issues remain unsolved and feelings about the issue may resurface inappropriately.

Smoothing is accomplished by complimenting one's opponent, downplaying differences, and focusing on minor areas of agreement, as if little disagreement exists. Smoothing may be appropriate in dealing with minor problems but, in response to major problems, it produces the same results as withdrawing.

Avoiding is similar to withdrawal, except the participants never acknowledge that a conflict exists. Avoidance is the conflict resolution technique often used in highly cohesive groups that are engaged in "groupthink." The group avoids disagreement because they do not want to do anything that may interfere with the good feelings they have for each other (Janis, 1972).

Forcing is a method that yields an immediate end to the conflict but leaves the cause of the conflict unresolved. A superior can resort to issuing orders, but the subordinate will lack commitment to the demanded action. Forcing may be appropriate in life or death situations but is otherwise inappropriate.

Competing is an all-out effort to win, regardless of the cost. Competing, like forcing, may be needed to prevail in situations involving unpopular or critical decisions.

Negotiation, collaboration, compromise, and confrontation are generally more effective modes of responding to conflict. *Negotiation* involves a give-and-take on various issues among the parties. It is used in situations in which consensus will never be reached. Therefore, the best solution is not often achieved. Negotiation often becomes a structured, formal procedure, as in collective bargaining.

Collaboration implies a mutual attention to the problem that utilizes the talents of all parties. In collaboration, the focus is on solving the problem, not defeating the opponent; the goal is to satisfy both parties' concerns. Collaboration is useful in situations where the goals of both parties are too important to be compromised.

Compromise is used to divide the rewards between both parties. Neither gets what he or she wants. Compromise can serve as a backup to resolve conflict when collaboration is ineffective. It is sometimes the only choice when opponents of equal power are in conflict over two or more mutually exclusive goals. Compromising is also expedient when a solution is needed rapidly.

The *confrontation* technique of resolving conflict is similar to the collaboration technique and is considered to be the most effective means for resolving conflicts. This is a very problem-oriented technique, where the conflict is brought out into the open and attempts are made to resolve it through knowledge and reason. Lawrence and Lorsch (1967) refer to this mode using aphorisms such as "by digging and digging the truth is discovered" and "seek 'til you find and you'll not lose your labor." The goal of this conflict resolution technique is to achieve win-win solutions.

Group Conflict Resolution

Filley (1975) identifies three basic strategies for dealing with conflict according to the outcome: *win-lose*, *lose-lose*, and *win-win*. In the *win-lose* outcome, one party exerts dominance, usually by power of authority, and the other party submits and loses. Forcing, competing, and negotiation are techniques that are likely to lead to win-lose competition. Majority rule is another example of the win-lose outcome, especially within groups. It may be a satisfactory method of resolving conflict, however, if various factions vote differently on different issues and the group functions over time so that members win some and lose some. Win-lose outcomes often occur between groups. A potential negative consequence of this is that frequent losing can lead to the loss of cohesiveness within groups and diminish the authority of the group leader.

In the *lose-lose* method, neither side wins. The settlement reached is unsatisfactory to both sides. Often, avoiding, withdrawing, smoothing, and compromising lead to lose-lose outcomes. One compromising strategy involves using bribes to influence another's cooperation in doing something he or she dislikes. For example, the nurse manager may promise a future raise in an attempt to coerce a staff member to work an extra weekend. Using a third party as arbitrator can lead to a lose-lose outcome. Since an outsider may want to give something to each side, neither gets what is desired. Often either a win-lose or a lose-lose outcome occurs. This is common in arbitration of labor-management disputes. Another strategy that may help a lose-lose or win-lose outcome is resorting to rules. The outcome is left to chance (whatever the rules say), and confrontation is avoided.

The win-lose and lose-lose methods share some common characteristics:

1. The conflict is a personal "we-they" conflict rather than a problem-centered focus. This is very likely to occur when two cohesive groups that do not share common values or goals are in conflict.

2. Parties direct their energy toward total victory for themselves and total defeat for the other. This can cause long-term problems for the organization.

3. Each sees the issue from her or his own point of view rather than as a problem in need of a solution.

4. The emphasis is on outcomes rather than definition of goals, values, or objectives.

5. Conflicts are personalized.

6. Conflict-resolving activities are not differentiated from other group processes.

7. There is a short-run view of the conflict, with settlement of the immediate problem as the goal rather than resolution of differences (Filley, 1975:25).

Win-win methods focus on goals and attempt to meet the needs of both parties. The common techniques of conflict resolution that lead to win-win outcomes are collaboration and confrontation. Two specific win-

win strategies are consensus and integrative decision making. Consensus involves attention to the facts and to the position of the other parties and avoidance of trading, voting, or averaging, where everyone loses something. The consensus decision is often superior to even the best individual one. This technique is most useful in a group setting.

Integrative decision-making methods focus on the means of problem solution rather than the ends and are most useful when the needs of the parties are polarized. Using integrative decision-making methods, the parties jointly identify the value needs of each, conduct an exhaustive search for alternatives that could meet these needs of each, and then select the best alternative. Like the consensus methods, integrative decision making focuses on defeating the problem, not each other.

The group consensus technique is sensitive to the seven characteristics of the win-lose and lose-lose outcomes listed above. If these factors are present as the parties attempt to resolve the issues, all of the involved parties will not be committed to the solution. In this situation, a win-win outcome is unlikely. True consensus occurs when the problem is fully explored, the needs and goals of the involved parties are understood, and a solution that meets these needs is agreed upon.

Integrative problem solving is a constructive process which emphasizes that the parties jointly identify the problem and their needs. They explore a number of alternative solutions and come to consensus on a solution. The focus of this group activity is to solve the problem and not to force, dominate, suppress, or compromise behaviors. The group works toward a common goal in an atmosphere that encourages the free exchange of ideas and feelings.

Personal Conflict Resolution Styles

Individuals have particular styles for resolving conflicts. Even though these might not be used in every situation, there are tendencies to behave in these ways. You can assess your own response to conflict by ranking the following questions. Place a five beside the sentence you think is most like yourself (your real you), a 4 beside the next, then 3, 2, and 1 respectively.

Conflict Questionnaire*

_____A. When conflict arises, I try to remain neutral.

_____B. I try to avoid generating conflict; but when it does appear, I try to soothe feelings to keep people together.

_____C. When conflict arises, I try to find fair solutions that accommodate others.

*Blake, Mouton & Tapper, 1981:9.

Figure 22–2 The Nurse Administrator Conflict Grid®

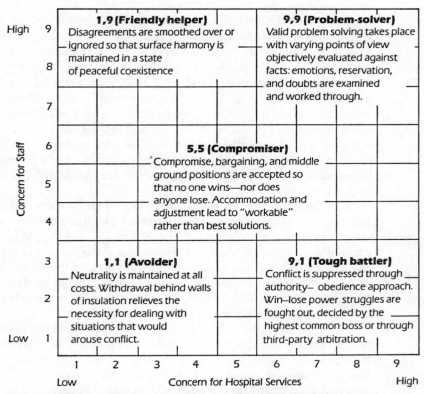

High 9

1,9 (Friendly helper)
Disagreements are smoothed over or ignored so that surface harmony is maintained in a state of peaceful coexistence

9,9 (Problem-solver)
Valid problem solving takes place with varying points of view objectively evaluated against facts: emotions, reservation, and doubts are examined and worked through.

5,5 (Compromiser)
Compromise, bargaining, and middle ground positions are accepted so that no one wins—nor does anyone lose. Accommodation and adjustment lead to "workable" rather than best solutions.

1,1 (Avoider)
Neutrality is maintained at all costs. Withdrawal behind walls of insulation relieves the necessity for dealing with situations that would arouse conflict.

9,1 (Tough battler)
Conflict is suppressed through authority— obedience approach. Win–lose power struggles are fought out, decided by the highest common boss or through third-party arbitration.

Concern for Staff

Low

1 2 3 4 5 6 7 8 9

Low   Concern for Hospital Services   High

Adapted from Blake, R., and Mouton, J. The fifth achievement. *Journal of Applied Behavioral Management*, 1970, 6, 413–426. Reproduced by permission.

_____D. When conflict arises, I try to cut it off or to win my position.

_____E. When conflict arises, I try to identify reasons for it and seek to resolve underlying causes.

These common styles of conflict resolution are shown in Figure 22–2, the nurse administrator grid. The five styles of conflict resolution used by nurse managers and the corresponding letter from the exercise above are avoider (A), friendly helper (B), compromiser (C), tough battler (D), and problem solver (E).

According to Blake, Mouton, and Tapper (1981:56) the nurse manager who uses the "avoider" style (1,1) in conflict situations tends to remain neutral, withdraws from the situation, delays responding to the conflict situation, or may even give the appearance of being busy to avoid others from bringing her into the conflict. Unfortunately, the issue doesn't go away and remains unresolved, and feelings about the issue may resurface inappropriately. Often this style leads to the conflict being taken to someone higher up.

The "friendly helper" nurse manager (1,9) dreads conflict because it threatens warmth and approval (Blake, Mouton & Tapper, 1981:39). Therefore, conflicts are smoothed over so that the nurse manager can get back into a closer supportive relationship with others.

Avoiding, withdrawing, and smoothing have been followed in the nursing profession, with its heritage of an emphasis on obedience and submissiveness. These strategies may still be useful techniques, such as when other issues are more important, and the current issue is trivial by comparison; the potential for disruption is greater than the benefits of resolution; or time is needed for emotions to stabilize and a perspective to be regained, but generally these techniques are not as useful as the techniques listed below.

The "tough battler" nurse manager (9,1) feels that she is losing control when conflict occurs and tends to respond with anger and attempts to use power to win any conflicts (Blake, Mouton & Tapper, 1981:20). This frequently causes suppression of the conflict, because others are denied any chance to react and wish to avoid the wrath of the nurse manager. There is some evidence to indicate that the tough battler tends to win frequently in conflicts with friendly helpers who want to smooth over the conflict quickly (See Figure 22–3).

The "compromiser" nurse manager (5,5) starts with the assumptions that no person or department ever has its exclusive way, extreme positions promote conflict and should therefore be avoided, and steady progress comes from compromising (Blake, Mouton & Tapper, 1981:72–74). This nurse manager uses tact and diplomacy, and seldom tries to confront conflict because that could cause someone to win and someone to lose. This technique involves a give-and-take on various issues among the par-

Figure 22–3 Estimated Outcomes in Dyadic Combinations of Conflict Style in Bargaining

	Tough battler	Friendly helper	Problem solver
Tough battler	Stalemate 80%	Battler wins 90%	Battler wins over 50%
Friendly helper	X	Stalemate 80%	Problem solver wins
Problem solver	X	X	Quick agreement

Adapted from Filley, A. C., House, R. J., Kerr, S.: *Managerial Process and Organizational Behavior.* Copyright © 1976 by A. C. Filley, University of Wisconsin, Madison, Wisconsin. Reprinted by permission.

ties. Often the solution selected is the one that is politically safe, salable, or workable.

The "problem solver" nurse manager (9,9) recognizes that conflict may delay or prevent the achievement of organizational and personal goals, but she also recognizes that conflict can frequently lead to innovation, creativity, and the development of new ideas (Blake, Mouton & Tapper, 1981:93). The nurse manager recognizes that though conflict may be inevitable, it might also be resolvable. Therefore, she tries to anticipate conflict, and when it does occur she confronts the conflict and tries to find out its causes and the optimal way to deal with it. Collaboration is often a technique used by the problem-solving nurse manager. Collaboration implies a mutual attention to the problem that utilizes the talents of all parties. In collaboration, the focus is on solving the problem, not defeating the opponent; the goal is to satisfy both parties' concerns. Collaboration is useful in situations where the goals of both parties are too important to be compromised.

Though problem solving is the preferred means by which nurse managers should deal with conflict, Figure 22–3 shows that the problem solver loses about 50% of the conflicts with the tough battler (Cummings, Harnett & Stevens, 1971). It is important for the organization to reward the problem-solving style of conflict resolution, train individuals in how to use this style, and discourage the tough battler style. As noted before, however, this technique is difficult to use by nurse managers because confrontation has been discouraged for women, and even more so for nurses, by society's traditional mores.

Conflict Intervention

Nurse managers may be involved in resolving conflict on several different levels. They may be participants in the conflict either as individuals, as supervisors, or as representatives of a unit. In fact, they must often initiate conflict by confronting staff, individually or collectively, when a problem develops. They may also serve as mediators or judges to conflicting parties. There could be a conflict within the unit, between parties from different units, or between internal and external parties (e.g., a nursing instructor from an outside school has a conflict with staff on a particular unit). Whatever the nurse manager's position in the conflict situation, the process needed to resolve conflict is essentially the same and is consistent with the problem-solving technique discussed before.

It is important for the nurse manager and other participants in conflict resolution to be realistic regarding the outcome. Often those inexperienced in conflict negotiation expect unrealistic outcomes. When there are two parties or more with mutually exclusive ideas, attitudes, feelings, or goals, it is extremely difficult, without the commitment and willingness of all concerned, to arrive at an agreeable solution that meets the needs of both.

Conflict resolution begins with a decision regarding if and when to intervene. The nurse manager should make sure the parties know when she is likely to intervene. Failure to intervene can allow the conflict to get out of hand, while early intervention may be demotivating to the parties, causing them to lose confidence in themselves and reduce risk-taking behavior in the future. Some conflicts are so minor, particularly if they are between only two people, that intervention is not necessary and may be better handled by the two people. This might provide a developmental experience and improve their abilities to resolve conflict in the future. On the other hand, where there is potential for considerable harm to result from the conflict, then the nurse manager must intervene.

Sometimes the nurse manager may postpone intervention purposely, to allow the conflict to escalate, since increased intensity can stimulate the participants to seek resolution. The manager can escalate the conflict even further by exposing the participants to each other more frequently without the presence of others and without an easy means of escape. Participants are then forced to face the conflict between them. Giving the participants a shared task or shared goals not directly related to the conflict may help them understand each other better and increase their chances to resolve their conflicts by themselves. Using a method such as this one is useful only if the conflict is not of high intensity, if the participants are not highly anxious about it, and if the manager believes that the conflict will not decrease efficiency of the department in the meantime.

If a nurse manager decides to intervene in a conflict between two or more parties, then mediation techniques are very applicable. She or he must make decisions as to when, where, and how the intervention should take place. Routine problems can be handled in either the superior's or subordinate's office, but serious conflicts should take place in a neutral location unless the parties involved in the conflict are of unequal power. In this case, the setting should favor the disadvantaged participant, thereby equalizing their power.

The time and place should be one where distractions will not interfere and adequate time is available. Since conflict resolution takes time, the manager must be prepared to allow sufficient time for all parties to explain their points of view and arrive at a mutually agreeable solution. A quick solution often resorted to by inexperienced managers is to impose positional power. This could result in a win-lose outcome, leading to feelings of elation and eventual complacency on the part of the winners and loss of morale on the part of the losers.

The following are some of the basic rules on how to mediate a conflict between two or more parties:

1. Protect each party's self-respect. Deal with a conflict of issues, not personalities.

2. Do not put blame or responsibility for the problem on the participants. The participants are responsible for developing a solution to the problem.

3. Allow open and complete discussion of the problem from each participant.

4. Maintain equity in the frequency and duration of each party's presentation. There is a tendency for a higher status person to speak more frequently and longer than a lower status person. If this occurs, the mediator should intervene and ask the lower status person for response and opinion.

5. Encourage full expression of positive and negative feelings within an accepting atmosphere. There is a tendency for the novice mediator to discourage expressions of disagreement.

6. Make sure both parties listen actively to each other's words. One way to do this is to establish the ground rule that requires each person to summarize the comments of the other prior to stating her or his own position.

7. Identify key themes in the discussion and restate these at frequent intervals.

8. Encourage the parties to provide frequent feedback to each other's comments. Each must truly understand the other's position.

9. Assist the participants in developing alternative solutions, selecting a mutually agreeable one, and developing a plan to carry it out. All parties must be agreeable to the solution for successful resolution to occur.

10. At an agreed-upon interval, follow up on the progress of the plan.

11. Give positive feedback to participants regarding their cooperation in solving the conflict.

Conflict resolution is a difficult process, consuming both time and energy. Management and staff must be concerned and committed to resolving conflict by being willing to listen to others' positions and to finding agreeable solutions.

Other Conflict Management Techniques

Many other techniques besides personal intervention can be used to resolve conflict and are consistent with the problem-solving approach. Some of these include changing or clarifying goals, developing superordinate goals, and holding confrontation meetings. In addition, other techniques that may be effective include appeals to the hierarchy, negotiating and providing cooling-off periods, establishing liaison persons, restructuring by buffering and decoupling, and dividing the resources so each party can partially achieve its goals (Hunger & Stern, 1976). These techniques are particularly useful in dealing with intergroup or intraorganizational conflict. Though the nurse manager frequently does not have direct responsibility for resolving these types of conflicts, it is important that she or he understand the nature of these conflicts and some of the techniques that can be used to resolve them.

Changing or clarifying goals, especially where a superordinate goal can be developed is a useful technique for reducing conflict in organizations. A superordinate goal is a goal "of high appeal value for (conflicting) groups . . . , but whose attainment is beyond the resources and efforts of any one group alone" (Sherif et al., 1961:202). Research by Hunger and Stern (1976) indicates that superordinate goals can be effective in reducing conflict between groups even though some of the underlying causes of the conflict remain unchanged. Health care institutions may have an advantage over other institutions in that a "natural" superordinate goal— *quality patient care*—is available to reduce conflict. When conflict does occur between groups, the nurse manager must focus on this issue in order to improve cooperation between the units. Similar to superordinate goals is finding a common enemy, such as a health care competitor. Focusing on this competitor may help units cooperate better.

The *confrontation meeting* developed by Beckhard (1967) is also a means for dealing with conflict. This is a one-day meeting of the entire administration of an organization in which they take a reading of the health of their organization. It includes seven steps. In Step 1, climate setting, the top administrator starts the session by stating her or his goals for the meeting and clarifying the issues to be addressed in the meeting. Step 2 involves small heterogeneous groups of five to seven members from the various functional units to work on the issues presented in Step 1. Step 3 involves the sharing of information from each of the small groups. In Step 4 the issues from the small groups are listed and priorities are set. The participants then meet in their functional work teams to identify and discuss the issues and problems related to their area, to decide on the priorities of these problems, and to determine action steps to be taken to remedy the problems that have been raised. This includes communicating the result of the confrontration meeting to their subordinates or others in their unit. Step 5 involves only the top administrative team, which meets after the rest of the participants have left to plan follow-up action steps. These are communicated to the rest of the administrative group after the meeting. Finally, Step 6 includes a progress review meeting where each group reports on progress in addressing the issues raised in the confrontation meeting and reviews the actions resulting from this meeting. This method is effective if problems are clarified, "hidden agendas" are brought out into the open, true dialogue is developed among the various units in conflict, and the various group members develop "ownership" of the problem (Brooten, Hayman & Naylors, 1980:92–93).

A liaison person or an integrating department can help manage conflict between units, especially highly differentiated units. Having such a person or group reduces the need for the units to deal directly with each other, in effect isolating the conflicting parties from each other. Buffering inventories might reduce the need to manage the relationship between units. Having extra inventories of commonly used supplies available on the floor or in the unit can also reduce the potential for conflict. Sometimes allowing units or persons to "blow off steam" can relieve the pressures from the conflict as well.

SUMMARY

- The nurse manager must recognize that conflict is inevitable in productive organizations.

- Conflict in health care organizations frequently results from different goals, different values and beliefs, competition for scarce resources, task interdependencies, and/or group processes.

- Conflict can be disruptive or can be used constructively to promote change.

- The nurse manager should ask whether the conflict is disruptive and, therefore, is keeping the conflicting parties from accomplishing organizational and/or personal goals.

- If the conflict is disruptive, then the nurse manager should ask what methods might be used to deal with the conflict.

- Should the nurse manager intervene in the conflict personally or should the nurse manager involve other parties, including her or his supervisor?

- The five styles of conflict resolution used by nurse managers to intervene in conflicts include the avoider, the friendly helper, the compromiser, the tough battler, and the problem solver. Though there are situations where each of these styles can be effective, the most effective style of conflict resolution is the problem solver style.

- Consistent with the problem-solving approach is the technique of mediation.

- Other means that can be used to resolve conflicts include superordinate goals, confrontation meetings, structural changes, negotiation and compromise, and buffering devices or dividing resources so each party can partially achieve its goals.

BIBLIOGRAPHY

Albanese, R. (1981). *Managing: Toward accountability for performance.* Homewood, IL: Irwin.

Beckhard, R. (1967). The confrontation meeting. *Harvard Bus R*, (March-April) 45:149–155.

Blake, R. R., Mouton, J. S., and Tapper, M. (1981). *Grid approaches for managerial leadership in nursing.* St. Louis: C. V. Mosby.

Brooten, D. A., Hayman, L., and Naylors, M. D. (1978). *Leadership for change: A guide for the frustrated nurse.* Philadelphia: J. B. Lippincott.

Cummings, L. L., Harnett, D. L., and Stevens, O. J. (1971). Risk, fate, conciliation and trust: An international study of attitudinal differences among executives. *Acad Mngmt J*, 14:285.

Douglass, L. (1983). *The effective nurse: Leader and manager*, 2nd ed. St. Louis: C. V. Mosby.

Feldman, D. C. (1984). The development and enforcement of group norms. *Acad Mngmt R*, 9:47–53.

Filley, A. C. (1975). *Interpersonal conflict resolution.* Glenview, IL: Scott, Foresman.

Filley, A. C., House, R. J., and Kerr, S. (1976). *Managerial process and organizational behavior.* Glenview, IL: Scott, Foresman.

Hunger, J. D. (1979). An analysis of intergroup conflict and conflict management. In: *Management pragmatics.* Webber, R. A. (editor). Homewood, IL: Irwin. Pp. 353–358.

Hunger, J. D., and Stern, L. W. (1976). An assessment of the functionality of the superordinate goal in reducing conflict. *Acad Mngmt J*, (December) 19(4): 591–605.

Janis, I. L. (1972). *Victims of group-think: A psychological study of foreign policy decisions and fiascos.* Boston: Houghton Mifflin.

Klein, S. M., and Ritti, R. R. (1984). *Understanding organizational behavior.* 2nd ed. Boston: Kent.

Lawrence, P. R., and Lorsch, J. W. (1967). Differentiation and integration in complex organizations. *Admin Sc Q*, (June) 12(1): 1–47.

Marriner, A. (1979). Conflict theory. *Superv Nurs*, (April) 10:12.

Sherif, M., Harvey, O. J., White, B. J., Hood, W., and Sherif, C. W. (1961). *Intergroup conflict and cooperation: The robbers' cave experiment.* Norman, OK: University Book Exchange.

Sherif, M., and Sherif, C. W. (1969). *Social Psychology.* New York: Harper and Row.

Silber, M. B. (1984). Managing confrontations: Once more into the breach. *Nurs Mngmt*, (April) 15(4): 54.

Thomas, K. W. (1976). Conflict and conflict management. In: *Handbook of Industrial and Organizational Psychology.* Dunnette, M. D. (editor). Chicago: Rand McNally. Pp. 889–935.

Thompson, J. D. (1967). *Organizations in action.* New York: McGraw-Hill.

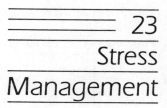

23
Stress
Management

NATURE OF STRESS

Stress is defined as the reaction of individuals to demands from the environment that pose a threat (Steers, 1984:506). The body's response to the conflict caused by two or more incompatible demands results in stress. Selye, who is considered the pioneer of stress research, suggests that the body's wear and tear results from its response to normal stressors (Selye, 1976). However, the rate and intensity of damage are increased when an organism experiences greater stress than it is capable of accommodating.

Selye maintains that response to stress is the same whether the stressor is positive or negative; for example, a promotion may be a stressful, though positive, event. In addition, a certain amount of stress is essential to sustain life, and moderate amounts serve as stimuli to performance. It is overpowering stress that causes one to respond in a maladaptive physiological or psychological manner.

Stress and the capability to handle it may be viewed as weights on a balance scale. Figure 23–1 depicts this balance in stress, which is essential for life. When the degree of stress is equal to the degree of ability to accommodate it, the organism is in a state of equilibrium and job performance and personal satisfaction tend to be high. Normal wear and tear occur, but sustained damage does not. When the degree of stress is greater (weighs more) than the ability to accommodate it, increased pres-

Figure 23–1 Stress Balance

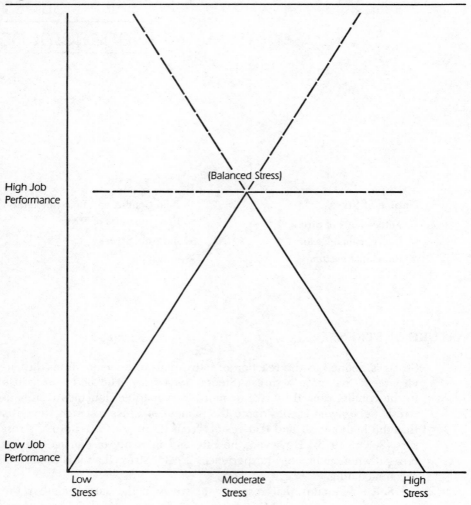

sure is applied to the organism. The situation is often described metaphorically through such statements as "He has a load on his shoulders" or "She bears a heavy burden." This often leads to physiological and psychological problems for the organism and poor performance for the organization. When the degree of stress is smaller (weighs less) than the ability to accommodate it, little pressure is applied to the organism (either internal or external) and lack of interest, apathy, boredom, low motivation, low performance, and even absenteeism can occur.

Figure 23–2 Stress Model

ANTECEDENTS	INTERVENING CONSTRUCTS	CONSEQUENCES
Organizational Factors		*Negative*
Job tasks		Stress
Physical environment		Health problems
Supervisor behavior		Marital problems/divorce
Institutional factors		Alcoholism/drug abuse
Changing environment		Lower performance
Societal/nursing traditions		Lower job satisfaction
Self-worth		Lower self-esteem
Intraprofessional divisiveness		Absenteeism/turnover
	Role Ambiguity	Career dissatisfaction/change
Interpersonal Factors		*Positive/Coping*
Role messages		
Trust/respect for senders		Role redefinition
Multiple roles		Share roles
(nurse, manager, parent, spouse)		Integrate roles
	Role Conflict	Confront role senders
Individual Factors		Redefine role
Rate of "life change"		Personal reorientation
Ability to perform roles		Reactive coping
Self-esteem/self-perception		Increased performance
Tolerance for ambiguity		Increased efficiency
Other personality traits		Prioritize tasks/goals

Source: Phillip J. Decker and Eleanor J. Sullivan. Used by permission.

An interesting aspect of stress is the individual perception of it. One person's stressful event is another's challenge. One person can experience an event, positive or negative, that would prove overwhelming for someone else.

Stress in the workplace and, specifically, for the nurse, can develop from several sources. Figure 23–2 shows a stress model and includes the antecedents of stress, the intervening variables of role ambiguity and role conflict, and the consequences of stress.

Antecedents of Stress

Stress resulting from *job tasks* and the *physical environment* develops from such conditions as task overload, conflicting tasks, inability to do the tasks assigned due to lack of preparation or experience, or from unclear or insufficient information regarding the assignment. Lack of training/education can contribute to role ambiguity and result in stress. Nurses' jobs are often performed in life or death situations. There may be periods of extreme overload caused by emergencies that are potentially stressful.

The *supervisor's behavior* can be a factor in stress. Close, punitive, and/or authoritarian supervisory behavior is closely related to stress. The degree to which supervisors clarify the goals of their subordinates and allow their subordinates to participate in decisions affecting their jobs are factors in how much stress the subordinate will perceive.

Institutional factors that can lead to stress include institutional norms and expectations that conflict with an individual's needs. Understaffing and the practice of assigning staff to unfamiliar units are examples. Some organizational norms dictate that an employee's primary loyalty be to the institution rather than to self, group, or profession. Events that challenge this norm can cause stress for both the individual and the institution. Multiple and conflicting bosses can also be a potential source of stress, especially where satisfying the requests of one authority figure makes it impossible to satisfy those of the other.

The rapidly *changing environment* of health care institutions has also been a contributor to stress in nursing. Rapid changes in technology, increased pressures from clients for service, liability issues, increased pressures for efficiency due to competition, and pressure from agencies such as Medicare have made the role of nurses more difficult, conflicting, and stressful.

Some *societal/nursing traditions* are a source of stress. Brooten, Hayman, and Naylors (1978) point out that of all the problems faced in nursing, the problem of self-worth is most basic. Since 98% of the nursing profession is female, many of the prevalent attitudes toward women in our society are reflected in nurses. Traditional concepts consider women to be passive, weak, intuitive, inconsistent, dependent, empathic, sensitive, and subjective. Yet male traits such as aggression, independence, competitiveness, rational thinking, self-discipline, and leadership ability are the traits our society values most. While some of the female traits such as empathy and sensitivity are valued nursing attributes, nurses are not typically described as aggressive, independent, analytical, and competitive. For these reasons, an image of nursing that closely associates nursing with female sex stereotypes has formed. As the role of women changes in our society, so does nursing, but a comparative lack of worth is still perceived by health care consumers, other health professionals, and even by nurses.

Nursing has seen tremendous changes over the years. Nurses are no longer expected to give their seats to physicians when physicians enter a nurses' station. Continuing education with emphasis on assertiveness training is encouraged by some nursing departments. Nursing administration is now seen as a specific specialty, with graduate nursing education dedicated to this purpose. Directors of nursing are now frequently seen on an equal administrative level with other senior hospital administrators at the vice-presidential or assistant administrator level (see Chapter 24 on working with higher management).

Interpersonal Factors

To add to the problem of self-worth, nurses must contend with division within the profession itself. This division begins with conflict regarding educational preparation, i.e., associate degree versus diploma versus baccalaureate. This division spawns the conflict over which education is the best preparation for practice and results in different role messages being sent to nurses. What is the current role of a nurse? Often different groups outside the nursing profession give different messages. Role messages from the administration of the health care institution relative to efficiency and protecting the organization are inconsistent with the messages that come from society relative to nursing as a helping and healing role. What is the perception of physicians concerning the role of the nurse? Does the role differ whether functional, team, or primary nursing is employed? Does the role differ depending on the type of health care institution? What perceptions do nurses have of these various role senders?

The lack of participation in professional associations by nurses also continues. Nursing associations are inhibited in lobbying for nursing issues due to the low percentage of member nurses. While specialty nursing organizations, such as those for critical care nurses and operating room nurses, have had greater success in recruiting members, the lobbying efforts of these organizations tend to support the specialty interests of their constituents. In fact, they can serve as a distancing mechanism between themselves and nurses not in the specialty group and thus contribute to differences in the role messages that nurses receive.

Multiple roles are a source of stress. For example, home-job conflict is a potential source of stress to nurses. Nurses perform a number of roles. Often they are a spouse and a parent. Given that a high percentage of nurses are women, this is a major source of stress, as expectations of the contributions women should make as a parent or spouse are much greater than those for males. Adding to this is the shift work and weekend work required by most nursing jobs. Most health care institutions must be staffed 24 hours a day, 7 days a week. Individuals who work on the evening or night shifts experience physiological problems if their spouse or children are on different shifts. This is especially a problem, if, periodically, they change shifts. Often it takes several weeks to adjust physiologically to a change in shifts (Levi, 1981:8–14).

In addition, conflict between the role of a nurse manager and the role of a nurse can be a source of stress. Doing and directing others are different jobs. Directing others is stressful, especially when the nurse manager believes she is a better nurse than those she is supervising. There is an old navy saying about the captain who is watching the ensign bring the ship into dock: the "captain bites his tongue until it bleeds."

Individual Factors

Stress can result from *individual factors*. One of these factors is "rate of life change." Researchers have shown that the rate of life change generates cumulative stress that, in turn, leads to the onset of disease or illness (Holmes & Rahe, 1967). These researchers assigned points for various life events based on the event's contribution to the amount of stress (see Figure 23–3). If an individual accumulated more than 150 points within a year's time, he or she had a 50% chance of developing serious illness the following year. For those individuals who scored 300 or more points, there was at least a 70% chance of contracting a major illness the following year.

Stress often results from an incongruence between one's expectations for one's performance and one's perception of the resulting performance. Past experience in coping with stress also is included in this category. People tend to repeat coping behaviors in similar situations, regardless of whether the initial behavior reduced stress or not. An individual's low self-esteem might make it difficult to cope with role conflict or role ambiguity. Individuals with high tolerances for ambiguity can deal better with the strains that come from role ambiguity and, therefore, are likely to be able to cope with this strain and perceive less stress from a given situation. The Type A behavior person is likely to create stress for herself or himself, while Type B persons are more relaxed, create less stress for themselves, and may cope better with stressful situations. Those individuals who perceive the locus of causality for factors in their life as being external to themselves may perceive less stress in a given situation. They are less likely to react negatively when they are controlled by surrounding events. Those who perceive factors as being internal react more negatively to situations that are beyond their control. But when internals have to react to situations that are within their control, they are more likely to be proactive and engage in positive coping behaviors to change the environment and reduce the stresses on themselves (Steers, 1984:519).

Role Conflict and Role Ambiguity

These antecedents manifest themselves in the *role-based stress* that results from role conflict and ambiguity. Role conflict occurs when the role messages a person receives are incompatible; role ambiguity occurs when there is a lack of clear, consistent information about the activities that must be performed and/or the goals that are to be pursued. Examples of role-based stress are the conflict between the role of the professional and the person or the conflict between the manager and staff member roles.

Figure 23–3 Social Readjustment Rating Scale

Forty-two common life changes are listed in the order in which Doctors Holmes and Rahe found them to be important precursors of illness. Total scores predict your chances of suffering serious illness within the next two years. If you score less than 150 within a year, you have only a 37% chance of getting sick within the next two years. But up your score to 150–300 and your chances increase to 51%. Hit 300 and you are, according to the doctors, in serious danger. Says Holmes, "If you have more than 300 life-change units and get sick, the probability is you will have cancer, a heart attack or manic-depressive psychosis rather than warts and menstrual irregularities." On the other hand, he adds, "There are worse things in this life than illness. It is worse to go on in an intolerable, dull, or demeaning situation."

Life Event	Your Value Score	Life Event	Your Value Score
1. Death of spouse	100 ____	23. Son or daughter leaving home	29 ____
2. Divorce	73 ____	24. Trouble with in-laws	29 ____
3. Marital separation	65 ____	25. Outstanding personal achievement	28 ____
4. Jail term	63 ____	26. Spouse begins or stops work	26 ____
5. Death of a close family member	63 ____	27. Starting or finishing school	26 ____
6. Personal injury or illness	53 ____	28. Change in living conditions	25 ____
7. Marriage	50 ____	29. Revision of personal habits	24 ____
8. Fired at work	47 ____	30. Trouble with boss	23 ____
9. Marital reconciliation	45 ____	31. Change in work hours, conditions	20 ____
10. Retirement	45 ____	32. Change in residence	20 ____
11. Change in family member's health	44 ____	33. Change in schools	20 ____
12. Pregnancy	40 ____	34. Change in recreation	19 ____
13. Sex difficulties	39 ____	35. Change in church activities	19 ____
14. Addition to family	39 ____	36. Change in social activities	18 ____
15. Business readjustment	39 ____	37. Mortgage or loan under $10,000	17 ____
16. Change in financial state	38 ____	38. Change in sleeping habits	16 ____
17. Death of close friend	37 ____	39. Change in number of family get-togethers	15 ____
18. Change to different line of work	36 ____	40. Change in eating habits	15 ____
19. Change in number of arguments with spouse	35 ____	41. Vacation	13 ____
20. Mortgage over $10,000	31 ____	42. Christmas	12 ____
21. Foreclosure of mortgage or loan	30 ____	43. Minor violation of law	11 ____
22. Change in work responsibilities	29 ____	Total ____	

Thomas H. Holmes and Richard H. Rahe, "The Social Readjustment Rating Scale," *Journal of Psychosomatic Research,* 1967, 11:213–218 gives complete wording of the items. Reprinted with permission from Pergamon Press, Ltd., copyright 1967.

Role conflict may be the most significant condition causing stress for nurses. A number of factors combine to create this situation. Such external factors as strife within the profession, differences in nurses' educational preparation, the structure of practice settings, and the role of labor and professional organizations contribute to the environment in which nurses must function. Within practice settings, relationships among various groups, such as physicians, patients, staff, and management, add varied expectations and role perceptions to the nurse's job.

Other types of role conflicts occur when an individual has two competing roles, such as when a nurse manager assumes a patient care assignment and is confronted with an emergency management meeting. More frequent is the conflict between a nurse's personal role as a parent or spouse versus her or his role as a professional nurse.

Individual role conflict is the result of an incompatibility between the individual's perception of the role and its actual requirements. A new nurse manager might experience this type of conflict when she or he finds that management expects primary loyalty to the organization and its goals, while the staff expects the nurse manager's first loyalty to be to their needs.

Role conflict within the profession places nursing at a distinct disadvantage in its relationship with other health care workers. This conflict has its roots in a perceived poor regard for nurses. The felt lack of worth is complicated by the division within the profession and the image nursing presents to others.

Role underload and underutilization can also be a consequence of the situation. Being underutilized or not having much responsibility may be very stressful to someone who has a high self-esteem and/or high achievement needs. On the other hand, underload or underutilization could lead to apathy and low productivity.

Consequences of Stress

What happens to a person when stress overload occurs? Both physiological and psychological responses occur that can cause both structural or functional changes or both. Warning signs of too much stress are (a) *undue, prolonged anxiety*, or a persistent state of fear or free-floating anxiety that seems to have many alternating causes; (b) *depression*, which causes people to withdraw from family and friends, to be unable to experience emotions, and to feel helpless to change the situation; (c) *abrupt changes in mood and behavior*, which may be exhibited as erratic behavior; (d) *perfectionism*, which is the setting of unreasonably high standards for one's self and thereby being under constant stress; and (e) *physical illnesses* such as peptic ulcer, arthritis, colitis, hypertension, myocardial infarction, and migraine headaches. Psychological disorders attributable to stress include anxiety reactions, depression, and phobias.

Attempts to reduce stress may include the excessive use of alcohol and other mood-altering chemicals, which can result in the development of chemical dependency. Some people become "workaholics" in an attempt to cope with real or imagined demands. "Burnout" results when the person has used up all available energy to perform the job and feels that this amount of energy is still inadequate for the job. At this point, he or she gives up the job and may drop out of the profession altogether.

The results of employee stress are increased absenteeism and turnover, and thus reduced quality of job performance. Although there are various causes of absenteeism and turnover (see Chapter 16), both may also result when the individual attempts to withdraw from a stressful situation. Job performance suffers during high stress times; so much energy and attention are needed to reduce the stress that little energy is available for performance. Such a situation may be financially costly in industry but may be more costly in human health and recovery in the hospital.

Positive coping responses to stressful situations include role redefinition. Individuals share their role expectations with others, clarifying these roles and attempting to integrate or tie together the various roles they have to play. Confronting the role senders by pointing out the conflicting role messages is also a positive means of coping with the situation. Requesting additional information regarding these roles from the role sender can reduce role ambiguity. Recognizing one's own tolerance for ambiguity and keeping out of conflicting situations is an adaptive coping response. Finally, increasing one's performance, being more efficient, and practicing good time-management techniques by prioritizing tasks and goals can be positive coping responses to stress.

MANAGING STRESS

It is obvious that stress (internal conflict) must be resolved if people are to pursue productive lives. A number of individual and organizational strategies can be used to reduce work-related stress (Steers, 1984). Nurse managers can use these strategies to help deal with their own stress, to help manage their unit, and to help their employees.

What can nurse managers do about their own stress?

1. Increase self-awareness. Nurses tend to think they can be "all things to all people." Acceptance of one's own limitations enables one to identify potential problems and plan for help before they develop further. One way to develop self-awareness is for the nurse manager to respond to the questionnaire shown in Figure 23–4.

2. Develop outside interests, such as hobbies, social groups, and recreational activities. The activity should provide diversion, relaxation, and enjoyment.

Figure 23—4 Stress Diagnostic Survey

Purpose

The following questionnaire is designed to provide you with an indication of the extent to which various individual level stressors are sources of stress to you.

Instructions

For each item, indicate the frequency with which the condition described is a source of stress. Next to each item write the appropriate number (1–7) which best describes how frequently the condition described is a source of stress.

Write 1 if the condition described is never a source of stress
Write 2 if it is rarely a source of stress
Write 3 if it is occasionally a source of stress
Write 4 if it is sometimes a source of stress
Write 5 if it is often a source of stress
Write 6 if it is usually a source of stress
Write 7 if it is always a source of stress

Stress Diagnostic Survey

_____ 1. My job duties and work objectives are unclear to me.
_____ 2. I work on unnecessary tasks or projects.
_____ 3. I have to take work home in the evenings or on weekends to stay caught up.
_____ 4. The demands for work quality made upon me are unreasonable.
_____ 5. I lack the proper opportunities to advance in this organization.
_____ 6. I am held accountable for the development of other employees.
_____ 7. I am unclear about whom I report to and/or who reports to me.
_____ 8. I get caught in the middle between my supervisors and my subordinates.
_____ 9. I spend too much time in unimportant meetings that take me away from my work.
_____ 10. My assigned tasks are sometimes too difficult and/or complex.
_____ 11. If I want to get promoted I have to look for a job with another organization.
_____ 12. I am responsible for counseling with my subordinates and/or helping them solve their problems.
_____ 13. I lack the authority to carry out my job responsibilities.
_____ 14. The formal chain of command is not adhered to.
_____ 15. I am responsible for an almost unmanageable number of projects or assignments at the same time.
_____ 16. Tasks seem to be getting more and more complex.
_____ 17. I am hurting my career progress by staying with this organization.
_____ 18. I take action or make decisions that affect the safety or well-being of others.
_____ 19. I do not fully understand what is expected of me.
_____ 20. I do things on the job that are accepted by one person and not by others.
_____ 21. I simply have more work to do than can be done in an ordinary day.
_____ 22. The organization expects more of me than my skills and/or abilities provide.
_____ 23. I have few opportunities to grow and learn new knowledge and skills in my job.

Figure 23–4   (continued)

_____ 24. My responsibilities in this organization are more for people than for things.
_____ 25. I do not understand the part my job plays in meeting overall organizational objectives.
_____ 26. I receive conflicting requests from two or more people.
_____ 27. I feel that I just don't have time to take an occasional break.
_____ 28. I have insufficient training and/or experience to discharge my duties properly.
_____ 29. I feel that I am at a standstill in my career.
_____ 30. I have responsibility for the future (careers) of others.

Source: John M. Ivancevich and Michael T. Matteson, _Stress and Work_ (Glenview, Ill.: Scott, Foresman and Company, 1980), pp. 118–19.

3. Maintain a program of regular physical exercise. Exercise has been shown to reduce stress. Any activity is appropriate as long as the activity does not become so much of a challenge that it adds stress.

4. Take regular vacations. A change of scene, even to the backyard, is essential. Again, regular intervals spent entirely away from the job help reduce stress.

5. Learn how to relax. For a person in a high stress job, this is not easy. Healthy methods for relaxing include listening to music, reading, socializing with friends, watching movies, and other activities that require little of the participant.

What can nurse managers do to decrease their subordinates' stress?

1. Identify whether the subordinates are under, adequately, or overly stressed. If the subordinates are not adequately stressed, they may be undermotivated. The nurse manager should consider assigning additional tasks or setting higher goals for the subordinates.

2. If the subordinates appear to be under a great deal of stress the nurse manager must identify the source(s) of the stress and decide how she or he can reduce or eliminate these sources.

3. Is role ambiguity or role conflict creating the stress? Can the nurse manager clarify the role(s) of the subordinate, what activities are to be performed and what goals are to be pursued, thereby reducing this conflict or ambiguity?

4. Is the nurse manager using the appropriate leadership style (see Chapter 10)? Has the nurse manager engaged in close and punitive supervision? Can this be changed? Does the nurse manager need to clarify the subordinates' goals and eliminate barriers that are interfering with goal (task) attainment? Is it appropriate to be directive, supportive, and/or participative? Involving subordinates in decision making is an excellent means of reducing stress.

5. Does the subordinate need counseling? Is it appropriate for the nurse manager to do so or are there counseling services available in the organization that could help the subordinate? Would additional training or education help reduce the stress?

6. Is the stress due to feelings of lack of self-worth? Can she or he positively reinforce (see Chapter 9) the subordinate, thereby helping the subordinate gain her or his self-confidence. Are there other sources of support, such as the work group, that can help the subordinate deal with the stress?

7. The nurse manager could also suggest that the subordinate try to deal with her or his personal stress by using some of the techniques suggested above for the nurse manager.

What can the health care institution do to manage stress in their employees? Institutional strategies can be developed that will reduce stress for employees. The nurse manager may be able to initiate a few of them or to encourage adoption by higher administration. Some institutional strategies include:

1. Attempt to match the job and the applicant during the selection and placement process (see Chapter 13).

2. Increase skills training, even for experienced personnel. Although costly, it pays in reduced stress, less turnover, and better performance. New equipment, procedures, and regulations require a training program. Although the programs may be presented by the department of education, the nurse manager should do a thorough follow-up to augment the formal program (see Chapter 14). Specific programs on stress management and on assertiveness training could be developed and offered.

3. Develop a program of job enrichment that is matched to the individual's goals and desires. Job enrichment may include increased autonomy and participation, support for advanced education, or a restructuring of assigned tasks across the unit (see Chapter 9).

4. Allow greater participation in decision making. Participation in decisions affecting work increases job involvement and commitment, thereby reducing stress.

5. Encourage a network of social support. Social support is critical to reducing stress. Team building within the unit and the organization is one way to encourage staff to build a network of support with others in their professional field.

6. Keep communication channels open both upward and downward. As discussed in Chapter 8, the grapevine is especially susceptible to mis-

information. Keeping personnel informed about what is going on in the organization helps reduce suspicion and rumor. In the other direction, receptivity to the concerns of subordinates promotes cooperation and reduces their stress.

7. Develop policies that reduce the stress from shift work. These include reducing the number of hours in the night shift, increasing rest time, and providing adequate dinner times (and providing adequate food during this period). A balance is needed between avoiding frequent changes in shift assignments while providing adequate opportunities for changing shifts for those already on the night shift (Levi, 1981:105). Fair policies should be set dealing with the assignment to weekend and/or holiday work.

Like external conflict resolution, internal conflict resolution takes planning, time, and energy. But the benefits in better health, a more enjoyable life style, and increased sense of self-esteem are well worth the effort.

SUMMARY

- Stress is the reaction of the individual to demands from the environment that pose a threat.

- Some of the antecedents of stress come from the job and organizational factors, from interpersonal factors, and from individual factors.

- Stress in nursing often results specifically from the nature of the work, from role conflict and role ambiguity, and from problems of self-worth and divisiveness within the profession.

- The consequences of stress are physiological and psychological problems for the individual, poor job performance, low job satisfaction, and high absenteeism.

- Strategies to help individuals as well as institutions reduce stress include clarifying goals and roles; providing support, including training and education on stress management; using participative management techniques; and practicing personal stress management techniques.

BIBLIOGRAPHY

Albanese, R. (1981). *Managing: Toward accountability for performance.* Homewood, IL: Irwin.

Brooten, D. A., Hayman, L., and Naylors, M.D. (1978). *Leadership for change: A guide for the frustrated nurse.* Philadelphia: J. B. Lippincott.

Douglass, L. (1983). *The effective nurse: Leader and manager.* 2nd ed. St. Louis: C. V. Mosby.

Holmes, T. H., and Rahe, R. H. (1967). The social readjustment rating scale. *J Psychosom Res, 11*:213.

Ivancevich, J. M., and Matteson, M. T. (1987). *Organizational behavior and management.* Plano, TX: Business Publications.

Ivancevich, J. M., and Matteson, M. T. (1980). *Stress and work.* Grenview, IL: Scott, Foresman.

Klein, S. M., and Ritti, R. R. (1984). *Understanding organizational behavior.* 2nd ed. Boston: Kent.

Levi, L. (1981). *Preventing work stress.* Reading, MA: Addison-Wesley.

Marriner, A. (1979). Conflict theory. *Superv Nurs,* (April) *10*:12.

Matteson, M. T., and Ivancevich, J. M. (1979). Organizational stressors and heart disease. *Acad Mngmt R, 4*:347–357.

Selye, H. (1978) (2nd ed) *The stress of life.* New York: McGraw-Hill.

Steers, R. M. (1984). *Introduction to organizational behavior,* 2nd ed. Santa Monica, CA: Goodyear.

Thomas, K. W. (1976). Conflict and conflict management. In: *Handbook of industrial and organizational psychology.* Dunnette, M.D. (editor). Chicago: Rand McNally. Pp. 889–935.

THE MAJOR EMPHASIS in this text so far has been on the various aspects of the relationships between the nurse manager and subordinates—relationships that are extremely important and consume a large portion of the nurse manager's day-to-day responsibilities. However, relationships with superiors are equally crucial. This chapter deals with the nurse manager's relationship with higher management; however, it cannot be discussed without integrating it with relations with peers, subordinates, and employees, as well as with the organization as a whole.

The nurse manager in the hospital is responsible for implementing and maintaining policies and standards for patients and staff and, at the same time, keeping higher management informed of issues and problems and gaining its support for needed changes. Effective downward, upward, and lateral communication is crucial to this process; and the nurse manager is in the key position to accomplish it. Subordinates often have difficulty in understanding the reasons for decisions made by higher management, and the nurse manager often feels like the person "caught in the middle." But the transmission of organizational goals down to the staff level is a responsibility of all nurse managers, and a very important aspect of their job is the relationship between them and their superiors and others in higher management.

Who the superior is will depend upon many variables, the most important one being the structure of the institution. A nurse manager's immediate superior may be another nurse one step higher in the administrative structure, such as a supervisor or an assistant director of nursing. In a highly decentralized or a matrix organization, however, the nurse manager may report to a physician, a divisional nursing director, or any combination thereof. No matter who the superior is, the skills needed to deal effectively with the person are essentially the same. There are some unique professional colleague issues related to reporting to a physician, and these will be discussed later.

STRUCTURAL AUTHORITY IN THE HEALTH CARE SYSTEM

Every organization has a system of authority to establish goals and to develop and maintain policies to carry out these goals. Hospitals and other health care organizations are no exception. Such a system is essential for the smooth operation of daily activities as well as for handling major crises.

Within the health care system, authority can be conceptualized as lay (nonprofessional) authority and professional authority. The administrator usually has lay authority, while the physician has professional authority. As a clinician, the nurse has professional authority, but as a manager, moves into the realm of lay authority.

While both lay and professional authorities agree that quality of patient care is their first priority, other concerns of each may be in conflict. A hospital administrator may be concerned with maintaining an adequate occupancy rate, while the physician's primary concern may be quality care for his or her patients. The nurse manager is often in a position that requires meeting the demands of both administration and physicians. The relationships that the nurse manager develops and the interactions that occur with all of the people in higher management are critical to the functioning of the unit as well as to success as a nurse manager.

Power and Politics

Nurse managers are an integral part of management. They are obligated to participate within the group and to carry out management decisions. They must understand the organizational structure, learn to function within it, identify how much input they have and how and where to use it. To do this, they need to learn about and to use power.

Politics is a reality in any organizational setting. Both politicians and managers need power—that is, the authority and ability to get things accomplished. Effective politicians sometimes compromise to accomplish personal and organizational goals. They also form personal alliances with others who can influence their own present and future success. This should not be seen as being manipulative or dishonest, but rather as using the situation, people, and resources in an astute but honest and ethical manner. Many respected leaders in nursing have written on the absolute necessity for nurses to learn how to develop and use power for the advancement of the profession. Nowhere is this more necessary than in nursing administration.

Yet nurses have been reluctant to recognize or use power. The traditional female characteristics that have inhibited nurses from dealing with conflict have also inhibited them from using power, either their own or that of others. However, in part due to the women's movement, nurses are becoming less reluctant to be assertive, to be political, and to use power. (See Chapter 8 for more on assertiveness.)

In a study comparing nursing administrators and first-level nurse managers, Heineken (1985) found that administrators believed more often than did first-level nurse managers that: (a) power is equated with political skill; and (b) control over others is necessary to acquire and retain power and autonomy. If top-level administrators and first-level managers differ in their perceptions of both the importance of politics and values about power, this difference will undoubtedly be reflected in distorted communication, conflict, and lack of unity. Such differences must be addressed if nursing personnel are to work together.

In any organization there are both formal and informal power structures. The formal structure is readily identifiable through the organizational chart, in which the chain of command depicts the hierarchy of power and responsibility. The hierarchy follows the channels shown on the organizational chart and shows who reports to whom.

Information flows through both formal and informal mechanisms (see Chapter 8). Going up through the hierarchy or the proper channels is the most common, and usually the most effective route, so pertinent information and problems should be communicated to one's immediate superior first. In the same way, a person's immediate subordinates are expected to bring their concerns to that person first.

Let's say, though, that you, as a nurse manager, do not feel that your superior handled your issue in an acceptable manner. Do not automatically take it a step higher. Instead, evaluate the situation to be sure you gave the superior adequate information and that you presented the issue in such a way that your desired outcome was clearly understood. If you still feel strongly about the situation, ask for another hearing. If the problem still cannot be worked out and you cannot live with it, tell your superior that you want to go higher in the chain of command. Don't go over your superior's head without first trying to resolve the problem with her. This is very rarely appropriate and can result in severe consequences for you.

It is important to clarify how much authority and autonomy you have to deal directly with your superior's peers, such as another department head or administrator. This will vary with the hospital's philosophy and the superior's management style. If your superior prefers to delegate as much as possible, you may be expected to handle interdepartmental problems directly with other department heads or administrators. Another supervisor, however, may want to be the only one to deal with her peers for interdepartmental issues. Even if your superior delegates this to you, keep her informed of the purpose and progress of the contact and negotiation with peers. For example, if you meet with the director of dietary to discuss patient and staff complaints about timely delivery of meals, your superior needs to know this, as she probably has responsibility for other nursing units that may be having similar problems. Keeping her informed will also allow her to determine the scope of the problem and to decide whether it is important to take the problem one more step up the ladder.

Informal communication channels, or "the grapevine," have been discussed in some detail in Chapter 8. Although "the grapevine" serves several purposes, information transmitted in this manner may or may not be accurate. In some organizations, however, the informal structures may be far more powerful and influential than the formal authorities—that is, one person may be able to influence others even though that person has little or no authority to do so.

Part of understanding the organizational structure is learning where the informal power is. Sometimes it rests with a secretary, an administrative assistant, a supervisor, or the director of nursing service. By paying attention to the person people take a problem to and to who helped them or did not, the novice nurse manager can determine the source of power. If the same person is continually facilitating or, conversely blocking, actions, it is fairly certain that he or she holds informal power. There may be several people in different areas in the organization with informal power. When you want something done, the people with the power can help.

Nurse managers have formal power and can develop informal power. By improving their interpersonal skills and developing positive relationships with others, they can influence other personnel, staff, and administrators, and help to improve the quality of patient care. Power is integral to the nurse manager's role as a leader and a follower.

One important caution regarding power. Power can be used to improve relationships, situations, and conditions. Everyone involved can benefit. However, if it is used primarily to further one person's or subgroup's self-interest, problems are sure to surface. Political power has sent some people to the moon and crushed others into servitude. It can do both. The ethical use of power is the responsibility of all.

IDENTIFICATION WITH MANAGEMENT

What happens when a good clinical nurse becomes a nurse manager? Take the following example. Nurses on Ms. Robbins' unit testify that when Ms. Robbins became nurse manager, "she changed." Ms. Robbins thinks "they" changed. They are both right. The relationship between them changed. No longer is Ms. Robbins responsible only for individual patient care, she is now responsible for the operation of an entire unit. She must see that patients on her unit receive the best care her staff can provide; that all staff are working to the best of their ability; and that adequate resources, such as equipment and supplies, are available. Further, she must identify with management so well that she can carry out organizational goals on her unit as if they were her own. Her responsibility has shifted to the organization as a whole.

It is not uncommon to hear a new supervisor say, "*They* want us to do . . ." or "*They* have interpreted the policy to mean . . ." The emphasis is on the pronoun "they" as opposed to the pronoun "we."

If Ms. Robbins identifies with management, she sees her problems as interlocked with those of her superior. When her superior makes a commitment, it will be Ms. Robbins' commitment, too. This does not mean she rubberstamps all of her supervisor's decisions. She may be very concerned about possible negative implications and may disagree with the superior about it in private. But when she comes out of the superior's office, it becomes a joint commitment, one to which she is firmly committed. Her follow-through and communication to those she manages will be based on an attitude that says, "We want this," not, "They want this." This is the foundation of nursing management and the nurse manager's most important assignment.

ROLE EXPECTATIONS

A position in an organization serves as a framework for performance of a role within that organization. Whoever fills that position is expected to perform it in essentially the same way as any other person. This is one of the ways in which organizations remain stable over time, even in the face of persistent turnover.

In real organizational life, however, each person's performance is unique. One aspect of the uniqueness is how the position holder responds to others' messages about how he or she should perform. These messages are often conflicting. For example, what the superior expects, what one's subordinates expect, what the nurse manager expects, and what one's family expects, may be mutually exclusive.

Staff nurses (clinicians) usually accept management positions only with great trepidation. First is the reluctance to leave clinical practice where, in spite of the problems, they considered themselves competent. Second is their lack of preparation for management. Most significant of all, though, is their perception of management. Many of them believe that management's goal is the antithesis of nursing's goal: the care of patients.

Most nurses have had little educational preparation for management positions. While they may have a great deal of commitment to the organization and know the system well, they are likely to be unskilled in management theory, research, and strategies. Today, however, most administrators prepare for hospital management like any other chief executive officer in business or industry.

Thus nurses move into management to fill a position (nurse manager) with ambiguous role expectations, their own as well as others', and with little preparation for the task. The same thing may be true of their superiors, the assistant director of nursing service, and so on.

Several management authorities suggest that "goodness of fit" between the organization's "personality" and that of the employee determines the latter's perception of higher management (Hershey & Blanchard, 1972; Katz & Kahn, 1978). The history and traditions of the organization, as well as the philosophies, personalities, goals, and objectives of the present management, determine the organization's philosophy and expectations. These interact with the personality of the employee, and when the two are compatible, the employee "fits" in the organization and, consequently, within management.

RELATIONSHIPS WITH SUPERIORS

Most of the management concepts related to dealing with subordinates also can be applied to relationships with one's superior. Working effectively with a superior is an important consideration for the nurse manager. A superior directly influences one's career and success with the organization.

It is safe to say that not all nurse manager positions are created equal. Just as the reporting relationships in the administrative hierarchy will differ among hospitals, so will the role and responsibilities of the nurse manager. Given the structure (centralized, decentralized, or matrix) and the philosophies of those in higher management, the amount of authority delegated to the nurse manager can range from a "charge nurse" role in one hospital to a full-blown department manager in another. The merits of these differing roles and responsibilities are not really relevant to this discussion. What is relevant is that in all situations there is a boss, a superior, and the relationship with that superior is important.

Superior/subordinate relationships are the responsibility of the subordinate as much as the superior. However, most subordinates act as if this were not the case. They allow the supervisor to control the relationship and refuse to accept responsibility for their part in developing and maintaining that relationship. However, any relationship between two persons requires participation by both and, in fact, both contribute to that relationship in either positive or negative, active or passive, ways. Nurse managers then, have a responsibility for their part of the relationship. They should remember that they can influence their boss!

What impedes these relationships? First is a person's reaction to authority which either inhibits or facilitates the relationship. One can "buck" it, avoid it, or try to circumvent it. A fourth reaction, however, is the effective, mature one: to work within the superior's value system as well as one's own. Studies have shown that people who want to become managers generally have positive feelings about those who have authority over them (Hegarty, 1982). They see that people in authority usually play a positive role and do not necessarily represent barriers. Perception of authority is extremely important in furthering one's career.

Second is self-esteem. A person with low self-esteem may react toward a superior in one of two ways: underwhelmed or belligerent (Hegarty, 1982). An underwhelmed response implies that the subordinate thinks her own ideas or suggestions are worthless and, possibly, that she herself is worthless. Such a person takes few initiatives, makes no suggestions, and may even fail to bring important matters to the superior's attention. A belligerent responder, on the other hand, argues with and fights every action the superior takes. This person causes dissension in a group, trying always to enhance her own self-esteem by reducing that of others, especially those with higher status positions.

Although most people with low self-esteem fall somewhere between these two extremes, they all tend to exhibit a high degree of sensitivity to any occurrence. For instance, assume you have proposed a new staffing pattern for your unit and it is turned down by higher administration. With low self-esteem, you would tend to take this rejection personally, yet there may be many reasons why your proposal was rejected: staffing is going to become centralized after installation of a computer system; the census on your unit has been low and your proposed staffing pattern will require additional personnel; or administration believes the suggested changes will not be cost-effective. There may be any number of reasons why your proposal was not selected, and probably it was not personal rejection.

Esteem of yourself simply means accepting yourself as you are with all of your assets and limitations. Self-esteem has nothing to do with performance or productivity. A person is more than that. Each person has *intrinsic* worth as a human being. Genuine self-esteem means that you view yourself as objectively as you view others. Evaluation of events is based on the facts, not just on their personal impact. Expectations of yourself and others are realistic.

In addition to response to authority and self-esteem, unrealistic expectations of what the superior can and should do for a subordinate are also impediments to the relationship. Some common beliefs held by subordinates are: (a) the supervisor should always like and/or love them; (b) the supervisor should take care of them; and (c) the supervisor should treat them like a pal. These expectations are obviously unrealistic but they are often the underlying assumptions that many subordinates have about their relationship with their superiors. The supervisor is *not* mother or father.

Subordinates may or may not like their superiors but this need not interfere with the quality of work they perform. Subordinates are responsible for their work and for their side of the relationship just as superiors are responsible for their side.

Superiors need the support of their subordinates, since their successes are tied directly to the types of relationships they have with subordinates, peers, and other superiors. Each person significantly influences each other's present job satisfaction and future job opportunities. Learning how to relate to one's superior, therefore, can create a work environment that is far more enriching than one in which conflict and stress perpetually exist.

Subordinate's Responsibility

First, subordinates must recognize that their superiors' sphere of responsibility is greater than their own. Just as the nurse manager is responsible for the functioning of an entire unit, the supervisor is responsible for all that happens on several units.

Second, nurse managers should remember that, like themselves, superiors have needs, too. However, some of these needs can interfere in the superior/subordinate relationship. For example, the superior may have a high need to be needed, to feel important, and may therefore be overwhelming to the subordinates she manages. If a superior comes to the rescue with every problem and seldom, if ever, delegates management of the problem, one can be fairly certain that that person has a significant need to be needed. This type of superior does not encourage the development of leadership qualities in subordinates. If subordinates want to learn leadership and management skills, they often must ask for this opportunity directly.

Suppose, for instance, that you are a nurse manager who wants to learn management skills. At an appropriate moment, tell Ms. Brennan, your supervisor, how much you have learned from her handling of problems and that you would like the opportunity to handle a problem yourself with some help from her. Ask if that is agreeable, provided you talk with her first and state that you would like to help her as well. Then the next time you call her with a problem, remind her that you've been wanting to handle a problem yourself and maybe you could handle this one with her help. Follow up on this, detail the outcome of your problem solving, and ask her advice for other ways to handle similar problems in the future. In this way, she remains a part of the process and you can develop some skills in management with her assistance.

It could be, though, that Ms. Brennan, the superior, needs to be liked or disliked. If she has an inordinate need to be liked, she will put personal popularity above the needs of the organization. She will be unwilling to make unpopular decisions, even though they may be necessary for the good of the group. For instance, if Ms. Brennan has been told that absenteeism in her area is higher than in any other, she may be unwilling to confront the offenders. Although she may be exceptionally well liked by her subordinates, the quality of her work may suffer and subordinates are left with unclear and ambiguous messages about expectations for the job.

One way to respond in this situation is to inform Ms. Brennan that you recognize that sometimes she has to make unpopular, though necessary, decisions. You can offer to announce those decisions yourself and tell her you will support them. As a boss yourself, you can tell her that you have learned that you cannot always be popular but you do hope that your subordinates will respect you. Supervisors who fail to learn to put the needs of the organization above their own need to be liked are not likely to survive very long in management roles.

On the other hand, the mythical Ms. Brennan may have a need to be disliked. She may think that if she does not exert control over her subordinates they will not do anything. Subordinates then become submissive, resist taking initiative and responsibility, and refer everything to her. A resistance-resentment-revenge cycle begins, and much of what the supervisor wants to accomplish gets sabotaged by those charged with carrying out orders.

There are ways to respond to a superior who needs to be disliked. Hegarty says to "ignore his rages and catch him doing something good" (Hegarty, 1982). When appropriate, tell Ms. Brennan how much you appreciate what she did and how it helps you with your job. Keep reinforcing her positive behavior. If you are still unsuccessful in changing her actions, you may have to leave either the institution or your particular position. Remember, you are only responsible for your part of the relationship with your supervisor. You are not responsible for her behavior.

Another type of relationship one might have with the superior is that of playing "politics" or gaining "brownie points." The nurse manager might feel that the only way to survive or to get ahead is to say what the supervisor wants to hear, rather than the truth. However, if you have to play such phony games or roles that disturb your conscience, you may be in the wrong organization—one with which your values are not compatible. If so, only you can decide if you can make the necessary compromises to work there.

As a new nurse manager, you may feel insecure and uncertain of your superior's expectations of you. In most cases, she has confidence in you or you would not have been appointed. Begin as soon as possible to discuss your responsibilities and to arrive at agreements regarding your role. Do not make the mistake of waiting too long for the supervisor to tell you what you can and cannot do. Assume you have the authority to proceed with the routine aspects of your job as defined in your job description. This assumes, of course, that you have the necessary skills and knowledge to do so. If not, begin quickly to learn from your superior or other experienced nurse managers.

Frequently new managers do not go ahead and make decisions because they fear they might make mistakes that would make them look bad to the supervisor. This may be because the supervisor has not created an atmosphere in which people can risk making decisions without the fear of punishment if the decisions are erroneous. But the nurse manager *must* make decisions. Not making them because of fear of mistakes is often a mistake in itself.

The extent of your responsibilities and authority may not be completely clear until you have worked with your superior for some time. You may be anxious about this temporary ambiguity, but with time, many collaborative decisions, and a spirit of cooperation in learning one another's expectations, many of the unclear points will be resolved.

The effective nurse manager accepts that the supervisor has strengths as well as limitations. To build on her strengths—that is, facilitating and supporting her activities—will make both of you effective. Trying to build on her weaknesses would be as frustrating and as foolish as trying to build on the weaknesses of a subordinate. As an effective nurse manager, therefore, ask: "What can my supervisor do really well?" "What has she done really well?" "What does she need to know to use her strength?" "What does she need from me to perform?"

In any job, you will need your superior's power and support so that together you can accomplish your tasks. You should strive to ensure that your superior's activities are productive because they are the key to your own effectiveness.

Rules for Working with Superiors

There are some basic principles that can help you work more effectively with your superior. By using these principles in your daily interactions, you can improve your part of the relationship (which usually improves the relationship).

Principle one. Always be polite. No matter what your superior says or does, remember you are responsible only for your own behavior. Never embarrass or ridicule her either in front of others or out of her presence. Good manners are catching and, even if the other person is not courteous, you have done your part.

Principle two. Praise positive behavior. Remember, the supervisor is human and needs rewards for positive behavior. A few words, such as, "I really appreciate your explaining why the administrator wants this report," lets the superior know that you recognized that she took time to explain details to you.

Ignore negative behavior unless it interferes with your work or endangers patient care. For instance, if your supervisor on evenings shows up intoxicated, it would be unsafe to ignore the danger to patients, and your first responsibility is to them. Allegiance to the superior is very important, but not at the risk of patient safety. In fact, reporting the incident might be the kindest action of all. If your superior is indeed an alcoholic, intervention may save her career and possibly her life.

However, many daily behaviors can be ignored. What your superior does is her responsibility, and negative behavior toward you probably is not meant personally. Superiors generally treat all their subordinates in the same way (Hershey & Blanchard, 1972). Whoever held the nurse manager position would probably have had the same treatment or experience as you.

If you think your supervisor's behavior is interfering with your work and you decide it is serious enough to confront her with it, by all means, do so. But be prepared for the consequences should the superior not change. Do you want to leave? Are you willing to accept her behavior and ignore it if she does not change?

Principle three. Learn how to handle conflict constructively. Whether you are a new or experienced nurse manager, conflict situations will invariably arise in the work situation. Sometimes nurse managers are tempted to take the path of least resistance and employ the "Yes, boss, anything you say" approach. This is a servile, condescending way of interacting with the superior. It could happen if you have not developed enough self-confidence or feel insecure around those in positions of authority. Or perhaps your supervisor is a dogmatic authoritarian who makes you think she wants you to be a yes-person. However, it is unlikely that this approach will gain your superior's respect. If you find yourself in this situation, seek a solution. Alternatives might be to take a course in assertiveness or conflict resolution (see Chapters 8 and 22) or practice by role playing with a confident nurse manager or peer the behavior you wish to use with your supervisor.

As a manager, you probably prefer to deal with subordinates who try to maintain positive relationships with you rather than those who seem perennially negative. You probably feel the same way about your superior, and she too, is likely to prefer positive relationships. This is not to say, however, that you should never have healthy and constructive differences of opinion.

One way to maintain a constructive relationship is to avoid arguments. Are you really likely to win an argument with your supervisor? Probably not. However, there will be occasions during which you may, and probably should, disagree with your superior. You will probably gain far more, however, if you learn how to disagree without arguing. Disagreements provide opportunities for drawing on your assertiveness, communication, and negotiation skills. Be certain, though, before airing any disagreement, that you weigh the advantages against the disadvantages of expressing your opposing views. You can often sense your supervisor's likely reaction.

Your purpose should be to try to accomplish or change something. If you are not going to be any better off as a result of your actions, then there may be little purpose in complaining. However, talking the situation out relieves your tension and frustration over the problem. If you sense that you need to "tell someone," seek out a friend or confidant instead of the supervisor. You probably will feel better and may gain some outside perspective that you would not otherwise have had.

Principle four. Keep the supervisor informed. Your position carries with it the obligation to keep the supervisor informed. Many new nurse managers experience conflict in following this principle. Their loyalties are divided; they want to keep the confidence of their staff yet they know they must keep their supervisor informed. These two loyalties may be in conflict occasionally but, most of the time, the information the supervisor needs is not confidential.

The nurse manager should keep the supervisor informed in several areas. One, she should alert her supervisor to problems that may result from the supervisor's decisions. You owe the supervisor your best estimate of both positive and negative outcomes. You are obligated to try to negotiate a settlement if you disagree with her ideas. If the superior makes a decision against your recommendation, however, you must implement and support it.

Also, the nurse manager is obligated to inform her superior of the facts the latter needs in order to make decisions. Supervisors need to know what goes on in individual units and it is the nurse manager's responsibility to provide the needed information. The nurse manager role gives you inside information about what would be effective at staff level. This is important input that should be provided to higher management if policies that are based on reality are to be developed.

The nurse manager is also obliged to inform the supervisor when problems do or may occur. Do not allow your supervisor to be surprised by events on your unit; remember, she is ultimately responsible for what happens there. Some problems can be resolved quickly if handled before they escalate into crises. If and when a crisis occurs, it must be handled at once. Usually this involves informing management.

Keeping the superior "too informed" can also happen. The supervisor has a variety of responsibilities and does not need to know every detail of your work. Consequently, you should become familiar with the boundaries of your decision-making authority. This understanding will come with time, trial and error, and honest and open communication with your superior. In some situations you may work for a person you see daily, such as a nursing supervisor who makes unit rounds. In other situations, you may work for someone who comes to your unit infrequently. If the latter, set up a scheduled time weekly to meet with her. Keep a list of the issues you wish to discuss. If you have nothing of substance to discuss, ask the supervisor if there is any reason to meet. If not, cancel the meeting; you can find many productive ways to use the time you have saved. In short, strive to reach the point where you are secure in making the routine day-to-day decisions. Require your superior's time only for exceptional situations that necessitate collaboration. In other words, be selective as to specifics shared with your supervisor.

Principle five. Admit your blunders. "To err is human," we often hear. It's safe to assume that you have made, and will continue to make, an occasional error.

There's a natural tendency, however, for people in management positions to be embarrassed by personal mistakes, especially those who suffer from the illusion that "managers aren't supposed to make mistakes." Rather than trying to cover up your mistakes or to "pass the buck" by blaming your subordinates or others for your actions, you are likely to gain far more of your superior's respect by admitting when you are wrong or when you do not know something. Most people do not expect you to be super-human, so they are not going to be surprised when you make an occasional error. When you do err, apologize sincerely and move on, so that you can resume business as usual.

In addition to admitting your errors, you should make every effort to maintain credibility. One way is to make only those commitments and take on only those assignments that you intend and will be able to fulfill. Keep track of your commitments, such as chairing a committee, doing special projects, or agreeing to pursue your formal education. Be sure to inform your superior in *advance*, when possible, if you will be unable to fulfill a prior commitment.

Principle six. Publicize your accomplishments. You may think that doing a good job is enough, that a job well done speaks for itself. It does if it is seen, but there are many people and events competing for your superior's attention. You must make your achievements visible, but in a subtle way. For example, suppose you were the nurse manager discussed in Chapter 21 who talked to a mother whose child was given an overdose of preoperative medication. You probably helped prevent a lawsuit against the hospital. However, your supervisor might not know about how you helped avert serious trouble for the hospital unless you let her know. It is inappropriate to blurt out, "I saved the hospital a lot of money." Rather, explain the circumstances and, in a matter of fact manner, describe your actions. Your superior can draw her own conclusions. You could also send her a copy of any correspondence you have with patients or their families.

Weekly reports are another way to state what you have accomplished. Merely state the circumstances without adding your own compliments. If you have difficulty stating your own accomplishments in this manner, review assertive techniques (Chapter 8).

Principle seven. Learn your supervisor's work style. Incongruent work styles between superior and subordinate often cause difficulties in their relationship. Work styles are sometimes diametrically opposed: for instance, an organized, formal style vs. an intuitive, informal one; task-oriented vs. relationship-oriented; written language preference vs. spoken language preference; or group activity vs. individual activity.

If one is task-oriented, for example, productivity is measured in terms of accomplishments and results. In clinical nursing, such an orientation results in high esteem for technical skill in patient care tasks and, in nursing management, high regard for the technical aspects of the job, such as reports completed on time. But a person who is relationship-oriented views interpersonal interactions and abilities—for example, one's ability to intervene effectively in a staff conflict—as most important. Most people have a combination of orientations but exhibit a preference for one style.

If your supervisor's style is task-oriented and you are oriented toward relationships, working with that particular supervisor may prove difficult; you will not fulfill each other's expectations. On the other hand, once you recognize this difference and accept it as a difference in work styles and not a personality conflict, you can turn it into an advantage for both of you. Previously, you were advised to build on a supervisor's strengths; you can also use your strengths to fill in for her weaknesses. If you are task-oriented and your supervisor is relationship-oriented, you can use that information in deciding how to divide some overlapping tasks in your respective workloads.

Principle eight. Learn how to avoid irritating your superior. Don't "push his or her buttons." Learn what words, phrases, topics, and approaches are irritants. Chances are, no matter what the discussion after that, your superior will have a negative response. Learning his or her likes and dislikes requires a sensitivity to the other's verbal and nonverbal communication, both during the time the two of you interact as well as during your observations of the superior's interactions with others. This knowledge also takes time. It behooves the manager to pay attention to these obvious irritants. One word of caution, though: Don't avoid giving your superior information he or she needs because it is unpleasant. Avoidance of irritants is related to your own style of approach.

Principle nine. Don't dominate your superior's time. Learn how to summarize information and emphasize the important points. Details are your job; be sure you have covered everything and then pull out the information related to your superior's actions. Ask: what does he or she need to know to make a decision, to report to *his or her* superior, to monitor change across units, or to intervene? There is a fine line between keeping your superior informed (principle four) and not dominating his or her time. Experience with each other and clear communication regarding responsibilities helps.

w to Influence Your Superior

Most textbooks and courses on nursing management are geared to teaching nursing managers how to influence the activities of their subordinates. Very little, however, has been written about how those same managers can constructively influence their supervisors. Many times nurse managers will need to approach their supervisors for support, influence, or approval for all sorts of things. You, for instance, might need your supervisor's support for the purchase of equipment or supplies; a change in staffing; a new procedure or policy; or a need for new information via an inservice or continuing education program.

Timing, rationale, possible objections, and choice of form and format are all important when preparing to make such a request. Timing is critical. Choose an opportunity when your supervisor has the time and appears to be in a receptive frame of mind to listen to your ideas. Also consider the impact of your ideas on other events occurring at that time.

Second, whatever you are asking for, you must provide a good reason for administration to support it. Be well prepared to present the necessary information in a concise form and to explain the benefits that will accrue to institution and staff. Explain future benefits, too, and give examples of possible outcomes. Be able to answer such questions as:

1. Why should administration accept your proposal?

2. What are the short- and long-term advantages?

3. What will be the consequences if this proposed idea is not accepted? What will have to be done later as a result?

4. What will it cost in time and money? Include recurring and one-time-only costs. Cost effectiveness is the single most persuasive argument.

5. How could it affect morale, turnover, or absenteeism? These cost money.

6. How long will it be before benefits are realized?

A third consideration is possible objections your superior may have to your proposal and some alternative suggestions. Even if you have to compromise, you may still achieve the goals you value and have set as a priority. In other words, think it through from all angles and consider all ways to approach what you want. Set priorities and know what give and take is possible.

Should you present your ideas in spoken or written form? Usually some combination of both is used. Even if you have a brief meeting and a relatively small request, it is a good idea to follow it up with a short memorandum detailing your ideas and the plans you both agreed to implement. Sometimes the procedure occurs in reverse. If a written proposal is read by the supervisor prior to a meeting, both of you are familiar with the idea at the start. In the latter case, careful preparation of the written material is essential to sell your ideas. For how to prepare a written proposal, see Chapter 8.

In spite of careful preparation, what can you do if the supervisor says no? First, think through the supervisor's objections and evaluate them. Ask yourself, "What new information did I get from the supervisor?" "What are the ways I can renegotiate?" "What do I need to overcome objections?" "Do I need more information?" Once these are answered, approach the supervisor again with the new material. This says that this proposal is a high priority with you, and possibly the new information may stimulate her to reevaluate your proposal. If it is important enough to you, you may want to take it higher. If so, tell your superior you would like that person's superior to hear the proposal. Keep an open mind, listen to objections, and try to meet the objections with suggestions as to how problems might be overcome. Keep in mind the possibility of compromise suggested earlier. Be prepared for a middle-of-the-road decision; it may be better than no movement at all.

Taking a Problem to the Supervisor

Many times subordinates (nurse managers) do not know how to approach their superiors, or how to get past verbal barriers. Most superiors probably *want* to help solve subordinate (nurse manager) problems, but may have developed some ineffective behaviors for conveying this message. Distractions such as the telephone, other people entering the office, or even the superior's scribbling on a pad can prevent the subordinate from feeling free to talk. Other superiors block good communication with subordinates by using commanding language, being sarcastic, or discounting the problem. Such a supervisor may well be avoided as a source for problem resolution.

Figure 24–1 Key Behaviors for Taking a Problem to Your Boss

1. State your desire to talk about a work-related problem and, if necessary, make an appointment to meet, identifying approximate amount of time needed.
2. If the suggested time is not convenient, ask when and where it would be convenient.
3. State the problem and explain its effect on work activities.
4. Listen for restatement of problem or for indication that problem has been understood.
5. State your willingness to cooperate in any solution to the problem and listen openly to supervisor's comments.

If necessary, continue:

6. State alternative or your preferred solution.
7. Agree on steps each of you will take to solve the problem.
8. Ask if there is a need to follow up the problem. If so, plan and record a specific follow-up date.

Taken from Decker, P. J. *Healthcare Management Microtraining.* 1983. Used with permission.

Certain steps or key behaviors are involved in taking a problem to the supervisor. Nurse managers can use these behaviors in taking a problem to *their* superiors and can also use the principles when subordinates come to them with problems. The behaviors are designed to facilitate problem-solving processes. By solving the problem together and, if necessary, by both taking active steps to solve the problem, the employee's and supervisor's acceptance of and commitment to the solution should be facilitated. Setting a specific follow-up date is also important, as it will prevent a solution from being delayed or forgotten.

Figure 24–1 presents steps in discussing a work-related problem with the supervisor.

By adhering to these steps, the nurse manager will ensure that the problem is addressed at a time when both she and her supervisor are able to devote attention to the problem. This should maximize the exchange of problem-relevant information, understanding, and solution-relevant ideas.

DEALING WITH PHYSICIANS

Historically, nurse/physician conflict can be traced to the fact that most nurses have been female and most physicians male in a society that has espoused male dominance and female subservience. Many changes in society have occurred in recent years, however, and some of these changes, such as the emergence of the women's movement, have not only had an impact on nursing but have also increased the conflict between nurse and physician (Morgan & McCann, 1983; Webster, 1985). Today it is relatively easy to ascribe sexist motives to many male/female interactions; those between physicians and nurses are no exception.

The socialization of physicians and nurses has encouraged dominant/submissive patterns of interaction. The physician's fear of an error that could cost a patient's life is very real. Kalisch and Kalisch (1977) suggest that by assuming a cloak of omnipotence, the physician reduces his anxiety about the heavy responsibility over life and death. This self-concept of invincibility is fostered throughout medical education as the student/intern/resident learns to adapt to the demands of making life-threatening decisions.

Compare this socialization with that of nursing students. The latter are rewarded for obedience, courtesy, and competent task performance but rarely for independent thinking or creative activities. In general, nurses come from a lower socioeconomic class than physicians, where male dominance is more commonly accepted, and they may unwittingly encourage dominant behavior in physicians.

Other factors also deter collaboration between nurses and physicians. One is the educational preparation of practitioners in each discipline. In today's society status is closely correlated with level of education, and physicians have completed considerably more education at entry to practice than have nurses. Moreover, the diversity of nurses' educational preparation and concomitant skills baffles both physicians and consumers. Although many remain opposed to the baccalaureate requirement for entry into nursing practice, increased educational requirements for entry afford any profession higher status. The status of the nursing profession will increase with additional education requirements for the professional, according to several nursing leaders (Booth, 1983; Christman, 1965).

Sheard (1980) describes differences in the structure of medical practice and nursing practice. The intensity and extensity of each practitioner's relationship with patients differ. The physician has a long-term (possibly life-time) relationship with the patient and deals with that patient individually. The nurse, on the other hand, has several patients at a time and usually for only a relatively short time. Additionally, she must be concerned with the functioning of her areas of responsibility (team, unit, floor) and how that functioning affects all patient care in the area. The physician usually has a private practice that is his primary concern, and hospital care of his patients is only a component of this practice. Therefore, the focus of care and the structure of work differ greatly between the two groups while responsibilities overlap. Conflict is inevitable.

The following are guidelines for dealing with physicians:

1. Consider yourself and the physician equal partners of a health care team.

2. Focus on the task to be accomplished or the problem to be solved, not personal differences.

3. Maintain the improvement of patient care as the goal of all collaborative efforts.

4. Establish clear roles and responsibilities for the physician, yourself, and the staff.

5. Always be prepared with *facts* when talking with physicians.

6. Respect the physician as a person—not as "just a doctor."

7. Serve as a role model to your staff exemplifying the above behaviors.

Implications for the Nurse Manager

The nurse manager is in a key position to influence nurse/physician relationships. She has frequent contact with physicians and can help both physicians and nursing staff to deal with each other.

First, the nurse manager should encourage an increase in interactions between physicians and nurses, both formally and informally. Research on discrimination has revealed that alienation between groups of people is reduced with increased contact between the individual members of the groups. The nurse manager should use every opportunity to include staff nurses in meetings that include physicians. Institution-wide committees whose decisions will affect patient care should include staff nurse representatives; if they do not, the nurse manager should request their inclusion.

Webster (1985) studied medical students' views of nurses' roles. She found that medical students seldom know what nurses' work is, have few interactions with them outside of specific patient problems (and even those interactions are brief and limited), and, when they do patient care tasks that they think nurses should be doing, they resent nurses. The general perception was that nurses' work is "invisible" and less important than physicians'. At best, it was perceived that nurses and physicians worked parallel to each other with little contact. However, nurses' roles were more accurately and positively depicted by medical students who spent time informally interacting with nurses in the work setting (for example, talking at the nurses' station). Thus, it seems that improving the opportunity for nurses and physicians (and nurses and medical students) to interact could have a positive effect on the relationships between the two professions.

Second, health care in an organizational setting is complex and utilizes a variety of professional specialties. Interdependent relationships among professionals is the norm, not the exception, so accountability is also shared. Consumers today believe that all providers are accountable. This is reflected by the increase in malpractice suits that include all health care participants as defendants.

Nurse managers can encourage involvement of staff and physicians in problem solving and decision making. They must be alert to opportunities to do this, both formally, as in appointment to collaboration committees, and informally, as in suggesting to either physician or nurse that either one might want to discuss an aspect of the patient's care with the other.

Nurse managers also serve as role models for their staffs. When staff see nurse managers collaborating with physicians, they will tend to emulate that behavior. An attitude of cooperation and collaboration rather than an adversarial one of "we" versus "they" encourages a similar response in staff members.

Nurse managers may also need to be mediators in a conflict between a staff nurse and a physician. The reader is referred to Chapter 22 on dealing with conflict for specific skills in conflict mediation. Special attention should be given to the imbalance of power and to techniques that can be utilized to reduce the imbalance.

In an effort to improve collaboration between physicians and nurses, nurse managers must remember that their staffs need support to participate in collaborative efforts. They must be assured, by words and actions, that they will be supported by their nurse manager, who is "on their side." This is critical for the nurse manager's success with staff and success in the organization.

SUMMARY

- Health care organizations have systems of structural organization designed to best carry out organizational goals. These systems may be centralized or decentralized depending on institutional philosophy of control and responsibility.

- Nurse managers are part of management with staff reporting to them and they, in turn, report to a superior.

- Informal, as well as formal structures, exist in all organizations; informal structures are generally considered to exert a great deal of power.

- Roles in organizations define the parameters of a job, remain constant regardless of the role occupier, and help maintain stability in the organization.

- Nurse managers are responsible for participation in the relationship with their superior. Nurse managers' negative reaction to authority, low self-esteem, and unrealistic expectations of the supervisor may interfere with development of positive, growth-enhancing relationships between nurse managers and their superiors.

- Supervisors' characteristics can interfere with the relationship; such as, the superior's need to be needed, need to be liked or need to be disliked. Nurse managers can deal constructively with these problems by accepting the supervisor's need and suggesting changes.

- Basic principles for working with superiors include being courteous, praising positive actions, learning how to handle conflict constructively, keeping the supervisor informed, admitting your mistakes, publicizing your accomplishments, and fitting into your supervisor's work style.

- Nurse managers need to learn how to influence their superiors when presenting new ideas and how to take problems to their superiors. Suggestions on both are included.

- Socialization, stereotyping, and the nature of each professional's work responsibilities account for the negative relationships that exist between physicians and nurses.

- Nurse managers serve as role models in exemplifying positive interactions with physicians and can assist their staff to encourage interactions where the focus is the patient and his or her problem.

BIBLIOGRAPHY

Booth, R. Z. (1983). Power: A negative or positive force in relationships. *Nurs Adm Quart*, 7:10.

Christman, L. (1965). Nurse-physician communications in the hospital. *J Am Med Assoc*, 194:539.

Decker, P. J. (1982). *Health care management microtraining*. St. Louis: Decker and Assoc.

Emery, K. R. (1987). Medical staff relations: An investment paying substantial dividends. *Health Care Supervisor*, 5(2): 54–64.

Gabarro, J., and Kotter, J. (1980). Managing your boss. *Harv Bus Rvw*, 58(1): 92–100.

Hegarty, C. (1982). *How to manage your boss*. Mill Valley, CA: Whatever Pub.

Heineken, J. (1985). Power: Conflicting views. *J Nurs Adm*, 15(11): 36–39.

Hershey, P., and Blanchard, K. H. (1972). *Management of organizational behavior*. 2nd ed. Englewood Cliffs, NJ: Prentice-Hall.

Johnston, P. F. (1983). Improving the nurse-physician relationship. *J Nurs Adm*, (March) 13(3): 19.

Kalisch, B. J., and Kalisch, P. A. (1977). An analysis of the sources of physician-nurse conflict. *J Nurs Adm*, (January) 7(1): 50–57.

Katz, D., and Kahn, R. L. (1978). *The social psychology of organizations*. New York: Wiley.

McConnell, C. R. (1987). Making upward communication work for your employees: Processes and people, with emphasis on people. (Part 3 of 3). *Health Care Supervisor*, 5(2): 71–80.

Morgan, A. P., and McCann, J. M. (1983). Nurse-physician relationships: The ongoing conflict. *Nurs Adm Quart*, 7:1.

Nurse-physician-administrator relationships. (1983). *Nurs Adm Quart*, (Summer). [Entire issue.]

Sheard, T. (1980). The structure of conflict in nurse-physician relations. *Superv Nurs*, 11:14.

Sheedy, S. G. (1984). Vice-president of medicine/vice-president of nursing: Collaboration or conflict? *J Nurs Adm*, 14(6): 38–41.

Stuart, G. W. (1986). An organizational strategy for empowering nursing. *Nurs Econ*, 4(2): 69–73.

Webster, D. (1985). Medical students' views of the role of the nurse. *Nursing Research*, 34(5): 313–317.

A Pragmatic View
of Nursing Management

THROUGHOUT THIS BOOK we have presented the most current knowledge available in nursing management today. Now, however, we offer you some practical advice—the kind of "hands-on" advice that is seldom found in a textbook but rather is the knowledge passed on by an experienced manager to the novice. We think you will find it useful and a fitting conclusion to the book.

TRANSITION

Transition from a clinical nursing role to that of a nurse manager calls for the learning and practicing of an entirely new set of skills. Imagine this: Your interview for the nurse manager job was a week ago and today is your first day on the job. You drive your car to work. You drive down a country road, through a little town, onto a major highway and into the city. You park your car in a maze of others and arrive at your work site. When you walk into the nursing administrator's office, she points out the window at an 18-wheel truck and says, "Drive it. Your trip will be 2,000 miles. It's a challenge. You'll feel achievement every day. You will have a seasoned driver to ride with you, but you must do the driving. Good luck."

Driving that truck and making a transition to a management position have much in common. You know the basic road rules, how a truck runs, how to read a road map, and you have a sense of the right direction. But learning the new skills, new knowledge, and new driving techniques is something else again.

So it is with nursing management. You know the basic concepts, you know generally how the organization runs, you know how to give good care. But the skills of management are different.

SOCIALIZATION

Clinical nursing is the focus of nursing education, and management courses that are offered usually do not have the needed depth to adequately prepare a nurse manager. Few nursing programs use professional management faculties to teach management at the baccalaureate level. At the associate degree level, even less management content is included. Yet the student graduates and within several weeks is managing a group of people. In a few years or so, she has joined the nursing management team.

The nursing student has been socialized toward clinical and academic values—toward autonomy in nursing practice, not teamwork and the common goal attainment necessary for management. Furthermore, resocialization into the managerial role all too often occurs within a day-to-day trial and error climate. Many hospitals do not yet provide a structured and comprehensive orientation to the new role. Consequently, health care, at its most critical management point, must frequently depend upon those least prepared to manage it. Some institutions have tried various nonnursing management systems, but these have generally proved less successful than systems with strong nurse managers. The power base for nursing within organizations has been eroded by this lack of management theory and know-how.

Fortunately, today, master's programs in nursing administration are educating better prepared managers. However, many still do not utilize management school courses sufficiently.

It is not uncommon for new nurse managers with baccalaureate and even master's degrees, but little management experience, to find themselves in a superior position to, or working for, other nurses without comparable academic credentials but with years of experience. This can create problems for both parties, and a new nurse manager must be sensitive to the possibly troublesome implications of this situation. It is similar to what is called the "boot ensign" relationship in the military, where a person who has just completed officers' training school and has had little practical experience finds himself working with, say, a highly seasoned, experienced enlisted man.

Problems will arise when the new nurse manager starts making changes and exercising authority without drawing on the backgrounds and experiences of the staff and those to whom she is subordinate. Both are going to resent the newcomer who makes such statements as, "I frankly don't see how you functioned before I got here." If you find yourself in this "boot ensign" position, try not to come on too strong with your superior, peers, or subordinates. Even if you see situations that are in dire need of changing, wait until you've gained the staff's confidence before making a lot of drastic changes. Never criticize or disparage anything the prior nurse manager did. Present yourself as simply wanting to build on her or his previous contributions. You will need your staff's and supervisor's respect and support to make improvements.

None of this is meant to imply that advanced education in nursing or management is not valued. Quite the contrary; one must continually acquire new knowledge just to survive and be effective in the complex and demanding field of health care. If you are fortunate enough to have advanced formal education or unique past experiences, treasure them. But use your knowledge in a way that does not offend or belittle others.

CAREER OR JOB?

Nurses who elect to be managers must reflect on the fact that while they have taken on a career that is clearly defined in a business sense, they must also retain their professional values. A career may be defined as any lifelong work characterized by commitment, personal growth, and increasing levels of responsibility. Careers are very different from jobs. One difference lies in the perception of how one is paid. A job pays for hours worked, while in a career one is paid for what one has accomplished.

A manager must internalize and value this career concept for both personal effectiveness and work satisfaction. Generally, nurses do not enter management with a well-defined sense of what is being asked of them or what this means in terms of a career.

Career effectiveness will emerge after one begins to think in this way, but a nurse manager must also have ambition, political savvy, and management skill. None of these qualities should be considered "bad" or morally reprehensible. Nurses must have *ambition* to be powerful. They must be *politically astute* to be effective managers, and they must be *managerially proficient* in dealing with corporate issues, people, and money. A career orientation to nursing management may well be the highest priority for nursing in the decades before us. It will certainly be a high priority for hospital administrators, boards, and consumers.

Astute hospital administrators and boards of trustees are beginning to realize that nurses are among the most significant controllers of cost. The effective nurse manager will make clear to staff the need for cost-containment measures and enlist their support in achieving them. Failure to inform them and elicit their cooperation will result in organizational failure.

KEEPING UP WITH TRENDS

For nurse managers, understanding trends and keeping track of them are essential skills. They need to develop a strong sense of where they are and where the world may be taking them.

Trends in three general areas—social, health care, and nursing—should be watched carefully, as they will generate a frame of reference for plotting one's course. In *Megatrends*, Naisbitt examines social changes and suggests that several states seem to be bellwether ones, leaders, in societal change (Naisbitt, 1982). California, Washington, Colorado, Connecticut, and Florida generally fall into this group, closely followed by Minnesota and North Carolina. Keep an eye on what nurses in these states are doing in relation to the following social trends or shifts in directions: movement from emphasis on sickness to one on prevention and wellness; from the small nuclear family to greater numbers of single-parent families and to dual-career families; to a more casual social style; more women working, more career options for women, and new definitions of role for both men and women; to faster communication; to a shift from mainstream economy to alternatives; to superorganizational structures; and to limited career mobility in organizations (people will hang onto jobs they now have).

These societal trends will profoundly affect changes in health care. Nurse managers must look upon the understanding and tracking of health care trends as a priority study. Here, for example, are some more current trends to keep an eye on:

1. rationing of care as a result of reimbursement issues and legislation

2. multihospital systems

3. extension of health care services originating in the organizational system

4. services once provided in the hospital setting now being "bled out" to others

5. complex legal and collaborative arrangements

6. an increasingly older population needing care

7. more attention to complex ethical issues such as "pulling the plug" or extension of life

There are likely to be significant changes in nursing during the next two decades, as trends in health care and social trends have their impact. For instance:

1. an awareness that the nurse is a major revenue producer in the hospital

2. growth in fees for service at both group and individual levels

3. major manpower distribution problems and patterns

4. third-party reimbursement for nurses and nursing services

5. joint practice issues between physicians and nurses being resolved

6. increasing demands for and on nursing managers

7. fewer care givers in proportion to the population and more health education for the public

8. increasing emphasis on basic and continuing education of high quality for the professional nurse

As a nursing manager you will be called upon by colleagues and others to translate these trends into action on a day-to-day basis. Careful and consistent reading in publications such as *Wall Street Journal, Harvard Business Review, Inc., Fortune,* and *Forum* will put you in a position to effect patient care of high quality by communicating needs efficiently in a futuristic perspective. To be on top of current trends, there are three more imperatives:

1. *You must know computers.* Managers cannot work without information.

2. *You must be business-oriented.* Health care is a business.

3. *You must think in long-range terms.* Before today is over, your world will have changed.

POLITICS

Politics—which is *not* a dirty word, by the way—refers to an inclusive complex of relationships within an organization, including the latter's norms, values, culture, the way things are done, and what is and is not acceptable. As a nursing manager on the way up the ladder, you must decide if you *want* to play. The process is the same as that of joining a new social group, church, or bowling league. There are ways to act and not to act within any given group. If you play, you're in; if not, you're out. Simple. You will never perfectly fit a given organization, but the closer the better. This means that you had better investigate such matters as:

1. *Who is chosen, and why,* to be promoted, to chair a committee, to be United Way chairman, or share lunch? Look into the personal qualities

of that individual, the social and business groups he or she belongs to, as well as the person's knowledge and skills.

2. *What is the "union card"* for your organization that guarantees positive impressions? Perhaps it is a BSN, or years of practice, or a degree in business. Find out the credential(s) you need for political acceptance.

3. *What has been the route to the top?* Investigate how most successful nurses got where they are. Consider their sponsors and mentors; consider yours.

Nurse managers who advance rapidly in their careers have usually discovered where the opportunities are in an organization. They know what the real power positions are and what is needed to take advantage of opportunities. They're aware, too, of what education is needed, what support groups are effective, and what image is acceptable. That's the political side. But it goes without saying that they also need to be committed nurses and effective, efficient managers.

From a practical point of view, successful nursing managers have learned that politics are played every day in every situation, especially at work. They are willing to become involved in this game. They become effective by:

1. *Having a face.* They join committees and work groups. They get to know lots of people. They "work the crowd."

2. *Preparing themselves.* They pursue educational programs that are highly directed toward their goals.

3. *Presenting a positive image.* They know the unwritten dress code and follow it. They have carriage and energy that proclaims confidence.

4. *Demonstrating an above-average grasp of written and oral communication skills.* They express themselves clearly, concisely, and with impact.

5. *Networking effectively.* They have a circle of people internally and externally from whom to draw information and support. They carry business cards so as to be ready to validate new liaisons.

6. *Having mentors and sponsors.* They are clear as to the responsibilities and obligations inherent in these types of relationships.

7. *Knowing organizational values.* They know where their organization is headed and why.

8. *Not wounding the lion or lioness.* They know the "hot buttons" and do not push them. They never publicly make moves that discredit themselves or others.

9. *Mobilizing resources.* They know who or what can be of help in given situations and how to activate these resources.

10. *Having vision.* They have a view of what may or could be and assume leadership in moving toward those goals.

MENTORS AND SPONSORS

As the nurse manager assesses her or his effectiveness, promotion potential, and security, one very crucial issue must be evaluated. Who is mentoring and who is sponsoring you? (They're not the same thing.) Mentors and sponsors are those very important guardian angels who provide support, advice, and depth to us in our career development. They provide the manager's informal system, which works something like this: Whenever you need advice or help, someone you know or have known over time assists you in reaching an objective. The relationship is generally based upon respect and trust between individuals. Your need is another person's opportunity to return a favor. The informal system frequently rests on personal relationships of long-standing and unspoken obligations. Informal systems are rarely openly discussed.

The three major players in an informal system are the managers, mentors, and sponsors.

Mentors give support. The relationship is characterized by a present orientation: it is for today and what must be done now. A mentor teaches the manager how to do a job. A mentor need *not* be a supervisor or one titled in the organization. Mentors tell you what you need to know and show you how to do it. They trust you with a job by giving assignments that are important, that test limits, and provide learning. Mentors help by talking to you. They introduce you to people with whom you will move. A manager/mentor relationship is an apprentice/teacher one. This relationship is rarely hidden.

Mentors are usually the same sex as the protégé, 8 to 15 years older, highly placed in the organization, powerful and with a need for power. They are knowledgeable individuals who are willing to share their expertise and are not threatened by the protégé's potential for equaling or surpassing them (Hunts & Michael, 1983). Protégés are selected by mentors for several reasons: good performance; the "right" social background or a social acquaintance with each other; they look well dressed; they are socially similar; they have the opportunity to demonstrate the extraordinary; and they have high visibility.

Mentor/protégé relationships seem to advance through several stages. The *initiation* stage usually lasts six months to a year, during which the relationship gets started. The *protégé* stage is that in which the protégé's work is not yet recognized for its own merit, but rather as a by-product of the mentor's instruction, support, and encouragement. The mentor thus buffers the protégé from criticism. (A *breakup* stage may occur from six months to two years after a significant change in the relationship, usually resulting from the protégé's taking a job in another department so that there is physical separation of the two individuals. It can also result when the mentor refuses to accept the protégé as a peer or when the relationship becomes dysfunctional for some reason.) The *lasting friendship* stage is the final phase of the relationship. This stage will occur if the mentor accepts the protégé as a peer or if the relationship is reestablished after a significant separation. The complete mentor process usually includes this latter stage.

The relationship with a sponsor is quite different. It is future- rather than present-oriented. This is the relationship that opens doors that are generally closed to the manager. A sponsor may be at any high-level position, formal or informal, in the organization or the community that affects the organization. A sponsor tells you not what you need to know nor how to do something, but what you *need* to do. Sponsors trust your ability. Sponsors trust you with inside information. They take you along to appropriate places, meetings, or gatherings. At first they may just silently make sure you are there. They help you by talking about you, especially to those who control your career moves. Sponsors make sure you know people who have influence. This relationship may be unidentifiable in that the sponsor chooses to remain silent and unknown. If open, it is a collegial relationship.

Both mentor and sponsor relationships are fragile and are based upon strong trust. Nursing managers, recognizing these relationships by identifiable points, can maximize their depth and effectiveness.

Some rules for the mentor or sponsor relationship:

1. Don't choose, or be chosen, by only one mentor or sponsor. Loss of power by that one individual can then mean loss of power for you.

2. Don't sit back and wait. Scout around senior management and search out relationships. Ask for advice.

3. Don't expect the relationship to give you all you need to do your job. Be realistic.

KNOWING THE SYSTEM

To know the system within which work is done may at first elude the new manager, then become a puzzle, and, with effort and tutoring, become a revelation. Complex organizational relationships, both formal and informal, bombard the new manager with deadly force. Traditional nursing and patient care values conflict with new information, and frequently the neophyte is ill prepared to cope with the results.

Having a sense of flow of information, approvals, and actions within a given health care organization takes energy and time. The nurse must know the pieces of the organization and how they fit together, yet each organization is different so it cannot be learned from a book. Success in plotting one's course depends upon reconnaissance. The manager must be excellent in environmental reconnaissance both within the hospital and outside of it. Rarely does a nurse manager enter a job having studied organizational dynamics in depth, desirable although the latter is.

A hospital system may be centralized or decentralized, for profit or not for profit, governmental or private. Each system deserves consideration and study. A system is the totality of elements or interactions that interact with each other to produce a product. It is your hospital.

Theories reflect macrocosmic understanding. Microcosmic efficiency—that is, how efficient a nurse manager is on her or his nursing unit—reflects macrocosmic understanding. Nursing managers must set out to learn all they can of management theory and then recognize that one theory cannot get them all the way. Managers must be eclectic, selecting the concepts that, when put into action in a particular situation, will yield the best results. Uni-theory people distort health care. Managers should seek out anything in psychology, business, accounting, anthropology, and so on that will help them identify direction. The effective manager is flexible!

With prospective reimbursement legislation, the person likely to emerge as the single most important controller of resources is going to be the nurse manager. Concern with total hospital cash flow is going to become critical for role effectiveness, and this may create problems for nurses who have been socialized to believe in a "best care possible" goal. The fact is that the "best" care may no longer be affordable. For health care professionals, the value conflict in this statement is awesome. Managers, however, must be able to validate the worth of the effort. We assume validity of our current system, but as funding sources become less consistent, it falls upon nurse managers to become leaders in care provision. They must be adept at defining (a) what the care system on the unit will look like; (b) what TEM (time, energy, and money) will be needed; and (c) what's the least expensive way to do what needs to be done and provide the best quality of care possible, given the available resources.

In order to provide cost-efficient services, the nurse manager must be able to maximize the one resource that is ultimately expandable—manpower. It is clear that performance is a function of the staff and the environment (culture of the nursing unit). If the manager is to produce desired results through people, then it follows that an appropriate work culture must be designed. This is a major part of a manager's job. For the nurse manager a good culture (environment) is generally one that facilitates performance; helps the nurse manager and staff to learn new things; compensates for weaknesses; provides promotion opportunity; supports risk taking; and reinforces successes.

GROUPS

People and group performance are critical issues in a nurse management position. Groups have not been studied enough and the new nurse manager, especially, does not have in-depth information about them. Yet, the organization's expectation is a unit staff that works together for maximum results. There is more about groups in Chapters 8 and 10, but here are some hints to keep in mind when leading group discussions:

- Set a warm, accepting, and nonthreatening climate.

- Define all terms and concepts.

- Foster cooperation in the group.

- Establish goals and identify major objectives.

- Allocate time for all decision-making steps.

- Lead/discuss so that all members have an opportunity to contribute.

- Help integrate the material and ideas that have been generated.

- Help group members identify the implications of the ideas.

- Help the group evaluate the quality of the discussion

BASIC SURVIVAL SKILLS

Necessary for survival in the world of nursing management are characteristics and style similar to those of business leaders. Successful nurse managers need to have:

A well-developed sense of self-awareness. Each nursing unit reflects the characteristics of the leader. Evaluation of your own idiosyncrasies, styles, and motivations will provide some insight into the climate of your unit. Nurse managers live in a world of false cues. Staff will be "dishonest" in an effort to please and to manipulate the climate. The manager is frequently told what she is perceived to want to know. The challenge is to make feedback, positive *or* negative, safe and OK.

The ability to manage work, personal, and family life. The higher you go in management and administration, the more involved you become. Organizations, especially health care, have no collective consciousness. Feeling as though you are juggling 25 Ping-Pong balls will wear you down. Decide which ones to drop. Set your priorities to accomplish what *you* do best—your professional work. Hire someone else to do the housework or yardwork. Give yourself time, also, to engage in activities that add to a sound, well-rounded life (and reduce the stress that accompanies management). A well-rounded life makes you more valuable.

Multiple interests and well-rounded experiences. Plan for a variety of educational, personal, and cultural experiences. Make opportunities for your staff to see units in other hospitals and other units in your own organization.

Interpersonal sensitivity. Listen to verbal and nonverbal cues from your staff. Chances are you are expert at listening to patients; do it with staff, also. Sense "vibes." Focus carefully on the total person who is communicating.

The courage to take risks. Don't worry about your job! Once managers become too cautious to take risks, their effectiveness is greatly diminished, thereby actually lessening job security. Begin early to network and, if possible, have a potential job offer in your pocket.

A competent assistant. Don't give up vacations or other opportunities to revitalize yourself. Develop staff who can run the show while you are away for vacation, a learning experience, or some other personal reason. One who is "indispensable" cannot be promoted, so always train your replacement.

A method for self-criticism and self-discipline. Nurse managers should design a method to move away from the "yearly" evaluation and create methods within the system that will provide accurate peer, medical staff, and consumer feedback as often as possible.

A great curiosity. Generally, in health care, we are governed by professional socialization to think in the scientific mode. Creative thinking is thereby greatly lessened. Learn the joy of a lively mind and play (creativity and play are the same) in your work setting.

An experiential attitude. Be optimistic. "Let us try" and "let us learn" should be often heard on your unit.

The tolerance for sustained work. Nursing is seldom if ever an eight-hour day. If that is your expectation or value, remove yourself from the position. Holding power is a winning strategy for your power position in the organization.

A sense of calling or mission. This may sound trite, but successful people have it. Others do not. There is a meaning to work that is a personal commitment.

THE FIRST WEEKS AS MANAGER

Here are some guidelines for your first weeks on the job, taken from Thompson and Wood's *Management Strategies for Women* (1980).

First Day on the Job

- Do a quick review of the budget. Collect any existing organizational planning documents.

- Meet the staff.

- Get your office set up for work. Decorate after hours.

- Start listing the things you think you want to accomplish for the organization.

- Mark all meetings or deadlines on your calendar.

- You're the boss. Get started.

Meeting and Dealing with Staff

- Learn names. Memorize them before you go "on tour."

- Meet as many people as possible on a one-to-one basis, starting with key staff.

- Invite people to your office so that they can learn more about you. Include potential antagonists to establish turf.

- When establishing relationships, it is 51% up to you and 49% up to your staff.

- Until you know how staff members operate, ask why they made the decisions they did.

- Ask for specific help and support. If it is not forthcoming and if your request is reasonable, lower the boom: firmly, calmly, and clearly.

- Take corrective action if your staff starts going over your head.

- Get involved in hiring key staff members.

- Immediately get on top of important issues. Establish a method for keeping track of them.

- Begin establishing informal grapevines. The sooner they're working, the better.

Initial Staff Meetings

- Don't meet in large groups until you are ready. But don't delay too long!

- Do not put substantive or complex problems on the first agenda if you are not ready to deal with them or cannot offer some solutions. Set the agenda yourself so that you stay in control.

- Be as certain as possible that you can deliver on any commitments you may make during the meeting.

- Postpone (tactfully) those issues raised by others that you are not prepared to handle. Set a definite time to deal with them, however.

- If possible, announce a major decision you've made or an important new policy or procedure.

- Don't be overly sentimental in your first remarks to the full group. Be pleasant, firm, and businesslike. At the same time, a little warmth will ease tension.

Strengthening Your Position in the Early Weeks

- Relax. You're going to mess up somewhere. Just keep the mistake small.

- If operational plans exist for your area of responsibility, become knowledgeable about them, pick up the reins, and move ahead. If they do not exist, begin planning activities so that you know where you are headed, why, and at what cost.

- Get your performance planning and appraisal processes underway as soon as possible. Help your staff to understand where they are headed, why, and at what cost.

- Don't be above asking for advice when you need it.

- Establish directions and priorities yourself and do the initial detailed work yourself. You can't turn the ship around with someone else doing the steering.

- Make a list of people you'll need to know outside the organization. Find ways to get to know them.

- If you delegate responsibility on an interim basis, delegate authority on the same basis.

- Analyze immediately why something failed.

- Study other people who you think are successful. Spend time with them. Talk with them. Borrow their good ideas. Try to figure out why they are successful in the eyes of others.

- If you hear about someone who has done something well, find out how he or she made it happen.

Dealing with Insecurities

- Don't jump headlong into tough situations without proper briefing and background. In the early weeks, move cautiously and carefully. It will build confidence for later on.

- If some individual really makes you feel insecure or anxious, get to know that person better.

- Don't spill your insecurities to everyone. Let them think you have it all together.

- Remember that people have greater respect for leaders who make mistakes with some degree of decisiveness than leaders who never make mistakes because they never lead.

Strategies with Your Superiors
(Also see Chapter 24 on working with higher management.)

- Always tell the truth to the one above you.

- Never let your superior get a surprise; keep him or her informed.

- If she or he asks you to do something, do it well and ahead of deadline if possible. If appropriate, add some of your own recommendations.

- After a time, take the initiative by suggesting solutions to important problems.

- When it is appropriate, be open about needs, problems, and information.

- Try to understand your superior's position and where you disagree. Keep your mouth shut until you know what you're talking about.

- If you find that your superior is making most of the decisions in your area of responsibility, address the problem head on.

- Make a conscious decision not to consult your superior any more than you have to. That way, when you do see her (or him), she will know you have something important to discuss.

HOW TO BE A SUCCESSFUL NURSE MANAGER

There are certain behaviors that can help you make a successful transition from practicing nurse to nurse manager. Go through this list and take some time for introspection, looking thoughtfully at your present behavior.

Vision. Great leaders in any field have always had vision. They have looked beyond today into tomorrow and, because of this, were able to move a group of people in a particular direction. An inhibitor of long-range vision is territoriality, or visualizing one's world in terms of a particular territory. Territoriality limits vision and it limits dreams.

Accompanying vision is the ability to dream, to dream about where you can go, where your unit can go, or where you can take that group of people that you lead. Another part of vision is having planning skills, one of the major functions of management. Then somehow translate those plans into action. Some people dream through their reading and in discussions with each other. Somebody has an idea, and you latch on to that idea, making it part of your own system of thinking by saying, "Hey, that sounds like a good idea" or "Yes, it may work this way," and then incubating it for a while and later translating it into action. You always steal a little. There are few new ideas in the world, mostly old ones that take on a new, fresh look.

See the big picture. This goes along with territoriality. You start with your unit or your area of work and you are able to see what goes on there, but you don't stop there, you move on to what is happening in your community, state, country, and the world. What do you do to look at the big picture? You read local newspapers, state newspapers, national newspapers, the *Wall Street Journal*, the *Harvard Business Review*, and the nursing and hospital journals. These publications enhance the scope of your knowledge. You attend seminars—local, state, and national—and you become involved in local and state politics. You develop a network.

Networking begins with trying to meet others who are "big picture" persons. You talk with people in a similar job, or you make a new contact, or a mentor somewhere else. They are going to have skills and interests that will enrich your particular big picture. In the hospital, seeing the big picture means moving away from territoriality into noting and understanding what exists outside of nursing service.

Know who you are. Know your good points and your bad ones; you know better than anyone else what they are. Sometimes a friend may be able to help you work through them. Say to yourself, "If I do have positives and negatives, what can I do about the negatives and what can I do to upgrade the positives?" Don't throw the baby out with the bathwater; identify those things that are fantastic and good so you don't lose them. Also look at deficits and try to remedy them. Identify what you can do about a problem and work on that. Do not try to change someone else's behavior, change your own.

Red flag sensitivity. That means you know—sometimes a day, week, or month in advance—that a problem is going to come, because you can see that things are beginning to happen. This sensitivity is almost indescribable. Just consider the number of times you have sensed that something is going to happen, forgotten it, and then have it surface and hit you in the face later. It is that bit of sensitivity that says, "Hey, this is a problem." React to the red flag by taking action or preparing to take action on whatever the red flag signals. This is basically prediction—an awareness that you develop once you develop a sensitivity to your surroundings.

Know trends or changes. What has happened and what is going on in relation to what has gone on before. In very specific language, what is the nosocomial rate on your division? How many hours of overtime? Is your budget over or under the estimate and in what categories? How does it compare with last month or the year to date? Why is it over or under?

What is the state of the quality assurance on your division? Is absenteeism up or down? Lateness? What is the morale on your division?

Those are just a few of the trends to mention; there are many others, all of them extremely important because you must make management judgments and you can't make them without knowing the trends. In terms of an entire nursing service, this is the director of nursing's job; for an entire hospital, it is the administrator's job. For your unit, it is your job.

Learn the tools of your trade. For management they are: communication skills; sensitivity; objectivity; assertiveness; budget awareness; time management; and the ability to counsel, motivate, teach, establish priorities, build a support system, and create a growth-enhancing environment. Those are the tools that have to do with people, but there are others: leadership ability, role modeling, and a knowledge of statistics if involved in projecting and forecasting, basic writing skills, basic reading, and speed reading. Focus on what tools you have and where you need some help. The bottom line is know what tools your trade has and use them.

Think continually. This is very important in nursing service. Do not think in tems of 8- or 12-hour shifts, but think on a continuous basis. Nursing services should flow. There should not be a start and stop time for tasks. In no way every single day will all the tasks for that day be completed at 3:30 P.M. or any other time. Sometimes they will be done at 1:00 P.M. and other times at 5:00 P.M., so if you begin to think continuously, you will instill that value in your staff. Then there will be less disgruntlement when Ms. A cannot get all the blood pressures taken within a given time, and Ms. B comes on at 7:00 A.M. and has to finish them. This is one of the most significant problems in nursing and it has to do with compartmentalization—"I've got my little set of tasks to do and I don't see further than that." The nurse manager must herself think continuously and then share that value with her staff.

Listen. Not only to your supervisors but to the physician, the administrator, the patients, and families. Develop active listening skills. These skills don't just happen, they have to be developed. You know someone is listening to you by watching their nonverbal communication, such as their eye contact, nodding their head, etc. You can notice these behaviors in others and yourself.

Know time and motion methods. One of the biggest problems in nursing is that we do not take measurements and we do not really know what we spend our time doing. A good example is a nurse making several trips from one side to the other to make a bed instead of completely making one side at a time. Evaluate your staff in relation to time and motion. Set up your division so that people do not waste time.

Learn the rules. But remember that rules are written in sand, not concrete; situations change, time changes, equipment changes, and people change. Consequently, rules change. Rules are guidelines. One of the biggest things that we can do for ourselves as nurses is to make sure that when a rule is made that we don't believe in, fight it. Then, once that rule is in place, we can make sure that it is not sabotaged because sabotage leads to disrespect of authority. This goes hand in hand with consensus decision making. Consensus is not majority rule. Consensus is that everybody agrees on something or at least agrees to support it actively and not sabotage it, even though they may not believe it to be a wise decision.

Develop a nondefensive stand and be nonemotional. Have your act together. It is best to hear comments that sound like, "Gee, there really is a problem here, but there are a few things I can do to help solve that problem. What can you do to work with me so that we can get it solved?" Interact either on a one-to-one level or with the whole group that is involved.

Avoid interpersonal putdowns. Some putdown behaviors are no eye contact, being late for a meeting or appointment, not being available, turning your back, and other behavior that says to another person, "You are not important."

Eye contact. Eye contact that says that you are in touch with a person is important. If you do not have a very positive image of yourself, it is one of the things you will not do. Eye contact is a very important power mechanism.

Escalation. What does escalate mean? Well, you have a problem; you don't like what is going on. You tell the supervisor or the director. You tell them over and over again, but they don't listen to you. Don't give up or let the matter ride. Instead, say, "Hey, I really feel so strongly about this, can we talk with someone else?" Escalate to higher levels until you are satisfied.

Look professional. Women, especially, and nurses in particular, have a tendency to lose power because of the way they look. In a managerial position, you must have power and one of the ways to gain and keep power is by the way you look. You can give away power in your body language and the way you dress. If you want to make a positive professional impression, then you will move toward a look that is both classic and professional, whether in uniform or street clothes.

Learn to live with a certain amount of discomfort. It is never comfortable for any manager, no matter how experienced, to say to an employee, "We have a problem and it has got to change." Nor is it comfortable to say, "I made a mistake." It is not comfortable to escalate, to confront, to admit your own mistakes. The more experience you have in doing those things, the more comfortable you may become, but it is never an easy job.

Enthusiasm and warmth. More positive things happen when you are enthusiastic. Your job is an exciting one. Let yourself enjoy it and let your enjoyment be visible. Don't be afraid to show warmth, either. It is one of the most important kinds of things that nurses have going for them, a real concern for other people.

Learn to trust. You have to build trust; delegation is built upon it. You have to make sure when you delegate that you trust the persons to whom you delegate. This means you must select them carefully. Also you have to build trust with others by carrying out your responsibilities to them.

View what you are doing as a career not a job. When you begin a career, you can think about enthusiasm and commitment, but when what you do becomes part of you (and not just for eight hours a day), then it becomes a career. You cannot forget what is a vital part of you when you walk out the door. Some people can do that, but those people have jobs, not a career. The time has passed, both from an economic and a self-fulfillment point of view, that you can say, "Well, I am working until it is quitting time." Write your own development plans and make sure that you follow through on them. You have power in your position. Think about the number of people a nurse manager is in charge of and how much she controls their day-to-day lives. Once you start thinking about that, then you realize your obligation to view yourself as a continually developing individual.

Don't give away your power. There are many ways we do that, as women and as nurses. How do you give away your power? You give it away by not using it, by the way you dress, by being afraid not to be alone, by being negative, by not caring, by not taking the option to make a decision when you can. You have got to take risks.

Get your priorities straight. To be successful you have got to get your priorities in order. Your health (mental and physical) comes first. Second, family or work. You decide, but think about it rationally.

Develop a support group. Many of us started our first jobs without having someone around who was a real support, someone who could tell us a lot about how to get the job done. Support groups turn complaining into goal setting, obstacles into opportunities, and defeat into growth. If you don't have a support group, you are out there all by yourself and you are scared to death. Turn it around. Find and cultivate supportive colleagues and friends.

Empathize. It is usually easy to empathize with patients and visitors, but when it comes to the human needs of co-workers, physicians, and administrators, it is harder. Empathize with all people you encounter.

Develop your self-esteem. If you don't feel important and worthwhile, you need to do something to help yourself. It takes a lot of work and sometimes it takes professional help to enhance your self-esteem, but it's worth it.

Avoid surprises. You do not want to be surprised by attending a meeting and hearing about an issue that you had not previously known about. Keep yourself informed. And don't give others surprises like that, either; it creates a defensive, nontrust kind of situation.

Have fun. Have fun with other people, have fun with the people on your unit, have fun because jobs and work are fun. Happy people make happy patients. Is there anything nicer than when you come on the unit and somebody smiles? It makes the world more pleasant.

Stretch toward excellence. Figure out what makes the best surgical, medical, neonatal, ICU area in the world and work for that. That is what dreams are made of and that is what excellence is made of. There are always new things happening; stretch for those things.

Be a boss. Be a manager. Be able to plan. Be able to implement and evaluate change. Be able to guide staff; be able to budget, communicate, make decisions, and develop positively. Articulate effectively with personnel in other disciplines. Command respect. That is a pragmatic view of management.

SUMMARY

- Transition from a clinical role to nurse manager calls for learning and practicing a new set of skills. Nurses are not educated for or socialized to management so they must learn these skills.

- Management is a career which takes ambition, political savvy, and management skills. It also requires keeping up with societal, business, and legal trends because these trends will affect health care.

- Nurse managers must understand and be willing to practice organizational politics, and know the route to success in their particular hospital.

- Successful nurse managers will network, find mentors, increase communication skills, and be visible to administration.

- Nurse managers must know the system in which they work: their hospital. What are its goals, values, priorities? Understanding organization theory and management theories is the key to understanding a hospital.

- Understanding group dynamics is also important. Nurses work in groups and group climate will determine productivity.

- Successful nurse managers need to have several survival skills: a sense of self-awareness, ability to manage work and personal/family life, interpersonal sensitivity, the courage to take risks, competent assistants, and curiosity.

- The first day on the job is critical. Several items need attention. Meeting staff and initial staff meetings are important considerations. Learning to deal with insecurities and discovering strategies to deal with one's supervisor are critical.

- Being a successful manager means knowing who you are, what your capabilities are, and working from there. It means growing, and gaining strength where you are weak.

- Being a successful manager means looking, acting, and thinking as a professional.

BIBLIOGRAPHY

Bowman, G. W., Warety, N. B., and Greepet, S. A. (1965). Are women executive people? *Harv Bus Rvw*, (July–August) 43:14.

Cavanaugh, D. E. Gamesmanship: The art of strategizing. *J Nurs Adm*, 15(4): 38–41.

Chenevert, M. (1985). *Pro-nurse handbook*. St. Louis: C. V. Mosby.

Darling, L. W., and McGrath, L. (1983). Minimizing promotion trauma. *J Nurs Adm*, 13(9): 14.

Dunn, J. M. (1982). The female administrator. In: *Contemporary nursing management*. Marriner, A. (editor). St. Louis: C. V. Mosby.

Gambacorta, S. (1983). Head nurses face reality shock, too! *Nurs Mngmt*, 14(7): 46.

Gleeson, S., Nestor, O. W., and Riddell, A. J. (1983). Helping nurses through the management threshold. *Nurs Adm Quart*, (Winter) 7(2): 11.

Hunts, D. M., and Michael, C. (1983). Mentorship: A career training and development tool. *Acad Mngmt Rvw*, 8:475.

Kanter, R. M. (1977). *Men and women of the corporation*. New York: Basic Books.

Levenstein, A. (1985). Caught in the middle. *Nurs Mngmt*, 16(2): 55–56.

Naisbitt, J. (1982). *Megatrends*. New York: Warner Books.

Persons, C. B., and Wieck, L. (1985). Networking: A power strategy. *Nurs Econ*, 3(1): 53–57.

Strasen, L. (1987). *Key business skills for nurse managers*. Philadelphia: J. B. Lippincott.

Thompson, A. M., and Wood, M. D. (1980). *Management strategies for women*. New York: Simon and Schuster.

Toffler, A. (1981). *The third wave*. New York: Bantam Books.

Veninga, R. L. (1987). When bad things happen to good nursing departments: How to stay hopeful in tough times. *J Nurs Adm*, 17(2): 35–40.

APPENDICES

American Nurses' Association
Standards of Nursing Practice

NURSING PRACTICE IS a direct service, goal directed and adaptable to the needs of the individual, family and community during health and illness. Professional practitioners of nursing bear primary responsibility and accountability for the nursing care clients/patients receive. The purpose of Standards of Nursing Practice is to fulfill the profession's obligation to provide and improve this practice.

The Standards focus on practice. They provide a means for determining the quality of nursing which a client/patient receives regardless of whether such services are provided solely by a professional nurse or by a professional nurse and nonprofessional assistants.

The Standards are stated according to a systematic approach to nursing practice: the assessment of the client's/patient's status, the plan of nursing actions, the implementation of the plan, and the evaluation. These specific divisions are not intended to imply that practice consists of a series of discrete steps, taken in strict sequence, beginning with assessment and ending with evaluation. The processes described are used concurrently and recurrently. Assessment, for example, frequently continues during implementation; similarly, evaluation dictates reassessment and replanning.

These Standards for Nursing Practice apply to nursing practice in any setting. Nursing practice in all settings must possess the characteristics identified by these Standards if clients/patients are to receive a high quality of nursing care. Each Standard is followed by a rationale and assessment factors. Assessment factors are to be used in determining achievement of the Standard.

STANDARD I

THE COLLECTION OF DATA ABOUT THE HEALTH STATUS OF THE CLIENT/PATIENT IS SYSTEMATIC AND CONTINUOUS. THE DATA ARE ACCESSIBLE, COMMUNICATED, AND RECORDED.

Rationale: Comprehensive care requires complete and ongoing collection of data about the client/patient to determine the nursing care needs of the client/patient. All health status data about the client/patient must be available for all members of the health care team.

Assessment Factors:

1. Health status data include:
   - Growth and development
   - Biophysical status
   - Emotional status
   - Cultural, religious, socioeconomic background
   - Performance of activities of daily living
   - Patterns of coping
   - Interaction patterns
   - Client's/patient's perception of and satisfaction with his health status
   - Client/patient health goals
   - Environment (physical, social, emotional, ecological)
   - Available and accessible human and material resources

2. Data are collected from:
   - Client/patient, family, significant others
   - Health care personnel
   - Individuals within the immediate environment and/or the community

3. Data are obtained by:
   - Interview
   - Examination
   - Observation
   - Reading records, reports, etc.

4. There is a format for the collection of data which:
   - Provides for a systematic collection of data
   - Facilitates the completeness of data collection

5. Continuous collection of data is evident by:
   - Frequent updating
   - Recording of changes in health status

6. The data are:
   - Accessible on the client/patient records
   - Retrievable from record-keeping systems
   - Confidential when appropriate

STANDARD II

NURSING DIAGNOSES ARE DERIVED FROM HEALTH STATUS DATA.

Rationale: The health status of the client/patient is the basis for determining the nursing care needs. The data are analyzed and compared to norms when possible.

Assessment Factors:

1. The client's/patient's health status is compared to the norm in order to determine if there is a deviation from the norm and the degree and direction of deviation.

2. The client's/patient's capabilities and limitations are identified.

3. The nursing diagnoses are related to and congruent with the diagnoses of all other professionals caring for the client/patient.

STANDARD III

THE PLAN OF NURSING CARE INCLUDES GOALS DERIVED FROM THE NURSING DIAGNOSES.

Rationale: The determination of the results to be achieved is an essential part of planning care.

Assessment Factors:

1. Goals are mutually set with the client/patient and pertinent others:
   –They are congruent with other planned therapies.
   –They are stated in realistic and measurable terms.
   –They are assigned a time period for achievement.

2. Goals are established to maximize functional capabilities and are congruent with:
   –Growth and development
   –Biophysical status
   –Behavioral patterns
   –Human and material resources

STANDARD IV

THE PLAN OF NURSING CARE INCLUDES PRIORITIES AND THE PRESCRIBED NURSING APPROACHES OR MEASURES TO ACHIEVE THE GOALS DERIVED FROM THE NURSING DIAGNOSES.

Rationale: Nursing actions are planned to promote, maintain and restore the client's/patient's well-being.

Assessment Factors:

1. Physiological measures are planned to manage (prevent or control) specific patient problems and are related to the nursing diagnoses and goals of care, e.g. ADL, use of self-help devices, etc.

2. Psychosocial measures are specific to the client's/patient's nursing care problem and to the nursing care goals, e.g. techniques to control aggression, motivation.

3. Teaching-learning principles are incorporated into the plan of care and objectives for learning stated in behavioral terms, e.g. specification of content for learner's level, reinforcement, readiness, etc.

4. Approaches are planned to provide for a therapeutic environment:
   –Physical environmental factors are used to influence the therapeutic environment, e.g. control of noise, control of temperature, etc.
   –Psychosocial measures are used to structure the environment for therapeutic ends, e.g. paternal participation in all phases of the maternity experience.
   –Group behaviors are used to structure interaction and influence the therapeutic environment, e.g. conformity, ethos, territorial rights, locomotion, etc.

5. Approaches are specified for orientation of the client/patient to:
   –New roles and relationships
   –Relevant health (human and material) resources
   –Modifications in plan of nursing care
   –Relationship of modifications in nursing care plan to the total care plan

6. The plan of nursing care includes the utilization of available and appropriate resources:
   –Human resources—other health personnel
   –Material resources
   –Community

7. The plan includes an ordered sequence of nursing actions.

8. Nursing approaches are planned on the basis of current scientific knowledge.

STANDARD V

NURSING ACTIONS PROVIDE FOR CLIENT/PATIENT PARTICIPATION IN HEALTH PROMOTION, MAINTENANCE AND RESTORATION.

Rationale: The client/patient and family are continually involved in nursing care.

Assessment Factors:

1. The client/patient and family are kept informed about:
   –Current health status
   –Changes in health status

-Total health care plan
-Nursing care plan
-Roles of health care personnel
-Health care resources

2. The client/patient and family are provided with the information needed to make decisions and choices about:
-Promoting, maintaining and restoring health
-Seeking and utilizing appropriate health care personnel
-Maintaining and using health care resources

STANDARD VI

NURSING ACTIONS ASSIST THE CLIENT/PATIENT TO MAXIMIZE HIS HEALTH CAPABILITIES.

Rationale: Nursing actions are designed to promote, maintain and restore health.

Assessment Factors:

1. Nursing actions:
-Are consistent with the plan of care.
-Are based on scientific principles.
-Are individualized to the specific situation.
-Are used to provide a safe and therapeutic environment.
-Employ teaching-learning opportunities for the client/patient.
-Include utilization of appropriate resources.

2. Nursing actions are directed by the client's/patient's physical, physiological, psychological and social behavior associated with:
-Ingestion of food, fluid and nutrients
-Elimination of body wastes and excesses in fluid
-Locomotion and exercise
-Regulatory mechanisms—body heat, metabolism
-Relating to others
-Self-actualization

STANDARD VII

THE CLIENT'S/PATIENT'S PROGRESS OR LACK OF PROGRESS TOWARD GOAL ACHIEVEMENT IS DETERMINED BY THE CLIENT/PATIENT AND THE NURSE.

Rationale: The quality of nursing care depends upon comprehensive and intelligent determination of nursing's impact upon the health status of the client/patient. The client/patient is an essential part of this determination.

Assessment Factors:

1. Current data about the client/patient are used to measure his progress toward goal achievement.

2. Nursing actions are analyzed for their effectiveness in the goal achievement of the client/patient.

3. The client/patient evaluates nursing actions and goal achievement.

4. Provision is made for nursing follow-up of a particular client/patient to determine the long-term effects of nursing care.

STANDARD VIII

THE CLIENT'S/PATIENT'S PROGRESS OR LACK OF PROGRESS TOWARD GOAL ACHIEVEMENT DIRECTS REASSESSMENT, RE-ORDERING OF PRIORITIES, NEW GOAL SETTING AND REVISION OF THE PLAN OF NURSING CARE.

Rationale: The nursing process remains the same, but the input of new information may dictate new or revised approaches.

Assessment Factors:

1. Reassessment is directed by goal achievement or lack of goal achievement.

2. New priorities and goals are determined and additional nursing approaches are prescribed appropriately.

3. New nursing actions are accurately and appropriately initiated.

American Hospital Association:
A Patient's Bill of Rights

The American Hospital Association Board of Trustees' Committee on Health Care for the Disadvantaged, which has been a consistent advocate on behalf of consumers of health care services, developed the Statement on a Patient's Bill of Rights, *which was approved by the AHA House of Delegates February 6, 1973. The statement was published in several forms, one of which was the S74 leaflet in the Association's S series. The S74 leaflet is now superseded by this reprinting of the statement.*

The American Hospital Association presents a Patient's Bill of Rights with the expectation that observance of these rights will contribute to more effective patient care and greater satisfaction for the patient, his physician, and the hospital organization. Further, the Association presents these rights in the expectation that they will be supported by the hospital on behalf of its patients, as an integral part of the healing process. It is recognized that a personal relationship between the physician and the patient is essential for the provision of proper medical care. The traditional physician-patient relationship takes on a new dimension when care is rendered within an organizational structure. Legal precedent has established that the institution itself also has a responsibility to the patient. It is in recognition of these factors that these rights are affirmed.

1. The patient has the right to considerate and respectful care.

2. The patient has the right to obtain from his physician complete current information concerning his diagnosis, treatment, and prognosis in terms the patient can be reasonably expected to understand. When it is not medically advisable to give such information to the patient, the information should be made available to an appropriate person in his behalf. He has the right to know, by name, the physician responsible for coordinating his care.

3. The patient has the right to receive from his physician information necessary to give informed consent prior to the start of any procedure and/or

treatment. Except in emergencies, such information for informed consent should include but not necessarily be limited to the specific procedure and/or treatment, the medically significant risks involved, and the probable duration of incapacitation. Where medically significant alternatives for care or treatment exist, or when the patient requests information concerning medical alternatives, the patient has the right to such information. The patient also has the right to know the name of the person responsible for the procedures and/or treatment.

4. The patient has the right to refuse treatment to the extent permitted by law and to be informed of the medical consequences of his action.

5. The patient has the right to every consideration of his privacy concerning his own medical care program. Case discussion, consultation, examination, and treatment are confidential and should be conducted discreetly. Those not directly involved in his care must have the permission of the patient to be present.

6. The patient has the right to expect that all communications and records pertaining to his care should be treated as confidential.

7. The patient has the right to expect that within its capacity a hospital must make reasonable response to the request of a patient for services. The hospital must provide evaluation, service, and/or referral as indicated by the urgency of the case. When medically permissible, a patient may be transferred to another facility only after he has received complete information and explanation concerning the needs for and alternatives to such a transfer. The institution to which the patient is to be transferred must first have accepted the patient for transfer.

8. The patient has the right to obtain information as to any relationship of his hospital to other health care and educational institutions insofar as his care is concerned. The patient has the right to obtain information as to the existence of any professional relationships among individuals, by name, who are treating him.

9. The patient has the right to be advised if the hospital proposes to engage in or perform human experimentation affecting his care or treatment. The patient has the right to refuse to participate in such research projects.

10. The patient has the right to expect reasonable continuity of care. He has the right to know in advance what appointment times and physicians are available and where. The patient has the right to expect that the hospital will provide a mechanism whereby he is informed by his physician or a delegate of the physician of the patient's continuing health care requirements following discharge.

11. The patient has the right to examine and receive an explanation of his bill regardless of source of payment.

12. The patient has the right to know what hospital rules and regulations apply to his conduct as a patient.

No catalog of rights can guarantee for the patient the kind of treatment he has a right to expect. A hospital has many functions to perform, including the prevention and treatment of disease, the education of both health professionals and patients, and the conduct of clinical research. All these activities must be conducted with an overriding concern for the patient, and, above all, the recognition of his dignity as a human being. Success in achieving this recognition assures success in the defense of the rights of the patient.

Canadian Nurses' Association
Code of Ethics

CARING AND THE PROFESSION

The nursing profession as a whole has ethical obligations to society as well as to its own membership. The profession has an obligation to examine its own goals and the service it offers in the light of existing health problems, and to design its programs in collaboration with other professionals which also provide health services within the society. Nursing, in keeping with its mandate as a service profession, is bound to see itself, not as an end to be promoted and served by society, but as a professional body, constituted and legitimized by society's approval, to offer a prescribed service required for the improvement of the health status of people.

In meeting its obligations to society, nursing has responsibility for monitoring the quantity and quality of persons entering the profession, and for identifying and implementing standards that promote the type and quality of nursing service dictated by society's needs. Nursing has a related responsibility to work for those conditions which will enable its members to provide the quantity and quality of service deemed necessary and desirable.

The nursing profession also has responsibilities to the international community. Since health is a basic condition for human development, and as no one nation or country can develop its potential in isolation, the interests of the profession transcend national boundaries. In fact, our credibility as a profession is called into question if we do not collaborate on an international level to promote the health of all peoples, and to work toward the relief of human suffering wherever it is experienced.

These broad obligations constitute the grounds for the ethical responsibilities of nursing's organized professional body, and include the following commitments:

1. In the context of existing health needs and problems, to identify Canada's need for nursing activities and services.

2. To establish relevant and realistic goals for the profession of nursing within Canadian society.

3. To foster collaboration with other health professions, political bodies, and other agencies in responding to the health needs of Canadians.

4. To collaborate with professional groups, institutions and agencies in promoting the welfare of peoples in other countries of the world.

5. To provide measures which will ensure that only those with the potential, motivation, and discipline required to function as caring persons are accepted into, and endorsed by the nursing profession.

6. To work for the realization of working conditions which enable nurses to function as caring persons with the required degree of autonomy.

7. To promote conditions for nurses which provide for legitimate personal, professional, and economic rewards.

8. To demonstrate, in its own transactions, accountability for the use of internal and external resources.

CARING AND THE INDIVIDUAL NURSE

The final test of the credibility of ethical standards in nursing lies in the behavior of the individual nurse-educator, practitioner, administrator, and researcher. Many of the responsibilities arising out of obligations of the profession as a whole, and the ethical demands of the caring community itself, are fulfilled only in the actions of the individual nurse. While the profession has the obligation to identify, promote, and monitor ethical standards, the execution of such standards is a personal responsibility, the final guarantee of which is in the conscience and commitment of the individual nurse.

GUIDELINES

The following guidelines include general principles, with statements of ethical responsibility which flow from these principles. They are intended to provide a guide for reflection and for the articulation of more specific ethical rules and standards applicable to concrete experiences. With the increasing complexity of ethical conflicts in nursing, and the potential for greater ethical concerns in the future, ethical discernment in nursing is an exciting challenge, requiring knowledge, skill, and great moral sensitivity. We have the capacity to meet this challenge—one which could be the greatest in the history of our profession.

A. General Principles

1. The human person, regardless of race, creed, color, social class, or health status, is of incalculable worth, and commands reverence and respect.

2. Human life has a sacred and even mysterious character, and its worth is determined not merely by utilitarian concerns.

3. Caring, the central and fundamental focus of nursing, is the basis for nursing ethics. It is expressed in compassion, competence, conscience, confidence, and commitment. It qualifies all the relationships in nursing practice, education, administration, and research including those between nurse-client; nurse-nurse; nurse-other helping professionals; educator-colleague; faculty-student; researcher-subject.

B. Statements of Ethical Responsibility

1. Caring demands the provision of helping services that are appropriate to the needs of the client and significant others.

2. Caring recognizes the client's membership in a family and a community, and provides for the participation of significant others in his or her care.

3. Caring acknowledges the reality of death in the life of every person, and demands that appropriate support be provided for the dying person and family to enable them to prepare for, and to cope with death when it is inevitable.

4. Caring acknowledges that the human person has the capacity to face up to health needs and problems in his or her own unique way, and directs nursing action in a manner that will assist the client to develop, maintain, or gain personal autonomy, self-respect, and self-determination.

5. Caring, as a response to a health need, requires the consent and the participation of the person who is experiencing that need.

6. Caring dictates that the client and significant others have the knowledge and information adequate for free and informed decisions concerning care requirements, alternatives, and preferences.

7. Caring demands that the needs of the client supersede those of the nurse, and that the nurse must not compromise the integrity of the client by personal behavior that is self-serving.

8. Caring acknowledges the vulnerability of a client in certain situations, and dictates restraint in actions which might compromise the client's rights and privileges.

9. Caring, involving a relationship which is, in itself, therapeutic, demands mutual respect and trust.

10. Caring acknowledges that information obtained in the course of the nursing relationship is privileged, and that it requires the full protection of confidentiality unless such information provides evidence of

serious impending harm to the client or to a third party, or is legally required by the courts.

11. Caring requires that the nurse represent the needs of the client, and that the nurse take appropriate measures when the fulfillment of these needs is jeopardized by the actions of other persons.

12. Caring acknowledges the dignity of all persons in the practice or educational setting.

13. Caring acknowledges, respects, and draws upon the competencies of others.

14. Caring establishes the conditions for the harmonization of efforts of different helping professionals in providing required services to clients.

15. Caring seeks to establish and maintain a climate of respect for the honest dialogue needed for effective collaboration.

16. Caring establishes the legitimacy of respectful challenge and/or confrontation when the service required by the client is compromised in incompetency, incapacity, or negligence, or when the competencies of the nurse are not acknowledged or appropriately utilized.

17. Caring demands the provision of working conditions which enable nurses to carry out their legitimate responsibilities.

18. Caring demands resourcefulness and restraint-accountability *for* the use of time, resources, equipment, and funds, and requires accountability *to* appropriate individuals and/or bodies.

19. Caring requires that the nurse bring to the work situation in education, practice, administration, or research, the knowledge, affective and technical skills required, and that competency in these areas be maintained and up-dated.

20. Caring commands fidelity to oneself, and guards the right and privilege of the nurse to act in keeping with an informed moral conscience.

Reprinted with the permission of the Canadian Nurses' Association, 50 The Driveway, Ottawa, Ontario.

Consumers' Association of Canada: Consumer Rights in Health Care

I Right to Be Informed

- about preventive health care including education on nutrition, birth control, drug use, appropriate exercise

- about the health care system including the extent of government insurance coverage for services, supplementary insurance plans, the referral system to auxiliary health and social facilities and services in the community

- about the individual's own diagnosis and specific treatment program including prescribed surgery and medication, options, effects and side effects

- about the specific costs of procedures, services and professional fees undertaken on behalf of the individual consumer

II Right to Be Respected as the Individual with the Major Responsibility for His Own Health Care

- right that confidentiality of his health records be maintained

- right to refuse experimentation, undue painful prolongation of his life or participation in teaching programs

- right of adult to refuse treatment, right to die with dignity

III Right to Participate in Decision Making Affecting His Health

- through consumer representation at each level of government in planning and evaluating the system of health services, the types and qualities of service and the conditions under which health services are delivered

- with the health professionals and personnel involved in his direct health care

IV Right to Equal Access to Health Care (Health Education, Prevention, Treatment and Rehabilitation) Regardless of the Individual's Economic Status, Sex, Age, Creed, Ethnic Origin and Location

- right to access to adequately qualified health personnel
- right to a second medical opinion
- right to prompt response in emergencies

Reprinted courtesy of the Consumers' Association of Canada. More consumer information is available in *Canadian Consumer* magazine—$18 a year: Consumers' Association of Canada, Box 9300, Ottawa, Ontario, K1G 3T9.

E
Computer Basics
Vicki L. Sauter

Learning to work with computers is just like learning to perform nursing tasks: if you do not know the jargon and technology, you cannot have a meaningful discussion with a professional. Before you became a nurse, for instance, the terms *blood gases* and *kidney dialysis* were probably as foreign to you as *chip* and *database* are to you now. Only after you learned the meaning of the terms and the procedures to be followed were you comfortable with providing patient care. Similarly, learning to adapt and cope with computers requires that you first learn to speak "computerese." This section is a brief introduction to the most commonly used terms and their interrelationships.

A *computer* is simply an electronic machine designed to perform a set of routine operations, thus freeing users to pursue more creative activities (Rees, 1978). In nursing, for example, computers can complete the tedious tasks of preparing morning reports or ordering medication, thus releasing the nurse to give more attention to patient care or, in the case of the nurse manager, to pursue other managerial and educational tasks. In addition, the computer can be helpful to nurses by providing another set of eyes for monitoring a patient's progress (such as vital signs) or for noticing patterns in a patient's response to care.

Different tasks require different types of machines. There are two basic types of computers: the *analog computer* and the *digital computer*. Nurses are most likely to interact with a digital computer on a daily basis. These computers perform numerical operations (similarly to a desk calculator) and manipulate strings of characters so they can be used for activities such as preparing and checking patient's charts, ordering and verifying medications, or preparing patient's bills. Nurses may also interact with analog (or *analog-digital hybrid*) computers. These computers use electrical circuits to simulate a physical function to make its measurement easier. Analog (or analog-digital hybrid) computers can be used to monitor vital signs, such as heart and respiratory rates.

The primary purpose for a computer in a hospital is to collect, analyze, and disseminate data. The collection of interrelated data that can be used to ensure the effectiveness and/or efficiency of the delivery of care to patients is referred to as a *database*. Databases existed, in principle, before computers existed: medical charts, admission forms, and nursing notes all provided information about a patient and they were all used at some stage of the process to facilitate the delivery of care.

Two principles distinguish computerized databases from those earlier ones: (a) computerized databases are integrated and (b) they are shared. *Integrated* means that a computerized database is one for which records are organized and maintained in such a way as to reduce redundancy in the information maintained about a patient. For example, in a noncomputerized system, the patient's name and address are kept in both the admissions office and the nurses' station (or, later, in the records office)—that is, in two places in the hospital. In a computerized system, the information is entered only once and is kept in only one place. However, the way in which the data are stored is not obvious to users because the information is *shared*. That is, the same information about a patient is available to all *qualified* users. For example, in a noncomputerized system, the pharmacist is not aware of the patient's condition or of other regimens being applied to the patient. However, in a computerized system, the pharmacist may be able to access much of the patient's medical chart; this puts him or her in a better position to evaluate whether undesirable consequences may occur as a result of the requested medication.

Databases are created and maintained by computers, which have two distinct components: *hardware* and *software*. As a general rule, one can distinguish between the two by remembering that hardware consists of all of those computer parts that are permanent and observable while software includes the parts that are changeable and that one cannot "see." More exactly, hardware refers to the computer itself, the associated machines, and its electronic components; software refers to the instructions that are provided to cause it to perform a specified set of instructions.

Hardware

Input/output devices. In order to perform its tasks, a computer must be able to capture or receive data and to release the processed information in a form that can be reused or retrieved *easily* by humans or other computers. The data that are made available to the machine are referred to as *input* and the results are referred to as *output*. For example, when a patient is admitted to the hospital, an admissions clerk asks certain questions such as name, address, age, previous illnesses, allergies to medication, and so on. These data, which constitute input into the system, are entered into the computer to create a patient record.

After being received, they are processed by the computer and put into a form that is usable as a patient chart. That chart, which will contain information to help the health care professionals provide better patient care, is considered output. Likewise, every time a nurse or physician requests a change in medication or regimen, he or she will enter it on the computerized patient chart; thus, it becomes input. The reports and printed results from the laboratory tests and the patient's bill are all considered outputs.

Those electronic parts through which data are received and translated for the computer are called *input devices*; the machines that translate and make available the results of the computer processing are called *output devices*. Collectively, they (along with storage devices, which will be discussed later) are referred to as *peripherals*. The different types of input and output devices are summarized in Figure E–1.

A wide range of input devices, each associated with a specific *input medium*, is available. The nurse manager is most likely to use a *terminal* similar to the one in Figure E–1. Most terminals look like a typewriter with a television on the top. The "typewriter" portion is referred to as the *keyboard* and the "television" is actually a *cathode ray tube* (generally referred to as a *CRT* or monitor). The terminal translates the information the nurse enters into electronic impulses that the computer can understand. In addition, the terminal has the capability of translating electronic impulses from the computer into text that appears on the screen of the CRT in a form the nurse can understand.

When a computer finishes processing data, it produces information that is usable by a person or another computer. The electronic and mechanical devices through which the computer translates the information into something that can be understood are called *output devices*. Just as there are options on how to provide information to a computer, there are also options on how to receive information from it. For example, the results from a computer may be observed on the CRT of a terminal, printed out in a report, or saved on magnetic tape or disk for use at a later time.

Nurse managers will generally either receive the information through a terminal or through a *line printer*. When one receives information on a terminal, it is generally referred to as *soft copy* because the information disappears from the CRT when a new task is begun. *Hard copy*, which one receives from a printer, can be saved for future reference, forwarded to other individuals, or taken from the computer for use elsewhere (such as during rounds).

Processing equipment. Every computer has three types of hardware that are used for data processing: (a) a storage or memory unit; (b) a control unit; and (c) an arithmetic/logic unit (ALU) (Piankian, 1978). The interrelationships among these types of hardware are illustrated in Figure E–2. Understanding the specifics of the processing equipment is not crucial for the nurse manager. However, understanding the implications of various types of processing equipment for her operations is important.

Figure E–1 Input/Output Components

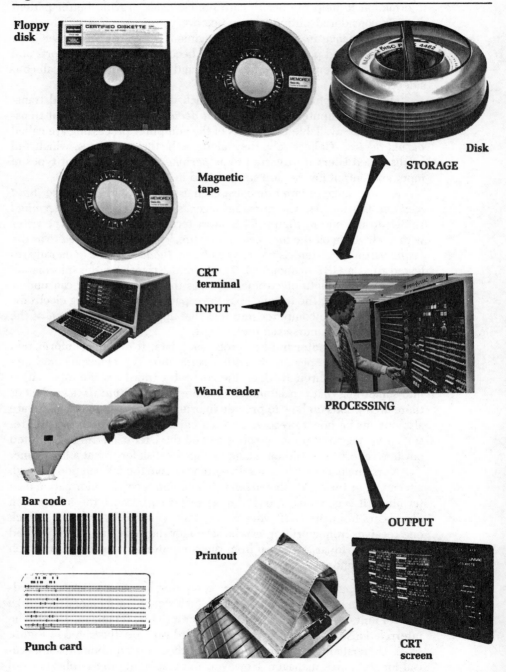

Clockwise from top right: Courtesy of Nashua Corporation (fig. 1); Unisys (fig. 2, 3, 8); Datagraphix (fig. 4); NCR Corporation (fig. 6 & 7); Memorex (fig. 9 & 11); 3M (fig. 10).

Figure E–2 Processing Components

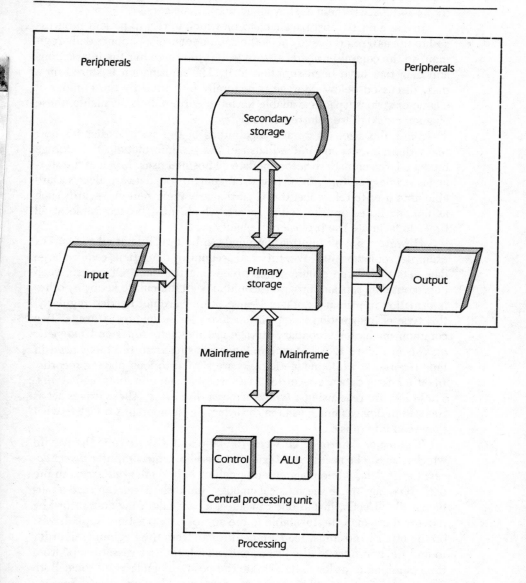

Hence, in this section, we will provide some simple definitions of the terms and discuss them as they affect nurse managers.

Just as a nurse must have a chart on which to record patient progress and to use as a reference to check the components of a patient's daily regimen, so the computer needs a *storage unit* to remember the instructions and data that have been supplied to it. The information is stored on a disk, discussed below. Storage is generally measured by the number of character strings (spaces available for letters or numbers) available; these character strings are referred to as *bytes*.

Since the size, or storage capabilities of the system, dictates how many departments and individuals can process information, this storage must be large enough to accommodate all hospital uses. Much of the storage is *primary storage*. In such an arrangement, the data are always available for a user to reference; this is particularly important for records such as nursing notes or the medical chart, which must be accessible at all times to facilitate the provision of quality care.

However, not all information needs to be available at all times. For example, some hospital inventory and accounting operations require large data sets with large programs for processing the data. Of course, such enormous data sets and programs could make it difficult to keep any other information in primary storage. Hence, if they are not needed regularly, this type of information is kept in *auxiliary* (or *secondary*) *storage*. Two common media for secondary storage are *magnetic tapes* and *magnetic disks* (see Figure E–1). Magnetic tapes are similar to the tapes used in tape recorders, while magnetic disks are similar to long-playing records. In either case, data are recorded as a series of magnetic spots, called *bits*. These bits are read using a *tape drive* or a *disk drive*. These drives act as translation devices much as tape recorders or phonographs translate what they read into music.

The major difference between the tape and disk drive is the way in which data can be accessed. Magnetic disks allow the computer *direct access* to the data, while magnetic tapes allow only *sequential access* to the data. If we again use the musical analogy, the disk drives can read a particular file directly, just as one can select a particular song on a record by moving the arm of the turntable to the appropriate position. Tape drives, on the other hand, must read a tape through from the beginning in order to find the appropriate file, just as one must listen to a cassette tape from the beginning in order to determine the position of a favorite song. Both tapes and disks are used to store large data sets. However, this difference in the ability to access information tends to result in different types of data being stored on the two media: magnetic tapes are used to store data that are not referenced frequently, while magnetic disks are used to store data that are needed regularly and quickly. In a hospital, a magnetic tape might be used to keep accounts data, inventory data, or past patient data that would be needed if a patient were readmitted. Magnetic disks, however, are used to store data on current patients that might be needed for diagnosis or accounting purposes.

The second type of hardware in a computer is the *control unit*. The role of the computer's control unit is similar to the role of a nurse manager in the delivery of patient care: each is responsible for directing the execution of instructions to others. The nurse manager examines activities assigned to her unit and instructs others in productive functioning. Similarly, the control unit analyzes each instruction in a program and directs other computer components to prepare for and execute those specific instructions.

All computations and comparisons, such as adding or comparing, are done in the *arithmetic/logic unit* (*ALU*). Each ALU component is responsible for a particular type of computation and performs that operation when directed to do so by the control unit. The ALU, when combined with the control unit, is referred to as the *central processing unit* (*CPU*) and is responsible for all processing activities.

Processing equipment is generally classified by its size and capabilities into one of three major divisions: *mainframes, minicomputers,* and *microcomputers.* Of these, mainframes are the most traditional and most powerful machines; they are capable of processing many users, with access to billions of characters of data at very fast speeds. Of course, they are also the most expensive of the three types, ranging from around $500,000 for a "small" and "slow" one to millions of dollars for the largest and fastest ones. Minicomputers are smaller, slower, and can serve fewer users at a time. They generally cost somewhere between $10,000 and $500,000, with peripherals and storage devices. Microcomputers, the newest of the three, can serve limited numbers of users (often only one at a time) who require limited access to data and limited processing capability. The cost of these machines can range from $300 to $10,000 depending on the size, capability, and attached devices desired.

Historically, hospitals have used mainframes, or mainframes supported by minicomputers, to perform accounting and other recordkeeping activities. Minicomputers have also been used to support specific functions such as laboratory analyses, while microcomputers have been used primarily for education and training. However, this trend is changing somewhat because of the increased power in the minicomputers and microcomputers and their cost relative to mainframe computers.

This trend of greater capabilities in smaller machines has had the most significant impact on the use of computers in nursing. Nursing no longer needs to convince other units within a hospital of the importance of functions they want computerized: they often can purchase a microcomputer and implement the function themselves. Further, with the increased reliance on microcomputers in general has come an increased availability of software for those machines to perform specific functions (the importance of this will be discussed in the next section).

Software

The set of instructions that tell the computer how to process the raw data into usable information is referred to as a *program*. Some programs are written to control the overall operations of the computer; these are referred to as *operating systems programs*. In addition, there are *database management systems (DBMS)* programs. DBMSs receive information that is entered at a terminal, determine how and where to store the data, manage it so as to best utilize the hardware, and control the access to it. These two types of programs are very important to the nurse and nurse manager because they are what makes the computerized system "easy" to use and reliable. However, the nurse and nurse manager are rarely aware that they are utilizing these systems. Generally, nurse managers will be more likely to be aware of *applications programs*, or programs that are intended to complete a specific function. In the hospital, there are programs that create a patient's chart and bill, programs that refer instructions to the appropriate department for action, and programs that prepare schedules as well as a wide variety of other operations (Aybalajobi, 1979). It is to these types of programs that the term *software* generally refers.

Software creation is generally initiated by a *systems analyst*, who examines the tasks the software is intended to complete. The systems analyst breaks down the tasks into specific activities, much as if the task were being done by hand, to determine the required steps and protocols. For example, in staff scheduling, one must first establish (a) how many nurses are available; (b) their schedule preferences; (c) hospital policies regarding staffing; (d) needs of the patients and their illnesses; and (e) other types of personnel available. After determining these five types of information, the systems analyst would determine the procedures the nurse manager would follow in order to derive the least expensive schedule that would satisfy the greatest number of nurses while still meeting the needs of the hospital. Furthermore, the systems analyst would attempt to determine if the nurse manager would like other issues (e.g., 8-hour shift vs. 12-hour shift) to be considered that she might not be able to consider when doing by hand. Finally, the systems analyst would determine if there are other activities with which this activity should be linked, such as the preparation of payroll.

A major function of the systems analyst is to determine not only the steps that are involved in the process, but also the interrelationships among those steps and other functions that are being computerized. After the systems analyst has completed the task analysis, the programmer must translate the resulting activities into a specialized language that the computer can understand. COBOL, BASIC, and MUMPS, for instance, are such languages; each has a special way of expressing thoughts and each specifies rules of grammar. The differences among the languages are generally due to the types of jobs they most commonly perform and the capabilities of the machines on which they are intended to run. For example,

COBOL is most commonly used for financial applications such as generating patients' bills and doing the payroll; hence, its structure and procedures were devised to make such operations easier. Similarly, MUMPS is most commonly used for clinical health applications; its structure and procedures were designed to handle large volumes of data on limited processing machines. Finally, the systems analyst must revise the code when it does not meet the needs of the users completely.

One reason for understanding the differences in hardware capabilities is to understand the wide range of software that is available for the different types of machines. The process that was described above is generally applicable to software on mainframe computers. It has advantages in that the hospital is able to request a complete system that meets the specific needs of the users at that particular site. Furthermore, it is the only way a hospital can get a system that is large enough and powerful enough to handle the processing needs of either the financial aspects or the patient record aspects of the hospital.

The process is not without its disadvantages, however. First of all, it can be long and time consuming, both for the systems analyst and for the hospital personnel. Furthermore, it is not always obvious that at the end of the process the users will get the system they thought they were getting; there are often communication problems between the hospital personnel and the analyst.

One way of getting around this problem is for the hospital to purchase a program that is already written to perform a specific function; this is generally referred to as a *canned package* or just a *package*. (Some computer manufacturers provide a similar type of product, called *firmware*. Firmware also performs a specified set of functions, but the program is stored on a computer chip, that is, on part of the hardware of the computer.) The difference between having software custom-built and using a package is similar to the choice beween having a home built to one's own specifications and buying a home that has already been built (or one for which there are limited options in building). In the former case, the new owner gets everything that he or she wants—assuming that the owner is able to adequately express those wishes to the architect and that the architect is willing or able to include them. Furthermore, the new owner probably spends a lot of time and energy making choices and communicating those choices. In the latter case, the new owner could examine some ready-made homes and decide whether they are close enough to what he or she wants to be happy. This new owner does not take the risks as to how his or her instructions and needs will be interpreted and does not expend as much effort in the process. However, this owner is unlikely to get exactly what he or she wants. Similarly, when a hospital purchases a package, it is committed to using a general set of procedures. If those are "close enough" to the desired procedures, this purchase is generally less time consuming, less expensive, and less difficult than purchasing software that is custom-written. However, the user loses most of his or her control over what that software actually does.

Historically, hospitals have been willing to consider packages for a limited number of applications, such as scheduling, accounting, inventory, and auditing, because these functions are similar from one hospital to another. However, because the more medical applications were hospital-specific (and because there were fewer packages from which to choose), many hospitals had at least part of their software custom-built.

This historical precedent is now changing, at least somewhat. First, there are more packages from which to choose. Second, more companies are willing to customize available packages to meet user needs. Furthermore, there has been a change in attitude about the type of computer that is appropriate to use. Hospitals, like most companies using computers, have historically relied only on mainframe computers. However, with the increasing capabilities and decreasing costs of microcomputers, along with the increasing capability to tie microcomputers together with a mainframe computer, more functions can be delegated to the microcomputer. Since this is a trend that many companies are experiencing, many packages are being developed to meet the needs of these users. Hence, there is an increasing marketplace of products from which to choose. For example, historically, if one wanted to use computer-aided instruction for nurses, one needed to purchase very expensive and complex packages for the mainframe computers. However, now there are many relatively cheap and relatively easy-to-use packages available for the microcomputer that can facilitate computer-aided instruction, such as NEMAS (Nursing Education Module Authoring System). Software availability is now a factor that affects the hardware purchase decision.

Index